RECENT ADVANCES IN IMMUNOLOGY TO TARGET CANCER, INFLAMMATION AND INFECTIONS

Edited by **Jagat R. Kanwar**

Recent Advances in Immunology to Target Cancer, Inflammation and Infections
Edited by Jagat R. Kanwar

Published by InTech

Janeza Trdine 9, 51000 Rijeka, Croatia

Publishing Process Manager Petra Nenadic

Technical Editor Teodora Smiljanic

Cover Designer InTech Design Team

Additional hard copies can be obtained from orders@intechopen.com

Recent Advances in Immunology to Target Cancer, Inflammation and Infections,
Edited by Jagat R. Kanwar
p. cm.
ISBN 978-953-51-0592-3

For EU product safety concerns:
IN TECH d.o.o., Prolaz Marije Krucifikse Kozulić 3, 51000 Rijeka, Croatia,
info@intechopen.com or visit our website at intechopen.com.

Meet the editor

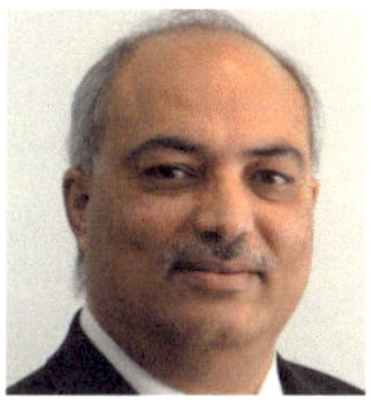

Professor Jagat R Kanwar is the Head of Nanomedicine-Laboratory of Immunology and Molecular Biomedical Research (LIMBR). He received his Master's degree in Medical Biochemistry and PhD in Molecular Immunology. He has an international reputation and expertise in investigating fundamental and applied molecular signaling aspects of pathogenesis of cancer and chronic inflammatory diseases, thereby, leading to the development of treatment strategies from bench to bedside. He has more than 110 publications in peer reviewed international journals, 17 book chapters and 3 edited books. He serves as an Editor, Reviewer and Editorial Advisory Board Member of more than 45 international journals, invited speaker in more than 50 conferences and chaired conferences sessions on Cancer, Immunology, Vaccines, Microbial infections, Nanotechnology, Nanomedicine and Biotechnology.

Contents

Preface

Immunology is a branch of biomedical sciences covering the broad concepts of immune system and its components of all the living beings. It is a study of the immune system physiology both in healthy and diseased states. In general, the immune system safeguards the human body from several infections and also evades the generation of cancerous cells and their attack. However, a hairline margin determines the actual mechanism of body defence termed as immunity and as autoimmunity characterised by the loss of tolerance. An imbalance in the immune cell regulation leads to the generation of several of the autoimmune diseases ranging from organ specific type to the systemic ones which also includes cancer. Though the precise pathogenic mechanisms behind the autoimmunity aren't yet identified, previous studies identified the genetic inheritance, infections and environmental pollutants as the major risk factors associated with the disease. The principle motto of this book is to serve the students, scholars and research personnel with up to date literature from the basics of immunology to the cutting edge techniques employed to counteract the diseased states. Added to the ease of access, peer review and open access will be one click away from the readers to have a complete understanding of the topic of their interest. I strongly hope that a majority of them will be benefitted from the books and find useful for applications into clinical research.

The first chapter by Dr. Butsch Kovacic Melinda covers the details of immune cell pathology involved in cervical cancer and its diagnostic importance, vaccines for therapy providing insights on the clinical studies conducted and evaluated. This will surely highlight the understanding of the disease and gap that needs to be filled. Computational studies lead to the development of a mathematical model that unmasked the secrets behind the adaptive immune system functioning and also for determining the optimum immunization. This chapter provided by Dr. De Castro Alexandre is interesting in explaining the simulations that found the dynamic behaviour and the antigen dependency for B-cell memory. It is followed by the review by Dr. Orozco-Suarez Sandra who explained the details of immune mediated CNS diseases along with therapeutic approaches for epilepsy. Plasma Exchange has attracted attention as new therapeutic intervention for the autoimmune neuromyelitis optica. The details of its pathology and treatment procedures are explained by Dr Bonnan Mickael. The novel findings of Pattern recognition receptors and their role in the cancer aetiopathogenesis is discussed in chapter by Dr. Kutikhin Anton substantiating the concepts of immunology and its importance for future therapeutics. Dr. Kuricova Miroslava dealt the aspects of Environmental xenobiotics and immunotoxicity as a separate chapter including the concepts of developing in vitro models for toxicity evaluation. The next chapter by Dr. Garcia-Munoz Ricardo, is about Chronic Lymphocytic Leukemia, a unique B-cell malignancy updates our current understanding with inclusions on its pathogenesis and immune dysregulation. The conceptual literature on neuroimmune regulators in brain disorders is covered by Dr. Neal James and the age related immune responses and alterations by Dr. Goriely Stanislas. Next chapters by Dr. Maier Olaf deal the interesting aspects of oligodendrocyte differentiation, its regulation and remyelination is followed by the explanations of Prof. Hahm Bumsuk on mechanistic viral ploy for escape from host immunity and its understanding for developing immunotherapeutic applications. Valuable information on early nutrition and its impact on immunity, mother and foetus immunological interactions are summarised as a separate chapter by Prof. Boehm Günther.

Prof. Cooper Edwin took efforts and provided exclusive information for comparing the adaptive immunity in prokaryotes and eukaryotes and the interesting outcomes will surely attract the readers in his chapter. Valuable additions are made by Dr. Robinson-Agramonte Maria on the detailed pathology of glial cells and axons in multiple sclerosis, its treatment and Dr. Sattler Susanne covered valuable information on the immunobiology of regulatory B-cells and their impact on the autoimmune and allergic disorders in her chapter. Chapter's by Prof. Mehrzad Jalil & Dr. Owais Mohammad will conclude covering the enthusiastic concepts of neutrophils, their interactions with pathogens along with the addressing of cutting edge techniques and the detailed biology of Toll-like receptor, its implications in various diseased states and its future therapeutic modulation. In chapter by Prof Kanwar covered the study of TH17 cells in cancer and inflammation. This field has been one of the fast-moving and exciting subject areas in immunology of immune-mediated chronic inflammatory diseases and autoimmunity, where the pathogenic role of TH17 cells has been well documented. Based on the evidence provided in this chapter from both human and clinical studies data, TH17 cells and TH17-associated cytokines/effector molecules have been shown to have both pro-tumorigenic and anti-tumorigenic functions. Lastly, chapter by Prof Sehgal and Prof Kanwar covered the immunology of leishmaniasis and its future prospective for the development of vaccines to leishmaniasis. Recent investigations have provided new insight into the role of cells of the innate immunity. Identification of new antigen candidates with broad species coverage, and a greater understanding of the immunology of protective immunity to leishmaniasis open new strategies in clinical vaccine to leishmaniasis.

Dr. Jagat R. Kanwar
Deakin University,
Australia

Section 1

Immunology of Viruses and Cancer

1

Cytokines and Markers of Immune Response to HPV Infection

Jill Koshiol[2] and Melinda Butsch Kovacic[1]
[1]*Cincinnati Children's Hospital Medical Center*
[2]*National Cancer Institute*
USA

1. Introduction

Cervical cancer is the third most commonly diagnosed cancer in women worldwide (Ferlay, Shin et al. 2010) and is a result of infection with cancer-causing types of human papillomavirus (HPV) (Bouvard, Baan et al. 2009). HPV is a very common infection, although in most circumstances, infection does not usually result in cervical disease (Trottier and Franco 2006). In fact, the natural history of HPV infection suggests that additional factors are required to drive progression from infection to the development of cancer. Most women are thought to clear their HPV infections within two years, but in approximately 10% of women, infection persists (Schiffman, Castle et al. 2007). Persistent HPV infection is, in effect, the strongest risk factor for progression to cervical precancer and cancer (Koshiol, Lindsay et al. 2008), and a dysfunctional immune response is likely to underlie the amplified risk that leads to HPV persistence and cervical cancer. Although efficacious prophylactic vaccines against the two types of HPV (16 and 18) that cause about 70% of cervical cancers (Munoz, Castellsague et al. 2006) are available, these vaccines are expensive, difficult to administer in poorer countries and will not protect women who have already been exposed to the virus (FUTURE II Study Group 2007; Hildesheim, Herrero et al. 2007) (Su, Wu et al. 2010). Thus, it is important to understand factors that predispose some women infected with a carcinogenic HPV infection to persist and progress.

HPV uses a variety of methods to avoid immune detection, such as maintaining an unobtrusive infectious cycle (e.g., non-viremic and non-cytolytic since replication occurs in cells already destined for natural cell death), suppressing interferon response, and down-regulating toll-like receptor (TLR)-9 (Stanley 2010). By employing such immune evasion tactics, HPV infection itself does not lead to a direct or obvious inflammatory response. Rather, inflammation due to other co-factors such as smoking, parity, oral contraceptive use, co-infection with other sexually transmitted diseases, multiple sexual partners etc. have long been hypothesized to lead to HPV incidence, persistence, and progression to cervical pre-cancer and cancer (Castle and Giuliano 2003). Studies that directly evaluate women's immune response to HPV infection may provide better insights into the role of inflammation and immunity in HPV persistence and cervical carcinogenesis.

Although humoral response to HPV infection has been well-characterized (Bhat, Mattarollo et al. 2011), cell-mediated response has not been well established. Numerous approaches have been used to characterize cell-mediated immune responses to HPV. Such approaches include measurement of cytokines and other immune markers that commonly lead to infiltration of immune cells. Cytokines are pleiotropic glycoproteins that regulate cell survival, proliferation, differentiation and activation at both local and systemic levels. During inflammation, their excessive release may lead to both chronicity and pathogenicity. The purpose of this review is to describe the current state of knowledge regarding these important regulators or other important immune markers of cell-mediated immune response in HPV infection. To this end, we have evaluated studies in plasma or serum from peripheral blood, in cervical secretions, in unstimulated and stimulated PBMCs (and cellular subsets thereof), and in cervical tissues themselves. Importantly, this chapter will highlight not only the large amount of knowledge gained from these studies, but also the many scientific gaps in knowledge that remain.

2. Methods

Relevant studies were identified by searching MEDLINE (via PubMed) using broad search term categories for cervix and immunity (Appendix 1). The search included studies identified through 3 November 2011. Studies that evaluated cell-mediated immune response immune response by HPV status (positivity, persistence, or clearance) were included if there were at least 10 women in each comparison group (usually HPV-positive versus HPV-negative; sometime HPV persistence versus clearance or difference by HPV type). To focus on more functional aspects of immune response, only studies of immune-related proteins and mRNA (evidence of expression) and studies with HPV DNA detection were included. Studies were excluded if the HPV status and disease status of the referent group was unclear or if they focused on DNA polymorphisms alone. Given the focus on HPV infection, studies were also excluded if they include cervical cancer patients, but no other groups [i.e. normal women, women with low-grade squamous intraepithelial lesions (LSIL) or cervical intraepithelial neoplasia (CIN)]. Studies that included some cervical cancer patients along with CIN or normal patients were retained. Post-treatment studies or studies involving mice, cell lines, or HPV at extra-cervical anatomical sites were excluded as well.

Data were abstracted on the study characteristics, HPV measurement, immune marker measurement, and results pertinent to this review. Study characteristics included the country in which the study was conducted, the method of cervical secretion collection, and descriptions of comparison groups relevant for this review (e.g., women with incident HPV versus no HPV). The assay used to detect HPV was also noted. Immune marker-related data included the assay used to measure the immune marker and the specific markers measured, along with the results. Approximately 50% of studies were double abstracted.

3. Literature review

In total, 35 studies met our inclusion criteria. These studies fell into four broad categories (Tables 1 to 4): circulating immune markers in plasma or serum (N = 7), those secreted locally in the cervix (N = 7), immune responses in patient-derived PBMCs (N = 10), and tissue-based immune markers (N = 12). One study contributed to both the circulating and PBMC-based immune marker categories.

Circulating Immune Markers in Plasma/Serum. Cytokines and soluble immune markers are increasingly being measured in readily accessible plasma and serum in the hope that they will provide useful diagnostic and prognostic information, as well as insight into the pathogenesis of numerous diseases. Further, the availability of inexpensive enzyme-linked immunosorbent assays (ELISAs), radioimmunoassays (RIAs), and other bioassays to reliably measure cytokines in these samples make them enticing targets for discovery. Currently, seven studies that met our inclusion criteria have directly examined HPV-infection-related immune responses in either serum or plasma (Table 1). All of these studies have focused on associations with carcinogenic infection using a Hybrid Capture assay. Hildesheim et al. (Hildesheim, Schiffman et al. 1997) was among the first to use plasma to evaluate markers of immunity. However, their comparison of carcinogenic HPV positive women with low-grade lesions to carcinogenic negative women with low-grade lesions failed to find a statistical difference in the soluble IL-2 receptor (sIL-2R; p=0.63). Adam et al. (Adam, Horowitz et al. 1999) similarly compared 10 women with high risk HPV infection to 10 HPV negative women and reported that high risk HPV infection was indeed associated with higher mean serum CSF-1 levels. Abike et al. (Abike, Engin et al. 2011) measured neopterin, often considered a marker of immune activation, and found lower concentrations in HPV-positive versus HPV-negative women with normal through high-grade histology. Unlike the earlier studies, Bais et al. (Bais 2005) measured numerous cytokines simultaneously (IL-2, IL-4, IL-10, IL-12, IFN-γ, TNF-α), as well as soluble markers (sTNFRI and sTNFRII) in plasma. They discovered that higher mean IL-2 levels alone were associated with carcinogenic HPV positivity. Baker et al. (Baker, Dauner et al. 2011) evaluated eleven circulating markers (adiponectin, resistin, tPAI-1, HGF, TNF-α, leptin, IL-8, sVCAM-1, sICAM-1, sFas, MIF) and found elevated levels of resistin [odds ratio(OR) for 3rd versus 1st tertile, 103.3; 95 confidence interval (CI), 19.3–552.8; P < 0.0001], sFas (OR, 4.2; 95% CI, 1.5–11.7; P = 0.003), IL-8 (OR, 59.8; 95% CI, 11.4–312.5; P < 0.0001), and TNA-α (OR, 38.6; 95% CI, 9.1–164.3, P < 0.0001) were in women with persistent HPV infection compared to HPV-negative women. Kemp et al. (Kemp, Hildesheim et al. 2010) evaluated an even broader spectrum of cytokines in their comparison of 50 HPV-positive women older than 45 years and 50 HPV-negative similarly aged women from their population-based cohort study in Guanacaste, Costa Rica. Plasma levels of IL-2, IL-4, IL-5, IL-6, IL-8, IL-10, IL-13, IL-17, IL-1α, IFN-γ, GM-CSF, TNF-α, MCP-1, MIP-1α, IP-10, RANTES, eotaxin, G-CSF, IL-12, IL-15, IL-7, and IL-1β were measured by Lincoplex assay, IFN-α was measured by bead array, and TGF-β1 was measured by ELISA. Their analysis revealed statistically significant differences between cases and controls in levels of IL-6, IL-8, TNF-α, and MIP-1α, GM-CSF, IL-1β (all P < 0.0001) and IL-1α (P = 0.02). However, it should be noted that this study was intentionally designed to explore differences between the extremes of the immunological spectrum. Thus, differences between these groups are likely to be biased away from the null (upward) in comparison to the general population. All six of these studies failed to concurrently evaluate potential confounders, and with the possible exception of TNF-α, none of their findings have been confirmed by other studies.

Unlike the other studies, Hong et al. (Hong, Kim et al. 2010) evaluated several potential confounders (parity, menopausal status, smoking, oral contraceptive use, histological findings of colposcopic-directed biopsy) in their recently published report of HPV persistence and clearance among 160 carcinogenic HPV positive Korean women (normal women or women with histologically confirmed mild dysplasia). While their univariate analysis revealed that the number of women who were serum negative for TNF-α was significantly higher in the carcinogenic HPV clearance group (N=107) than their persistence group (N=53, P = 0.0363), their multivariate logistic regression analysis indicated that none of the four cytokines measured (IFN-γ, TNF-α, IL-6, and IL-10) had a significant association with clearance of the carcinogenic HPV infection, pointing to the importance of these factors in future study design. In fact, they found that only age was significantly associated with clearance of carcinogenic HPV infections (OR, 0.95; 95% CI, 0.92- 0.98; P = 0.001).

Author & Year	Study source (Origin Country)	Immune Marker	HPV -/+ N (Measurement Method)	Major Conclusions
Hildesheim 1997	Kaiser Permanente clinics (US)	CellFree IL-2R test kits for sIL-2R from plasma recovered by centrifugation of peripheral blood	45/60 (Hybrid Capture)	No statistically significant association between sIL-2R and high risk HPV positivity in plasma.
Adam 1999	Centers for Disease Control collection (United States and Panama)	ELISA for Macrophage colony-stimulating factor (CSF-1) in serum	10/10 (ViraPap + ViraType dot blot hybridization assay for screen positives)	High-risk HPV infection is associated with higher mean serum CSF-1 levels.
Bais 2005	Outpatient GYN clinic (The Netherlands)	ELISA for IL-2, IL-4, IL-10, IL-12, IFN-γ, TNF-α, sTNFRI, sTNFRII in plasma and leucoctye count for leucocytes, neutrophils, monocytes, and lymphocytes in peripheral venous blood	11/10 (GP5+/GP6+ PCR)	High-risk HPV infection is associated with higher mean plasma IL-2 levels.
Hong 2010	University hospital and women's health center (Korea)	ELISA for IFN-γ, IL-6, IL-10, TNF-α in serum	0/160* (Hybrid Capture 2)	Based on univariate analysis, the number of women that were serum negative for TNF-α was significantly higher in the high risk HPV clearance group than the persistence group (P = 0.0363). Based on multivariate logistic regression, none of the 4 cytokines had a significant association with clearance of the high risk HPV infection. Only age was significantly associated with clearance of the high risk HPV infection (OR, 0.950; 95% confidence interval, 0.92-0.98; P = 0.001).**
Kemp 2010	Population-based cohort (Costa Rica)	Linco-plex assay for IL-2, IL-4, IL-5, IL-6, IL-8, IL-10, IL-13, IL-17, IL-1α, IFN-γ, GM-CSF, TNF-α, MCP-1, MIP-1α, IP-10, RANTES, eotaxin, G-CSF, IL-12, IL-15, IL-7, and IL-1β; ELISA for TGF-β1; single analyte in a bead array for IFN-α.	50/50 (MY09/11 PCR, dot blot hybridization for genotyping)	Persistent HPV infection in older women with evidence of immune deficit is associated with an increase in systemic inflammatory cytokines and weak lymphoproliferative responses.
Abike 2011	GYN Department (Turkey)	ELISA for neopterin in serum	78/44 (Amplisense HPV multiplex PCR typing kit)	Neopterin levels were lower in women with HPV than women without HPV.
Baker 2011	Population-based cohort (Costa Rica)	Millipore Multiplex Bead Assay for adiponectin, resistin, tPAI-1, HGF, TNF-α, leptin, IL-8, sVCAM-1, sICAM-1, sFas, MIF in PBMCs from heparinized blood	50/50 (MY09/11 PCR, dot blot hybridization for genotyping)	Resistin, sFas, IL-8, and TNA-α were elevated in women with persistent HPV infection compared to HPV-negative women.

* Compared HPV persistence and clearance. Thus, all were HPV-positive at baseline. **Adjusted for age, parity, menopause, oral contraception, histological findings of colposcopic-directed biopsy, and cytokines. Abbreviations: US = United States, HPV = human papillomavirus, DNA = deoxyribonucleic acid, GYN = Gynecology, PCR = polymerase chain reaction, ELISA = enzyme-linked immunosorbent assay, PBMCs = peripheral blood mononuclear cells

Table 1. Studies of circulating immune markers in plasma and serum.

Local Immune Marker Secretions in the Cervix. It is believed that measurement of cytokines in cervical secretions may better reflect local cytokine production relevant to cervical carcinogenesis than circulating cytokines. Currently, seven studies that met our inclusion criteria have measured immune responses in cervical secretions (Table 2). Unlike the studies of circulating cytokines above, most of these studies have tested for a broad range of HPV types, although one (Guha and Chatterjee, 2009) only tested for carcinogenic HPV types using the Hybrid Capture 2 assay, and another only analyzed results for women with carcinogenic HPV infection compared to women without carcinogenic HPV infection (Marks, Viscidi et al. 2011). Scott et al. (Scott, Stites et al. 1999) evaluated RNA expression of IL-4, IL-12, IFN-γ, and TNF and found that a T-helper type 1 (TH1) cytokine expression pattern (as defined by IFN-γ and TNF positivity and IL-4 negativity, with variable IL-12 expression) preceded HPV clearance. Crowley-Nowick et al. (Crowley-Nowick, Ellenberg et al. 2000) measured IL-2, IL-10, and IL-12 cytokine levels in HIV-positive and HIV-negative adolescents recruited from 16 clinical care settings in 13 US cities. Crowley-Nowick et al. found that HPV-positive girls had higher IL-12 concentrations compared to HPV-negative women ($P = 0.01$). Race, age, SIL status, smoking, other vaginal infections, and CD4 count were considered as potential confounders, but all were dropped out of the backwards regression model. Tjiong van der Vange et al. (Tjiong 2001) evaluated IL-12p40, IL-10, TGF-β1, TNF-α, and IL-1β levels by HPV status in CIN patients referred to an outpatient gynecology department. Similar to Crowley-Nowick et al., Tjiong van der Vange et al. found higher levels of IL-12 in HPV-positive compared to HPV-negative patients ($P=0.04$) (Tjiong 2001). However, no attempts were made to adjust for potential confounders. Unlike Crowley-Nowick et al. (Crowley-Nowick, Ellenberg et al. 2000) and Tjiong van der Vange et al. (Tjiong 2001), Gravitt et al. (Gravitt, Hildesheim et al. 2003) found no statistical differences in IL-10 and IL-12 concentrations by HPV-positivity versus HPV-negativity in women selected from a population-based cohort study in Guanacaste, Costa Rica, after adjusting for stage of menstrual cycle, recent oral contraceptive use secretion volume, and pH. Lieberman et al. (Lieberman, Moscicki et al. 2008) used a multiplex immunoassay kit to measure IL-1β, IL-2, IL-4, IL-5, IL-6, IL-8, IL-10, IL-12 (p40/p70), IL-13, IFN-γ in young women attending a family-planning clinic or university health center, or their friends. Although no significant differences were observed for women with incident or persistent HPV infections compared to women without HPV, there was some suggestion that IL-1β and IL-13 levels were reduced in women with incident or persistent HPV infections and that IL-6 and IL-2 levels were reduced in women with incident infections. Guha et al. (Guha and Chatterjee 2009) measured IL-1β, IL-6, IL-10, and IL-12 cytokine levels in commercial sex workers or spouses of HIV-positive men coming in for an HIV test. After taking HIV status into account, IL-1β, IL-10, and IL-12 seemed to be elevated in HPV-positive women compared to HPV-negative women. IL-6 was also higher in HPV-positive women compared to HPV-negative women ($P < 0.0004$). After stratifying by HIV status, however, IL-6 was only notably elevated in in women positive for both HPV and HIV, making the association with HPV less clear. This study also evaluated cytokine levels by abnormal versus normal cervical cytology and found that only IL-6 was related to abnormal cytology ($P = 0.03$). Finally, a recent study by Marks et al. (Marks, Viscidi et al. 2011) evaluated 27 different cytokines in a multiplex assay in cervical secretions from 35–60-year-old women attending outpatient obstetrics and gynecology clinics for routine examination. Similar to Gravitt et al. (Gravitt, Hildesheim et al. 2003) and Lieberman et al. (Lieberman, Moscicki et al. 2008), this study found no association between IL-12p70 and HPV status. However, IL-5 ($p = 0.03$), IL-9 ($p = 0.04$), IL-13 ($p = 0.01$), IL-17 ($p = 0.003$), EOTAXIN ($p = 0.04$), GM-CSF ($p = 0.01$), and MIP-1α ($p = 0.005$) levels were elevated in women with carcinogenic HPV infection compared to those without carcinogenic HPV. In addition, T-cell and pro-inflammatory cytokines tended to be correlated with EOTAXIN in women with carcinogenic HPV, while they were correlated with IL-2 in women without carcinogenic HPV. The authors conclude that this shift from IL-2 to EOTAXIN may reflect a shift away from antigen-specific adaptive responses toward innate responses.

Author & Year	Study source (Origin Country)	Immune Marker Measurement	HPV -/+ N (Measurement Method)	Major Conclusions
Scott 1999	Family planning clinics (US)	RT-PCR of cDNA from total RNA for IL-4, IL-12, IFN-γ, TNF	13/22 (MY09/11 PCR)	HPV-positive subjects (especially those who cleared) tended to be IFN-γ positive, TFN positive, and IL-4 negative ("Th1 cytokine pattern").
Crowley-Nowick 2000	16 clinical care settings in 13 cities (United States)	ELISA for IL-2, IL-10, IL-12 in Weck-cel sponges	18/20 (PCR)	"Coinfection with HIV, human papillomavirus, and other STIs predicted the highest IL-12 concentrations."*
Tjiong 2001	GYN department (The Netherlands)	ELISA for IL-12p40, IFN-γ, IL-10, TGF-β1, TNF-α and IL-1β in cervical washes	13/50 (HPV-16-specific PCR; negative samples confirmed by CPI and CPIIG)	IL-12 was more often detected than in the HPV-DNA negative CIN patients (P=0.04, Chi Square test). No other significant associations between cytokine levels and the detection of HPV-DNA were found.
Gravitt 2003	Population-based cohort (Costa Rica)	ELISA for IL-10 & IL12 in Weck-cel sponges	194/51 (MY09/11 + reverse-blot hybridization	No significant association between HPV and IL-10 or IL-12.**
Lieberman 2007	Family-planning clinic or university health center or friends (US)	Protein Multiplex Immunoassay kits for IL-1β, IL-2, IL-4, IL-5, IL-6, IL-8, IL-10, IL-12 (p40/p70), IL-13, IFN-γ in Merocel sponges	34/33 (PGMY09/11 PCR)	Although there were no significant differences between groups, IL-1β and IL-13 seemed to be depressed in women with incident or persistent HPV infections. IL-6 and IL-2 also seemed to be depressed in women with incident infections.
Guha 2009	Commercial sex workers or spouses of HIV+ men (India)	ELISA for IL-1β, IL-6, IL-10, IL-12 in lavage samples	28/17 (Hybrid Capture 2)	Taking HIV status into account, IL-1β, IL-10, and IL-12 seemed elevated in HPV+ vs. HPV- women. IL-6 seemed elevated when HIV was not taken into account (16.6 vs. 4.5 pg/ml, p≤0.0004), but otherwise was only notably elevated in women positive for both HPV and HIV.†
Marks 2011	Outpatient OB/GYN clinics (US)	Bio-Rad multiplex assay for BASIC FGF, EOTAXIN, GCSF, GMCSF, IFN-γ, IL-1β, IL-1ra, IL-2, IL-4, IL-5, IL-6, IL-7, IL-8, IL-9, IL-10, IL-12p70, IL-13, IL-15, IL-17, IP-10, MCP-1, MIP-1α, MIP-1β, PDGF-BB, RANTES, TNF-α, VEGF in Merocel sponges	44/34 (Roche HPV Linear Array)	Carcinogenic HPV associated with elevated IL-5, IL-9, IL-13, IL-17, EOTAXIN, GM-CSF, and MIP-1α levels and a shift from IL-2 to EOTAXIN compared to no carcinogenic HPV, possibly reflecting a shift away from antigen-specific adaptive responses toward innate responses.

*Considered potential confounders, but all were dropped through backwards modeling. †Stratified by HIV status, but did not evaluate additional confounders. Abbreviations: US = United States, HPV = human papillomavirus, HIV = human immunodeficiency virus, CIN = cervical intraepithelial neoplasia, GYN = gynecology, OB/GYN = obstetrics and gynecology, PCR = polymerase chain reaction, qRT-PCR = quantitative reverse transcriptase PCR, STI = sexually transmitted infection

Table 2. Studies of immune markers in cervical secretions.

There is little consistency in the cytokines evaluated in these seven studies, but where there is overlap, the results tend to be contradictory. For example, one study found evidence that IL-6 levels were reduced in women with incident HPV infections (Lieberman, Moscicki et al. 2008), while another found that IL-6 levels tended to be elevated in HPV-positive women (Guha and Chatterjee 2009). Similarly, one study found no evidence that IL-12 levels varied by HPV status (Gravitt, Hildesheim et al. 2003), while two others (Crowley-Nowick, Ellenberg et al. 2000; Tjiong, van der Vange et al. 2001) observed higher levels of IL-12 in HPV-positive versus HPV-negative women. In addition, results from the study by Guha et al. (Guha and Chatterjee 2009) suggested a tendency toward increased levels of IL-1β in HPV-positive women versus HPV-negative women, while the results from Lieberman et al. (Lieberman, Moscicki et al. 2008) showed a trend toward decreased levels of IL-1β in women with incident or persistent HPV infection compared to HPV-negative women. These inconsistencies are not yet resolved.

Cytokine Responses in Patient-derived PBMCs. There is evidence that cell-mediated immune responses play an important role in the control of HPV infections. Cell-mediated immune responses are regulated by T lymphocytes [T-helper (Th) lymphocytes and cytotoxic lymphocytes (CTLs)] in cooperation with antigen-presenting cells such as monocytes and dendritic cells. These cells all are modulated by and release cytokines that can influence one another's synthesis. Characterization (including quality and quantity) of lymphocytes directed against HPV epitopes has been examined with the goal of providing insights into the clinical outcomes of HPV-positive patients. To this end, analyses of cytokines and concurrent lymphoproliferative and CTL responses in patient-derived peripheral blood mononuclear cells (PBMCs), T-cell fractions isolated from PBMCs or whole blood cultures after stimulation with several antigens and/or HPV peptides has been evaluated in 10 publications (Table 3).

Tsukui et al. (Tsukui, Hildesheim et al. 1996) was one of the first to measure IL-2 levels in culture supernatants of PBMCs stimulated with predominantly 15mer overlapping peptides from HPV-16 E6 and E7 oncoproteins. The HPV early proteins E2, E6 and E7 are among the first of proteins that are expressed in HPV-infected epithelia. Stimulation with influenza served as a specificity control, and stimulation with phytohemagglutinin (PHA) served as a positive control since it is known to activate lymphocytes and induce rapid cell proliferation as well as lead to the release of inflammatory and immune cytokines. While the report itself focused on associations with IL-2 and disease progression, the study included both HPV typing data and IL-2 response data for each subject included in the study. Interestingly, by using the data presented in the paper for statistical calculation, we found that IL-2 levels were significantly increased in a group of 32 HPV positive healthy women and women with LSIL compared to a group of 51 HPV negative healthy women and women with LSIL ($P=0.006$). Among 18 women with HSIL with HPV typing and adequate IL-2 data, only 2 women had positive IL-2 levels (1 HPV positive, 1 HPV negative).

Several other studies also attempted to evaluate IL-2 levels in a similar manner. deGruijl et al. (de Gruijl, Bontkes et al. 1998) examined IL-2 reactivity in PBMCs stimulated with HPV16 E7 and sorted by anti-CD4 or anti-CD8 antibodies. They found that positive CD4+ T helper cell IL-2 reactivity was restricted to patients infected by HPV16 and related types and that reactivity was strongly associated with HPV persistence. Further, women with cervical carcinoma showed IL-2 responses at a significantly reduced rate [7 of 15 (47%); $P = 0.014$].

Author & Year	Study source (Origin Country)	Immune Marker Measurement	HPV -/+ N (Measurement Method)	Major Conclusions
Tsukui 1996	Kaiser Permanent or Simmons Cancer Center (US)	IL-2 was measured by radioimmunoassay in culture supernatants of PBMCs from whole blood that were stimulated with 15mer HPV16 peptides to E6 and E7, or stimulated with FLU or PHA	56/40 (ViraPap: Hybrid Capture with HPV-16-specific Hybrid Capture for +samples. Tumors: GP5+/GP6+ PCR)	IL-2 is signficantly increased in healthy HPV+ women and HPV+ women with LSIL. Few women with HSIL or cancer have detectable IL-2 levels.
Kadish 1997	Colposcopy clinic (US)	Measured lymphocyte proliferation in HPV16 E6 and E7 peptide stimulated cultures of PBMCs from heparinized blood	26/51 (PCR and Southern Blot assay; typing by dot blot for 39 types)	Lymphoproliferative responses to specific HPV16 E6 and E7 peptides are significantly associated with the clearance of HPV infection.
de Gruijl 1998	Non-intervention cohort follow-up study of patients with cervical dysplasia plus follow-up study of HPV-positive women with normal cervical cytology (Netherlands)	IL-2 was measured by IL-2 bioassay in culture supernatants of PBMCs from heparinized blood that were stimulated with 14 different 20mer HPV16 peptides to E7, or stimulated with PHA; T cell subsets were depleted by magnetic bead sorting and anti-CD4 and anti-CD8 antibodies	15/51 (GP5+/GP6+ PCR)	Positive CD4+ T helper cell IL-2 reactivity was restricted to patients infected by HPV-16 and related types and showed a strong association with viral persistence. Women with cervical carcinoma showed IL-2 responses at a significantly reduced rate [7 of 15 (47%); P = 0.014].
Bontkes 1999	Non-intervention cohort follow-up study of patients with cervical dysplasia (Netherlands)	IL-2 was measured by IL-2 bioassay in culture supernatants of PBMCs from heparinized blood that were stimulated with HPV16 N-terminal and C-terminal E2 protein fragments or with PHA.	22/52 (GP5+/GP6+ PCR)	HPV16 infection was not associated with IL-2 responsiveness against the N-terminal domain of E2, but HPV clearance was associated with IL-2 responsiveness against the C-terminal E2 domain
de Gruijl 1999	Non-intervention cohort follow-up study of patients with cervical dysplasia (Netherlands)	IL-2 was measured by IL-2 bioassay in culture supernatants of PBMCs from heparinized blood that were stimulated with HPV16 L1-VLP or synthetic L1-derived 15-mer peptides P1 (amino acids 311-325) and P2 (amino acids 321-335), or stimulated with PHA; T cell subsets were depleted by magnetic bead sorting and anti-CD4 or CD8 antibodies. HPV-16 L1-VLP-speciic plasma IgG was measured by ELISA.	15/49 (GP5+/GP6+ PCR)	IgG responses were significantly associated with HPV16 persistence but CD4 T helper IL-2 responses were significantly associated with both HPV clearance and persistence. Neither cell-mediated nor humoral immune responses against HPV16 L1 seemed adequate for viral control.

Abbreviations: US = United States, HPV = human papillomavirus, DNA = deoxyribonucleic acid, GYN = Gynecology, PCR = polymerase chain reaction, ELISA = enzyme-linked immunosorbent assay, PBMCs= peripheral blood mononuclear cells, FLU= influenze, PHA = phytohemagglutinin, LSIL = low grade squamous intraepithelial lesion, HSIL = high grade squamous intraepithelial lesion, mCTLp= memory cytotoxic T-cell precursor

Table 3. Part 1. Cytokine Responses in Patient-derived PBMCs.

Author & Year	Study source (Origin Country)	Immune Marker Measurement	HPV -/+ N (Measurement Method)	Major Conclusions
Bontkes 2000	Non-intervention cohort follow-up study of patients with cervical dysplasia (Netherlands)	HPV16-specific mCTLp activity was measured in cultured PBMCs from heparinized blood stimulated with both HPV16 E6 and E7 peptides. IL-2 was measured by IL-2 bioassay in culture supernatants of PBMCs that were stimulated with 14 different 20mer HPV16 peptides to E7, or stimulated with PHA.	11/20 (GP5+/GP6+ PCR)	mCTLp activity was significantly associated with persistent HPV16 infection but not observed in HPV negative women or women with viral clearance. HPV 16 E7-specific mCTLp activity was associated with previously published IL-2 release in response to HPV 16 E7-derived peptides at the end of follow-up.
Molling 2007	Non-intervention cohort follow-up study of patients with cervical dysplasia (Netherlands)	Cultured PBMCs taken from heparinized blood were stimulated with 14 different 20mer HPV16 E7 peptides or with PHA. IL-2 levels were determined by bioassay. CTL activity determined by chromium release assay. iNKT and Treg counts were measured by FACS. FoxP3 staining was performed using an available kit. Lymphocytes were characterized by staining with monoclonal antibodies.	24/58 (GP5+/GP6+ PCR and type specific PCR for 27 types)	Treg frequencies significantly increased in women with persistent HPV16 infection. Treg frequencies were increased in patients who had detectable HPV16 E7 specific IL-2 producing T-helper cells, suggesting HPV may affect Treg development. No evidence that iNKT cells affect persistence of HPV16 infection.
Seresini 2007	Healthy donors and women with cervical lesions (Italy)	CD4+ T cells were purified from cultured PBMCs from perifpheral blood stimulated with HPV18 E6 peptides or PHA and CTL activity was measured by chromium release assay as well as IL-4, IL-5, IL-10 and IFN-γ levels using cytometric bead array kits. The immune infiltrates in cervical lesions were also evaluated.	25/37 (Hybrid Capture 2 and typing by reverse hybridization assay)	One or more HPV18 E6 peptides were observed to be able to induce a response in 40-50% of the women evaluated. Response percentages increased to 80-100% when HPV18+ women alone were considered. Levels of IFN-γ released were shown to predict HPV persistence and/or disease relapse after surgery. A higher number of infiltrating CD4(+) and T-bet(+) T cells were observed in the lesions which correlated with favorable clinical outcomes.
Sharma 2007	Outpatient department or cancer clinic (India)	IL-2, IFN-γ, IL-4, and IL-10 was measured by ELISA in cultured PBMCs from heparinized blood stimulated with PHA	30/84 (HPV16 and HPV 18 PCR)	Increasing levels of IL-4 and IL-10 levels were significantly associated with HPV infection. Decreasing levels of IL-2 and IFN-γ were associated with HPV status.
Kemp 2010	Population-based cohort (Costa Rica)	Linco-plex assay for IL-6, IL-8, TNF-α, MIP-1α in unstimulated and PHA stimulated PBMCs	50/50 (MY09/11 PCR, dot blot hybridization for genotyping)	IL 6, TNF-α, MIP-1α levels were significantly higher in unstimulated PBMCs from HPV+ and HPV- women; IL-6, IL-8, TNF-α and MIP-1α levels were significantly lower in PHA stimulated PBMCs between HPV+ and HPV- women

Abbreviations: US = United States, HPV = human papillomavirus, DNA = deoxyribonucleic acid, GYN = Gynecology, PCR = polymerase chain reaction, ELISA = enzyme-linked immunosorbent assay, PBMCs = peripheral blood mononuclear cells, FLU = influenze, PHA = phytohemagglutinin, LSIL = low grade squamous intraepithelial lesion, HSIL = high grade squamous intraepithelial lesion, mCTLp = memory cytotoxic T-cell precursor

Table 3. Part 2. Cytokine Responses in Patient-derived PBMCs.

These findings are consistent with Tsukui et al. (Tsukui, Hildesheim et al. 1996) and suggest that IL-2 responsiveness may differ by cytological and/or disease stage. In 1999, deGruijl et al. (de Gruijl, Bontkes et al. 1999) again evaluated IL-2 levels, as well as IgG responses, in this same population. This time, they used HPV16 L1-VLP or synthetic L1-derived 15-mer peptides P1 (amino acids 311-325) and P2 (amino acids 321-335) to stimulate the PBMCs and sorted them as before. Importantly, they found IgG responsiveness was significantly associated with HPV16 persistence alone, but that CD4 T helper IL-2 responsiveness was significantly associated with both HPV clearance and persistence. Further, they reported that neither cell-mediated nor humoral immune responses against HPV16 L1 seemed adequate for viral control. In another publication, this group took their study one step further and measured IL-2 levels in response to HPV E2 N-terminal and C-terminal protein fragments (Bontkes, de Gruijl et al. 1999). They reported that HPV16 infection was not associated with IL-2 responsiveness against the N-terminal domain of E2, but HPV clearance was associated with IL-2 responsiveness against the C-terminal E2 domain. The following year, Bontkes et al. (Bontkes, de Gruijl et al. 2000) evaluated HPV 16 E6- and E7-specific memory cytotoxic T-cell precursor (mCTLp) activity in the same cohort of patients with cervical dysplasia. They found that activity was significantly associated with persistent HPV16 infection but not observed in HPV negative women or women with viral clearance. Kadish et al. (Kadish, Ho et al. 1997) had previously observed a similar phenomenon. Subjects with positive lymphoproliferative responses to E6 and/or E7 peptides were more likely to be HPV negative at the same clinic visit than were nonresponders ($P = 0.039$). Subjects who were negative for HPV and those with a low viral load were also more likely to respond than were those with a high viral load (P for trend = 0.037). These data suggest that lymphoproliferative responses to specific HPV 16 E6 and E7 peptides appear to be associated with the clearance of HPV infection.

In 2007, three additional reports evaluating patient-derived PBMCs were published. Sharma et al. (Sharma, Rajappa et al. 2007) focused on IL-2, IFN-g, IL-4, and IL-10 levels in PBMCs stimulated with PHA. They observed that increasing levels of IL-4 and IL-10 levels were significantly associated with HPV infection and that decreasing levels of IL-2 and IFN-γ were associated with HPV status. Seresini et al. (Seresini, Origoni et al. 2007) measured lymphoproliferative responses and IL-2, IFN-g, IL-4, and IL-10 levels in PBMCs stimulated not with HPV16 peptides, but rather with HPV18-specific E6 peptides. Their analyses revealed that one or more HPV18 E6 peptides were able to induce a response in 40-50% of the women evaluated. Response percentages increased to 80-100% when HPV18-positive women alone were considered. Levels of IFN-γ released were also shown to predict HPV persistence and/or disease relapse after surgery. In addition, they showed that a higher number of infiltrating CD4(+) and T-bet(+) T cells in lesions correlated with favorable clinical outcomes. Finally, Molling et. al. (Molling, de Gruijl et al. 2007) evaluated cultured PBMCs again stimulated with 14 different 20mer HPV16 E7 peptides or with PHA and measured both IL-2 levels and CTL activity. Importantly, they also measured invariant natural killer T-cells (iNKT) and FoxP3+ regulatory T cells (Tregs) levels by flow cytometry (FACSCalibur). While iNKT cells did not appear to be associated with HPV persistence, Treg frequencies were significantly increased in women with persistent HPV16 infection; and the Tregs were significantly more common in women who had detectable HPV16 E7 specific IL-2 producing T-helper cells. These data suggest that HPV infection may affect Treg development - a finding that opens the door for a whole new avenue of research related to HPV-related immune research.

Immune Markers in Cervical Tissues PBMC responses and circulating or secreted cytokines can be useful indicators of immune response, but the best indications may come from the actual site of interaction between HPV infection and the immune system: tissue. A number of studies have attempted to measure immune markers in HPV-positive compared to HPV-negative women in different ways. Among studies included in this review, these markers fall into three major categories: immune presentation molecules, cytokines or cytokine receptors, and immune cells.

Several studies used immunohistochemistry (IHC) to stain for major histocompatibility complex (MHC) proteins in cervical tissue (Table 4). MHC class I molecules present endogenous antigens (cytoplasmic proteins) to cytotoxic (CD8+) T cells and are typically present on all nucleated cells (Murphy, Travers et al. 2011). In contrast, MHC class II molecules present exogenous antigens from outside the cell to helper (CD4+) T cells and are typically present only on antigen presenting cells, such as dendritic cells and macrophages. Thus, normal cervical epithelial cells should be MHC class I positive and MHC class II negative. In humans, MHC class I consists of major human leukocyte antigens (HLA) A, B, and C and minor antigens E, F, and G, while MHC class II consists of HLA-DM, -DO, -DP, -DQ, and -DR.

Using a polyclonal stain specific for HLA-A, -B and -C heavy chains in formalin-fixed, paraffin-embedded (FFPE) tissue from biopsies and resection specimens from women with CIN1-3 or cancer, Cromme et al. (Cromme, Meijer et al. 1993) found that normal MHC class I expression, defined positive staining in ≥75% of cells, was reduced in women with HPV16, 18, or 31 infection versus HPV-negative women (p=0.04). MHC class II expression, as measured through a polyclonal HLA-DR antigen stain, was also altered, with normal staining (<25% positively stained cells) in 42% of women with HPV16, 18, or 31 infection versus 64% of HPV-negative women. This alteration was not statistically significant, however (p=0.14). Gonclaves el al (Goncalves, Le Discorde et al. 2008) also examined MHC class I expression in FFPE biopsy blocks, but in women with normal through cancerous histology. They found that HLA-A/B/C expression was not significantly elevated in HPV-positive compared to HPV-negative women (OR, 2.29; 95% CI, 0.77- 11.00; P = 0.14). Strangely, HPV16/18 infection was inversely associated with HLA-A/B/C expression (OR, 0.12; 95% CI, 0.02- 0.79; P = 0.04), but as reported, it was unclear whether this association was based on comparison to HPV-negative women, or a combination of both HPV-negative women and women with HPV infections other than HPV16 and 18. HLA-E expression tended to be increased in HPV-positive versus HPV-negative women (OR, 3.83; 95% CI, 0.49-30.10; P = 0.22), especially for HPV16/18 infections (OR, 11.25; 95% CI: 2.32-55.47; P = 0.003). Similarly, Dong et al. (Dong, Yang et al. 2010) stained for HLA-G in FFPE blocks from CIN1-3 patients and found higher HLA-G expression in HPV16/18-positive patients than HPV16/18-negative patients (P = 0.02).

In addition to interaction with an antigen MHC complex, T-cells require costimulation with an antigen nonspecific molecule to be full activated. T cells that encounter antigen MHC complex without costimulation may be come anergic and thus tolerant to the presence of HPV. To investigate this possibility, Ortiz-Sanchez et al. (Ortiz-Sanchez, Chavez-Olmos et al. 2007) evaluated expression of the CD80 and CD86 MHC class II costimulatory molecules through immunohistochemistry (IHC), quantitative reverse transcriptase PCR (qRT-PCR), and RNA in situ hybridization (ISH) in FFPE biopsies from histologically normal HPV-negative women and HPV16-positive women with LSIL. They found that CD86, but not CD80, was expressed in all HPV-negative normal cervical epithelial samples, while CD86

Author & Year	Study source (Origin Country)	Immune Marker Measurement	HPV -/+ N (Measurement Method)	Major Conclusions
Cromme 1993	Oncological GYN oupatient department (Netherlands)	IHC for MHC-I & MHC-II expression in FFPE tissue from biopsies & resection specimens	14/107 (GP 5/6 PCR + TS PCR for HPV6, 11, 16, 18, 31, 33; RNA ISH for HPV16 E7)	Normal MHC-I expression reduced in women with HPV16, 18, or 31 vs. HPV-negative women (p=0.04). MHC-II expression was also altered with HPV16/18/31, but not significantly.
Fernandes 2005	Outpatient GYN Clinic (Brazil)	Double-sandwich ELISA for IFN-γ, TNF-α, IL-10 in snap frozen cervical biopsies	0/42 (GP5/6, MY09/11, HPV16E7.667/HPV16E7.774, HPV18E7.696/HPV18E7.799 PCRs)*	HPV16 associated with higher IL-10 and IFN-γ intralesional levels than other HPV types, but HPV18 was associated with reduced TNF-α and INF-γ levels. Thus, immune response may vary by HPV type.
Ortiz-Sanchez 2007	Women undergoing a routine hysterectomy due to uterine myomatosis and women with LSIL (Mexico)	IHC, qRT-PCR, ISH for CD80 and 86; IHC for IL10 in FFPE biopsies	30/30 (MY09/11 and p16-1 and p16-2R primer PCR. HPV typing by sequence comparison. Only the HPV-16 samples included in CD86 expression analysis.)	CD86 expression was decreased in patients with HPV16 positive LSIL versus normal women, independent of IL-10. Expression of CD86 on normal cervical keratinocytes could indicate the ability to activate cytotoxic T cells, while the shut-off of this molecule in HPV-16 positive lesions could be a mechanism for evading host immune surveillance, resulting in the persistent HPV infection and probable progression of cervical lesions.
Song 2007	OB/GYN clinic (Republic of Korea)	qRT-PCR for IL-6, IL-10, IFN-γ, TNF-α in frozen tissue biopsies	0/67 (Hybrid Capture 2 + HPV DNA Chip)*	IFN-γ was significantly associated with HPV-16 E6, E7, and high-risk HPV viral load among HPV-positive women.**
Bermudez-Morales 2008	Instituto Nacional de Cancerolog´ıa (National Cancerology Institute, Mexico)	RT-PCR for IL-10 in cervical scraping and biopsies (storage not specified)	28/47 (PCR-RFLPs)	Strong association between HPV positivity and IL10 mRNA levels
Butsch Kovacic 2008	The ASCUS/LSIL Triage Study for Cervical Cancer (ALTS) trial (US)	Visual counting of lymphocytes, neutrophils, macrophages, plasma cells, and eosinophils in 3 H&E sections per biopsy (stromal and epithelial sections of hematoxylin and eosin stain slides from FFPE biopsy tissue evaluated)	228/288 (Hybrid Capture 2 and PCR)	These data suggest that cervical inflammation varies with type of human papillomavirus infection, risk of persistence and progression and HPV cofactors.**

*Evaluated cytokine expression by HPV type in HPV-positive women. **Study adjusted for confounding factors in regression models. †Compared HPV persistence and clearance. Thus, all were HPV-positive at baseline. Abbreviations: HPV = human papillomavirus, CIN = cervical intraepithelial neoplasia, FFPE = formalin-fixed paraffin-embedded, GYN = gynecology, ISH = in situ hybridization, IHC = Immunohistochemistry, OB/GYN = obstetrics and gynecology, qRT-PCR = quantitative reverse transcriptase PCR, STI = sexually transmitted infection, TIL = tumor infiltrating lymphocytes, RFLPs= Restriction Fragment Length Polymorphisms, ASCUS = Atypical Squamous Cells of Undetermined Significance, LSIL = low grade squamous intraepithelial lesion, HSIL = high grade squamous intraepithelial lesion, US = United States

Table 4. Part 1. Immune Markers in Cervical Tissues.

Author & Year	Study source (Origin Country)	Immune Marker Measurement	HPV -/+ N (Measurement Method)	Major Conclusions
Gonclaves 2008	GYN Reference Services (Brazil)	IHC for HLA-A/B/C and HLA-E in RNA from FFPE biopsy blocks	19/55 (GP5+/6+, MY09/11, HPV16E7.667/ HPV16E7.774, HPV18E7.696/ HPV18E7.799)	Some evidence that HPV infection was associated with increased HLA-E expression, especially HPV16/18 infection. Association with HLA-A/B/C was less clear.
Song 2008	OB/GYN clinic (Republic of Korea)	qRT-PCR for IL-6, IL-10, IFN-γ, TNF-α from frozen tissue biopsies	0/57 (Hybrid Capture 2)†	IFN-γ correlated with high-risk HPV clearance.**
Tirone 2009	Women with CIN or normal women with hysterectomies due to uterine myoma (Brazil)	RT-PCR for IFNAR 1, IFNAR 2, 2'5'OAS, IFN-α from cervical tissue biopsies	31/14 (Hybrid Capture 2)	Lower IFN-α receptor expression with HPV infection.
Brismar Wendel 2010	Healthy volunteers at Karolinska Division of Obstetrics and Gynecology (Sweden)	qRT-PCR for CD3, CD4, CD8, CD19, CD27, CCR5, CCL5/Rantes, IL-2, IL-4, IL-10, IL-12a, IL-17a, IL-7R, HLA-DRα, IFN-γ, TNF-β, PD-1, CTLA-4, LAG3, IgA, IgG from frozen biopsy of ectocervix outside the transformation zone	13/11 (Roche Linear Array)	HPV not associated with a local inflammatory immune response as measured by qRT-PCR.
Dong 2010	Department of Pathology (China)	IHC for HLA-G and visual counting of TILs in 5 high-power fields from FFPE blocks	22/33 (ISH for HPV16 & 18 in FFPE tissue section)	HLA-G elevated in HPV16/18+ lesions and associated with lower TIL counts, suggesting inhibition of immune response against HPV.
Øvestad 2011	Women refered to a hospital for abnormal Papanicolaou tests (Norway)	IHC for CD4, CD8, CD25, from RNA isolated from paraffin blocks of punch biopsies CD138, FOXp3	0/45 (AMPLICOR and Linear Array)*	HPV16 and related types were correlated with lower CD8-positive cell counts in the stroma compared to other HPV types.**

*Evaluated cytokine expression by HPV type in HPV-positive women. **Study adjusted for confounding factors in regression models. †Compared HPV persistence and clearance. Thus, all were HPV-positive at baseline. Abbreviations: HPV=human papillomavirus, CIN=cervical intraepithelial neoplasia, FFPE=formalin-fixed paraffin-embedded, GYN=gynecology, ISH=in situ hybridization, IHC=Immunohistochemistry, OB/GYN= obstetrics and gynecology, qRT-PCR=quantitative reverse transcriptase PCR, STI=sexually transmitted infection, TIL=tumor infiltrating lymphocytes, RFLPs=Restriction Fragment Length Polymorphisms, ASCUS=Atypical Squamous Cells of Undetermined Significance, LSIL=low grade squamous intraepithelial lesion, HSIL=high grade squamous intraepithelial lesion, US=United States

Table 4. Part 2. Immune Markers in Cervical Tissues.

expression was lower (73% by IHC) in HPV16-positive LSIL samples. This decrease in CD86 expression in HPV-positive women could represent and immune evasion mechanisms through the down-regulation of costimulatory molecules.

The next major category of immune markers measured in cervical tissue includes cytokines and their receptors. In addition to testing for MHC costimulatory molecules, Ortiz-Sanchez et al. (Ortiz-Sanchez, Chavez-Olmos et al. 2007) used IHC to stain for IL-10, which inhibits CD86 expression. IL-10 detection was likewise poor in both HPV-negative normal tissue and HPV16-positive LSIL tissue, but detection was higher in a high-grade SIL (HSIL) control sample. Fernandez et al. 2005 tested for IFN-γ, TNF-α, and IL-10 protein from snap frozen cervical biopsies from HIV-positive or HIV-negative LSIL and HSIL patients infected with HPV using a double-sandwich ELISA approach. They reported that HPV16 was associated with higher IL-10 (P = 0.03) and IFN-γ (P = 0.04) intra-lesional levels than other HPV types, but HPV18 was associated with reduced TNF-α (P = 0.009) and INF-γ levels (P = 0.01) suggesting that immune responses may vary by the infecting HPV type.

The majority of studies measured cytokines with quantitative reverse transcriptase PCR (qRT-PCR). Bermudez-Morales et al. (Bermudez-Morales, Gutierrez et al. 2008) found a strong association between HPV positivity and IL10 mRNA levels, especially for HPV16. Song et al. evaluated IL-6, IL-10, IFN-γ, and TNF-α and both HPV16 positivity (Song, Lee et al. 2008.) and HPV clearance versus persistence (Song 2008) among women positive for carcinogenic HPV. They found that IFN-γ was associated with HPV-16 *E6* (OR, 28.20; 95% CI, 2.66-299.11) and *E7* (OR, 19.62; 95% CI, 2.14-180.25) expression (Song, Lee et al. 2007), as well as with clearance of carcinogenic HPV (OR, 8.26; 95% CI: 1.24-54.94) (Song, Lee et al. 2008.). Tirone et al. (Tirone, Peghini et al. 2009) found some evidence that the IFN-α receptor subunits IFNAR 1 and IFNAR 2 were under-expressed in HPV-positive women with CIN1-3 compared to HPV-negative women with normal through CIN3 histology. Brismar Wendel et al. (Brismar Wendel, Kaldensjo et al. 2010) measured a number of different cytokines and other immune markers and found no difference between HPV-positive and HPV-negative healthy volunteers (22/24 with normal cytology).

Another major category of immune markers is the immune cells themselves. Two studies in this review evaluated infiltrating immune cells in cervical tissue by visually counting the cells. Butsch Kovacic et al. (Butsch Kovacic, Katki et al. 2008) counted lymphocytes, neutrophils, macrophages, plasma cells, and eosinophils among women with typical squamous cells of undetermined significance or LSIL and found that cervical inflammation varies with type of HPV infection, as well as risk of persistence and progression. Women with carcinogenic HPV infections also had more severe epithelial inflammation and less severe stromal inflammation than HPV-negative women. These associations were limited to carcinogenic and not the non-carcinogenic HPV types. Dong et al. (Dong, Yang et al. 2010) determined that among HPV16/18-positive CIN lesions, moderate to strong HLA-G expression was associated with weak immune response, as measured by few tumor infiltrating lymphocytes (TIL), whereas weak HLA-G expression was associated with strong immune response (high numbers of TIL). HLA-G expression was not associated with TIL in HPV-negative women, suggesting that the increased HLA-G expression in HPV-positive lesion may reflect an inhibition of immune response against HPV. Brismar Wendel et al. (Brismar Wendel, Kaldensjo et al. 2010) used qRT-PCR to measure CD3, CD4, CD8, CD19, and CD27 expression but found no difference by HPV status. Finally, Øvestad et al. (Ovestad, Vennestrom et al. 2011) used IHC to stain for cell surface marker in biopsies from CIN2-3 patients and found that HPV16 and related types were correlated with lower CD8-positive cell counts in the stroma compared to other HPV types ($P = 0.02$).

4. Conclusions and future perspectives

Taken together, these studies support the role of cell-mediated immune response in HPV-related carcinogenesis although their findings, particularly for those measuring cytokines, are largely inconsistent. There are many potential explanations. There has been a real lack of consistency in sample collection methods, cytokine measurement methods and even the outcome definitions used for analyses.

For example, some studies assessed HPV positivity, regardless of timing and/or disease state, while others evaluated incident HPV infection or HPV persistence or clearance. Further, these studies more than often focused on HPV 16, on carcinogenic HPV types, or any HPV type infection together. However, those few studies that did evaluate immune markers by individual HPV type found evidence that immune responses vary by HPV type (Fernandes, Gonçalves et al. 2005; Butsch Kovacic, Katki et al. 2008; Ovestad, Vennestrom et al. 2011). Thus, HPV type is an important consideration. Moreover, while we chose to focus on immune markers' associations with HPV infection, most of the studies reviewed in this chapter predominantly assessed associations between immune markers and disease state (LSIL, HSIL, cancer or CIN1-3 and cancer). Ideally, future studies would evaluate differences by individual HPV type and better consider the timing of disease.

There are also other notable differences in the study populations considered by these studies (e.g., sample size, young versus old women, inclusion of HIV-positive women). Many studies used convenience samples of women. In fact, there is a general lack of consideration for factors that could confound or modify both cytokine production and the infectious outcomes. Only eight of the 35 studies made any attempt to account for co-factors that may influence cytokine level. The importance of adjusting for such potential confounders was recently highlighted at an international workshop that addressed best practices for sampling techniques and assessment of mucosal immune responses. The workshop identified a number of characteristics that should be considered when studying female genital tract immunity, including age, race, body mass index, sexually transmitted infections, other genital tract infections, vaginal flora, alcohol or substance use, recent immunization, pregnancy, phase of menstrual cycle, genital inflammation, recent douching, gynecologic procedures, recent intercourse/semen, and contraception (Anderson and Cu-Uvin 2011). The number of women included in each study is another important consideration in the evaluation of these studies. Twenty-two of the 32 (69%) studies meeting our criteria included less than 30 women in one or more groups (e.g., the HPV-positive or HPV-negative group). Fifteen (47%) included less than 20 in one or more groups. Small numbers of women in the comparison groups can lead to unstable results and may help explain why results for individual immune markers are so inconsistent.

Most studies have measured only a few cytokines, and few have evaluated infiltrating immune cells concurrently with cytokines, making it challenging to explore the activation pathways of cells involved in the immune response against HPV. One research group has made extensive use of their study population to characterize several aspects of immune response as measured in PBMCs (de Gruijl, Bontkes et al. 1998; Bontkes, de Gruijl et al. 1999; de Gruijl, Bontkes et al. 1999; Bontkes, de Gruijl et al. 2000; Molling, de Gruijl et al. 2007). However, few studies have been so thorough. In fact, more than half of the studies of PBMCs (five of nine studies), have come from this same research group with the same study population. Additional studies characterizing many aspects of immune response in different study populations would help clarify whether the results are broadly applicable.

Many studies focused on T-helper type 1 (TH1) versus T-helper type 2 (TH2) polarization, using a single cytokine (or small group of cytokines) to characterize the T-helper phenotype. However, advances in immunology have led to the shift of the TH1/TH2 paradigm to the TH1/TH2/TH17/T-reg hypothesis, a multi-lineage commitment from the same T-helper precursor cells. TH17 cells, in fact, have been shown to inhibit both TH1 and TH2 cells, and therefore are likely to play a critical role in HPV-related immune responses as well. Few studies have evaluated TH17 or Treg cells. The recent study by Molling et al. (Molling, de Gruijl et al. 2007) is among the few that have measured these cells. Using flow cytometry in HPV16 E7 stimulated PBMCs, they determined that Treg frequencies were significantly greater in women with persistent HPV16 infection and in women with detectable HPV16 E7 specific IL-2 producing T-helper cells, suggesting that HPV infection may affect Treg development. These findings may also be supported by tissue-based studies of MHC class II expression. Although data are limited, one study found evidence of increased MHC class II expression in HPV-positive versus negative patients (Cromme, Meijer et al. 1993), while another found reduced expression of the CD86 MHC class II costimulatory molecule (Ortiz-Sanchez, Chavez-Olmos et al. 2007). It could be hypothesized that HPV upregulates MHC class II expression and down-regulates MHC class II costimulatory molecules in order to increase T-cell anergy through incomplete signaling. Additional studies are needed to better understand these relationships.

For studies of cervical secretions, the collection method can have a large impact on the results. Of the seven cervical secretion studies included in this review, two collected cervical secretions through cervicovaginal lavage (Tjiong, van der Vange et al. 2001; Guha and Chatterjee 2009), four used Weck-cel® (Crowley-Nowick, Ellenberg et al. 2000; Gravitt, Hildesheim et al. 2003) or Merocel® (Lieberman, Moscicki et al. 2008; Marks, Viscidi et al. 2011) ophthalmic sponges, and one used cytobrush sample suspensions (Scott, Stites et al. 1999). Cervicovaginal lavages may not be specific enough to the cervix and may overly dilute the specimen. Even studies that used ophthalmic sponges tended to use Weck-cel® sponges (Gravitt, Hildesheim et al. 2003; Moscicki, Ellenberg et al. 2004), which may not provide adequate cytokine recovery, especially compared to Merocel® sponges (Castle et al.(Castle, Rodriguez et al. 2004).

Studies evaluating tissue have seldom considered both stroma and epithelium. In this chapter, only two studies examined inflammation in both stroma and epithelium (Butsch Kovacic, Katki et al. 2008; Ovestad, Vennestrom et al. 2011). One study found opposite inflammatory patterns by HPV status ((Butsch Kovacic, Katki et al. 2008)). This study also found that neutrophils tended to be found only in the superficial epithelial layers, whereas mononuclear cells were found mainly near the basement membrane, suggesting that inflammatory patterns in the stroma and the epithelium may depend on the specific cell type. The second study only reported differences by CD8 in the stroma (Øvestad 2011).

Tissue-based studies of cytokines are also heterogeneous. Only two studies evaluated cytokine proteins in tissue (Fernandes, Gonçalves et al. 2005; Ortiz-Sanchez, Chavez-Olmos et al. 2007). It is not surprising that few studies have evaluated cytokine proteins in tissue since it can be challenging to find an appropriate antibody and optimize the assay. For example, antibodies that perform well in western blots may not work for staining since staining requires fixation, which can change the confirmation of the cytokine protein, thereby preventing antibody binding (Sachdeva and Asthana 2007). Most tissue-based studies of cytokines in this review measured RNA expression, but accurate measurement of RNA expression requires high quality tissue. If the tissue was not snap frozen immediately after surgery and well maintained, endogenous RNases may have degraded the RNA. RNA quality is rarely addressed. Although the presence of cytokine transcripts in tissue may be meaningful, the absence is not given the short-lived nature of RNA, even for high quality tissues (Sachdeva and Asthana 2007).

To clarify the role of immune response in cervical carcinogenesis, future studies should be conducted in well-characterized epidemiologic studies that can address most or all of the characteristics and considerations described above. Studies should include large numbers of women, evaluate a broader spectrum of cytokines/immune markers and measure and adjust for potential confounders concurrently. Possible usefulness of tissue microarrays and multiplex arrays with well-defined phenotypes should be considered as they are likely to make these studies more feasible. Emerging results must be repeated in different study populations and specimen types, but are encouraging. Accumulating evidence indicates that there is a cell-mediated immune response to HPV. As technologies improve, it should become possible to better characterize these responses to distinguish between women at risk of developing cervical cancer and women who can effectively resolve their HPV infections.

5. Appendix 1. Search strategy for immune function in cervical carcinogenesis

("humans"[MeSH Terms] AND "female"[MeSH Terms] AND English[lang]) AND ("cervix uteri"[MeSH Terms] OR "Uterine Cervical Neoplasms/immunology"[Mesh] OR "Uterine Cervical Neoplasms/pathology"[Mesh] OR "Uterine Cervical Neoplasms/blood" [Mesh] OR "Cervical Intraepithelial Neoplasia/metabolism"[Mesh] OR "Mucus/metabolism" [Mesh]) AND ("Cytokines/blood*"[Mesh] OR "Cytokines/metabolism"[Mesh] OR "Immunity, Innate"[Mesh] OR "Adaptive Immunity"[Mesh] OR "Immunity, Cellular"[Mesh] OR "Immunity, Humoral"[Mesh] OR "Immunity, Mucosal"[Mesh] OR "Immunity, Innate/immunology"[Mesh] OR "immune infiltrates" OR immunity OR "immune response" OR "immune cells" OR "immune cell" OR inflammation OR infiltration OR "Lymphocyte Subsets/immunology"[Mesh] OR "TH1 Cells/ immunology" [Mesh] OR "TH2 Cells/ immunology" [Mesh]) NOT (mice OR mouse OR "cell line" OR "cell lines" OR "mouth" OR "oropharynx" OR "Antiretroviral Therapy, Highly Active"[Mesh] OR "Models, Theoretical"[Mesh] OR "Papillomavirus Vaccines/administration & dosage"[Mesh] OR "Premature Birth/immunology"[Mesh] OR "HIV Infections/immunology"[Mesh] OR "Combined Modality Therapy"[Mesh] OR "Complementary Therapies"[Mesh] OR "Blood Vessels/chemistry"[Mesh] OR "Laser Therapy"[Mesh] OR "Labor Stage, First/physiology"[Mesh] OR "Foreign-Body Reaction/pathology"[Mesh] OR "Postoperative Complications/pathology"[Mesh] OR "Male"[Mesh] OR "Labor, Obstetric/metabolism"[Mesh])

6. References

FUTURE II Study Group (2007). "Quadrivalent vaccine against human papillomavirus to prevent high-grade cervical lesions." *N Engl J Med* 356(19): 1915-1927.

Abike, F., A. B. Engin, et al. (2011). "Human papilloma virus persistence and neopterin, folate and homocysteine levels in cervical dysplasias." *Arch Gynecol Obstet* 284(1): 209-214.

Adam, R. A., I. R. Horowitz, et al. (1999). "Serum levels of macrophage colony-stimulating factor-1 in cervical human papillomavirus infection and intraepithelial neoplasia." *Am J Obstet Gynecol* 180(1): 28-32.

Anderson, B. L. and S. Cu-Uvin (2011). "Clinical parameters essential to methodology and interpretation of mucosal responses." *American journal of reproductive immunology (New York, N Y : 1989)* 65(3): 352-360.

Bais, A. G. (2005). "A shift to a peripheral Th2-type cytokine pattern during the carcinogenesis of cervical cancer becomes manifest in CIN III lesions." *Journal of Clinical Pathology* 58(10): 1096-1100.

Baker, R., J. G. Dauner, et al. (2011). "Increased plasma levels of adipokines and inflammatory markers in older women with persistent HPV infection." *Cytokine* 53(3): 282-285.

Bermudez-Morales, V. H., L. X. Gutierrez, et al. (2008). "Correlation between IL-10 gene expression and HPV infection in cervical cancer: a mechanism for immune response escape." *Cancer investigation* 26(10): 1037-1043.

Bhat, P., S. R. Mattarollo, et al. (2011). "Regulation of immune responses to HPV infection and during HPV-directed immunotherapy." *Immunological reviews* 239(1): 85-98.

Bontkes, H. J., T. D. de Gruijl, et al. (1999). "Human papillomavirus type 16 E2-specific T-helper lymphocyte responses in patients with cervical intraepithelial neoplasia." *J Gen Virol* 80 (Pt 9): 2453-2459.

Bontkes, H. J., T. D. de Gruijl, et al. (2000). "Human Papillomavirus Type 16 E6/E7-Specific Cytotoxic T Lymphocytes In Women With Cervical Neoplasia." *Int. J. Cancer* 88: 92-98.

Bouvard, V., R. Baan, et al. (2009). "A review of human carcinogens--Part B: biological agents." *Lancet Oncol* 10(4): 321-322.

Brismar Wendel, S., T. Kaldensjo, et al. (2010). "Slumbering mucosal immune response in the cervix of human papillomavirus DNA-positive and -negative women." *International journal of oncology* 37(6): 1565-1573.

Butsch Kovacic, M., H. A. Katki, et al. (2008). "Epidemiologic analysis of histologic cervical inflammation: relationship to human papillomavirus infections." *Human Pathology* 39(7): 1088-1095.

Castle, P. E. and A. R. Giuliano (2003). "Chapter 4: Genital tract infections, cervical inflammation, and antioxidant nutrients--assessing their roles as human papillomavirus cofactors." *J Natl Cancer Inst Monogr*(31): 29-34.

Castle, P. E., A. C. Rodriguez, et al. (2004). "Comparison of ophthalmic sponges for measurements of immune markers from cervical secretions." *Clin Diagn Lab Immunol* 11(2): 399-405.

Cromme, F. V., C. J. Meijer, et al. (1993). "Analysis of MHC class I and II expression in relation to presence of HPV genotypes in premalignant and malignant cervical lesions." *Br J Cancer* 67(6): 1372-1380.

Crowley-Nowick, P. A., J. H. Ellenberg, et al. (2000). "Cytokine profile in genital tract secretions from female adolescents: impact of human immunodeficiency virus, human papillomavirus, and other sexually transmitted pathogens." *The Journal of infectious diseases* 181(3): 939-945.

de Gruijl, T. D., H. J. Bontkes, et al. (1999). "Immune responses against human papillomavirus (HPV) type 16 virus-like particles in a cohort study of women with cervical intraepithelial neoplasia. I. Differential T-helper and IgG responses in relation to HPV infection and disease outcome." *J Gen Virol* 80 (Pt 2): 399-408.

de Gruijl, T. D., H. J. Bontkes, et al. (1998). "Differential T helper cell responses to human papillomavirus type 16 E7 related to viral clearance or persistence in patients with cervical neoplasia: a longitudinal study." *Cancer Res* 58(8): 1700-1706.

Dong, D.-d., H. Yang, et al. (2010). "Human leukocyte antigen-G (HLA-G) expression in cervical lesions: association with cancer progression, HPV 16/18 infection, and host immune response." *Reproductive sciences (Thousand Oaks, Calif)* 17(8): 718-723.

Ferlay, J., H. R. Shin, et al. (2010). GLOBOCAN 2008, Cancer Incidence and Mortality Worldwide: IARC CancerBase No. 10 Lyon, France: International Agency for Research on Cancer. Available from: http://globocan.iarc.fr.

Fernandes, A. P. M., M. A. G. Gonçalves, et al. (2005). "HPV16, HPV18, and HIV infection may influence cervical cytokine intralesional levels." *Virology* 334(2): 294-298.

Goncalves, M. A. G., M. Le Discorde, et al. (2008). "Classical and non-classical HLA molecules and p16(INK4a) expression in precursors lesions and invasive cervical cancer." *European journal of obstetrics, gynecology, and reproductive biology* 141(1): 70-74.

Gravitt, P. E., A. Hildesheim, et al. (2003). "Correlates of IL-10 and IL-12 concentrations in cervical secretions." *Journal of Clinical Immunology* 23(3): 175-183.

Gravitt, P. E., A. Hildesheim, et al. (2003). "Correlates of IL-10 and IL-12 concentrations in cervical secretions." *J Clin Immunol* 23(3): 175-183.

Guha, D. and R. Chatterjee (2009). "Cytokine levels in HIV infected and uninfected Indian women: Correlation with other STAs." *Experimental and Molecular Pathology* 86(1): 65-68.

Hildesheim, A., R. Herrero, et al. (2007). "Effect of human papillomavirus 16/18 L1 viruslike particle vaccine among young women with preexisting infection: a randomized trial." *JAMA* 298(7): 743-753.

Hildesheim, A., M. H. Schiffman, et al. (1997). "Immune activation in cervical neoplasia: cross-sectional association between plasma soluble interleukin 2 receptor levels and disease." *Cancer Epidemiol Biomarkers Prev* 6(10): 807-813.

Hong, J. H., M. K. Kim, et al. (2010). "Association Between Serum Cytokine Profiles and Clearance or Persistence of High-Risk Human Papillomavirus Infection." *International Journal of Gynecological Cancer* 20(6): 1011-1016.

Kadish, A. S., G. Y. Ho, et al. (1997). "Lymphoproliferative responses to human papillomavirus (HPV) type 16 proteins E6 and E7: outcome of HPV infection and associated neoplasia." *J Natl Cancer Inst* 89(17): 1285-1293.

Kemp, T. J., A. Hildesheim, et al. (2010). "Elevated Systemic Levels of Inflammatory Cytokines in Older Women with Persistent Cervical Human Papillomavirus Infection." *Cancer Epidemiology Biomarkers & Prevention* 19(8): 1954-1959.

Koshiol, J., L. Lindsay, et al. (2008). "Persistent human papillomavirus infection and cervical neoplasia: a systematic review and meta-analysis." *Am J Epidemiol* 168(2): 123-137.

Lieberman, J. A., A. B. Moscicki, et al. (2008). "Determination of Cytokine Protein Levels in Cervical Mucus Samples from Young Women by a Multiplex Immunoassay Method and Assessment of Correlates." *Clinical and Vaccine Immunology* 15(1): 49-54.

Marks, M. A., R. P. Viscidi, et al. (2011). "Differences in the concentration and correlation of cervical immune markers among HPV positive and negative perimenopausal women." *Cytokine.*

Molling, J. W., T. D. de Gruijl, et al. (2007). "CD4(+)CD25hi regulatory T-cell frequency correlates with persistence of human papillomavirus type 16 and T helper cell responses in patients with cervical intraepithelial neoplasia." *International journal of cancer Journal international du cancer* 121(8): 1749-1755.

Moscicki, A. B., J. H. Ellenberg, et al. (2004). "Risk of high-grade squamous intraepithelial lesion in HIV-infected adolescents." *J Infect Dis* 190(8): 1413-1421.

Munoz, N., X. Castellsague, et al. (2006). "Chapter 1: HPV in the etiology of human cancer." *Vaccine* 24 Suppl 3: S3/1-10.

Murphy, K., P. Travers, et al. (2011). *Janeway's Immunobiology*, Garland Publishing (Taylor & Francis Group).

Ortiz-Sanchez, E., P. Chavez-Olmos, et al. (2007). "Expression of the costimulatory molecule CD86, but not CD80, in keratinocytes of normal cervical epithelium and human papillomavirus-16 positive low squamous intraepithelial lesions." *International journal of gynecological cancer : official journal of the International Gynecological Cancer Society* 17(3): 571-580.

Ovestad, I. T., U. Vennestrom, et al. (2011). "Comparison of different commercial methods for HPV detection in follow-up cytology after ASCUS/LSIL, prediction of CIN2-3 in follow up biopsies and spontaneous regression of CIN2-3." *Gynecol Oncol* 123(2): 278-283.

Sachdeva, N. and D. Asthana (2007). "Cytokine quantitation: technologies and applications." *Front Biosci* 12: 4682-4695.

Schiffman, M., P. E. Castle, et al. (2007). "Human papillomavirus and cervical cancer." *Lancet* 370(9590): 890-907.

Scott, M., D. P. Stites, et al. (1999). "Th1 cytokine patterns in cervical human papillomavirus infection." *Clin Diagn Lab Immunol* 6(5): 751-755.

Seresini, S., M. Origoni, et al. (2007). "IFN-gamma produced by human papilloma virus-18 E6-specific CD4+ T cells predicts the clinical outcome after surgery in patients with high-grade cervical lesions." *Journal of immunology (Baltimore, Md : 1950)* 179(10): 7176-7183.

Sharma, A., M. Rajappa, et al. (2007). "Cytokine profile in Indian women with cervical intraepithelial neoplasia and cancer cervix." *International Journal of Gynecological Cancer* 17(4): 879-885.

Song, S. H., J. K. Lee, et al. 2008. "Interferon-γ (IFN-γ): A possible prognostic marker for clearance of high-risk human papillomavirus (HPV)." *Gynecologic Oncology* 108(3): 543-548.

Song, S., J. Lee, et al. (2007). "The relationship between cytokines and HPV-16, HPV-16 E6, E7, and high-risk HPV viral load in the uterine cervix." *Gynecologic Oncology* 104(3): 732-738.

Stanley, M. (2010). "HPV - immune response to infection and vaccination." *Infect Agent Cancer* 5: 19.

Su, J. H., A. Wu, et al. (2010). "Immunotherapy for cervical cancer: Research status and clinical potential." *BioDrugs* 24(2): 109-129.

Tirone, N. R., B. C. Peghini, et al. (2009). "Local expression of interferon-alpha and interferon receptors in cervical intraepithelial neoplasia." *Cancer Immunology, Immunotherapy* 58(12): 2003-2010.

Tjiong, M. Y., N. van der Vange, et al (2001). "Cytokines in Cervicovaginal Washing Fluid from Patients with Cervical Neoplasia." *Cytokine* 14(6): 357-360.

Trottier, H. and E. L. Franco (2006). "The epidemiology of genital human papillomavirus infection." *Vaccine* 24 Suppl 1: S1-15.

Tsukui, T., A. Hildesheim, et al. (1996). "Interleukin 2 production in vitro by peripheral lymphocytes in response to human papillomavirus-derived peptides: correlation with cervical pathology." *Cancer Res* 56(17): 3967-3974.

2

Viruses Strive to Suppress Host Immune Responses and Prolong Persistence

Curtis J. Pritzl, Young-Jin Seo and Bumsuk Hahm
Departments of Surgery and Molecular Microbiology & Immunology
University of Missouri – Columbia
USA

1. Introduction

Viruses regulate host immune responses to propagate their progeny. Indeed, certain viruses successfully establish viral persistence for long periods of time even in the immunocompetent host. Many viruses seem to have developed clever tactics to elude, utilize, or suppress host innate and adaptive immune systems. Unlike the parental strain, the clone 13 (Cl 13) strain of lymphocytic choriomeningitis virus (LCMV) has been shown to persist in mice for 60 - 100 days by nullifying the function of the host immune system. Multiple findings obtained from this mouse model have held true in humans chronically infected with viruses including human immunodeficiency virus (HIV) and hepatitis viruses. These viruses have evolved a repertoire of mechanisms to suppress and evade the host immune system. By utilizing the model for the LCMV infection of mice, this review will focus on the viral mechanisms for inhibition or escape of host immunity, in particular the host dendritic cell (DC) and T cell responses. Investigating the viral strategies will help us better understand the virus-host interplay and design new immunotherapeutic approaches.

1.1 The lymphocytic choriomeningitis virus model of chronic viral infection

The Cl 13 strain of LCMV is a variant isolated from the spleens of mice infected neonatally with the prototypic LCMV strain, Armstrong 53b (Arm) (Ahmed, Salmi et al. 1984). Mice infected with LCMV Arm develop a robust acute immune response of cytotoxic T lymphocytes (CTLs) that rapidly clears the virus from its host (within 10 days). In contrast, the infection of adult mice with LCMV Cl 13 induces a profound suppression of the host immune system leading to viral persistence (60-100 days following the start of infection) (Figure 1) (Borrow, Evans et al. 1995; Sevilla, Kunz et al. 2003). The clinical importance of virus-induced altered or suppressed immune responses is reflected by several human virus infections that inhibit the immune response such as HIV and hepatitis C virus (HCV) (Steinman, Granelli-Piperno et al. 2003; Liu, Woltman et al. 2009). Thus, the system of LCMV Cl 13 infection of its natural host, the mouse, serves as an excellent model for the mechanistic study of virus-induced immunosuppression and for the development of novel targets controlling viral persistence.

Immunosuppression caused by LCMV Cl 13 is associated with the inhibition of DC function and the reduced frequency and impaired activation (exhaustion) of virus-specific T cells

(Borrow et al. 1995; Sevilla et al. 2003; Barber, Wherry et al. 2006; Trifilo, Hahm et al. 2006). Exhausted T cell responses are characterized by the cells' inability to produce antiviral and immune stimulatory cytokines, destroy virus-infected cells, or proliferate, and have been documented following multiple infections including HIV, HCV, and hepatitis B virus (Yi, Cox et al. 2010).

LCMV Cl 13 differs from Arm by only two amino acids (aa); a Leu in the viral glycoprotein at aa 260 in Cl 13 as compared to Phe in ARM is responsible for DC infection and immunosuppression (Salvato, Borrow et al. 1991). LCMV Cl 13 preferentially replicates in the white pulp of the spleen and infects DCs in spleen and bone marrow (BM) of the mice via the receptor α-dystroglycan (Cao, Henry et al. 1998; Smelt, Borrow et al. 2001; Sevilla et al. 2003). The modulation of immuno-regulatory proteins expressed on DCs was reported to explain the failure of DC function to stimulate or maintain T cell responses upon LCMV Cl 13 infection. Such modulation included the downregulation of MHC molecules and co-stimulatory proteins (Sevilla, McGavern et al. 2004), preferential production of the immunosuppressive cytokine, IL-10 (Brooks, Trifilo et al. 2006; Ejrnaes, Filippi et al. 2006; Brooks, Ha et al. 2008), and increased expression of the negative regulator, programmed death-ligand 1 (PD-L1) on DCs for enhanced PD-L1-PD1 interaction leading to T cell exhaustion (2, 11).

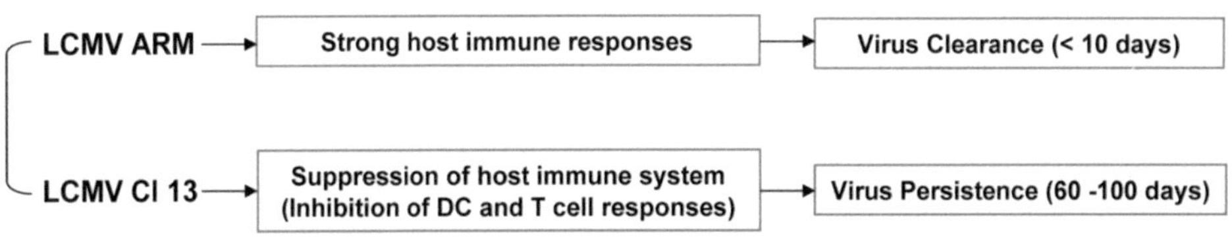

Fig. 1. Characteristics of the different LCMV infection models. LCMV ARM infection of adult mice rapidly generates a strong CD8 T cell response in the host which can clear the virus within 10 days, while an LCMV Cl 13 infection suppresses the host immune responses which leads to a prolonged viral persistence lasting 60 – 100 days.

Furthermore, following LCMV Cl 13 infection, virus-specific CD4+ T cells were functionally dysregulated, which contributes to the inability to sustain CTL function and facilitates viral persistence (Matloubian, Concepcion et al. 1994; Brooks, Teyton et al. 2005). Virus-specific CD4+ T cells were functionally inactivated early during the transition into viral persistence and failed to produce effector cytokines such as IL-2 and TNF-α. Recently, IL-21 was identified as an essential component of CD4+ T cell help to sustain CD8+ T cell effector activity and resolve persistent infection (Elsaesser, Sauer et al. 2009; Frohlich, Kisielow et al. 2009; Yi, Du et al. 2009). The detailed underlying molecular mechanism and intracellular signaling path for the virus-induced immunosuppression and viral persistence, however, are unclear.

2. Chronic viral infections inhibit innate and dendritic cell responses

It is generally thought that a robust CD8+ T cell response is responsible for clearing an acute LCMV infection (Byrne and Oldstone 1984; Fung-Leung, Kundig et al. 1991). However, a strong innate immune response is important for the generation of an effective adaptive response against viral infections (Jung, Kato et al. 2008; Rahman, Cui et al. 2008; Zucchini,

Bessou et al. 2008). Moreover, DCs are indispensible for the generation of the CD8+ effector T cells. The innate immune response provides stimulatory signals, such as type I interferons and IL-12 that promote the priming of CD8+ T cells and favor the T-helper 1 phenotype of CD4+ T cells. DCs are the key intermediate between the innate immune response and the adaptive immune response. DCs are the major professional antigen presenting cell subset that provides the necessary primary and secondary signals to induce the activation and proliferation of virus-specific CTL. A virus that can actively suppress these two responses has a significant advantage over the host immune system and the opportunity to establish a persistent infection.

2.1 Chronic LCMV infections suppress type I interferon expression

Type I interferons (IFN) and inflammatory cytokines are key to the initiation of anti-viral immune responses (Seo and Hahm 2010). Type I IFN is a family of cytokines comprised of IFN-α, IFN-β, IFN-ε, IFN-κ, and IFN-ω. These molecules have been shown to be potent antiviral cytokines by the deletion of the common receptor subunit (IFNAR1). Transgenic mice lacking IFNAR1 have been demonstrated to the lose ability to interfere with the replication of many different viruses (Muller, Steinhoff et al. 1994; Goodman, Zeng et al. 2010; Kolokoltsova, Yun et al. 2010). High levels of type I IFN have been detected at early time points during an acute, LCMV Arm infection (Montoya, Edwards et al. 2005). Zhou et al. have demonstrated that this induction of type I IFN is due at least in part to the recognition of the LCMV RNA genome by retinoic acid-inducible gene I (RIG-I) and melanoma differentiation-associated gene 5 (MDA5) pathway along with toll-like receptor (TLR) 2 and 6 (Zhou, Kurt-Jones et al. 2005; Zhou, Cerny et al. 2010). Similarly, DCs from LCMV Cl 13-infected mice have also been shown to produce type I IFN at early time points of virus infection (Dalod, Salazar-Mather et al. 2002; Diebold, Montoya et al. 2003; Zuniga, Hahm et al. 2007). However, several days later, these cytokines are no longer detectable in the sera of LCMV Cl 13-infected mice (Martinez-Sobrido, Emonet et al. 2009), which suggests that the virus is actively suppressing the host type I IFN response. This observation was confirmed by Zuniga et al. who specifically examined the production of type I IFN by plasmacytoid DCs during an LCMV CL 13 infection (Zuniga, Liou et al. 2008). Plasmacytoid DCs (pDC) are a specialized subset of DCs that rapidly produce large amounts of type I IFN in response to viral infection (Asselin-Paturel and Trinchieri 2005; Delale, Paquin et al. 2005). In response to certain stimulation conditions, these cells have been observed to dedicate 50% of their cellular transcription to the production of type I IFN (Liu 2005; Lee, Lund et al. 2007). Because of this high level of type I IFN, it is suggested that these cells play a key role in the orchestration of antiviral immune responses. In the case of an LCMV Cl 13 infection, the number of pDCs in LCMV Cl 13-infected mice was reduced by 50% compared to mice infected with LCMV Arm at 30 days post-infection (Zuniga et al. 2008). Moreover, the production of type I IFN in response to TLR9 activation was severely impaired in pDCs isolated from LCMV CL 13-infected mice, which suggests that the virus is severely limiting the potential of these cells to respond not only to LCMV, but also additional, unrelated pathogenic stimulation (Zuniga et al. 2008).

Indeed, it has been shown that LCMV Cl 13 utilizes specific molecular mechanisms to inhibit type I IFN production by the host cells. Martinez-Sobrido et al. have shown that the nucleoprotein of LCMV is responsible for the blockade of the host type I IFN response

(Martinez-Sobrido, Zuniga et al. 2006). This inhibition of cytokine production is due to the interaction of the viral protein with the interferon regulatory factor-3 (IRF-3) activation pathway. The data demonstrated that LCMV nucleoprotein (NP) impaired the nuclear translocation of IRF-3, which is involved in the upregulation of type I IFN synthesis. More specifically, amino acid residue 382 of LCMV NP was sufficient to inhibit the host type I IFN response (Martinez-Sobrido et al. 2009).

Additional studies have been carried out to investigate the mechanisms behind the LCMV-mediated blockade of the host type I IFN response. LCMV NP blockade of the IRF-3 pathway also affects the response to RIG-I and MDA5 (Zhou et al. 2010). Moreover, this same study demonstrated that LCMV NP physically interacts with both RIG-I and MDA5. Mutations in LCMV NP that prevented the inhibition of type I IFN however did not affect this interaction, which suggests that there are additional inhibitory mechanisms (Zhou et al. 2010).

This suppression of type I IFN not only affects the host response against LCMV, but it may also reduce the effectiveness of responses against other opportunistic pathogens whose clearance requires type I IFN (Zuniga et al. 2008). The effects of chronic LCMV Cl 13 infections also lead to disruptions in the ability of the host's pDCs to produce type I IFN in response to other unrelated infections such as vesicular stomatitis virus (VSV) or murine cytomegalovirus (MCMV). In addition, LCMV Cl 13 infection had deleterious consequences on the host's natural killer cell population which may be important in the immune response to other viral, bacterial, or parasitic infections such as HIV, influenza virus, *Mycobacterium tuberculosis* (Vankayalapati, Garg et al. 2005), and *Plasmodium falciparum* (Alter, Malenfant et al. 2004; Byrne, McGuirk et al. 2004; Siren, Sareneva et al. 2004; Korbel, Newman et al. 2005; Zuniga et al. 2008). Pre-infection with LCMV Cl 13 was also demonstrated to prevent the host from counteracting the early spread of MCMV and therefore preventing viral clearance (Zuniga et al. 2008).

2.2 Suppression of dendritic cell functions

DCs are key mediators of adaptive immune responses. This group of cells can efficiently present endogenously and exogenously synthesized viral antigens to CD8+ T cells. In addition, these cells provide the necessary co-stimulatory signals to CTL for activation. The effect of chronic LCMV Cl 13 infections on the production of type I IFN by pDCs is only one aspect of the virus-induced restrictions of the host's DC responses. Not only do chronically infecting viruses suppress cytokine production by host DCs, but it has also been shown that they can suppress the development of dendritic cells from hematopoietic precursor cells, inhibit the maturation of DCs following exposure to activation signals, and also lead to the destruction of these cells that are critical for effective anti-viral immune responses.

One major mechanism that LCMV Cl 13 uses to suppress DC responses is to suppress their development from hematopoietic precursor cells (Hahm, Trifilo et al. 2005; Trifilo et al. 2006). The cytokines fms-like tyrosine kinase receptor-3 ligand (Flt3-L) and granulocyte macrophage-colony stimulating factor (GM-CSF) are major signals in the development of DCs from hematopoietic stem cells and can be used to induce the differentiation of DCs both *in vitro* and *in vivo* (Sevilla et al. 2004; Hahm et al. 2005). When Flt3-L is administered to mice, it dramatically increases the number of splenic DCs (Drakes, Lu et al. 1997). When bone marrow is cultured *in vitro* with GM-CSF, the stem cells differentiate into CD11c+

dendritic cells. It has been demonstrated that LCMV Cl 13-infected mice do not respond to Flt3-L treatment, suggesting that the virus induces an Flt3-L-refractory state in the hematopoietic precursor cells (Sevilla et al. 2004; Hahm et al. 2005). Moreover, *in vitro* culture of bone marrow cells infected by LCMV Cl 13 with GM-CSF induced the development of significantly fewer CD11c+ DCs compared to uninfected bone marrow cells (Sevilla et al. 2004; Hahm et al. 2005). Collectively these data indicate that one mechanism that chronic LCMV infection utilizes to evade the immune system is to prevent the development of DCs which are critical to a successful adaptive immune response.

Although LCMV Cl 13 does inhibit the differentiation of DCs from their hematopoietic progenitors, functional DCs do develop. However, the virus employs additional strategies to suppress the responses induced by these cells. Our laboratory and others have demonstrated that LCMV Cl 13 infection of DCs inhibits their ability to upregulate major histocompatibility complex class I (MHC-I) molecules and co-stimulatory molecules such as B7-2 (Figure 2A) (Sevilla et al. 2004). Moreover, the LCMV Cl 13 infection in our studies not only prevented the upregulation of MHC-I and B7-2 but reduced the levels of their expression to below baseline levels. This suppression of MHC-I and co-stimulatory molecule expression renders the DCs unable to efficiently prime CD8+ T cells, which are necessary to clear the infecting virus. Although the inhibition of type I IFN expression may be the cause of this downregulation, there may be additional unknown mechanisms for this phenomenon. Further, the infected DCs were impaired in the ability to synthesize IL-12, a critical cytokine for T cell stimulation, in response to TLR9 ligation (Figure 2B). The results also support the functional abrogation of host immunity in LCMV Cl 13-infected mice upon the invasion of a secondary microbe that contains TLR9 ligand components such as DNA viruses or bacteria.

The final postulated mechanism for LCMV evasion of dendritic cell responses is the targeted killing of these cells. It has been shown that persistently infecting strains of the virus have a mutation in the glycoprotein that affects their tropism and increases the infectivity of DCs (Borrow et al. 1995; Sevilla, Kunz et al. 2000). This dendritic cell-specific infection leads to increased antigen load and therefore makes these cells ideal targets for activated CD8+ T cells. Indeed, a loss of splenic DCs has been observed in the spleens of LCMV Cl 13-infected mice although, the ability of these infected DCs to act as targets has not yet been confirmed. However, DCs are efficient antigen presenting cells and because they are preferentially infected during an LCMV Cl 13 infection, it has been speculated that they are targeted for destruction by activated CD8+ T cells (Odermatt, Eppler et al. 1991; Borrow et al. 1995).

These multiple findings have been recapitulated when DCs were infected with human-tropic viruses. For instance, measles virus (MV) suppressed DC generation from bone marrow progenitor cells under the GM-CSF or Flt3-L-supplemented culture system (Hahm et al. 2005). Further, MV could kill DCs or strongly inhibit the ability of DCs to stimulate anti-viral T cells (Hahm 2009). The decrease in the DC population was also observed in the bloodstream of HCV or HIV-infected patients (Donaghy, Pozniak et al. 2001; Pacanowski, Kahi et al. 2001; Kanto and Hayashi 2004; Kanto, Inoue et al. 2004; Siavoshian, Abraham et al. 2005). Functional abrogation of professional antigen presenting DCs has been reported in multiple cases of patients who were chronically infected with pathogenic viruses.

Like the inhibition of type I IFN, DCs have been shown to play a key role in the host response and elimination of viral infections. Because of this, LCMV and other chronically

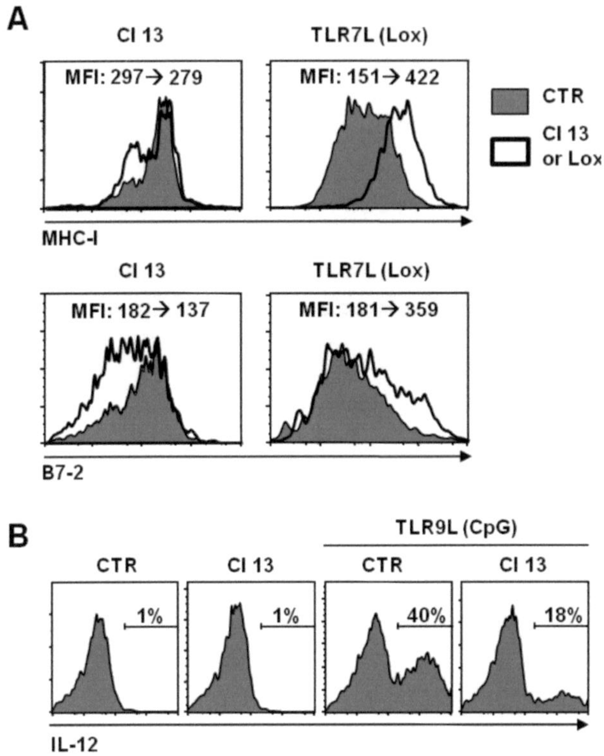

Fig. 2. LCMV Cl 13 suppresses DC responses. (A) Bone marrow-derived DCs were untreated (control, CTR), infected with LCMV Cl 13 (Cl 13), or treated with loxoribine (TLR7 ligand, 0.5mM). DCs were analyzed for the expression levels of MHC-I and B7-2 by flow cytometry on the following day. Mean fluorescent intensities (MFIs) for each molecule are shown. (B) DCs were uninfected (CTR) or infected with LCMV Cl 13. At one day post-infection (dpi), these cells were untreated or treated with CpG (TLR9 ligand, 200 ng/ml) and the synthesis of IL-12 was assessed by flow cytometry.

infecting viruses have developed multiple strategies to counteract and evade the dendritic cell responses. Although a great deal of effort has been focused on these evasion tactics, the underlying mechanisms that the viruses use to suppress these responses are still not yet fully elucidated.

3. Virus-mediated T cell exhaustion

CD8+ Cytotoxic T lymphocytes (CTLs) are a critical line of defense against viral infections. These cells are responsible for the recognition and subsequent killing of virus-infected cells. During an acute virus infection, CTLs recognize antigenic peptides displayed on the surface of professional antigen presenting cells (Carbone, Moore et al. 1988). This recognition, along with co-stimulatory signals activate the CTLs to proliferate and gives them license to kill virus infected cells through their effector functions including the release of the cytotoxic molecules perforin and granzyme B (Lancki, Hsieh et al. 1991). In addition, activated CTLs also upregulate inflammatory cytokines including IFN-γ and TNF-α (Murray, Lee et al. 1990; Martin, Vallbracht et al. 1991; Brehm, Daniels et al. 2005). Following the resolution of the infection this large population of effector CTLs contracts into a small pool of memory cells which are able to quickly respond to subsequent infections by the same pathogen.

Because CTLs are able to eliminate replicative reservoirs, persisting viruses have evolved methods for the evasion of these immune responses. Although the suppression of CTL responses begins with the disruption of dendritic cell responses as described previously, persistently infecting viruses such as LCMV and HIV have developed several mechanisms to specifically perturb CTL responses. The first method involves the exhaustion of CTLs in which the cells lose their ability to kill infected cells, while the other involves the modulation of dominant CTL epitopes, allowing the virus to escape immune recognition. These escape mechanisms give the viruses an additional advantage over the host immune system and allow for chronic viral infections.

3.1 Exhaustion of CD8+ T cells by LCMV Cl 13

3.1.1 Exhaustion of cytotoxic CD8+ T lymphocytes during chronic viral infection

Exhaustion of CTL has been described in multiple viral infections including both LCMV and HIV as the loss of effector functions by antigen-specific CD8+ T cells. The presence of both acutely-infecting and chronically-infecting strains of LCMV have made this virus an outstanding model for determining both the effects of the virus on CTLs as well as the mechanism by which the virus induces T cell exhaustion. During a chronic LCMV infection, the virus-specific CD8+ T cell response is activated and peaks similar to an acute viral infection (Figure 3). However, instead of clearing the virus, the CTLs lose effector functions (Figure 3). The loss of CTL functionality occurs in a stepwise manner. Individual effector functions are lost at distinct time points over the course of the infection (Wherry, Blattman et al. 2003). Initially, the CTLs lose the ability to proliferate and produce IL-2 in the case of most chronic viral infections (Wherry et al. 2003). As the infection continues, the CTLs become dysfunctional in their ability to produce and secrete the inflammatory cytokine TNF-α (Sakuishi, Apetoh et al. 2010). At later time points of the persistent infection, the cells also fail to produce IFN-γ and lose their cytotoxic potential (Wherry et al. 2003; Jin, Anderson et al. 2010). In certain cases, the end result of T cell exhaustion is the death of T cells which leads to the reduction of the total virus-specific T cell population. The culmination of these dysfunctions is the inability of antigen-specific CTLs to kill virus infected cells, thereby allowing the virus to persist. The mechanisms LCMV Cl 13 uses to exhaust CTLs are not yet fully understood. It is known however that the virus activates inhibitory molecules that are involved in the regulation of normal immune responses to exhaust CTLs.

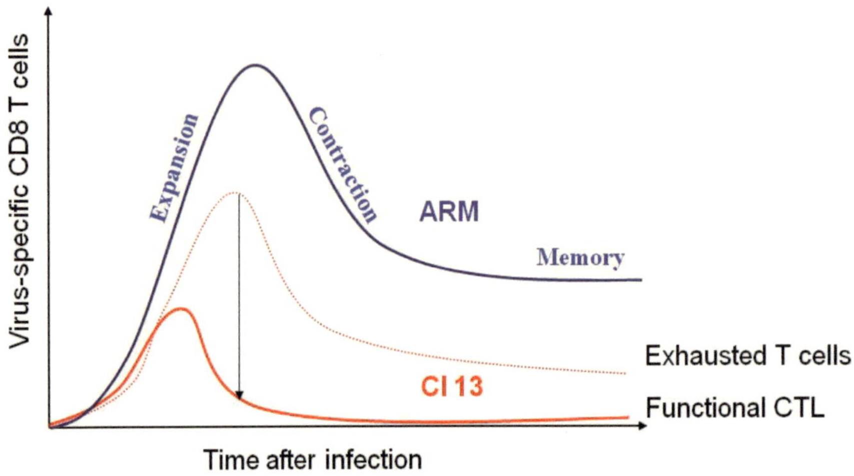

Fig. 3. CD8 T cell response to acute and persistent LCMV infections over time. In response to an acute LCMV infection (ARM, blue line), CD8 T cells rapidly expand until approximately day 7. Following this expansion, the cells contract leaving a small population of memory cells. During a chronic infection (Cl 13, red line), CD8 T cells expand in a similar fashion however quickly lose effector functions (dotted red line) and leave only a small population of functional CTL that are unable to resolve the infection (solid red line).

3.1.2 Inhibitory receptors involved in T cell exhaustion

The inhibitory receptor programmed death - 1 (PD-1) is the most extensively characterized molecule associated with LCMV Cl 13-mediated T cell exhaustion (Wherry, Ha et al. 2007; Blackburn, Shin et al. 2009; Jin et al. 2010; Vezys, Penaloza-MacMaster et al. 2011). PD-1 is a negative immuno-regulatory molecule in the CD28/CTLA-4 family that is expressed on the surface of activated CD8+ T cells. PD-1 has two ligands, PD-L1 and PD-L2 which could be upregulated on the surface of activated DCs and macrophages, although PD-L1 is expressed on multiple cell types (Yamazaki, Akiba et al. 2002; Brown, Dorfman et al. 2003). The expression of this inhibitory receptor has been directly linked to type I IFN production (Terawaki, Chikuma et al. 2011). The role of the PD-1 activation in non-persistent viral infections is the attenuation of T cell responses to prevent unnecessary immunopathology (Freeman, Long et al. 2000). PD-1 is thought to play a critical role in the LCMV-mediated exhaustion of CTLs as virus-specific CD8+ T cells express significantly higher levels of this molecule during chronic LCMV infections. The mechanisms behind the LCMV-mediated upregulation of PD-1 have yet to be fully elucidated. However, the blockade of the PD-1 pathway restores functionality of these cells and leads to clearance of the persistent virus infection (Barber et al. 2006).

Another molecule that has been implicated in the exhaustion of CD8+ T cells during chronic LCMV infections is lymphocyte activated gene - 3 (LAG-3) (Wherry et al. 2007; Grosso, Goldberg et al. 2009). This molecule belongs to the immunoglobulin superfamily and has been shown to be immunomodulatory in the prevention of autoimmune disorders (Workman, Dugger et al. 2002). The expression of LAG-3 does not change on CD8+ T cells during acute infections with LCMV, but is upregulated on CD8+ T cells in LCMV Cl 13-

infected mice (Richter, Agnellini et al. 2010). It has been suggested that LAG-3 functions in a similar fashion to PD-1 during chronic LCMV Cl 13 infections (Blackburn et al. 2009). Although mice deficient in LAG-3 do not demonstrate improved CD8+ T cell responses during persistent LCMV infections (Richter et al. 2010), the simultaneous blockade of both the PD-1 and LAG-3 pathways leads to significant improvements in the CTL responses of LCMV Cl 13-infected mice compared to PD-1 blockade alone (Blackburn et al. 2009).

Multiple other immunomodulatory molecules have been suggested to be involved in the attenuation of virus-specific CD8+ T cell responses. An extensive study by Wherry et al. has shown that the expression of many different genes from multiple cellular processes is affected during CD8+ T cell exhaustion. These markers include natural killer cell marker 2B4 (2B4), which has since been shown to be involved in the regulation of memory CD8+ T cells during chronic LCMV infections (West, Youngblood et al. 2011), T cell Ig- and mucin-domain-containing molecule-3 (Tim-3), CD160, paired Ig-like receptor-B (PIR-B), and GP49B. All of these molecules have been shown to have inhibitory functions during immune responses (Wherry et al. 2007; Jin et al. 2010; Vezys et al. 2011). Although Tim-3 has been shown to act in cooperation with PD-1 in the exhaustion of CD8+ T cells during persistent LCMV infections (Jin et al. 2010), no specific mechanisms in the loss of function of CD8+ T cells have been attributed to these additional markers of T cell exhaustion. Until these markers are investigated individually or in conjunction with the known inhibitory molecules, they are only guilty by association.

The markers and mechanisms that have been described by comparing the persistent and acute LCMV infections are by no means the only ones involved in the suppression of CD8+ T cell responses. Other immunosuppressive molecules have been shown to either be involved in the exhaustion of CD8+ T cell responses or upregulated on exhausted T cells in other persistent viral infections. CTLA-4, among the others discussed above, has been shown to be important in serious human infections such as HIV and HCV (Hryniewicz, Boasso et al. 2006; Kaufmann, Kavanagh et al. 2007; Nakamoto, Cho et al. 2009).

3.1.3 Transcription factors involved in T cell exhaustion

Several transcription factors have also been identified as modulators of the CD8+ T cell response during a persistent LCMV Cl 13 infection (Shaffer, Lin et al. 2002; Agnellini, Wolint et al. 2007). Nuclear factor of activated T cells (NFAT) is a transcription factor that regulates multiple genes involved in the cytotoxicity and inflammatory cytokine production by CD8+ T cells, including IL-2, the loss of which is a hallmark of T cell exhaustion (Wherry et al. 2003). NFAT expression and phosphorylation are unperturbed in the CD8+ T cells from mice persistently infected with LCMV. However, the translocation of NFAT molecules from the cytoplasm to the nucleus is disrupted during chronic LCMV infections which prevents the transcription factor from upregulating genes necessary for complete CTL function (Agnellini et al. 2007). The transcription factor B-lymphocyte-induced maturation protein-1 (Blimp-1) which is known to govern the fate decision of B-cells has also been associated with the exhaustion of CD8+ T cells (Shaffer et al. 2002; Calame 2006). Blimp-1 expression was shown to be dramatically increased in T cells during chronic viral infections (Shin, Blackburn et al. 2009). In this same series of experiments, a conditional knockout of Blimp-1 resulted in significant decreases of the inhibitory receptors PD-1 and LAG-3 in CD8+ T cells during a chronic LCMV Cl 13 infection. Moreover, this conditional knockout resulted in increased cytotoxicity of

LCMV-specific CTL and improved viral control (Shin et al. 2009). Although the research into these transcriptional regulators has revealed another level of immune evasion by LCMV Cl 13, they have not completely elucidated the pathway by which the virus induces T cell exhaustion. Therefore more research is still required to fully understand these mechanisms.

3.1.4 Role of chronic antigen stimulation on T cell exhaustion

One possible mechanism that has been postulated to be involved in the upregulation of these markers and the subsequent exhaustion of virus-specific CD8+ T cells is the prolonged presence of viral antigens. In a study by Bucks et al., repeated exposure to influenza antigen was shown to induce the exhaustion of antigen-specific CTLs. In these experiments, repeated exposure to antigen reduced both the frequency and number of virus specific CD8+ T cells, and significantly impeded the ability of the remaining cells to produce IFN-γ (Bucks, Norton et al. 2009). In support of these findings, a more recent study has investigated the epigenetic regulation CD8+ T cells during a chronic LCMV infection (Youngblood, Oestreich et al. 2011). The results of this study indicate that long-term antigen exposure results in prolonged demethylation of the PD-1 gene locus, leading to extended PD-1 expression which has been observed during chronic LCMV infections. In addition, this demethylation does not resolve rapidly in exhausted T cells due to a downregulation of methyltransferases. Consequently, these exhausted CD8+ T cells have the potential for rapid upregulation of PD-1 upon subsequent antigen encounters (Youngblood et al. 2011).

3.1.5 Cytokines implicated in T cell exhaustion

Another potential inducer of CD8+ T cell exhaustion is the anti-inflammatory cytokine IL-10. IL-10 has been shown to be a potent inhibitor of inflammatory and adaptive immune responses. Two different studies have implicated IL-10 in chronic viral infections (Brooks et al. 2006; Ejrnaes et al. 2006). In these studies it was shown that IL-10-deficient mice chronically infected with LCMV have higher frequencies of virus-specific CTLs and antibody-mediated blockade of the IL-10 receptor can restore the function of exhausted, virus specific CD8+ T cells (Brooks et al. 2006; Ejrnaes et al. 2006). Furthermore, the IL-10 receptor blockade also led to accelerated viral clearance in both studies (Brooks et al. 2006; Ejrnaes et al. 2006). The source of the IL-10 involved in the immune suppression as well as the mechanisms by which IL-10 is induced is still under investigation.

Although the inflammatory cytokine IL-21 has not been shown to be directly involved in the induction of T cell exhaustion, its requirement in the clearance of the virus has been clearly demonstrated. IL-21 is produced primarily by CD4+ T cells and has been shown to induce the proliferation of CD8+ cytotoxic T-lymphocytes in a fashion similar to that of IL-2 (Kasaian, Whitters et al. 2002). Because IL-2 production is lost quickly during a chronic LCMV infection, it is thought that IL-21 may act in a compensatory fashion. The requirement of IL-21 in the clearance of LCMV CL 13 was demonstrated in IL-21 receptor-deficient mice. These mice failed to clear the virus while the wild-type control mice had cleared the infection by day 60 post-infection. (Elsaesser et al. 2009). In the same study by Elsaesser et al., it was shown that IL-21 is produced by CD4+ T cells throughout an LCMV Cl 13 infection (Elsaesser et al. 2009). However, in parallel experiments by Yi et al., it was shown that the number of IL-21-producing CD4+ T cells is 7.8 times lower than in an acute LCMV infection. Therefore, this loss of IL-21-producing, CD4+ T cells may be another critical factor in the rapid exhaustion of CD8+ T cells during a persistent LCMV infection.

The topic of T cell exhaustion is a major focus in the field of viral immunity. It is still not clear if the expression of these markers is due to the presence of a persisting viral infection, or if viruses have evolved specific mechanisms to activate these immunosuppressive pathways. However, multiple studies have demonstrated that the targeting of certain molecules relieves the suppression and allows the host CTL response to reassert control over the infection and accelerate viral clearance. If the mechanisms behind the virus-mediated upregulation of these molecules and CD8+ T cell exhaustion can be determined, the many new targets for immune-based therapies can be designed, giving medicine a much needed advantage in the treatment of chronic viral infections.

3.2 Dysfunction of CD4+ T cells during chronic LCMV infection

CD4+ T cells have been shown to not play a major role in the clearance of an acute, LCMV Arm infection. Experiments conducted with mice deficient in CD4+ T cells demonstrate that they are able to clear the infection as efficiently as their wild-type counterparts (Matloubian et al. 1994). However in the case of a chronic LCMV Cl 13 infection, CD4+ T cells appear to play a more significant role, as depletion of CD4+ T cells prevents mice from clearing the virus (Matloubian et al. 1994). One of the major contributions these cells make is the production of IL-21, which as described above appears to be critical for viral clearance (Elsaesser et al. 2009; West et al. 2011). In addition, there is evidence that CD4+ T cells also become exhausted during an LCMV Cl 13 infection. Brooks et al. have demonstrated that CD4+ T cells begin to lose the ability to make inflammatory cytokines such as IFN-γ and TNF-α as well as IL-2 as early as day 9 post-infection (Brooks et al. 2005). Moreover, an increase in the production of the anti-inflammatory cytokine IL-10 by virus-specific CD4+ T cells was also observed during the chronic LCMV infection (Brooks et al. 2005). There was however no increase in the number of T regulatory CD4+ T cells observed during the course of the viral infection (Brooks et al. 2005). Similar to exhausted CD8+ T cells, exhausted CD4+ T cells have also been shown to upregulate the expression of PD-1 (Day, Kaufmann et al. 2006; Kasprowicz, Schulze Zur Wiesch et al. 2008). In addition, recent evidence suggests that viral persistence actually reprograms the differentiation of CD4+ T cells from the T-helper 1 phenotype to a T-follicular helper cells (Fahey, Wilson et al. 2011).

System Targeted	Disruption of Cellular Function	Phenotype/Mechanism
Type I Interferon	Inhibition of type I IFN production	LCMV NP - Inhibition of IRF3 - Inhibition of MDA5 and RIG-I Inhibition of plasmacytoid DCs
Dendritic Cells	Inhibition of DC development	Decrease in the frequency of CD11c+ cells
	Inhibition of DC maturation	MHC-I and B7-1/B7-2 upregulation impaired following PAMP ligation Loss of IL-12 production Increased IL-10 synthesis
T cells	Suppression of T cell function (exhaustion)	PD-1↑, LAG-3↑, Tim-3↑, Blimp-1↑, NFAT↑ IFN-γ↓, TNF-α↓, IL-2↓, Proliferation↓, Cytotoxic activity ↓

Table 1. Immunological Effects of Persistent LCMV Cl 13 Infections.

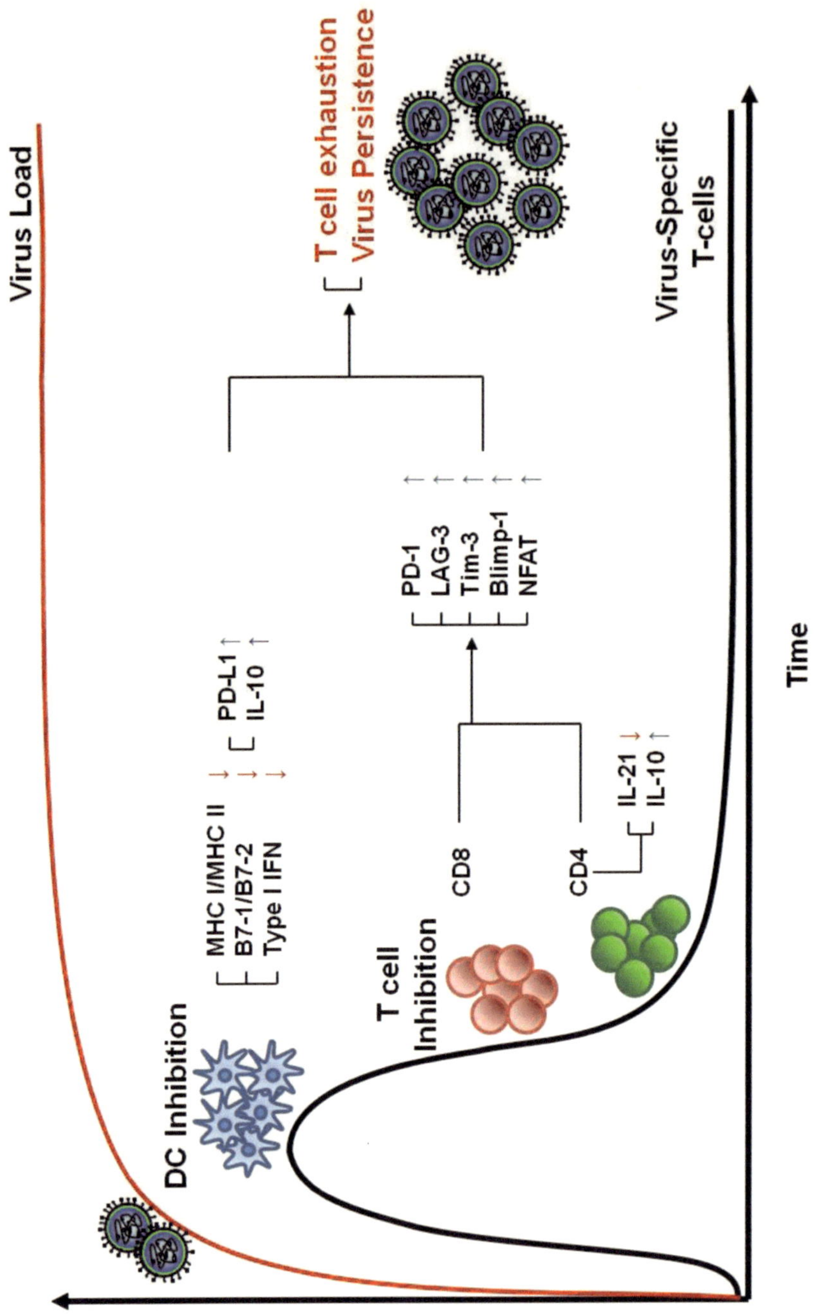

Fig. 4. Schematic representation of the immune cell phenotypes during a chronic LCMV infection. Viral load over time is represented by the red line. The functional T cell response is illustrated using the black line. Alterations in cell surface molecule and cytokine expression is noted with each cell type.

4. Perspectives

Chronic viral infections continue to be a tremendous burden on human health. Many years of research, especially with LCMV Cl 13, has led to a large body of knowledge as to how these viruses subvert and evade both innate and adaptive immune responses (Figure 4 and Table 1). Although there is still a great deal of research needed, several potential molecular immunotherapeutic treatment options have been developed through these studies. First, findings by Brooks *et al.* and Ejarnes *et al.* have clearly demonstrated that the blockade of IL-10 signaling could be used as a potential treatment to restore functionality to exhausted CD8+ T cells. This has been examined recently and it was found that CD8+ T cells from HIV positive patients could be restored using an IL-10-specific antibody (Brockman, Kwon et al. 2009). Similarly, clinical trials are being conducted to evaluate a treatment consisting of inhibition of the PD-1/PD-L1 interaction to recover exhausted CD8+ T cells during HIV infection and certain types of cancer (Sakthivel, Gereke et al. 2011). Other treatment options have been explored including multiple therapeutic vaccination strategies such as DNA vaccines (Martins, Lau et al. 1995), recombinant virus vectors (Wherry, Blattman et al. 2005), and lipo-peptide vaccines (von Herrath, Berger et al. 2000). Finally, the use of IFN-α for the treatment of chronic virus infections was introduced in 1986 for the treatment of hepatitis C virus infections (Hoofnagle, Mullen et al. 1986). However, some evidence suggests that therapeutic vaccination post-infection may not be as effective as hoped because of the immunosuppressed state of the host caused by the infection (Wherry et al. 2005).

In addition to the molecular therapies, immune cell-based therapeutic approaches have been developed. Since CD8+ CTLs are principal players for the eradication of viruses, the CD8+ T cell-based therapy has been implemented (Gottschalk, Bollard et al. 2006; Kapp, Tan et al. 2007). However, the requirement of CD4+ T cells for the maintenance of CTL activity has prompted the use of combined T cell therapies. Further, owing to the extraordinary ability of DCs to serve as natural adjuvants, the potential of antigen-mounted, activated DCs for the treatment of infectious diseases has been confirmed in multiple experimental models (Inaba, Metlay et al. 1990; Fajardo-Moser, Berzel et al. 2008). If DCs are suppressed by chronic viral infections for T cell exhaustion or deletion, provision of active, modulatory DCs presenting viral epitopes could overcome virus-induced suppressive environments and initiate vigorous anti-viral T cell immunity. The proper use of DC subtypes, DC modulation methodology and the way to activate intracellular class I MHC antigen presenting pathways as well as MHC class II pathways need to be considered to maximize the efficacy of DC-based immunocytotherapy.

Collectively, there is a great deal of understanding the mechanisms behind LCMV-induced immunosuppression (Figure 4 and Table 1) that has had practical applications for serious chronic human viral infections and have led to clinical trials for therapeutic interventions. However, many of the underlying causes have yet to be determined and further investigations are needed. In conjunction with molecular mechanistic studies, the approach to subvert the immunosuppressive environment caused by chronic viral infections could aid the development of immune-therapeutic drugs and treatments to combat many viral diseases.

5. Acknowledgements

We thank the editors for invitation of this review. This work was supported by NIH/NIAID grants AI088363 and AI091797 (B.H.).

6. References

Agnellini, P., P. Wolint, et al. (2007). "Impaired NFAT nuclear translocation results in split exhaustion of virus-specific CD8+ T cell functions during chronic viral infection." *Proc Natl Acad Sci U S A* 104(11): 4565-4570.

Ahmed, R., A. Salmi, et al. (1984). "Selection of genetic variants of lymphocytic choriomeningitis virus in spleens of persistently infected mice. Role in suppression of cytotoxic T lymphocyte response and viral persistence." *J Exp Med* 160(2): 521-540.

Alter, G., J. M. Malenfant, et al. (2004). "Increased natural killer cell activity in viremic HIV-1 infection." *J Immunol* 173(8): 5305-5311.

Asselin-Paturel, C. and G. Trinchieri (2005). "Production of type I interferons: plasmacytoid dendritic cells and beyond." *J Exp Med* 202(4): 461-465.

Barber, D. L., E. J. Wherry, et al. (2006). "Restoring function in exhausted CD8 T cells during chronic viral infection." *Nature* 439(7077): 682-687.

Blackburn, S. D., H. Shin, et al. (2009). "Coregulation of CD8+ T cell exhaustion by multiple inhibitory receptors during chronic viral infection." *Nat Immunol* 10(1): 29-37.

Borrow, P., C. F. Evans, et al. (1995). "Virus-induced immunosuppression: immune system-mediated destruction of virus-infected dendritic cells results in generalized immune suppression." *J Virol* 69(2): 1059-1070.

Brehm, M. A., K. A. Daniels, et al. (2005). "Rapid production of TNF-alpha following TCR engagement of naive CD8 T cells." *J Immunol* 175(8): 5043-5049.

Brockman, M. A., D. S. Kwon, et al. (2009). "IL-10 is up-regulated in multiple cell types during viremic HIV infection and reversibly inhibits virus-specific T cells." *Blood* 114(2): 346-356.

Brooks, D. G., S. J. Ha, et al. (2008). "IL-10 and PD-L1 operate through distinct pathways to suppress T-cell activity during persistent viral infection." *Proc Natl Acad Sci U S A* 105(51): 20428-20433.

Brooks, D. G., L. Teyton, et al. (2005). "Intrinsic functional dysregulation of CD4 T cells occurs rapidly following persistent viral infection." *J Virol* 79(16): 10514-10527.

Brooks, D. G., M. J. Trifilo, et al. (2006). "Interleukin-10 determines viral clearance or persistence in vivo." *Nat Med* 12(11): 1301-1309.

Brown, J. A., D. M. Dorfman, et al. (2003). "Blockade of programmed death-1 ligands on dendritic cells enhances T cell activation and cytokine production." *J Immunol* 170(3): 1257-1266.

Bucks, C. M., J. A. Norton, et al. (2009). "Chronic antigen stimulation alone is sufficient to drive CD8+ T cell exhaustion." *J Immunol* 182(11): 6697-6708.

Byrne, J. A. and M. B. Oldstone (1984). "Biology of cloned cytotoxic T lymphocytes specific for lymphocytic choriomeningitis virus: clearance of virus in vivo." *J Virol* 51(3): 682-686.

Byrne, P., P. McGuirk, et al. (2004). "Depletion of NK cells results in disseminating lethal infection with Bordetella pertussis associated with a reduction of antigen-specific Th1 and enhancement of Th2, but not Tr1 cells." *Eur J Immunol* 34(9): 2579-2588.

Calame, K. (2006). "Transcription factors that regulate memory in humoral responses." *Immunol Rev* 211: 269-279.

Cao, W., M. D. Henry, et al. (1998). "Identification of alpha-dystroglycan as a receptor for lymphocytic choriomeningitis virus and Lassa fever virus." *Science* 282(5396): 2079-2081.

Carbone, F. R., M. W. Moore, et al. (1988). "Induction of cytotoxic T lymphocytes by primary in vitro stimulation with peptides." *J Exp Med* 167(6): 1767-1779.

Dalod, M., T. P. Salazar-Mather, et al. (2002). "Interferon alpha/beta and interleukin 12 responses to viral infections: pathways regulating dendritic cell cytokine expression in vivo." *J Exp Med* 195(4): 517-528.

Day, C. L., D. E. Kaufmann, et al. (2006). "PD-1 expression on HIV-specific T cells is associated with T-cell exhaustion and disease progression." *Nature* 443(7109): 350-354.

Delale, T., A. Paquin, et al. (2005). "MyD88-dependent and -independent murine cytomegalovirus sensing for IFN-alpha release and initiation of immune responses in vivo." *J Immunol* 175(10): 6723-6732.

Diebold, S. S., M. Montoya, et al. (2003). "Viral infection switches non-plasmacytoid dendritic cells into high interferon producers." *Nature* 424(6946): 324-328.

Donaghy, H., A. Pozniak, et al. (2001). "Loss of blood CD11c(+) myeloid and CD11c(-) plasmacytoid dendritic cells in patients with HIV-1 infection correlates with HIV-1 RNA virus load." *Blood* 98(8): 2574-2576.

Drakes, M. L., L. Lu, et al. (1997). "In vivo administration of flt3 ligand markedly stimulates generation of dendritic cell progenitors from mouse liver." *J Immunol* 159(9): 4268-4278.

Ejrnaes, M., C. M. Filippi, et al. (2006). "Resolution of a chronic viral infection after interleukin-10 receptor blockade." *J Exp Med* 203(11): 2461-2472.

Elsaesser, H., K. Sauer, et al. (2009). "IL-21 is required to control chronic viral infection." *Science* 324(5934): 1569-1572.

Fahey, L. M., E. B. Wilson, et al. (2011). "Viral persistence redirects CD4 T cell differentiation toward T follicular helper cells." *J Exp Med* 208(5): 987-999.

Fajardo-Moser, M., S. Berzel, et al. (2008). "Mechanisms of dendritic cell-based vaccination against infection." *Int J Med Microbiol* 298(1-2): 11-20.

Freeman, G. J., A. J. Long, et al. (2000). "Engagement of the PD-1 immunoinhibitory receptor by a novel B7 family member leads to negative regulation of lymphocyte activation." *J Exp Med* 192(7): 1027-1034.

Frohlich, A., J. Kisielow, et al. (2009). "IL-21R on T cells is critical for sustained functionality and control of chronic viral infection." *Science* 324(5934): 1576-1580.

Fung-Leung, W. P., T. M. Kundig, et al. (1991). "Immune response against lymphocytic choriomeningitis virus infection in mice without CD8 expression." *J Exp Med* 174(6): 1425-1429.

Goodman, A. G., H. Zeng, et al. (2010). "The alpha/beta interferon receptor provides protection against influenza virus replication but is dispensable for inflammatory response signaling." *J Virol* 84(4): 2027-2037.

Gottschalk, S., C. M. Bollard, et al. (2006). "T cell therapies." *Ernst Schering Found Symp Proc*(4): 69-82.

Grosso, J. F., M. V. Goldberg, et al. (2009). "Functionally distinct LAG-3 and PD-1 subsets on activated and chronically stimulated CD8 T cells." *J Immunol* 182(11): 6659-6669.

Hahm, B. (2009). "Hostile communication of measles virus with host innate immunity and dendritic cells." *Curr Top Microbiol Immunol* 330: 271-287.

Hahm, B., M. J. Trifilo, et al. (2005). "Viruses evade the immune system through type I interferon-mediated STAT2-dependent, but STAT1-independent, signaling." *Immunity* 22(2): 247-257.

Hoofnagle, J. H., K. D. Mullen, et al. (1986). "Treatment of chronic non-A,non-B hepatitis with recombinant human alpha interferon. A preliminary report." *N Engl J Med* 315(25): 1575-1578.

Hryniewicz, A., A. Boasso, et al. (2006). "CTLA-4 blockade decreases TGF-beta, IDO, and viral RNA expression in tissues of SIVmac251-infected macaques." *Blood* 108(12): 3834-3842.

Inaba, K., J. P. Metlay, et al. (1990). "Dendritic cells pulsed with protein antigens in vitro can prime antigen-specific, MHC-restricted T cells in situ." *J Exp Med* 172(2): 631-640.

Jin, H. T., A. C. Anderson, et al. (2010). "Cooperation of Tim-3 and PD-1 in CD8 T-cell exhaustion during chronic viral infection." *Proc Natl Acad Sci U S A* 107(33): 14733-14738.

Jung, A., H. Kato, et al. (2008). "Lymphocytoid choriomeningitis virus activates plasmacytoid dendritic cells and induces a cytotoxic T-cell response via MyD88." *J Virol* 82(1): 196-206.

Kanto, T. and N. Hayashi (2004). "Distinct susceptibility of dendritic cell subsets to hepatitis C virus infection: a plausible mechanism of dendritic cell dysfunction." *J Gastroenterol* 39(8): 811-812.

Kanto, T., M. Inoue, et al. (2004). "Reduced numbers and impaired ability of myeloid and plasmacytoid dendritic cells to polarize T helper cells in chronic hepatitis C virus infection." *J Infect Dis* 190(11): 1919-1926.

Kapp, M., S. M. Tan, et al. (2007). "Adoptive immunotherapy of HCMV infection." *Cytotherapy* 9(8): 699-711.

Kasaian, M. T., M. J. Whitters, et al. (2002). "IL-21 limits NK cell responses and promotes antigen-specific T cell activation: a mediator of the transition from innate to adaptive immunity." *Immunity* 16(4): 559-569.

Kasprowicz, V., J. Schulze Zur Wiesch, et al. (2008). "High level of PD-1 expression on hepatitis C virus (HCV)-specific CD8+ and CD4+ T cells during acute HCV infection, irrespective of clinical outcome." *J Virol* 82(6): 3154-3160.

Kaufmann, D. E., D. G. Kavanagh, et al. (2007). "Upregulation of CTLA-4 by HIV-specific CD4+ T cells correlates with disease progression and defines a reversible immune dysfunction." *Nat Immunol* 8(11): 1246-1254.

Kolokoltsova, O. A., N. E. Yun, et al. (2010). "Mice lacking alpha/beta and gamma interferon receptors are susceptible to junin virus infection." *J Virol* 84(24): 13063-13067.

Korbel, D. S., K. C. Newman, et al. (2005). "Heterogeneous human NK cell responses to Plasmodium falciparum-infected erythrocytes." *J Immunol* 175(11): 7466-7473.

Lancki, D. W., C. S. Hsieh, et al. (1991). "Mechanisms of lysis by cytotoxic T lymphocyte clones. Lytic activity and gene expression in cloned antigen-specific CD4+ and CD8+ T lymphocytes." *J Immunol* 146(9): 3242-3249.

Lee, H. K., J. M. Lund, et al. (2007). "Autophagy-dependent viral recognition by plasmacytoid dendritic cells." *Science* 315(5817): 1398-1401.

Liu, B., A. M. Woltman, et al. (2009). "Modulation of dendritic cell function by persistent viruses." *J Leukoc Biol* 85(2): 205-214.

Liu, Y. J. (2005). "IPC: professional type 1 interferon-producing cells and plasmacytoid dendritic cell precursors." *Annu Rev Immunol* 23: 275-306.

Martin, R., A. Vallbracht, et al. (1991). "Interferon-gamma secretion by in vivo activated cytotoxic T lymphocytes from the blood and cerebrospinal fluid during mumps meningitis." *J Neuroimmunol* 33(3): 191-198.

Martinez-Sobrido, L., S. Emonet, et al. (2009). "Identification of amino acid residues critical for the anti-interferon activity of the nucleoprotein of the prototypic arenavirus lymphocytic choriomeningitis virus." *J Virol* 83(21): 11330-11340.

Martinez-Sobrido, L., E. I. Zuniga, et al. (2006). "Inhibition of the type I interferon response by the nucleoprotein of the prototypic arenavirus lymphocytic choriomeningitis virus." *J Virol* 80(18): 9192-9199.

Martins, L. P., L. L. Lau, et al. (1995). "DNA vaccination against persistent viral infection." *J Virol* 69(4): 2574-2582.

Matloubian, M., R. J. Concepcion, et al. (1994). "CD4+ T cells are required to sustain CD8+ cytotoxic T-cell responses during chronic viral infection." *J Virol* 68(12): 8056-8063.

Montoya, M., M. J. Edwards, et al. (2005). "Rapid activation of spleen dendritic cell subsets following lymphocytic choriomeningitis virus infection of mice: analysis of the involvement of type 1 IFN." *J Immunol* 174(4): 1851-1861.

Muller, U., U. Steinhoff, et al. (1994). "Functional role of type I and type II interferons in antiviral defense." *Science* 264(5167): 1918-1921.

Murray, L. J., R. Lee, et al. (1990). "In vivo cytokine gene expression in T cell subsets of the autoimmune MRL/Mp-lpr/lpr mouse." *Eur J Immunol* 20(1): 163-170.

Nakamoto, N., H. Cho, et al. (2009). "Synergistic reversal of intrahepatic HCV-specific CD8 T cell exhaustion by combined PD-1/CTLA-4 blockade." *PLoS Pathog* 5(2): e1000313.

Odermatt, B., M. Eppler, et al. (1991). "Virus-triggered acquired immunodeficiency by cytotoxic T-cell-dependent destruction of antigen-presenting cells and lymph follicle structure." *Proc Natl Acad Sci U S A* 88(18): 8252-8256.

Pacanowski, J., S. Kahi, et al. (2001). "Reduced blood CD123+ (lymphoid) and CD11c+ (myeloid) dendritic cell numbers in primary HIV-1 infection." *Blood* 98(10): 3016-3021.

Rahman, A. H., W. Cui, et al. (2008). "MyD88 plays a critical T cell-intrinsic role in supporting CD8 T cell expansion during acute lymphocytic choriomeningitis virus infection." *J Immunol* 181(6): 3804-3810.

Richter, K., P. Agnellini, et al. (2010). "On the role of the inhibitory receptor LAG-3 in acute and chronic LCMV infection." *Int Immunol* 22(1): 13-23.

Sakthivel, P., M. Gereke, et al. (2011). "Therapeutic intervention in cancer and chronic viral infections: Antibody mediated manipulation of PD-1/PD-L1 interaction." *Rev Recent Clin Trials.*

Sakuishi, K., L. Apetoh, et al. (2010). "Targeting Tim-3 and PD-1 pathways to reverse T cell exhaustion and restore anti-tumor immunity." *J Exp Med* 207(10): 2187-2194.

Salvato, M., P. Borrow, et al. (1991). "Molecular basis of viral persistence: a single amino acid change in the glycoprotein of lymphocytic choriomeningitis virus is associated with suppression of the antiviral cytotoxic T-lymphocyte response and establishment of persistence." *J Virol* 65(4): 1863-1869.

Seo, Y. J. and B. Hahm (2010). "Type I interferon modulates the battle of host immune system against viruses." *Adv Appl Microbiol* 73: 83-101.

Sevilla, N., S. Kunz, et al. (2000). "Immunosuppression and resultant viral persistence by specific viral targeting of dendritic cells." *J Exp Med* 192(9): 1249-1260.

Sevilla, N., S. Kunz, et al. (2003). "Infection of dendritic cells by lymphocytic choriomeningitis virus." *Curr Top Microbiol Immunol* 276: 125-144.

Sevilla, N., D. B. McGavern, et al. (2004). "Viral targeting of hematopoietic progenitors and inhibition of DC maturation as a dual strategy for immune subversion." *J Clin Invest* 113(5): 737-745.

Shaffer, A. L., K. I. Lin, et al. (2002). "Blimp-1 orchestrates plasma cell differentiation by extinguishing the mature B cell gene expression program." *Immunity* 17(1): 51-62.

Shin, H., S. D. Blackburn, et al. (2009). "A role for the transcriptional repressor Blimp-1 in CD8(+) T cell exhaustion during chronic viral infection." *Immunity* 31(2): 309-320.

Siavoshian, S., J. D. Abraham, et al. (2005). "Hepatitis C virus core, NS3, NS5A, NS5B proteins induce apoptosis in mature dendritic cells." *J Med Virol* 75(3): 402-411.

Siren, J., T. Sareneva, et al. (2004). "Cytokine and contact-dependent activation of natural killer cells by influenza A or Sendai virus-infected macrophages." *J Gen Virol* 85(Pt 8): 2357-2364.

Smelt, S. C., P. Borrow, et al. (2001). "Differences in affinity of binding of lymphocytic choriomeningitis virus strains to the cellular receptor alpha-dystroglycan correlate with viral tropism and disease kinetics." *J Virol* 75(1): 448-457.

Steinman, R. M., A. Granelli-Piperno, et al. (2003). "The interaction of immunodeficiency viruses with dendritic cells." *Curr Top Microbiol Immunol* 276: 1-30.

Terawaki, S., S. Chikuma, et al. (2011). "IFN-alpha directly promotes programmed cell death-1 transcription and limits the duration of T cell-mediated immunity." *J Immunol* 186(5): 2772-2779.

Trifilo, M. J., B. Hahm, et al. (2006). "Dendritic cell inhibition: memoirs from immunosuppressive viruses." *J Infect Dis* 194 Suppl 1: S3-10.

Vankayalapati, R., A. Garg, et al. (2005). "Role of NK cell-activating receptors and their ligands in the lysis of mononuclear phagocytes infected with an intracellular bacterium." *J Immunol* 175(7): 4611-4617.

Vezys, V., P. Penaloza-MacMaster, et al. (2011). "4-1BB signaling synergizes with programmed death ligand 1 blockade to augment CD8 T cell responses during chronic viral infection." *J Immunol* 187(4): 1634-1642.

von Herrath, M. G., D. P. Berger, et al. (2000). "Vaccination to treat persistent viral infection." *Virology* 268(2): 411-419.

West, E. E., B. Youngblood, et al. (2011). "Tight regulation of memory CD8(+) T cells limits their effectiveness during sustained high viral load." *Immunity* 35(2): 285-298.

Wherry, E. J., J. N. Blattman, et al. (2005). "Low CD8 T-cell proliferative potential and high viral load limit the effectiveness of therapeutic vaccination." *J Virol* 79(14): 8960-8968.

Wherry, E. J., J. N. Blattman, et al. (2003). "Viral persistence alters CD8 T-cell immunodominance and tissue distribution and results in distinct stages of functional impairment." *J Virol* 77(8): 4911-4927.

Wherry, E. J., S. J. Ha, et al. (2007). "Molecular signature of CD8+ T cell exhaustion during chronic viral infection." *Immunity* 27(4): 670-684.

Workman, C. J., K. J. Dugger, et al. (2002). "Cutting edge: molecular analysis of the negative regulatory function of lymphocyte activation gene-3." *J Immunol* 169(10): 5392-5395.

Yamazaki, T., H. Akiba, et al. (2002). "Expression of programmed death 1 ligands by murine T cells and APC." *J Immunol* 169(10): 5538-5545.

Yi, J. S., M. A. Cox, et al. (2010). "T-cell exhaustion: characteristics, causes and conversion." *Immunology* 129(4): 474-481.

Yi, J. S., M. Du, et al. (2009). "A vital role for interleukin-21 in the control of a chronic viral infection." *Science* 324(5934): 1572-1576.

Youngblood, B., K. J. Oestreich, et al. (2011). "Chronic Virus Infection Enforces Demethylation of the Locus that Encodes PD-1 in Antigen-Specific CD8(+) T Cells." *Immunity* 35(3): 400-412.

Zhou, S., A. M. Cerny, et al. (2010). "Induction and inhibition of type I interferon responses by distinct components of lymphocytic choriomeningitis virus." *J Virol* 84(18): 9452-9462.

Zhou, S., E. A. Kurt-Jones, et al. (2005). "MyD88 is critical for the development of innate and adaptive immunity during acute lymphocytic choriomeningitis virus infection." *Eur J Immunol* 35(3): 822-830.

Zucchini, N., G. Bessou, et al. (2008). "Cutting edge: Overlapping functions of TLR7 and TLR9 for innate defense against a herpesvirus infection." *J Immunol* 180(9): 5799-5803.

Zuniga, E. I., B. Hahm, et al. (2007). "Type I interferon during viral infections: multiple triggers for a multifunctional mediator." *Curr Top Microbiol Immunol* 316: 337-357.

Zuniga, E. I., L. Y. Liou, et al. (2008). "Persistent virus infection inhibits type I interferon production by plasmacytoid dendritic cells to facilitate opportunistic infections." *Cell Host Microbe* 4(4): 374-386.

3

T_H17 Cells in Cancer Related Inflammation

Rupinder K. Kanwar and Jagat R. Kanwar
Nanomedicine-Laboratory of Immunology and Molecular Biomedical Research (LIMBR), Centre for Biotechnology and Interdisciplinary Biosciences (BioDeakin), Institute for Technology & Research Innovation, Deakin University, Geelong, Technology Precinct, Waurn Ponds, Geelong, Victoria, Australia

1. Introduction

Until 2005, T helper (CD4+) cells were proposed to be a binary system, consisting of T_H1 and T_H2 cells (Mosmann TR *et al.*,1986) , when a third T helper -cell subset, known as T_H17 (interleukin-17 (IL-17) expressing cells), was identified (Harrington LE *et al.*, 2005, Park H *et al.*, 2005). This was followed up by the another independent discovery in three different laboratories of the differentiation factors cytokines such as interleukin (IL)-6 and transforming growth factor beta (TGF-β), that simplified *in vitro* analysis of this T cell subset to a large extent (Veldhoen M *et al.*, 2006, Bettelli E *et al.*, 2006, Mangan *et al.*, 2006). The discovery of these unique T_H17 cells has opened up exciting new avenues for research into the etiology and therapeutics of a broad spectrum of human diseases and data on the biology of these cells have emerged at an astounding pace in just 5 years. The reason for these cells to receive considerable attention in these recent years is their emerging involvement as principal mediators of pathogenesis in several autoimmune and chronic inflammatory disorders. Many reviews of the field have already highlighted the important role of T_H17 cells in the diverse group of human autoimmune and inflammatory diseases (Tesmer *et al.*, 2008, Sallusto and Lanzavecchia 2009, Torrado and Cooper 2010, Kimura and Kishimoto 2011, Cosmi *et al.*, 2011).

With regards to cancer, the involvement of T_H17 cells in tumour immunology has raised their status as a target for cancer therapy. However based on the reported evidence on the potential anti-tumourigenic and pro-tumourigenic activities of T_H17 cells, their role as friends or foes, respectively is still under debate; could be because of a few studies have focused on primary T_H17 cells in the human tumour microenvironment (Wilke *et al.*, 2011). The link between cancer development and inflammation is now widely accepted and cancer patients have local and systemic changes in inflammatory parameters (Chechlinska, *et al.*, 2010). Tumours frequently display the characteristics of chronically inflamed tissue, including immune cell infiltration and an activated stroma (Kanwar *et al.*, 2008, Mantovani *et al.*, 2008). Indeed inflammation has been proposed as the seventh trait of cancer by supplementing Hanahan and Weinberg's model that identifies six hallmarks of cancer (Mantovani 2009). This chapter focuses on the role of T_H17 cells in cancer by understanding its links with chronic inflammation.

2. Association of cancer with inflammation

Inflammation is the first line of defence against various extracellular stimuli (microbes, trauma, chemicals, heat or any other phenomenon) and can be acute or chronic. Acute or physiological inflammation is when body cells respond to external stimuli for short periods of time. Normal inflammation, for example, inflammation associated with acute infections, injury, wound healing is usually self-limiting; however, dysregulation of any of the involved factors leads to abnormalities. If the stimulus sustains for longer time, it results in a pathological state known as chronic or pathological inflammation as seen in autoimmune and chronic inflammatory diseases such as atherosclerosis, multiple sclerosis, rheumatoid arthritis, allergic inflammation of the lung leading to asthma (Kanwar *et al.*, 2001a, Kanwar 2005, Kanwar *et al.*, 2008, Kanwar *et al.*, 2009, Barreiro *et al.*, 2010). Chronic inflammation is also the case during tumour progression in cancer. The patients with chronic inflammatory conditions have a greatly increased risk of cancer in the affected organs. Also chronic inflammation resulting from viral or bacterial infections can often lead to or hasten the development of malignancy (Coussens and Werb 2002, Kanwar *et al.*, 2011). Table 1 summarizes the chronic inflammatory conditions associated with cancer.

Inflammatory Condition	**Associated Cancer(s)**
AIDS	Non-Hodgkin's lymphoma, squamous cellcarcinomas, Kaposi's sarcoma
Asbestosis, silicosis	Mesothelioma, lung carcinoma
Barrett's oesophagus	Oesophageal carcinoma
Bronchitis	Lung carcinoma
Chronic cholecystitis	Gall bladder cancer
Chronic pancreatitis, hereditary pancreatitis	Pancreatic carcinoma
Coeliac disease	Lymphoma
Gingivitis	Oral squamous cell carcinoma
Helicobacter pylori infection	Gastric cancer
Hepatitis B or C	Hepatocellular carcinoma
Inflammatory bowel disease, Crohn's disease, chronic ulcerative colitis	Colorectal carcinoma
Lichen sclerosus	Vulvar squamous cell carcinoma
Mononucleosis	B-cell non-Hodgkin's lymphoma, Burkitts lymphoma,
Obesity related inflammation	Liver cancer
Opisthorchis, Cholangitis	Cholangiosarcoma, colon carcinoma
Osteomyelitis	Sarcoma
Pelvic inflammatory disease, chronic cervicitis	Ovarian carcinoma, cervical/anal carcinoma
Prostate inflammatory atrophy	Prostate cancer
Rheumatoid arthritis	Lymphoma
Shistosomiasis, bladder inflammation	Bladder carcinoma
Sialadenitis	Salivary gland carcinoma
Sjögren syndrome, Hashimoto's thyroiditis	MALT lymphoma
Skin inflammation	Melanoma

Modified from Coussens and Werb, 2002, Conro y *et al.*, 2010

Table 1. Chronic inflammatory conditions and infections associated with cancer.

When the control of cell proliferation, growth and cell death (apoptosis) is lost, we obtain a clone of cells known as benign tumour. By growing its own blood supply (angiogenesis), the tumour feeds itself, grows indefinitely and spreads (metastasizes) in the body thereby leads to malignant cancer. Tumour cells are known to produce various pro inflammatory cytokines such as IL-1β, IL-6, IL-23 and tumour necrosis factor (TNF)-αand chemokines that attract inflammatory leukocytes which include neutrophils, dendritic cells, macrophages, eosinophils, mast cells and lymphocytes (Coussens and Werb 2002, Kanwar *et al.,* 2008,). These cells further produce growth factors, various cytokines, chemokines, cytotoxic mediators like reactive oxygen species, matrix metalloproteinases (MMPs), membrane-perforating agents and soluble mediators of cell killing such as TNF-α, interleukins and interferons (Wahl *et al.,* 1998, Kuper *et al.,* 2000, Coussens and Werb 2002, Kanwar *et al.,* 2008). The recruitment of dendritic cells capture antigen and stimulate anti-tumour immunity by T lymphocyte activation which kill cancer cells via cell mediated cytotoxicity (Kanwar *et al.,* 1999). According to the immune surveillance theory, tumours arise only if cancer cells are able to escape immune surveillance, yet sometimes a robust immune response might result in a favourable effect that might be due to CD8+ cytotoxic T cells which have the capacity to kill tumour cells (Kanwar *et al.,* 2001b) CD4+ T cell responses are also important as they help recruiting CD8+ cytotoxic T cell and generate an inflammatory response that chains the function of CTLs activity (Kanwar *et al.,* 2003). The growth factors asnd cytokines released by inflammatory cells can also have pro-tumour actions. They can lead to proliferation, survival and migration of the tumour by promoting angiogenesis and lymphanogenesis, remodelling extracellular matrix to facilitate invasion, coating tumour cells to make available receptors for spreading cells via lymphatics and capillaries, and evading host mechanisms (Coussens and Werb 2002, Rigo *et al.,* 2010). In this context tumour-associated macrophages (TAMs) have a significant role. After migration the monocytes, recruited largely by monocyte chemotactic protein (MCP) chemokine become the significant component of inflammatory infiltrates as TAMs in neoplastic tissues, and has a dual role in neoplasms. TAMs may kill neoplastic cells following activation by IL-2, interferon and IL-12 or potentiate neoplastic progression through the production of a number of potent angiogenic and lymphangiogenic growth factors, cytokines and proteases, all of which are mediators for tumour growth (Brigati *et al.,* 2002, Tsung *et al.,* 2002). Further TAMs and tumour cells also produce IL-10, which effectively blunts the anti-tumour response by cytotoxic T cells, and prevent maturation of anti-tumour dendritic cells *in situ* leading to immunosuppression and immune evasion (Coffelt *et al.,* 2009). Increasing evidences have suggested that many types of cancer are closely associated with inflammation (Table 1). Thus, inflammation is a process used by immune cells to eliminate cancer and by cancer cells to promote tumour progression and metastasis.

3. CD4+ T cell subsets as essential regulators of immune responses and inflammatory diseases

Immune system consists of innate and adaptive immunity. Adaptive immunity is mediated by T and B cells. T helper cells/CD4+ cells are the key actors in establishing an immune response. Naive $CD4^+$ T cells differentiate into different types of effector cells depending upon the combination of cytokines in milieu, antigen and the antigen presenting cell (APC). There are four types known so far (Figure 1) and include T_H1, T_H2, T- regulatory (Treg) and T_H17. T_H1 cells, induced by IL-12, express T_H1 specific Transcription factors (T-bet) and produce IFN-γ as their signature cytokine and evoke cell-mediated immunity and phagocyte-dependent inflammation. Vigorous pro-inflammatory activities of T_H1 cells has been seen to cause tissue damage and elicit unwanted T_H1-dominated responses in the pathogenesis of organ-specific autoimmune/inflammatory disorders, Crohn's disease, sarcoidosis, acute kidney allograft rejection, and some unexplained recurrent abortions (Romagnani, 2000).

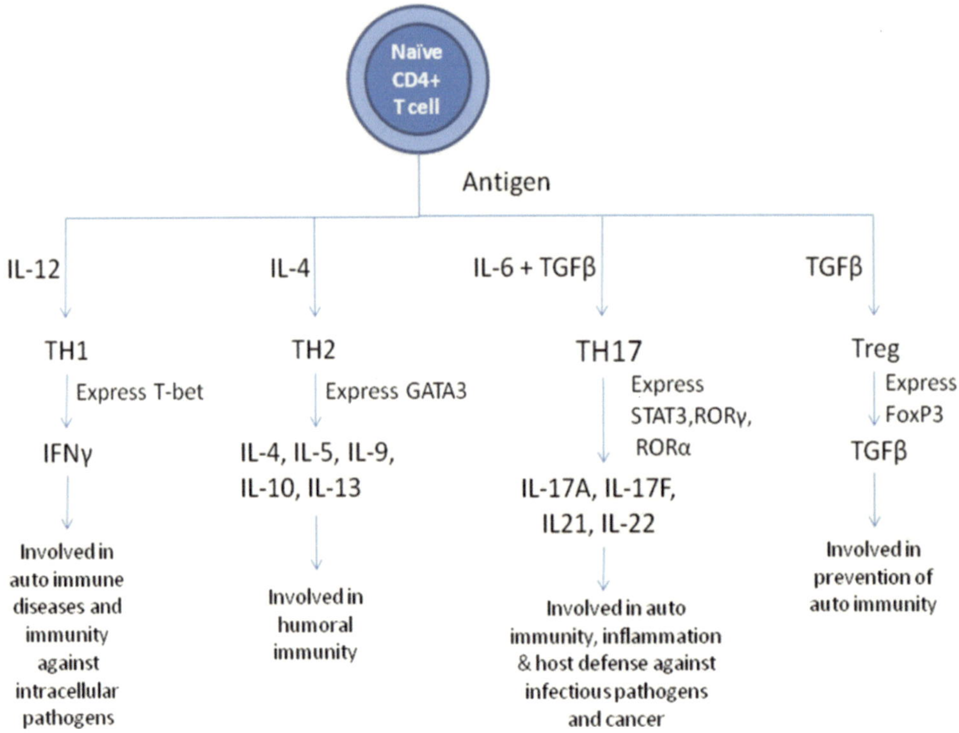

Fig. 1. CD4+ T- Cell differentiation: Naive CD4+ T cells differentiate into different effector cells under the influence of the pool of cytokines present in the surroundings. There are four known types of effector T_H cells which have different functions based on the expression of unique transcription factors and characteristic cytokines.

T_H2 cells are induced by IL-4, express GATA 3 and produce IL-4, IL-5, IL-9, IL-10 and IL-13. These are associated with the humoral immunity and resistance against extracellular forms of pathogens. T-regulatory (Treg) cells, characterized by expression of FoxP3 (forkhead/winged helix transcription factor), produce TGF-β (transforming growth factor-β1). These distinct regulatory T cell subsets suppress adaptive T cell responses, have anti-inflammatory role and are involved in maintaining tolerance to self components (prevent autoimmunity).

T_H17 cells, a newly defined lineage of CD4+ cells, are not only distinct from other T_H cells in their gene expression and regulation, but also in terms of their biological function (Dong 2008) T_H17 cells are characterized in particular through the production of IL-17 and IL-17F, and have functions in autoimmune diseases, inflammation and host defence against infectious pathogens. Recently accumulating evidence suggests that T_H cells possess functional 'plasticity' (Bettelli *et al.*, 2006, Yang *et al.*, 2008a, Crome *et al.*, 2010a) i.e. they can be converted into other types of T_H cells under *in vitro* as well as *in vivo* conditions. This property seems to be certainly beneficial to mount different and varied responses for combating immunological insults given at short notices.

T_H17 cells: a new lineage of effector T_H cells Discovery: The presence of T_H17 cells as a specific lineage was recognized when it was demonstrated that lipopeptides from the spirochete *Borrelia burgdorferi* triggered the increased levels of IL-17A mRNA in T cells to produce IL-17 (member of IL-17 family composed of 6 cytokines, IL-17A-F), TNF-α and GM-CSF while these cells were negative for IFN-γ or IL-4, revealing a novel cytokine phenotype distinct from T_H1 or T_H2. (Infante-Duarte *et al.*, 2002). This was the first report to establish the link between bacterial infection and a new effector T cell phenotype later to become T_H17 while foretelling the description of a factor later identified as critical to T_H17 development: IL-6 (Weaver *et al.*, 2007) . Further hint came when, Aggarwal *et al.* 2003, who demonstrated that IL-23 stimulates murine CD4+ T cells to secrete IL-17 following stimulation of the T- cell receptor (TCR). These crucial findings that IL-23 but not IL-12, stimulated memory, but not naive, CD4 T cells to produce IL-17A and IL-17F, were consistent with a unique effector CD4 T cell population similar to that previously reported by Infante-Duarte and colleagues in 2002. Then the findings that IL-17 secreting CD4+ T cells arise in the absence of T_H1 and T_H2 induced transcription factors and cytokines solidified the lineage separation between T_H1/T_H2 and T_H 17 cells (Harrington *et al.*, 2005; Park *et al.*, 2005).

Differentiation and transcriptional regulation: Although early studies by Aggarwal and colleagues in 2003 implicated IL-23 in driving T_H17 expression and generation , it was later on demonstrated that IL-23 receptor (IL-23R) is not expressed on naïve T cells. Instead, IL-23, as well as TNF-α, acts as survival signals for T_H17 cells. It is apparent now as reviewed recently (Weaver *et al.*, 2007, Torchinsky and Blander 2010, Kimura and Kishimoto 2011) that IL-23 is important only for T_H17 cells' expansion, survival and pathogenicity. The key cytokines required for T_H17 differentiation, surprisingly, are a combination of pro-inflammatory and anti-inflammatory cytokines; i.e, IL-6 and TGF-β respectively (Veldhoen M *et al.*, 2006, Mangan *et al.*, 2006, Betteli *et al.*, 2006). The studies by Betteli and colleagues identified TGF-β as a critical factor for T_H17 commitment while IL-6 acted to deviate TGF-β-driven development of Foxp3-expressing Tregs toward T_H17 (Betteli *et al.*, 2006).

Further attempts were made to delineate the precise signalling mechanisms through which IL-6 and TGF-β cooperate to induce T_H17 differentiation. Studies have shown that the key transcription factors in determining the differentiation of the T_H17 lineage are retinoid-related orphan receptor γt (RORγt) and RORα which can be induced by the combination of IL-6 and TGF-β (Ivanov *et al.*, 2006, Yang *et al.*, 2008b). RORγt was shown to be specifically expressed by mouse and human T_H17 cells (Ivanov *et al.*, 2006, Wilson *et al.*, 2007). Further a central role for IL-6-induced STAT3 activation was made evident. Although IL-6 activates both STAT3 and STAT1, it has been demonstrated that STAT3 activation is maintained while STAT1 activation is suppressed in T_H17 cells (Kimura *et al.*, 2007). Interferon regulatory factor (IRF) 4 and T-bet are other players in the scene of transcriptional regulation, which act as positive and negative regulators of $T_H17$commitment, respectively (Brüstle *et al.*, 2007, Rangachari *et al.*, 2006). Further Aryl hydrocarbon receptor (Ahr) was shown to be induced under T_H17-polarizing conditions such as in the presence of TGF-β plus IL-6, and promotes T_H17 cell development through inhibiting STAT1 and STAT5 activation. More recently, an AP-1 transcription factor, BATF was shown to also play a role in T_H17 differentiation. BATF-/- mice had a defect specifically in differentiation of T_H17 cells, and were resistant to autoimmune encephalomyelitis (Schraml *et al.,* 2009). IL-1 (Chung *et al.,* 2009) and IL-21 (Korn *et al.,* 2007) have also been shown to be required for their differentiation. And certain studies have shown that IL-10 released by Treg cells and IL-2 inhibit T_H17 cell development (Weaver et al., 2007). - Apart from IL-17 as its major cytokine, T_H17 cells also release IL-21 and IL-22 (Wei *et al.,* 2007, Dong 2008). As IL-21 is required for T_H17 cells' differentiation as well as is produced by them, it may be acting as a positive feedback loop to amplify the production of these cells (Torchinsky and Blander 2010). T_H17 cells also express CCR6, CXCR4, CD49 integrins and CD161 (Kryczek, *et al.,* 2009). Crome *et al.,* 2010b established a novel method to isolate *in vivo* differentiated T_H17 cells from peripheral blood by sorting CD161+CCR4+CCR6+CXCR3-CD4+T cells. These authors also suggested low expression of granzyme A and B as another distinguishing feature of T_H17 cells. T_H17 cells also express IL-23R at high levels. There exists also a negative regulatory system for T_H17 cell differentiation and IL-27 was shown to important role in curbing T_H17 responses by limiting development of T_H17 effectors (Batten *et al.,*2006, Stumhofer *et al.,* 2006). Thus, various cytokines and transcription factors can either enhance or inhibit T_H17 differentiation (Figure 2). Very recently, Martinez *et al.* in 2010 suggested that Smad2 positively regulates the generation of T_H17 cells *in vivo* and *in vitro* (Figure 3).

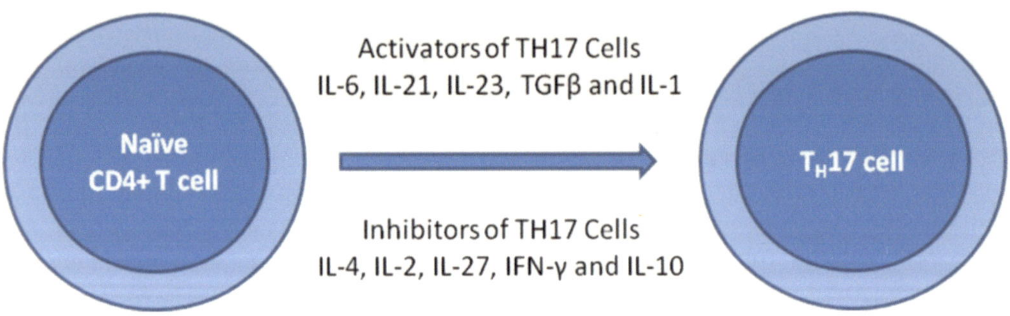

Fig. 2. Activators and inhibitors of T_H17 differentiation: The figure below shows the different activators and inhibitors which promote or inhibit the differentiation of T_H17 cells.

Cytokine production: The T_H17 lineage was originally defined by the production of hallmark cytokines interleukin-17 (also known as IL-17A) and IL-17F, members of IL-17 family (Aggarwal *et al.,* in 2003) as homodimers or heterdimers (Liang *et al.,* 2007). Later on studies have shown that $T_H17$cells are also characterized by the production of IL-10 family cytokine, IL-22 (Liang *et al.,* 2006). IL-21, besides acting in concert with TGF-β to promote T_H17 differentiation, is also produced by T_H17 cells (Korn *et al.* ,2007). T_H17 cells are also known to produce certain cytokines that are expressed by other T helper cell lineages, including TNF-α and lymphotoxin-β, and the T_H17 subset can be characterized by expression of chemokine receptor CCR6 and the CCR6 ligand, CCL20 (Hirota *et al.,* 2007, Torchinsky and Blander 2010). A subset of T_H17 cells is reported to co-expresses IFN-γ in humans where as many as half of all the IL-17+ cells also express IFN-γ. It is not yet clear if these cells represent a stable phenotype or a transitional phase, undergoing a switch from T_H17 to T_H17 or vice versa (reviewed by Tesmer *et al.,* 2008) (Figure 3).

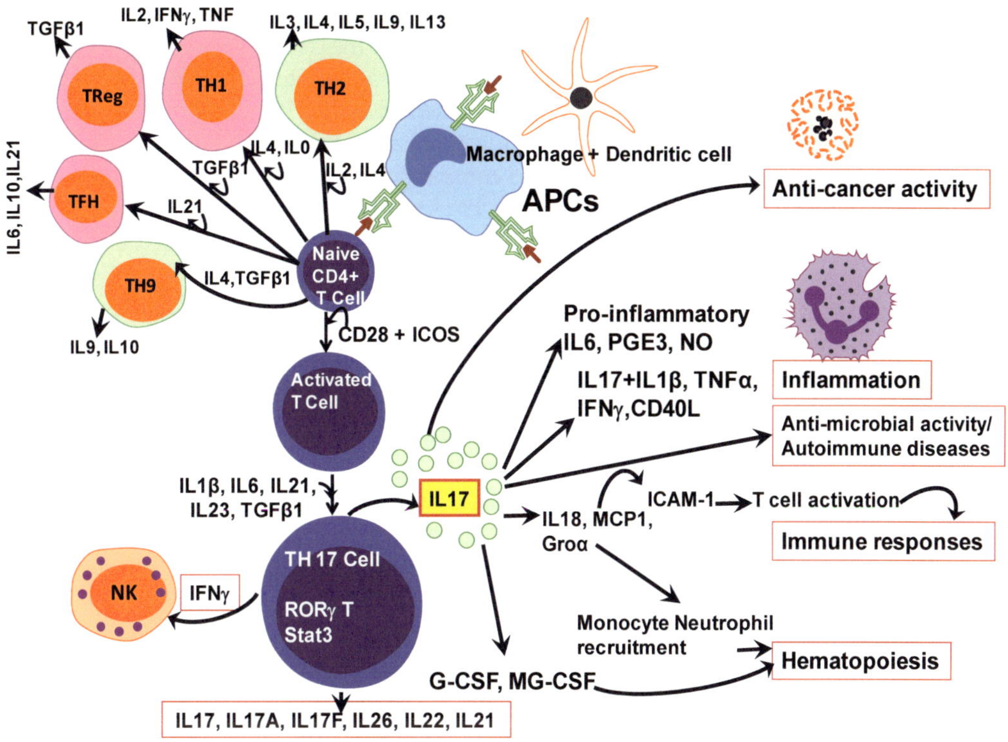

Fig. 3. T_H17 differentiation and activation of immune cells for immune responses, inflammation, anti-cancer activity and hematopoiesis.

Biological activities/functions: The important roles of IL-17 in host defence against many extracellular and intracellular pathogens have already been established (reviewed by Torchinsky and Blander 2010). IL-17A, F released by T_H17 cells, is involved in the recruitment, activation and migration of neutrophils which help the body to fight against infection with various bacterial and fungal species (Yang *et al.*, 2008c). Non-immune cells are major targets for the effector functions of T_H17 cells. Specifically, cytokines produced by T_H17 cells act on cells such as fibroblasts and keratinocytes (Chrome *et al.*, 2010) and thereby contribute to immunity in barrier tissues such as the skin and gut. T_H17 cells have also been involved with tissue repair functions through their production of the cytokine IL-22 along with IL-10 (Dong C 2008). Further the anti-infective and anti-inflammatory roles of IL-22 are associated with its functions in maintaining the integrity of epithelial barriers (Torchinsky and Blander 2010). More interestingly, it was shown that TGF-β and IL-6 from antigen presenting dendritic cells, that recognized apoptotic cells carrying TLR ligands, were able to drive differentiation of naı¨ve CD4+ T cells to the T_H17 lineage (Torchinsky *et al.*, 2009). Thus T_H17 cells may be uniquely suited to serve in host response against pathogens causing significant apoptosis and tissue damage (Figure 3).

There are effector molecules as discussed above (cytokines, chemokines and integrin α3) associated with T_H 17 cells that act as pro-inflammatory mediators of inflammation and upregulate the expression of adhesion molecules thereby mediating the migration of circulating mixed leukocytes, such as monocytes, neutrophils, T cells and natural killer (NK) cells. The infiltrated leukocytes further augment the ongoing inflammation, indirectly by secreting an elaborated number of chemokines and cytokines, including IL-1, IL-6, TNF-α, monocyte chemoattractant protein-1(MCP-1), keratinocyte-derived chemokine (KC), IFN-γ, IL-17, and IL-23 (Coussens and Werb 2002, Kryczek *et al*, 2009a, Barreiro *et al.*, 2010),. When these inflammatory signals are altered or misprocessed, the inflammation can become chronic, causing extensive tissue damage. To combat chronic inflammation in autoimmune diseases, novel therapeutic strategies targeting T_H17 cells and their effector molecules thus represent opportunities for therapeutic intervention.

4. Association of T_H17 cells with chronic inflammation

Earlier, T_H1 phenotype was associated with inflammation and autoimmunity and now the T_H17 subset has also been described as pro-inflammatory to play a role in autoimunity and chronic inflammation. The findings that IFN-γ and IFN-γ receptor-deficient mice and mice lacking IL-12p35 and other molecules involved in T_H1 differentiation were not protected from experimental autoimmune encephalomyelitis (EAE), but rather developed more severe disease have challenged the concept that autoimmunity is a T_H1 driven disease process (Gran B *et al.*, 2002, Torchinsky and Blander 2010). The suggestion about another subset of T cells, distinct from the T_H1 lineage that might be required for the induction of EAE and other organ-specific autoimmune diseases has recently established role and importance of T_H17 cells in the pathogenesis of organ-specific autoimmune inflammation based on animal studies and clinical findings. The topic on the broad implications of T_H17 cells in the pathogenesis of number of immune-mediated diseases such as psoriasis, rheumatoid arthritis, multiple sclerosis, inflammatory bowel disease, and asthma is beyond the scope of this chapter, but readers are referred to excellent recent reviews (Tesmer *et al.*, 2008, Dong C 2008, Torchinsky and Blander 2010, Cosmi *et al.*, 2011) (Figure 1).

Inflammation and pathogenesis induced by T_H17 cells is a result of the pro-inflammatory cytokines, chemokines and chemokine receptors these cells produce and express, respectively. Recently, T_H17 polarized cells have been shown to be associated with cancers. Cancer and inflammation are now considered to be inextricably linked. Inflammatory mediators and cellular effectors are important constituents of the local environment of tumours. Many cancers arise from the sites of infection, chronic irritation and inflammation as shown in Table 1, the inflammatory conditions are present before a malignant change occurs. To understand the kinetics and targets of inflammation in a discussion of T_H17 cells and cancer, the relationship between T_H1-derived IFNγ, T_H17 cells and antigen-presenting cells (APCs) in humans was recently studied (Kryczek *et al.*, 2008a). These authors demonstrated in a cutting edge study that IFNγ could rapidly induce elevated B7-H1 expression on APCs and stimulate their production of IL-1 and IL-23. B7-H1 signaling resulted in abrogation of the T_H1-polarizing capacity of APC, whereas IL-1 and IL-23 directed them toward a memory T_H17-expanding phenotype. These findings thus suggest that in the course of inflammation, that the acute T_H1-mediated response is attenuated by IFNγ-induced B7-H1 on APCs and is subsequently evolved toward T_H17-mediated chronic inflammation by APC derived IL-1 and IL-23. This study in addition to challenging the dogma that IFNγ suppresses T_H17 and enhances T_H1 development, also strengthens the notion that T_H17 kinetics depends strongly on the context of the ongoing immune reactions and the constituents of the cytokine milieu, both of which are influenced by disease progression (Figure 3).

5. T_H17 cells in cancer

Various studies have been carried out in the recent years with rapid progress on different cancer types to investigate the association of cancer and T_H17 cells. It has been seen that, T_H17 cells, might either promote tumour growth or regulate antitumour responses. This may be due to the irregular conflicting data based on the studies in humans versus those in mice and contradictory data from experiments in immunocompetent versus immunodeficient mice (Wilke *et al.,* 2011). There is, however, a strikingly high frequency of tumour-infiltrating T_H17 cells in patients with diverse cancer types. These cells when examined in cancer patients, the findings reveal that human tumour-associated T_H17 cells express minimal levels of human leukocyte antigen (HLA)-DR, CD25 and granzyme B, suggesting that they are not a 'conventional' effector cell population (Wilke *et al.,* 2011). On examining the associated mechanisms and clinical significance of T_H17 cells in 201 ovarian cancer patients, it was found that T_H17 exhibited a polyfunctional effector T-cell phenotype, were positively associated with effector cells, and were negatively associated with tumour-infiltrating Treg cells (Kryczek *et al.,* 2009a). The study authors further reveal that for homing molecules, tumour-associated T_H17 highly express chemokine receptors CXCR4 and CCR6, c-type lectin receptor CD161 and the CD49 integrin isoforms c, d and e, while CCR2, CCR5 and CCR7 are not present on these cells (Figure 3).

Several biological activities of T_H17 cells are directly or indirectly linked to human tumour pathogenesis. Tumour-associated T_H17 cells have the ability to influence the tumour immune response through the action of their cytokines products in cancer patients which reportedly include high levels of pro inflammatory granulocyte-macrophage colony stimulating factor (GM-CSF), TNF-α, IL-2 and IFNγ, but negligible levels of anti-inflammatory IL-10 . This phenotype was observed in six types of human cancers which include ovarian, colon, liver, skin, pancreatic and renal (Kryczek *et al.,* 2009a). 50% of T_H17 cells, in patients with hepatocellular carcinoma (HCC) produced IFNγ-IFNγ, a typical T_H1-type cytokine (Zhang *et al.,* 2009, Kryczek *et al.,* 2009, Wilke *et al.,* 2011). Further, on *in vitro* expansion, the T_H17cells from tumour-infiltrating lymphocyte populations in melanoma, breast and colon cancers secrete elevated amounts of IL-8 and TNF-α, but no IL-2 (Su *et al.,* 2010). Since this profile has been seen previously in T_H17 cells isolated from healthy donors (Liu and Rohowsky-Kochan 2008) and patients with autoimmune diseases (Kryczek *et al.,* 2008b), it may indicate a possible difference in the phenotypes of freshly isolated T_H17cells and those expanded or induced *in vitro* from tumour-associated populations (Figure 3). Earlier information reviewed from both experimental animal systems and human cancer patients suggested that IL-17 and IL-23 are generally favourable to the growth of tumours thus overshadowing their roles in the generation of T-cell anti-tumour immunity (Tesmer *et al.,* 2008).

Still the role of IL-17 producing T_H17 cells in cancer is elusive as different immunopathological implications of these cells have been observed in different malignancies. Analysis of tumour-derived naive and memory $CD4^+$ T cells revealed that IL-17 producing T cells are in memory phase as they are positive for CD45RO, but negative for CD45RA, CD62L, and CCR7 (Miyahara *et al.,* 2008). These authors also indicated that tumour cells may secrete key cytokines required for the expansion of T_H17 cells. Further Su *et al.*, 2010 demonstrated elevated CD4+ T_H17 cell populations in the tumour-infiltrating lymphocytes (TILs) and suggested development of tumour-infiltrating T_H17 cells may be a general feature in cancer patients, when they extended their studies from ovarian cancers to melanoma, breast and colon cancers. Their study further demonstrated that tumour cells and tumour-derived fibroblasts, mediate the recruitment of T_H17 cells by secreting chemokines RANTES (regulated upon activation, normal T cell expressed and secreted) and MCP-1 in the tumour microenvironment. The tumour microenvironments produce a pro-inflammatory cytokine milieu and provide cell–cell contact engagement that facilitates the generation and expansion of T_H17 cells. They also showed that inflammatory TLR and nucleotide oligomerization binding domain (Nod2) 2 signalling promote the attraction and generation of T_H17 cells and that this was induced by tumour cells and tumour-derived fibroblasts.

6. Dynamic interaction between T_{reg} and T_H17 cells

Levels of both T_{reg} and T_H17 cells increase synchronically following tumour development and are inversely associated. TGF-β promotes T_{reg} development and both TGF-β plus IL-6 are required for T_H17 differentiation (Veldhoen M *et al.*, 2006, Mangan *et al.*, 2006, Betteli *et al.*, 2006). Although, both the cytokines needed for T_H17 cell development have been seen to be present in high levels in tumours (Zhou 2005), yet the levels of T_{reg} cells and other T subsets are more than T_H17 cells in both mouse and human tumours (Kryczek *et al.*, 2007). So there must be something that prevents differentiation of T_H17 cells. An interesting study by Kryczek and colleagues in 2009 from ovarian cancer patients, raised concerns on the roles of IL-6 an TGF-β, where it has been reported that inhibition of IL-1β, but not IL-6 or TGF-β, decreased T_H17 cell induction by myeloid APCs isolated from patients, and the levels of IL-17 and numbers of T_H17 cells did not correlate with the levels of IL-6 and TGF-β in these patients' samples. These observations hinted a crucial role of only IL-1β, but not of IL-6 or TGF-β, for T_H17 cell development in the ovarian cancer microenvironment. Similar support for a crucial role of IL-1β in promoting T_H17 cell development has been reported in mouse studies (Chung *et al.*, 2009, Gullen *et al.*, 2010).

According to few studies, IL-10 released by T_{reg} cells negatively regulates differentiation of T_H17 cells and IL-2, a growth factor for most T cells promote FoxP3 expression in T_H17 cells and inhibit cellular differentiation to T_H17 cells (Wilson *et al.*, 2007). Retinoic acid has been found to enhance TGF-β signalling and decrease IL-6 signalling, thus, it might also be affecting the balance between T_H17 and T_{reg} cells. Apart from this, it has also been seen that mouse peripheral mature T_{reg} can be converted to T_H17 cells favoured by inflammation and IL-6 ('plasticity') (Yang *et al.*, 2008a). The role of TGF-β in the differentiation of both induced T_{reg} cells as well as T_H17 cells, along with the documented interactions between RORα and FoxP3 that influence the two subsets, suggest a system that balances inflammation with tolerance (Figure 3).

7. Evidences for the negative and positive roles of T_H17 in anti-tumour Immunity

Though reports have addressed the presence of T_H17 cells in experimental and human tumours but they lack regarding the clear indication about either a pro-tumoural or antitumoural activity of these cells (Bronte 2008).There are various biological functions of T_H17 cells and their effector molecules as mentioned earlier in the chapter that could be on the basis of experimental and clinical data, suggest T_H17 cells might either be positively or negatively co-related with cancer.

Negative role of T_H17 cells in anti-cancer

IL-17 produced by T_H17 cells is an angiogenic factor (Numasaki *et al.*, 2003) which stimulates the migration and cord formation of vascular endothelial cells *in vitro* and elicits vessel formation *in vivo* which in turn promotes tumour growth and metastasis through *de novo* carcinogenesis and neovascularisation via STAT3 signalling. Another cytokine, IL-23 required for T_H17 activity has been identified as a cancer-associated cytokine because it promotes tumour incidence and growth (Langowski *et al.*, 2006). It has been seen that T_H17 cells produce negligible levels of HLA- DR, CD 25, granzyme B, PD1 and FoxP3, all of which are involved in effector functions suggesting that they do not contribute to immune suppression in the tumour environment. Thus, as T_H17 cells produce pro-inflammatory cytokines and have been found to accumulate in tumour microenvironment and as inflammation is linked to cancer development and progression, it is reasonable to predict a positive relation between these cells and cancer progression. Also, the data from experiments on ovarian cancer suggest that T_H17 cells through TNF-α are involved in the development or progression of cancer in mice and humans(Charles *et al.*, 2009).

Further T_H17 cells might increase their own frequency in the tumour by both direct and indirect mechanisms (Zou and Restifo 2010). The induction of T_H17 cells in the human tumour microenvironment through IL-1β production by the myeloid APCs may in turn promote dendritic cell trafficking into tumour-draining lymph nodes and the tumour environment by producing CCL20 (Kryczek *et al.*, 2009a). Further as CCR6+ T_H17 cells are known to efficiently migrate towards CCL20 (Kryczek *et al.*, 2008b, Kryczek *et al.*, 2009a), and CCL20 can then lead to the recruitment of dendritic cells to the tumour-draining lymph nodes and tumour itself in a CCR6-dependent manner (Martin-Orozco *et al.*, 2009). Compared with corresponding non-tumour regions, the levels of T_H17 cells were found to be significantly increased in tumours of HCC patients. Most of these intratumoural T_H17 cells exhibited an effector memory phenotype with increased expression of CCR4 and CCR6. Furthermore, the intratumoural cell density of T_H17 correlated with poor survival in HCC patients (Zhang *et al.*, 2009). A study from Kuang and colleagues in 2010, has demonstrated predominantly enriched levels of IL-17 producing cells in peritumoural stroma of murine HCC tissues, where their levels correlated with monocyte/macrophage density. The level of murine hepatoma-infiltrating CD4+ IL- 17+ cells as well as the tumour growth was reduced significantly when monocyte/macrophage inflammation in liver was inhibited via treatment with a Kupffer cell toxicant (gadolinium chloride).

Similar to humans, healthy mice has limited populations of T_H17 cells but these cells expanded in the blood, bone marrow and spleens but not in the tumour draining lymph nodes and largest populations were seen in tumour itself of mice with the aggressive B16 melanoma, fibrosarcoma and advanced head and neck cancers, The number of CD4+IL-17+ T cells gradually increased in the tumour microenvironment during tumour development but interestingly, the number of these cells remained limited during tumour development in the tumour draining lymph nodes, including advanced tumour stages. (Kryczek *et al.*, 2007).On the other hand in nasopharyngeal carcinoma, data from human samples demonstrated no correlation of T_H17 cells with patient clinicopathological characteristics or survival outcomes (Zhang *et al.,* 2010). Studies with patient samples from lung adenocarcinoma or squamous cell carcinoma revealed that malignant pleural effusion from these patients was chemotactic for T_H17 cells, and this activity was partially abrogated by CCL20 and/or CCL22 blockade (Ye *et al.,* 2010). Interestingly, higher infiltration of T_H17 cells in malignant pleural effusion predicted improved patient survival.

Positive role of T_H17 cells in anti-tumour immunity

Both human and mouse tumours study data suggest several lines of evidence about the protective role of T_H17 cells with the induction of protective anti-tumour immune response.T_H17 cells have been seen to positively co-relate with effector immune cells like $IFN\gamma^+$ effector T cells, cytotoxic $CD8^+$ T cells and natural killer (NK) cells in the tumour microenvironment which might be to produce an anti- tumour response against cancer cells to kill them by promoting cell mediated cytotoxicity (Kryczek *et al.,* 2009a). Various experimental studies have shown that IL-17 overexpression or exogenous T_H17 cell induction lead to decreased tumour growth, for example; Muranski and colleagues in 2008, through a first functional study showed that T_H17-polarized CD4+ T cells (following treatment with TGF-β and IL-6), induced potent tumour eradication of large established melanoma in mice. The study provides a support for a clinical trial involving the adoptive transfer of T_H17-polarized, tumour-specific CD4+ T cells to patients with cancer. A year later, another interesting functional study, revealed for the first time that T_H17-polarized CD8+ T cells induce potent tumour eradication in mice, and provided again support for a clinical trial involving the adoptive transfer of T_H17-polarized, tumour-specific CD8+ T cells to cancer patients (Hinrichs *et al.,* 2009). Once *in vivo,* T_H17-polarized CD8+ T cells might be converted to an IFNγ-producing phenotype, induced tumour regression and persisted in the host longer than non-polarized cells. tumourIL-17 deficient mice (IL-17A knockout (IL-17A -/-) have accelerated tumour growth and more lung metastasis than wild-type mice (Kryczek *et al.,* 2009b, Martin-Orozco *et al.,* 2009, Wei *et al.,* 2010). Transgenic expression of human or murine IL-17 in tumour cells suppresses or slows tumour growth and increases tumour-specific cytotoxic responses (Hirahara *et al.,* 2001, Benchetrit *et al.,* 2002). However, contrasting results were shown by Wang *et al.,* 2009 who have reported that transferred tumours of B16 and bladder carcinoma MC49 grew more slowly in IL-17-/- mice.

In prostate cancer patients, a significant inverse correlation was seen between T_H17 cell differentiation and tumour progression (Sfanos *et al.,* 2008). In addition to these evidences, it is known that IL-17 released by T_H17 cells promote dendritic cell maturation which might allow for better tumour antigen presentation and thereby leading to a stronger T cell response. Furthermore, direct mechanistic and functional evidence that T_H17 cells mediate antitumour immunity by promoting dendritic cell trafficking to tumour-draining lymph nodes, and to the tumour itself has also been provided (Martin-Orozco *et al.,* 2009). tumourtumourMore recently, CTLA4 (cytotoxic T lymphocyte antigen 4) blockade was shown to increase T_H17 cells in patients with metastatic melanoma and IL-17 levels in tumour-associated ascites positively predicted patient survival (von Euw *et al., 2009).* To summarize the above data, there is strong evidence that T_H17 cells can have protective roles in tumour immunity but the exact nature of T_H17 cells in anti-tumour immunity remains to be explored.

8. Conclusions

Rapid and large advances in understanding the development, regulation and function of these cells have been made since T_H17 cells are originally identified as a third lineage of effector T helper cells in 2005. The study of T_H17 cells has been one of the fast-moving and exciting subject areas in immunology. This has been particularly true in the context of a diverse group of immune-mediated chronic inflammatory diseases and autoimmunity, where the pathogenic role of T_H17 cells has been well documented. With regards to cancer, T_H17 cells are found to be present in the tumour microenvironment though not as a predominant T cell subset within the tumour. Based on the evidence provided by both human and clinical studies data, T_H17 cells and T_H17-associated cytokines/effector molecules have been shown to have both pro-tumorigenic and anti-tumorigenic functions. On one hand it seems that the pro-inflammatory T_H17 cells might engineer the microenvironment around tumours, and contribute to the proliferation, migration and survival of cancer cells. On the other hand, it is possible that inflammatory cells and molecules play roles to initiate and maintain protective anti-tumour immunity as seen in the case of infectious diseases (Punj *et al.*, 2003). The IL-17 dependent pro-tumorigenic or anti-tumorigenic activity might be due to inherent technical limitations for example source and dose of exogenous versus endogenous IL-17, in each of the studies (Zou and Restifo 2010). Further, based on the results from recent murine model studies, employing T_H17-polarized T cells for cancer therapy may appear to be to be a promising approach for translational research. It is also important to study futher the specific nature of inflammatory response and the tissue context, so that the positive or negative effects of T_H17 cells on tumour immunopathology can be determined. Equally important to understand is i) how the effector functions of $T_H17$cells are regulated?, ii) how do the regulators of T_H17-cell differentiation work? iii), do T_H17 play same role in different types and stages of cancer?, and iv) how T_{reg} cells can be suppressed in chronic inflammatory or large tumour burdens to increase the T_H17 cells and later activation and proliferation of cytotoxic T cells to clear tumour cells? The answers will, help in designing future novel therapeutic vaccine approaches; specifically targeting inflammatory T_H17 cells for cancer therapy.

9. Abbreviations

CD	Cluster of Differentiation
IL	Interleukin
IFN	Interferon
TNF	Tumour Necrosis Factor
TGF	Tumour Growth Factor
MMP	Matrix Metalloproteinase
APC	Antigen Presenting Cells
FoxP3	Forkhead Box P3
MAPK	Mitogen-Activated Protein Kinases
TRAF6	Tumour Necrosis Factor Receptor-Associated Factor-6
TLR	Toll-like Receptors

10. References

[1] Aggarwal S, Ghilardi N, Xie MH, de Sauvage FJ, Gurney AL (2003). Interleukin-23 promotes a distinct CD4 T cell activation state characterized by the production of interleukin-17. J. Biol. Chem. 278:1910–1914.

[2] Barreiro O, Martín P, González-Amaro R, Sánchez-Madrid F (2010). Molecular cues guiding inflammatory responses. Cardiovasc Res 86:174-182.

[3] Batten M, Li J, Yi S, Kljavin NM, Danilenko DM, Lucas S et al. (2006). Interleukin 27 limits autoimmune encephalomyelitis by suppressing the development of interleukin 17-producing T cells. Nat Immunol 7: 929–936.

[4] Benchetrit F, Ciree A, Vives V, Warnier G, Gey A, Sautes-Fridman C et al. (2002). Interleukin-17 inhibits tumor cell growth by means of a T-cell-dependent mechanism. Blood 99: 2114–2121.

[5] Bettelli E, Carrier Y, Gao W, Korn T, Strom TB, Oukka M et al. (2006). Reciprocal developmental pathways for the generation of pathogenic effector T_H17 and regulatory T cells. Nature 441:235–238.

[6] Brigati C, Noonan DM, Albini A, Benelli R. (2002). Tumors and inflammatory infiltrates: friends or foes? Clin Exp Metastasis 19:247–258.

[7] Bronte V. Th17 and cancer: friends or foes?. Blood 112: 214.

[8] Brüstle A, Heink S, Huber M, Rosenplänter C, Stadelmann C, Yu P, et al. (2007). The development of inflammatory T(H)-17 cells requires interferon-regulatory factor. Nat Immunol 8:958–966.

[9] Charles KA, Kulbe H, Soper R, Escorcio-Correia M, Lawrence T, Schultheis A et al. (2009). The tumor-promoting actions of TNF-alpha involve TNFR1 and IL-17 in ovarian cancer in mice and humans. J Clin Invest 119: 3011–3023.

[10] Chechlinska M, Kowalewska M, Nowak, R. (2010). Systemic inflammation as a confounding factor in cancer biomarker discovery and validation. Nat Rev Cancer 10: 2-3

[11] Chung Y, Chang SH, Martinez GJ, Yang XO, Nurieva R, Kang HS et al. (2009). Critical regulation of early Th17 cells differentiation by interleukin-1 signaling. Immunity 30(4):576-587.

[12] Coffelt SB, Hughes R, Lewis CE. (2009). Tumor-associated macrophages: Effectors of angiogenesis and tumor progression. Biochim et Biophys Acta 1796:11–18.

[13] Crome SQ, Wang AY, Levings MK. (2010a). Translational mini-review series on Th17 cells: function and regulation of human T helper 17 cells in health and disease. Clin Exp Immunol 159: 109–119.

[14] Crome S Q, Clive B, Wang AY, Kang CY, Chow V, Yu J et al. (2010b). Inflammatory effects of *ex vivo* human Th17 cells are suppressed by regulatory T cells. J Immunol 185:3199-3208.

[15] Cosmi L, Liotta F, Maggi E, Romagnani S, Annunziato F. (2011). Th17 cells: new players in asthma pathogenesis. Allergy 66:989-998.

[16] Coussens LM and Werb Z. (2002). Inflammation and cancer. Nature 420(6917):860-867.

[17] Dong C. (2008). T_H17 cells in development: An updated view of their molecular identity and genetic programming. Nat Rev Immunol 8:337-348.

[18] Gran B, Zhang GX, Yu S, Li J, Chen XH, Ventura ES et al. (2002). IL-12p35-deficient mice are susceptible to experimental autoimmune encephalomyelitis: evidence for redundancy in the IL-12 system in the induction of central nervous system autoimmune demyelination. J Immunol. 169:7104–7110.

[19] Gulen MF, Kang Z, Bulek K, Youzhong W, Kim TW, Chen Y, et al. (2010). The receptor SIGIRR suppresses Th17 cell proliferation via inhibition of the interleukin-1 receptor pathway and mTOR kinase activation. Immunity 32, 54–66.

[20] Harrington LE, Hatton RD, Mangan PR, Turner H, Murphy TL, Murphy KM, Weaver CT. (2005). Interleukin 17-producing CD4+ effector T cells develop via a lineage distinct from the T-helper type 1 and 2 lineages. Nat Immunol 6:1123-1132.

[21] Hinrichs CS, Kaiser A, Paulos CM, Cassard L, Sanchez-Perez L, Heemskerk B, Wrzesinski C, Borman ZA, Muranski P, Restifo NP. (2009). Type 17 CD8+ T cells display enhanced anti-tumour immunity. Blood 114: 596–599.

[22] Hirahara N, Nio Y, Sasaki S, Minari Y, Takamura M, Iguchi C, Dong M, Yamasawa K, Tamura K.. (2001). Inoculation of human interleukin-17 gene transfected Meth-A fibrosarcoma cells induces T cell-dependent tumor specific immunity in mice. Oncology 61: 79–89.

[23] Hirota K, Yoshitomi H, Hashimoto M, Maeda S, Teradaira S, Sugimoto N, et al. (2007) Preferential recruitment of CCR6-expressing Th17 cells to inflamed joints via CCL20 in rheumatoid arthritis and its animal model. J Exp Med 204:2803–2812.

[24] Infante-Duarte C, Horton HF, Byrne MC, Kamradt T (2000). Microbial lipopeptides induce the production of IL-17 in Th cells. J. Immunol. 165:6107–6115.

[25] Ivanov II, McKenzie BS, Zhou L, Tadokoro CE, Lepelley A, Lafaille JJ, et al.(2006). The orphan nuclear receptor RORγt directs the differentiation program of proinflammatory IL-17+ T helper cells. Cell 126:1121–1133.

[26] Kanwar JR. (2005). Anti-inflammatory immunotherapy for multiple sclerosis/experimental autoimmune encephalomyelitis (EAE) disease. Curr Med Chem. 12(25):2947-2962.

[27] Kanwar JR, Berg RW, Lehnert K, Krissansen GW. (1999). Taking lessons from dendritic cells: multiple xenogeneic ligands for leukocyte integrins have the potential to stimulate anti-tumor immunity. Gene Ther 6:1835–1844.

[28] Kanwar JR, Berg RW, Yang Y, Kanwar RK, Ching LM, Sun X, Krissansen GW. (2003). Requirements for ICAM-1 immunogene therapy of lymphoma. Cancer Gene Ther 10 :468-476.

[29] Kanwar RK, Kanwar JR, Wang D, Ormrod D and Krissansen GW (2001a).Temporal expression of heat shock proteins 60 and 70 at lesion prone sites during atherogenesis in the apolipoprotein E-deficient mouse. Arterioscler Thromb and Vas Biol 21: 1991-1997.

[30] Kanwar JR, Kanwar RK, Burrow H, Baratchi S. (2009). Recent advances on the roles of NO in cancer and chronic inflammatory disorders. Curr Med Chem 16(19):2373-2394.

[31] Kanwar RK, Macgibbon AK, Black PN, Kanwar JR, Rowan A, Vale M et al. (2008). Bovine milk fat enriched in conjugated linoleic and vaccenic acids attenuates allergic airway disease in mice. Clin Exp Allergy 38: 208-218.

[32] Kanwar JR, Palmano KP, Sun X, Kanwar RK, Gupta R, Haggarty N et al. (2008). 'Iron-saturated' lactoferrin is a potent natural adjuvant for augmenting cancer chemotherapy. Immunol Cell Biol 86: 277-288.

[33] Kanwar JR, Shen WP, Kanwar RK, Berg RW, Krissansen GW. (2001b). Effects of survivin antagonists on growth of established tumors and B7-1 immunogene therapy. J Natl Cancer Inst 93:1541-1552.

[34] Kanwar RK, Singh N, Gurudevan S, Kanwar JR (2011). Targeting Hepatitis B Virus and Human Papillomavirus Induced Human Viral Carcinogenesis: Novel Patented Therapeutics. Recent Patents on Anti-Infective Drug Discovery, May 6(2):158-74.

[35] Kimura A and Kishimoto T (2011). Th17 cells in inflammation. Internat Immunopharmacol 11:319-322.

[36] Kimura A, Naka T, Kishimoto T (2007). IL-6-dependent and -independent pathways in the development of interleukin 17-producing T helper cells. Proc Natl Acad Sci USA 104:12099–12104.

[37] Korn T, Bettelli E, Gao W, Awasthi A, Jager A, Strom TB, et al. (2007). IL-21 initiates an alternative pathway to induce proinflammatory TH17 cells. Nature 448:484-487.

[38] Kryczek I, Wei S, Zou L, Altuwaijri S, Szeliga W, Kolls J, Chang A et al. (2007). Cutting Edge: T_H17 and regulatory T cell dynamics and the regulation by IL-2 in the tumor microenvironment. J Immunol 178: 6730-6733.

[39] Kryczek, I. Wei S, Gong W, Shu X, Szeliga W, Vatan L, Chen L, Wang G, and Zou W (2008a) Cutting edge: IFN-gamma enables APC to promote memory Th17 and abate Th1 cell development. J. Immunol., 181,5842–5846.

[40] Kryczek I Banerjee M, Cheng, P, Vatan L, Szeliga W, Wei S et al. (2009). Phenotype, distribution, generation, and functional and clinical relevance of Th17 cells in the human tumour environments. Blood 114: 1141–1149.

[41] Kryczek I. Bruce AT, Gudjonsson JE, Johnston A, Aphale A, Vatan L, Szeliga W, Wang Y, Liu Y, Welling TH, Elder JT, Zou W. (2008b) Induction of IL-17+ T cell trafficking and development by IFN-gamma: mechanism and pathological relevance in psoriasis. J. Immunol 181:4733–4741.

[42] Kryczek I. Wei S, Szeliga W. Vatan L. Zou W. (2009b). Endogenous IL-17 contributes to reduced tumor growth and metastasis. Blood 114: 357–359.

[43] Kuang DM, Kuang DM, Peng C, Zhao Q, Wu Y, Chen MS, Zheng L(2010) Activated monocytes in peritumoral stroma of hepatocellular carcinoma promote expansion of memory T helper 17 cells..Hepatology, 51:154–164.

[44] Kuper H, Adami HO, Trichopoulos D. (2000). Infections as a major preventable cause of human cancer. J Intern Med 248:171–183.

[45] Langowski JL, Zhang X, Wu L, *et al.* (2006). IL-23 promotes tumour incidence and growth. Nature 442: 461 - 465.

[46] Liang SC, Long AJ, Bennett F, Whitters MJ, Karim R, Collins M et al. (2007). An IL-17F/A heterodimer protein is produced by mouse Th17 cells and induces airway neutrophil recruitment. J Immunol 179:7791–7799.

[47] Liang SC, Tan XY, Luxenberg DP, Karim R, Dunussi-Joannopoulos K, Collins M et al. (2006). Interleukin (IL)-22 and IL-17 are coexpressed by Th17 cells and cooperatively enhance expression of antimicrobial peptides. J Exp Med 203:2271–2279.

[48] Liu H, Rohowsky-Kochan C. (2008) Regulation of IL-17 in human CCR6+ effector memory T cells. J. Immunol 180: 7948–7957.

[49] Mangan PR, Harrington LE, O'Quinn DB, Helms WS, Bullard DC, Elson CO et al. (2006). Transforming growth factor-beta induces development of the T(H)17 lineage. Nature 441:231–234.

[50] Mantovani, A. (2009). Inflaming metastasis. Nature 457:36–37.

[51] Mantovani A, Allavena P, Sica, A, Balkwill F. (2008). Cancer-related inflammation. Nature 454:436-444.

[52] Martinez GJ, Zhang Z, Reynolds JM, Tanaka S, Chung Y, Liu T et al. (2010). Smad2 positively regulates the generation of th17 cells. J Biol Chem. 285(38): 29039-29043.

[53] Martin-Orozco N, Muranski P, Chung Y, Yang XO, Yamazaki T, Lu S, Hwu P, Restifo NP, Overwijk WW, Dong C. (2009). T helper 17 cells promote cytotoxic T cell activation in tumour immunity. Immunity 31, 787–798.

[54] Miyahara Y, Odunsi K, Chen W, Peng G, Matsuzaki J, Wang. (2008). Generation and regulation of human CD4+ IL-17-producing T-cells in ovarian cancer. Proc Natl Acad Sci USA 105(40):15505-15510.

[55] Mosmann TR, Cherwinski H, Bond MW, Giedlin MA, Coffman RL. (1986). Two types of murine helper T cell clone. I. Definition according to profiles of lymphokine activities and secreted proteins. J Immunol 136:2348–2257.

[56] Muranski P, Boni A, Antony PA, Cassard L, Irvine KR, Kaiser A, Paulos CM, Palmer DC, Touloukian CE, Ptak K, Gattinoni L, Wrzesinski C, Hinrichs CS, Kerstann KW, Feigenbaum L, Chan CC, Restifo NP. (2008) Tumor specific Th17-polarized cells eradicate large established melanoma. Blood 112: 362 –373.

[57] Numasaki M, Fukushi J, Ono M, Narula SK, Zavodny PJ, Kudo T et al. (2003). Interleukin-17 promotes angiogenesis and tumor growth. Blood 101: 2620–2627.

[58] Park H, Li Z, Yang XO, Chang SH, Nurieva R, Wang YH, et al. (2005). A distinct lineage of CD4 T cells regulates tissue inflammation by producing interleukin 17. Nat Immunol 6(11):1133-1141.

[59] Punj V, Saint-Dic D, Daghfal S, Kanwar JR. (2004). Microbial-based therapy of cancer: a new twist to age old practice. Cancer Biol Ther 3-:708-714.

[60] Rangachari M, Mauermann N, Marty RR, Dirnhofer S, Kurrer MO, Komnenovic V et al. (2006). T-bet negatively regulates autoimmune myocarditis by suppressing local production of interleukin 17. J Exp Med 203:2009–2019.

[61] Rigo, A., Gottardi, M., Zamo, A., Mauri, P., Bonifacio, M, Kramper M et al. (2010). Macrophages may promote cancer growth via a GM-CSF/HB-EGF paracrine loop that is enhanced by CXCL12. Mol Cancer 9: 273.

[62] Romagnani S (2000). T-cell subsets (Th1 versus Th2). Ann Allerg, Asthma Immunol 85: 9-18.

[63] Sallusto F, Lanzavecchia A. (2009). Human Th17 cells in infection and autoimmunity. Microb Infect / Institut Pasteur 11: 620-624.

[64] Schraml BU, Hildner K, Ise W, Lee WL, Smith WA, Solomon B (2009). The AP-1 transcription factor Batf controls T(H)17 differentiation. Nature 460:405–409.

[65] Sfanos KS, Bruno TC, Maris CH, Xu L, Thoburn CJ, DeMarzo AM et al. (2008). Phenotypic analysis of prostate-infiltrating lymphocytes reveals TH17 and Treg skewing. Clin Cancer Res 14:3254-3261.

[66] Stumhofer JS, Laurence A, Wilson EH, Huang E, Tato CM, Johnson LM et al. (2006). Interleukin 27 negatively regulates the development of interleukin 17-producing T helper cells during chronic inflammation of the central nervous system. Nat Immunol 7:937–945.

[67] Su X, Ye J, Hsueh EC, Zhang Y, Hoft DF, Peng G. (2010). Tumor microenvironments direct the recruitment and expansion of human Th17 cells. J Immunol 184: 1630-1641.

[68] Torrado E and Cooper AM. (2010). IL-17 and Th17 cells in tuberculosis. Cytokine Growth Factor Rev 21:455-62.

[69] Torchinsky MB and Blander JM. (2010). T helper 17 cells: discovery, function, andphysiological trigger. Cell. Mol. Life Sci 67:1407–1421.

[70] Torchinsky MB, Garaude J, Martin AP, Blander JM (2009). Innate immune recognition of infected apoptotic cells directs T(H)17 cell differentiation. Nature 458:78–82.

[71] Tsung K, Dolan JP, Tsung YL, Norton JA. (2002). Macrophages as effector cells in interleukin 12-induced T cell-dependent tumor rejection. Cancer Res 62:5069–5075.

[72] Veldhoen M, Hocking RJ, Atkins CJ, Locksley RM, Stockinger B. (2006). TGF beta in the context of an inflammatory cytokine milieu supports de novo differentiation of IL- 17 producing T cells. Immunity 24: 179-89.

[73] Euw, E. et al. (2009). CTLA4 blockade increases Th17 cells in patients with metastatic melanoma. J. Transl. Med. 7: 35.

[74] Wahl LM, Kleinman HK. (1998). Tumor-associated macrophages as targets for cancer therapy. J Natl Cancer Inst 90: 1583–1584.

[75] Wang L, Yi T, Kortylewski M, Pardoll DM, Zeng D, Yu H. (2009). IL-17 can promote tumor growth through an IL-6- Stat3 signaling pathway. J Exp Med 206:1457–1464.

[76] Weaver CT, Hatton RD, Mangan PR, Harrington LE. (2007). IL-17 family cytokines and the expanding diversity of effector T cell lineages. Annu Rev Immunol 25:821-852.

[77] Weaver CT, Murphy KM. (2007). T-cell subsets: the more the merrier. Curr Biol 17:61-63.

[78] Wei L, Laurence A, Elias KM, O'Shea JJ (2007). IL-21 is produced by Th17 cells and drives IL-17 production in a STAT3- dependent manner. J Biol Chem 282:34605-34610.

[79] Wei S. Kryczek I, Namm J, Szeliga W, Vatan L, Chang A. et al. (2010) Endogenous IL-17, tumor growth, and metastasis. Blood 115: 2256–2257.

[80] Wilke CM, Kryczek I, Wei S, Zhao E, Wu K, Wang G, Zou W. (2011). Th17 cells in cancer: help or hindrance? Carcinogenesis 32: 643-649.

[81] Wilson NJ, Boniface K, Chan JR, McKenzie BS, Blumenschein WM, Mattson JD et al. (2007). Development, cytokine profile and function of human interleukin 17-producing helper T cells. Nat Immunol 8:950–957.

[82] Yang XO, Nurieva R, Martinez GJ Kang HS, Chung Y, Pappu BP. et al. (2008a). Molecular antagonism and plasticity of regulatory and inflammatory T cell programs. Immunity 29:44–56.

[83] Yang XO, Pappu BP, Nurieva R, Akimzhanov A, Kang HS, Chung Y et al. (2008b). T helper 17 lineage differentiation is programmed by orphan nuclear receptors RORα and ROR γ. Immunity 28:29–39.

[84] Yang XO, Chang SH, Park H, Nurieva R, Shah B, Acero L, et al. (2008c). Regulation of inflammatory responses by IL-17F. J Exp Med 205: 1063–1075.

[85] Ye ZJ, Zhou Q, Gu YY, Qin SM, Ma WL, Xin JB, Tao XN, Shi HZ. (2010) Generation and differentiation of interleukin-17-producing CD4+ T cells in malignant pleural effusion. J. Immunol, 185: 6348–6354.

[86] Zou, W (2005). Immunosuppressive networks in the tumour environment and their therapeutic relevance. Nature Rev. Cancer 5:263–274.

[87] Zou W, Restifo NP. (2010). T_H17 cells in tumor immunity and immunotherapy; Nat Rev Immunol 10: 246-256.

[88] Zhang JP Yan J, Xu J, Pang XH, Chen MS, et al. (2009) Increased intratumoral IL-17-producing cells correlate with poor survival in hepatocellular carcinoma patients. J. Hepatol 50:980–989.

[89] Zhang YL. Li J, Mo HY, Qiu F, Zheng LM, Qian CN. et al. (2010) Different subsets of tumor infiltrating lymphocytes correlate with NPC progression in different ways. Mol. Cancer 9: 4.

4

Is Chronic Lymphocytic Leukemia a Mistake of Tolerance Mechanisms?

Ricardo García-Muñoz[1], Judit Anton-Remirez[2], Jesus Feliu[3], María Pilar Rabasa[1], Carlos Panizo[4] and Luis Llorente[5]
[1]Hematology Service, Hospital San Pedro, Logroño, La Rioja,
[2]Rehabilitation Service, Complejo Hospitalario de Navarra, Pamplona, Navarra,
[3]Hematology Service, Complejo Hospitalario de Navarra, Pamplona, Navarra,
[4]Hematology Service, Clínica Universidad de Navarra, Pamplona, Navarra,
[5]Department of Immunology and Rheumatology, Instituto Nacional de Ciencias Médicas y Nutrición Salvador Zubirán, Mexico City
[1,2,3,4]Spain
[5]México

1. Introduction

Chronic Lymphocytic Leukemia (CLL) is a chronic lymphoproliferative disorder of the B lymphocytes. Small lymphocytic lymphoma (SLL) is considered to be the same disease in a non-leukemic form. CLL remains as an incurable tumour and clinical features have very variable presentation, course, and outcome. The progressive accumulation of monoclonal B lymphocytes leads to leukocytosis, lymphadenopathy, hepatosplenomegaly and marrow failure, and is sometimes associated with autoimmune manifestations.

It has been suggested that CLL cells are defective in apoptosis, which leads to the accumulation of malignant B cells. Furthermore, patients with proliferation rates greater than 0.35% per day have been found to have a more aggressive disease[18,19]. Proliferation of CLL cells is most prominent in proliferative centers that include specific areas in lymph nodes and bone marow[20,21]. Numerous CD4 T cells and dendritic cells are in close contact with CLL B cells [22], and micro environmental interactions like BM stromal cells are able to extend the survival of CLL upon direct contact[21]. Thus, the CLL population may originate from a clone with few or no V- domain mutations, or from a more mature clone whose V-domains have undergone the hypermutation process. This creates two separate pools of B cells, both of which originate from antigen-stimulated B lymphocytes. Additionally, IGHV unmutated CLL B cells expressing polyreactive antibodies whereas most IGHV mutated CLL´s did not. However, reversion of the IGHV mutated sequences to germline counterparts restored the polyreactivity (Herve et al 2005). Despite these features, the biological etiology of the divergent natural histories of IgVH unmutated vs mutated CLL and the origin of this type of leukemia/lymphoma remains unknown. For this reason we review the immunologic aspects that can help to understand this complex disease based in the findings that suggest that both unmutated and mutated subgroups of patients originally derive from autoreactive clones.

2. Diagnosis

The diagnosis of CLL requires the presence of at least 5000 B lymphocytes/μL in the peripheral blood (Hallek, et al 2008). CLL/SLL can be identified by the immunophenotype CD5+, CD10–, CD19+, CD20+, dim expression of surface immunoglobulin, CD23+, CD43 +/–, and cyclin D1– (Matutes, et al 2007). The absence of cyclin D1 is critical in distinguishing CLL/SLL from MCL. Bone marrow involvement is characteristically more than 30% of the nucleated cells in the aspirate are lymphoid.

Prognostic Markers and Genomic Aberrations

A favorable prognosis in CLL/SLL is associated with the presence of a mutated immunoglobulin heavy chain variable region, and low CD38 and zeta-chain–associated protein kinase 70 protein expression(Damle et al 1999;Kröber et al 2002;Hamblin et al 1999; Tobbin et al 2002; Crespo et al 2003). Chromosomal aberrations in CLL include del 6q, del 11q, del 13q, trisomy 12, and del 17p (Döhner et al 2000). Importantly, specific genomic aberrations have been associated with disease characteristics such better survival for patients with 12q trisomy and 13q deletion, poor survival and massive lymphadenopathy in 11q deletion and resistance to therapy in the group of patients with 17p deletion and p53 abnormalities (Döhrner et al 2000; Döhrner et al 1995; Döhrner et al 1997;Krober et al 2006). In addition, two miRNA (miR-15a and miR-16-1) were recently identified to be located in the critical region of the 13q14 deletion and their absence in CLL appears to be a major factor in preventing apoptosis and progression through the cell cycle (Aqeilan et al 2010; Cimmino et al 2005; Callin et al 2004; Mertens et al 2006).

Pathophysiology and cell of origin/normal counterpart of CLL

Different from other types of malignancies derived from mature B cells, the pathogenesis of B-CLL/SLL is much less understood. Notwithstanding extensive searching it is not known whether there is an equivalent normal cell in which the CLL arise. However, several cell types have been suggested as giving rise to chronic lymphocytic leukemia included memory, transitional, B1 and marginal zone B cells (Chiorazzi and Ferrarini 2011; Griffin et al 2011). In addition, it is not certain at what stage in lymphocyte maturation the CLL cell arises, since roughly equal numbers seem to come from pre-germinal center B lymphocytes (unmutated group) and post-germinal center B lymphocytes (mutated group). However, the comparison of CLL gene expression profiles with those of purified normal B cell subpopulations indicates that the common CLL gene expression profile is more related to memory B cells than to those derived from naïve B cells, CD5+ B cells, or germinal center centroblasts and centrocytes (Klein et al 2001; Rosenwald et al 2001, Klein and Dalla-Favera 2005). Interestingly, unmutated and mutated chronic lymphocytic leukemias derive from self reactive B cell precursors despite expressing different antibody reactivity (Herve et al 2005). This similar expression profile also suggest that the consequences or even the mechanism of transformation may be similar, irrespective of IGHV mutations status. This too suggests that rather than having a cellular origin or cellular subtype, CLL is originated by a coordinated normal immunologic tolerance mechanism to destroy self-reactive B cells and to avoid autoimmunity during their process of differentiation. This point of view is supported by the fact that some CLL mutated and unmutated cases derive from self-reactive B cells (Herve et al 2005) had evidence of multiple, related rearranged heavy and light chain immunoglobulin genes (Volkheimer et al 2007; Hadzidimitriou et al 2009, Stamatopoulos et al 1996); some express more than one functional Ig heavy chain (Rassenti et al 1997), some had been anergized (Mockridge et al 2007; Muzio et al 2008), edited (Hadzidimitriou et al 2009, Stamatopoulos et al 1996), switched (Cerutti et al 2002) and/or had progressive immunoglobulin gene mutation (Volkheimer et al 2007; Roudier et al 1990; Ruzickova et al 2002).

Hypothesis: Autoimmunity as origin of CLL

The basic hypothesis of the origin of autoimmune disease depends of the emergence of a clone or a small number of clones of T and B lymphocytes capable of damaging interaction with normal cells of organ or tissue involved. Each clone is initiated from a cell which has developed an immune receptor adequately reactive with an accessible self antigen as a result of a V/D/J gene recombination in bone marrow (unmutated) or during somatic mutations in germinal centers (mutated). Importantly, this newly self-reactive cell ("forbidden clone") is anomalously resistant to inactivation by central and peripheral tolerance check points (Burnet 1972). Similar to an autoimmune disease, some lymphoproliferative diseases (marginal zone lymphomas and chronic lymphocytic leukemia) depends of the emergence of a clone capable of interact with an (auto) antigen and with other normal cells and an specific microenvironment to proliferate and survive. In a parallel way, newly malignant B cells are anomalously resistant to apoptosis and proliferate as result of acquisition of genetic damage during V/D/J gene recombination, somatic mutations, class switching and receptor edition/revision. Importantly, with the exception of class switching, the other mechanisms to increase the diversity of B cell receptors might induce both self-reactivity and/or DNA damage.

B cell development and autoimmunity

The current model of the pathogenesis of CLL suggest that stimulation by (self) antigens provides a pro-survival and possibly pro-proliferative advantage for CLL (precursor) cells, most likely leading initially to oligoclonal and subsequently monoclonal selection of malignant cells (Mertens et al 2011)

In humans, B cells develop from progenitors within the bone marrow (Fig1). The stages of B cell ontogeny from pro-B to pre-B to early B to mature B cells are marked by phenotypic changes, the most important of which is expression of the BCR for antigen on the cell surface at the early B cell stage of development (van Lochem et al 2004; Fuda et al 2009) . During the course of ontogenesis, B cells mature in the bone marrow according to the evolution of the Ig chain synthesis. Starting with the rearrangement of the V/D/J genes for the heavy chain at the pre-B stage, the recombination process continues through the VJ gene rearrangements for kappa light chain or for the lambda light chain at the immature stage. Thus, the resulting receptor (BCR) comprised of randomly selected heavy and light chains have an unpredictable specificity that could include ability to bind "self". However, there are tolerance check points at every stage of B cell activation and maturation (table 1 and 2). This tolerance mechanisms in bone marrow include receptor editing, clonal deletion, clonal anergy and differentiation to B1 cells (Goodnow et al 2005; Radic et al 1993; Tiegs et al 1993; Nemazee et al 2000; Luning Prak et al 2011) Notably, current evidence suggest that anergy, receptor edition and differentiation to B1 B cells could be implicated in the generation of CLL B cells (Herve et al 2005; Chu et al 2010; Mockridge et al 2007; Hadzidimitriou et al 2009, Stamatopoulos et al 1996; Ghia et al 2008a; Rassenti & Kipps 1997; Murray et al 2008;

Griffin et al 2011). Additionally , hematopoietic stem cells sorted from a CLL patient´s bone marrow produce CLL like disease when transplanted into immunosuppresed mice (Kikushige et al 2011). Importantly, autoreactive B cells may suffer receptor editing and anergy in bone marrow. At the same, recent evidence shows that L chain receptor editing occurs not only in bone marrow with a pre-B/immature B cell phenotype but also in immature/transitional splenic B cells. Nevertheless, editing at the H chain locus appears to occur exclusively in bone marrow cells with pro-B phenotype (Nakajima et al 2009).

Repertoire analyses of antibodies cloned from B cells derived from bone marrow and peripheral blood of healthy donors provide evidence for both a central tolerance check point in the bone marrow and a second peripheral checkpoint, as evidenced by a decrease in the frequency of autoreactive antibodies from 75% in bone marrow to 20% in the circulating naïve compartment (Yurasov, et al. 2005). Other tolerance mechanisms and peripheral check points include memory development check points (Tsuiji et al 2006) CD5+ expression (Morikawa et al 1993; Gary-Gouy et al 2002; Hillion et al 2005; Hippen et al 2000, Gary-Gouy et al 2002b, Dallou et al 2008), germinal centre exclusion (Cappione et al 2005; Pugh-Bernard et al 2001), receptor edition/revision (Luning Prack et al 2011), antibody feedback (Ravetch & Bolland 2001), anti-idiotypic network (Jerne 1974; Jerne 1984; Forni et al 1980) and all contribute to maintain tolerance and avoid autoimmune diseases.

The contribution of this mechanism in the development of CLL remain unknown, however, Ghia et al describe that CLL expressing IGHV3-21/IGVL3-21 most likely were derived from B cells that had experienced somatic mutation and germinal center maturation in an apparent antigen driven immune response previous to undergoing Ig receptor editing and after germinal-center leukemogenic selection (Ghia et al 2008b). This suggest that peripheral tolerance mechanism also contribute to the shape of self reactive CLL B cells generated and selected after somatic hypermutation. Other mechanisms as germinal centre exclusion, defects in antibody feedback and anti-idiotypic network in lymphoproliferative disorders remain unsolved, however some conjectures about their role have been proposed (García-Muñoz 2009a; García-Muñoz et al 2009b).

The fact that unmutated and mutated chronic lymphocytic leukemias derive from self reactive B cell precursors despite expressing different antibody reactivity (Herve et al 2005) suggest that this B cells escape from tolerance mechanisms. Even more Chiorazzi and Ferrarini suggest that CLL derives from competent B lymphocytes selected for clonal expansion and eventual transformation by multiple encounters and responses to (auto)antigen(s) (Chiorazzi and Ferrarini 2003). This two characteristics of CLL B cells guide us to think that CLL is the product of the selective pressure of tolerance check points in an auto-reactive B cell.

Development of Unmutated CLL B cells

Tumors displaying unmutated V genes have a shorter median survival, in one study of 99 months vs 293 months in the mutated cases (Hamblin et al 1999). Here, a cut-off of $\geq$98% homology to donor germline gene has been used to define unmutated tumor V genes to allow for a low degree of polymorphic allelic variation. There is an association between unfavorable cytogenetic aberrations (del 17p and del 11q) and unmutated CLL, although 13q- is more frequent in mutated CLL. However, there are discrepancies with many cases having some high-risk and other low-risk molecular features and more than 50% of IgVH unmutated cases have no unfavorable cytogenetics (Krober et al 2006). Prominently unmutated CLL B cells are self reactive or polyreactive (Herve et al 2005) and seem that they are resistant to several tolerance mechanism.

Are unmutated CLL B cells invulnerable to anergy?

Low BCR signaling induced by weak reactivity to self antigens induce B cells to enter a tolerized but alive state referred to as anergy (Gauld et al 2006; Getahun et al 2009) . In most cases, anergic B cells are characterized by chronic low level BCR signaling and exhibit reduced surface IgM levels but can express high levels of IgD (Getahun et al 2009; Goodnow et al 1998; Dolmetsh et al 1997). Interestingly, anergy depends on the degree of BCR occupancy and require constant transduction of a BCR signal (Goodnow et al 1989; Benshop et al 2001;Gauld et al 2005). Although it is clear that stimulation through the BCR occurred during the natural history of all types of CLL, it is quite peculiar that unmutated CLL cells retain the capacity to transmit signals through the BCR via surface IgM (Lanham et al 2003). The low expression of the BCR is the hallmark of CLL cells and anergic B cells, and appears to contribute towards producing poorer responses to BCR stimulation. Despite low levels of surface expressed immunoglobulin, signalling through the B cell receptor is possible. ZAP-70 expression has shown to augment signalling via IgM ligation in CLL cells as measured by phosphorylation of downstream mediators such as Syk, BLNK and PLC and calcium influx (Chen et al 2005) This increased signalling might lead to enhanced proliferation or survival of the leukemic cell (Bernal et al 2001). Significantly, a number of studies have shown a strong association between ZAP-70 expression and unmutated IGHV genes. This findings could imply that if an immature self-reactive B cell recognize an auto-antigen and also express ZAP-70 survival and activating signals prevail over anergy. In this case a self reactive CLL B cell selected by a self-antigen during B cell development in bone marrow might mature despite they undergo an anergy process and likely to progress to transitional and mature B cell.

Unmutated CLL cases are more frequently CD38 (66-77%) and ZAP-70 (93%) positive, exhibit IgM+ and IgD+ surface immunoglobulin, express higher amounts of BCR and response better to stimulation compared with mutated CLL´s (Wiestner et al 2003, Hamblin et al 2002; Thumberg et al 2001; Döhner et al 2000; Mockridge et al 2007; Guarini et al 2008). This characteristics suggest that this unmutated CLL B cells where resistant to anergy and progress to mature autoreactive naive B cells.

Receptor editing be unsuccessful to avoid self-reactivity and might induce polyreactive BCR in unmutated CLL B cells

Immature B cells expressing self-reactive IgM antibodies may undergo repeated rounds of light chain rearrangement to lessen the self specificity of the antibody, a process termed receptor editing (Nemazee et al 2000; Luning Prak et al 2011). Evidence of receptor editing in CLL is provided by the fact that a number of CLL´s have multiple light chain rearrangements (Hadzidimitriou et al 2009). B cell receptor of CLL B cells react with recurrent self antigens in vitro including IgG, thyroglobulin, DNA, actin, cardiolipin and others as well as microbial antigens and epitopes exposed on cell surface as a result of apoptosis and also could be stimulated by stroma-derived antigens (Sthoeger et al 1989; Dighiero et al 1991; Chiorazzi et al 2005; Lanemo Myhrinder et al 2008). Sustained or repetitive BCR signaling promotes survival in CLL cells (Petlickovsky et al 2005; Bernal et al

2001). Notably, unmutated CLL B cells are self reactive or polyreactive (Herve et al 2005). Interestingly, 79.3% of unmutated CLL antibodies are polyreactive (Herve et al 2005), and reactivity with a particular form of apoptotic cells is a common feature of this subset (Chu et al 2010). Even more, recently Rozcova et al revealed that Toll like receptor 9 (TLR-9) agonists are a potent stimulus from CLL B cells and induce proliferation, expression of CD38 and secretion of cytokines (Rozcova et al 2010). Outstandingly, TLR-9 recognition of self-molecules (nucleic acids in apoptotic cells) of the host, which are not easily distinguishable from those of no-self (infectious organisms) has the potential to provoke autoimmune diseases. Intriguingly, the unmutated CLL subset expresses antibodies with long heavy and light chain CDR3 (Herve 2005) and some cases of unmutated CLL with 100% of IGHV identity have multiple light chain rearrangements (Hadzidimitriou et al TS25 2009), associated with receptor edition. This suggest that receptor editing mechanisms could be not working well in this subset, even more is possible that increase polyreactivity (Luning Prak et al 2011; Binder et al 2010) and promote survival of self-reactive (Sandel et al 1999) CLL B cells. Consequently, BCRs that react with diverse epitopes may be more prone to sustained signaling. As a result, some unmutated CLL B cells expressing multireactive BCR have a more aggressive course than CLLs expressing less reactive BCRs (Binder et al 2010).

Are unmutated CLL B cells insensitive to CD5 action?

Induction of CD5 by autoantigen might be a mechanism by which the production of autoantibodies is avoided and also maintains tolerance in anergic B cells (Berland et al 2002; Hippen et al 2000). Recently, a very interesting observation was made that many CLL leukemia antibodies recognize non-muscle myosin heavy chain IIA exposed apoptotic cells (MEACs) and that natural antibodies from human serum also react with MEACs. In this study 15 of 16 MEAC-reactive CLL mAbs carried unmutated IGVH genes (Chu et al 2010). Several mechanisms are involved in the tolerance associated with expression of CD5. Likewise, CD5 expression prevents B lymphocytes from uncontrolled self reactivity increasing the BCR signalling threshold[51], and is associated with reexpresion of RAG, receptor edition/revision, and lack of responsiveness to BAFF in some cells outside bone marrow and germinal centres (Lee et al 2009; Hippen et al 2000, Hillion et al 2005). Along this line, the fact that anergic autoreactive B cells may express CD5+ and that immunoglobulin secreted by unmutated B-CLL cells is often autoreactive and react with a variety of autoantigens (including Fc portion of IgG, DNA, histones, cardiolipin, cytoskeletal proteins and insulin) support the notion that unmutated self-reactive B CLL cells are under check to avoid pathogenic autoimmunity (Broker et al 1988; Caligaris-Cappio et al 1996; Morbach et al 2006). We speculate that the expression of ZAP-70 and CD38 could encourage the stimulation of unmutated CLL B cells and overcome the inhibition induced by CD5. In addition, CD5 does not inhibit properly the BCR mediating signalling in leukemic B cells and in some cases provide viability signals or/and promote CLL B cell survival (Perez-Chacon et al 2007; Perez-Chacon 2007b; Gary-Gouy et al 2007; Gary-Gouy et al 2002; Gary-Gouy et al 2002).

Are unmutated CLL B cells transformed human B1 cells?

Similarities between normal human B1 cells and malignant chronic lymphocytic leukemia (CLL) cells, include that both are CD20+CD27+CD43+CD70-; most normal B1 cells express CD5, as do malignant CLL cells; and, both express relatively nonmutated IGHV. In addition, normal human B1 cells are ZAP-70+ like unmutated CLL cells. As a final point, in respect to pathophysiology, Griffin et al propose that the chronically activated phenotype of normal B1 cells may predispose to malignant transformation (Griffin et al 2011).

Are unmutated CLL naïve self-reactive B cells efficiently excluded by germinal centres?

In order to prevent autoimmunity, censoring mechanisms, including anergy and sequestration into the marginal zone, ultimately forbid the participation of mature autoreactive B cells in productive germinal centres reactions, thereby precluding their expansion into the long-lived IgG memory and plasma cell compartments. Importantly, most self reactive and polyreactive IgG antibodies originate from non self-reactive B cells that acquired reactivity by somatic hypermutation (Tiller et al 2007). Significantly, somatic hypermutation does not appear to occur uniformly among CLL IGHV genes(Chiorazzi et al 2005; Fais et al 1998; Tobin et al 2002; Ghia et al 2005) and might suggest the effect of germinal centre exclusion and tolerance mechanisms to maintain the self-reactive BCR in a germ line state and avoid the participation of unmutated CLL cases in germinal centres reactions.

Development of Mutated CLL B cells

Fifty percent of CLL patients have undergone somatic hypermutation in IGHV, and these patients have a more indolent clinical course and longer survival than those without somatic hipermutation (Hamblin et al 1999; Damle et al 1999). The majority of cases of mutated CLL fail to signal via IgM in vitro (Lanham et al 2003; Chen et al 2002). Interestingly, CLL B cells that express only IgD+ are linked to mutated IGHV genes, negative or low CD38 expression, and 50% of mutated CLL cases unable to signal via IgM were able to signal via IgD (Stevenson et al 2004). Muzio et al, showed that CLL B cells (typically IGH-mutated cases) that do not respond to BCR ligation show activation cellular pathways that suggest anergy (Muzio et al 2008). Essentially, mutated CLL cases derive from B cells with self-reactive receptors that were anergized, edited or regulated to avoid autoimmunity. This is supported by the fact that when mutated non autoreactive immunoglobulin sequences of mutated CLL cases were reverted to their germline counterparts, they encoded polyreactive and autoreactive antibodies (Herve 2005). Despite somatic hypermutation had been proposed as a mechanism to change original BCR self reactivity (germ line) towards some non-self BCR (Murray et al 2008), this is an eccentric mode to loss self reactivity because, self reactive naive B cells are efficiently excluded from germinal centres (Tsuji et al 2006; Cappione A 3rd et al 2005; Pugh-Bernard et al 2001) and if this check point is bypassed B cells progress to plasmatic cells that produce auto-antibodies. Still, a significant fraction of self-reactive BCR fail to be edited or trigger deletion in primary lymphoid tissues, either because the self-antigen are bound with only low avidity or because they are not sufficiently abundant in primary lymphoid organs. For receptors with intermediate avidity for self antigens, the risk they pose for autoimmunity may not overshadow their potential use in fighting infection. B cells with receptors that fall into this zone undergo a conditional type of clonal deletion that is extrinsically regulated through competition with B cells bearing less self reactive BCR (Cyster et al 1994; Lanemo Myhrinder et al 2008). This also can explain that unmutated CLL cases and mutated CLL cases express different antibody repertoires and different VH genes (Fais et al 1988; Johnson et al 1997). Current data support that CLL cells are in active (auto) antigen driven receptor editing, presumably by keeping away from autoreactivity associated with preferential autoimmune linked IGHV gene utilization in CLL patients like IGHV3-21, IGHV4-34, IGKV1-17 (Foreman et al 2007; Hadzidimitruiou et al 2009) and also IGHV5-51 and IGHV1-69 in unmutated IgVH genes (Chapal et al 2000; Vanura et al 2008). Interestingly, highly polyreactive antibodies are expressed frequently by unmutated CLL, but only rarely by mutated cases, supporting the view that the receptor editing mechanism is significantly active to try to elude autoimmunity in CLL.

In mutated CLL cases quite a lot of cellular strategies are used to regulate self-reactive receptors at different points during B cell differentiation.

1. The receptor is edited to one that is less self reactive by V(D)J recombination (Hadzidimitriou et al 2009; Rassenti et al 1997 Ghia et al 2008b; Kalinina et al 2011).
2. Regulation by BCR downregulation and anergy (Muzio et al 2008).
3. Induction of inhibitory receptors as CD5 by self-reactive BCR (Hippen et al 2000; Morikawa et al 1993; Dallou et al 2008; Hillion et al 2005).

Table 1. BCR tolerance mechanisms in central lymphoid organs (bone marrow) include receptor edition, anergy and induction of inhibitory receptors as CD5.

Regulation of self reactive receptor in follicles

Each of the checkpoints described above deal with self-reactive receptor generated by V(D)J recombination in the primary lymphoid organs; however, self-reactive BCRs are also generated in a second wave of receptor-gene-diversification through somatic hypermutation in germinal centre follicles of peripheral lymphoid tissues (Shiono et al 2003; Radic et al 1994; Ray et al 1996). Despite somatic hypermutation could produce modifications in BCR to ablate self-reactivity (Murray et al 2008) also might produce new self-reactive BCR. In addition somatic hypermutation poses a particular severe threat of autoimmunity for the reason that increase the affinity of antibodies for self-antigens, the follicular pathway of B cell differentiation generates long lived plasma and memory cells and numerous apoptotic cells be present in germinal centres with self components that are trapped and displayed as immune complexes on follicular dendritic cells. For these reasons the immune system contain a number of mechanisms to elude the maturation of self-reactive B cells that encourage an autoimmune disease. Self-reactivity of mutated CLL cases may derive from immature self-reactive B cells that suffer somatic hypermutation or by non-self reactive B cells that acquire self-reactive BCR during somatic hypermutation in germinal centres. In humans two types of memory B cells have been described: IgM+ memory B cells and class-switched memory B cells (Agematsu et al 1997; Klein et al 1998; Tangye et al 1998). Transition from naive B cells into circulating IgM+ memory B cells is accompanied by efficient counter selection against self reactive naive B cells before the onset of somatic hypermutation and that self reactive IgM+ memory B cells present in the circulation of healthy humans gain self-reactivity as a result of somatic hypermutation (Tsuji et al 2006).

The increase in self-reactivity during transition between mature naive and IgG+ memory B cells might be due to selective advantage for pre-existing self-reactive cells, or selection for cells with self reactive antibodies produced by somatic hypermutation. (Tiller et al 2007) This mechanisms could contribute to generate the IgG+ CLL cases (Ghiotto F, et al 2004).

1. Germinal centre exclusion (Tsuji et al 2006; Cappione A 3rd et al 2005; Pugh-Bernard et al 2001).
2. The receptor is modified to one that is less self reactive by BCR hypermutation (Murray et al 2008, Tiller et al 2007).
3. Receptor edition/revision (Hadzidimitriou et al 2009; Kalinina et al 2011; Rochas et al 2007)
4. CD5 expression (Hillion et al 2005).
6. Absence of T cell help (Shokat et al 1995)
7. Competition for follicular niches (Cyster et al 1994)

Table 2. Tolerance mechanisms in peripheral lymphoid organs.

Tolerance induced by absence of T-cell help:

A substantial portion of the activated B cells migrate to germinal centers where they undergo the process of somatic hypermutation. These B cells first remove the BCR from their surface, then undergo several rounds of division, and finally re-express mutated immunoglobulin receptors. The cells then undergo a negative selection process similar to that of transitional B cells. The antigen is provided from antigen-antibody complexes on follicular dendritic cells. Survival requires the receptor to be of high enough affinity to out-compete the already circulating antibody and allow B cell uptake and processing of antigen For display peptides to primed helper T cells, which have also moved into the germinal centers (Kearneay et al 1994). If the B cell receives T cell-help it survives and is stimulated to undergo another round of expansion and differentiation. If T cell help is not received, the B cell can become anergized or die by apoptosis (Shokat, et al 1995).

We suggest that in CLL with mutated Ig genes, the proliferating B cells is likely to have traversed a germinal center and acquire "*de novo* self-reactivity" originated in the process of somatic hypermutation mechanism or by receptor editon revision. After this "*de novo* autoreactivity" a normal CD5- B cell can theoretically be transformed into a "*de novo* autoreactive memory B cell" that express CD5+ (increase the threshold for BCR activation), suffer receptor revision (change light chains to evade autoimmunity), down regulate surface Ig (to avoid activation), and remain under check by germinal center exclusion (to diminish the chance to progress in the maturation and become plasma cells that produce autoantibodies). Finally, all this tolerance mechanism converts this B CD5- B cell into an "anergic-edited-CD5+CD27+ memory B cell" excluded from germinal centres. These "*de novo* autoreactive" memory B cells could retain a process of "self-renewal", a specificity that changes (receptor editing-revision) and/or that can not be activated because this "new malignant cell" is an "anergic cell" excluded from germinal centres. This speculation could explain why mutated IGVH CLL susbsets ("anergic cells") have an indolent course related to the absence of BCR signalling activation.

IGVH gene usage in CLL is highly selective, and often associated with autoantibody reactivity (Oscier et al 1987). The fact that almost 30 % of CLL patients share BCRs with restricted, quasi-identical immunoglobulins sequences should aid the understanding of the functional interplay between CLL cells and the microenvironment. On the one hand, unmutated IGVH CLL subsets recognizes apoptotic cells in bone marrow and spleen and express a functionally competent BCR, as shown by the fact that most of it can be stimulated following Ig ligation *in vitro*. On the other hand, CLL mutated that has acquired "*de novo*" autoreactivity induced by somatic hypermutation recognizes apoptotic cells in germinal centres; however they become anergic and are unresponsive throughout BCR stimulation. In a CLL mutated subset the "memory-anergic" B cell returns to bone marrow in the same way that normal memory B cells.

Other immunologic alterations that theoretically might predispose the lost of CLL clone control: Impaired immunologic synapses

CD4 and CD8 T cells of patients with CLL show impaired immunological synapse formation with antigen presenting cells (APC)(Ramsay et al 2008). This dysfunction is in part induced by the CLL B cells. This impaired immunological synapse within T cells and APC could contribute to the failure to mount an effective immune response in patients with CLL. Moreover, it may also add other immunological abnormalities like hipogammaglobulinemia (impaired T cell – B cell interactions), autoimmunity (impaired regulatory T cell control), and second tumours (diminished immunosurveillance mediate by NK and CD8 T cells). Interestingly, lenalidomide, an immunomodulatory drug, could repair this synapses with an enhancement of immune cell function. This effect is clinically observed during treatment of CLL patients with this agent because lenalidomide probably induces a strong activation of the immune system complicated by swelling of involved lymph nodes and fever named tumour flare reaction (Chanan-Khan et al 2006; Aue et al 2009)

Antibody mediated immunoregulation:

The antigen-antibody complexes are also likely to be responsible for the phenomenon known as original antigenic sin, in which memory B cells, generated during a prior exposure to a cross-reacting antigen, present or down-regulate the response to these unique new determinants on the antigen[70]. Memory B cells seem to have an advantage for rapid activation and this produces antibodies that feed back to inhibit the priming of naïve B cells possessing receptors that are specific to unique determinants of the second immunogen. This feedback mechanism is most likely mediated through antigen-antibody complexes that interact with FcγRIIb on the naïve B cells and inhibit signal transduction through their IgM receptors (Ravetch et al 2001). In patients with hipogammaglobulinemia this feedback mechanism is impaired and might contribute to expansion of autoreactive B cells (García-Muñoz 2009b) , and in patients with CLL it may add an additional risk to uncontrolled proliferation of CLL clones.

Anti-idiotypic B cell regulation: In 1974 Jerne proposed that antibody production could be regulated by other antibodies that recognized unique idiotypic determinants in the V regions of the first antibody. He postulated that an increase in the production of the first antibody could negatively regulate the production of anti-idiotypic antibodies, and vice versa. Because of the interconnected pathways in such a network, perturbation of one segment would be dampened by the presence of others segments and thus the original steady state would be buffered (Jerne 1984; Jerne 1970; Forni et al 1980).

Patients with CLL have an increased proportion of autoimmune haemolytic anemia (AIHA) and idiopatic autoimmune thrombocytopenia (ITP) and infections. It is probable that the idiotypic network is disrupted in CLL patients and that this could lead to an increased risk of autoimmunity on one hand and immunodeficiency on the other. Treatment with intravenous immunoglobulins (IVIg) could in theory restore idiotypic network and antigen-antibody-complexes feedback in CLL B cells. Remarkably, patients with AIHA treated with IVIg experiment a reduction of the size of lymph nodes and spleen (Diehl et al 1998). This suggests that immune-complexes feedback and idiotypic network could contribute indirectly in the control of CLL.

MYD88 Mutation

Interestingly, mutations in MYD88 and KLHL6 genes have been reported recently in patients with mutated CLL patients (Puente et al 2011). Significantly, similar to CLL patients, patients with MYD88-deficiency do not secrete autoantibodies (Isnardi et al 2008). We speculate that if mutations in MYD88 gene were acquired during germinal center reaction, is possible that self-reactive B cells cannot progress to plasmatic cells but retain some features or memory B cells. Even more, TLR-9 acts via MYD88 and might induce proliferation of CLL B cells. However, mutations in MYD88 might disturb the function of this TLR-9 and contribute to the biology and better prognosis of mutated CLL cases.

IGHV gene usage in CLL is highly selective, and often associated with autoantibody reactivity. The fact that almost 30 % of CLL patients share BCRs with restricted, quasi-identical immunoglobulins sequences should aid to the understanding of the functional interplay between CLL cells and the microenvironment. On the one hand, unmutated *IGHV* CLL subsets recognizes apoptotic cells in bone marrow and spleen and express a functionally competent BCR, as shown by the fact that most of it can be stimulated following Ig ligation *in vitro*. On the other hand, CLL mutated that has acquired "*de novo*" autoreactivity (¿mutations in MYD88?) induced by somatic hypermutation recognizes apoptotic cells in germinal centres; however they become anergic and are unresponsive throughout BCR stimulation. In a CLL mutated subset the "memory-anergic" B cell returns to bone marrow in the same way that normal memory B cells.

3. Conclusion

Chronic lymphocytic leukemia can be separated into cases that harbour somatic mutation in their IGVH genes, or cases without somatic mutations. IGVH gene usage in CLL is highly selective, and often associated with autoantibody reactivity. Despite the fact that the cell surface markers and gene expression of CLL cells suggest that both subsets originate from a precursor cell of the same developmental stage, these findings could be only the result of several immunologic mechanisms that try to destroy or avoid the persistence of self-reactive CLL B cells. CLL is characterized by multiple immune deficiencies and autoimmune phenomena associated with persistent tolerance mechanism trying to control self-reactive CLL B cells growth.

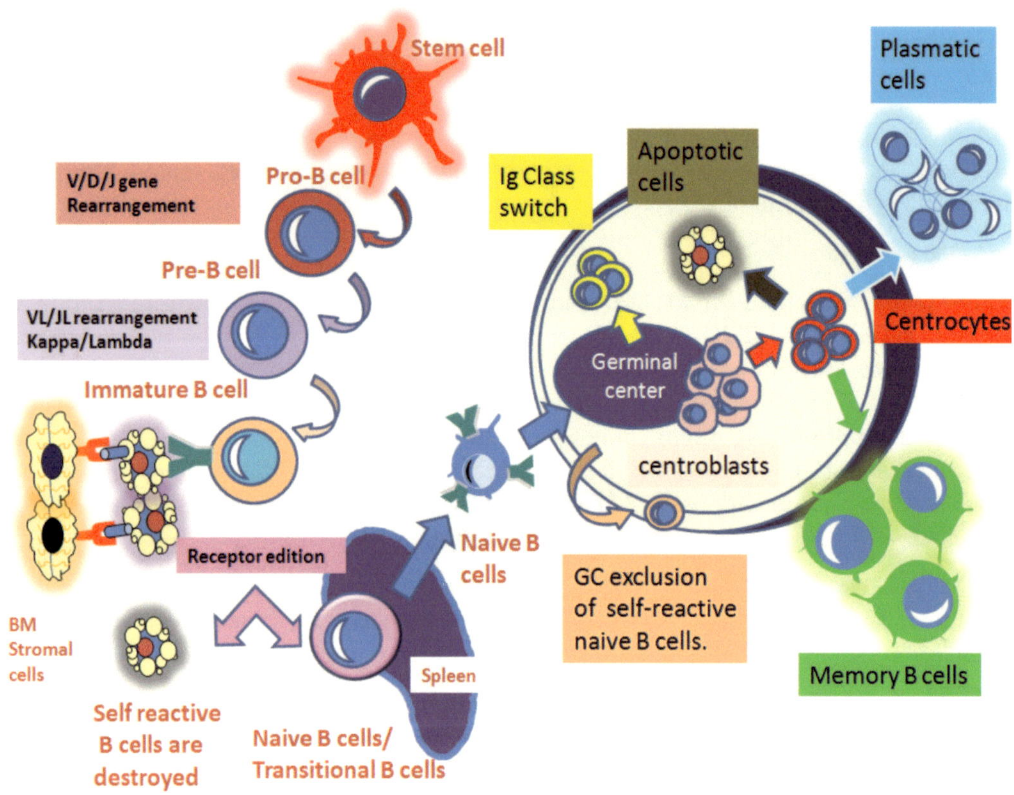

B-cell development occurs initially in the bone marrow and subsequently in lymphoid organs. In bone marrow, hematopoietic progenitor cells (HSC) differentiate into the earliest identifiable cell type committed to the B-cell lineage, the pro-B cell. The pro-B cell undergoes a rearrangement of its immunoglobulin (Ig) heavy chain genes and is called a pre-B cell. Subsequent rearrangement of the light chain enables the cell to express surface IgM and the cell becomes an immature transitional B lymphocyte. These cells leave the bone marrow and are called naïve B cells. They are arrested in the G0 phase of the cell cycle. These naïve B cells enter the lymphoid tissue, where they are exposed to antigen-presenting cells, become activated and differentiate into plasma cells or memory B cells. Through activation by an antigen, B cells differentiate into centroblasts, resulting in Ig isotype switching and somatic mutations in the variable region of the Ig with the generation of high-affinity antibodies. Centroblasts then progress to the centrocyte stage and re-express surface Ig. The centrocytes with high-affinity antibodies differentiate into either memory B cells or plasmablasts, which subsequently move to the bone marrow and terminally differentiate into plasma cells.

Fig. 1. Normal B cell development.

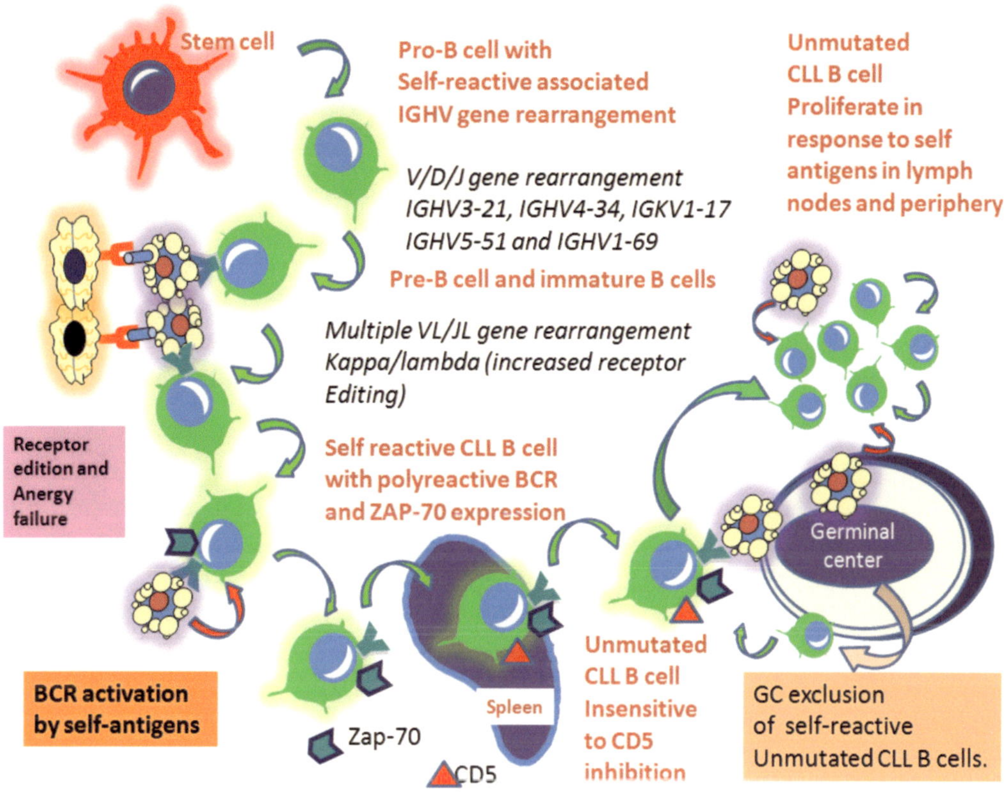

Unmutate CLL B-cell development occurs initially in the bone marrow and subsequently in lymphoid organs. In bone marrow, hematopoietic progenitor cells (HSC) differentiate into the pro-B cell that use IGHV genes related with autoimmunity. The pro-B cell undergoes a rearrangement of its immunoglobulin (Ig) heavy chain genes and is called a pre-B cell. Subsequent rearrangement of the light chain enables the cell to express surface self reactive BCR that fail to be corrected by several rounds of receptor edition. This self-reactive B cells acquire Zap-70 or other alterations that induce increased BCR activation. This is the way in which this self-reactive CLL B cells pass up tolerance mechanisms as anergy and inhibition exerted by CD5. These cells leave the bone marrow as unmutated polyreactive CLL B cells. These unmutated polyreactive CLL B cells enter in the lymphoid tissue, where they are exposed to antigen-presenting cells and self-antigens, however, they cannot be converted into plasma cells or memory B cells with mutations because they are efficiently excluded by germinal centers.

Fig. 2. Hypothesis about generation of unmutated B cells (García-Muñoz et al. Ann Hematol. Accepted).

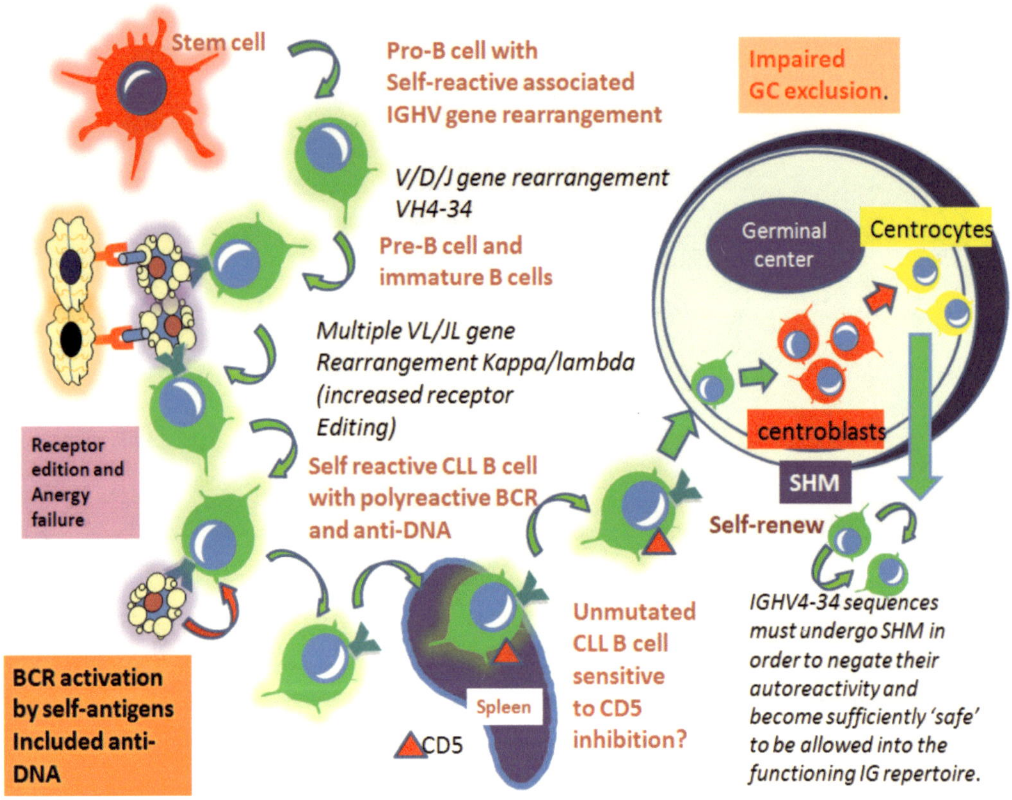

Mutated CLL B-cell development occurs initially in the bone marrow and subsequently in lymphoid organs. In bone marrow, hematopoietic progenitor cells (HSC) differentiate into the pro-B cell that use IGHV genes related with autoimmunity. The pro-B cell undergoes a rearrangement of its immunoglobulin (Ig) heavy chain genes and is called a pre-B cell. Subsequent rearrangement of the light chain enables the cell to express surface self reactive BCR that fail to be corrected by several rounds of receptor edition. This self-reactive B cells enter in germinal centres and undergo somatic hypermutation in order to negate their autoreactivity. This is the way in which this self-reactive CLL B cells pass up tolerance mechanisms as germinal centre exclusion, however, fortunately they suffer some mutations to reverse their self reactivity and avoid autoimmune diseases as SLE. These cells leave the germinal center as mutated CLL B cells memory like cells.

Fig. 3. "Impaired Germinal Centre exclusion model for development of mutated CLL cases wiht VH4-34.

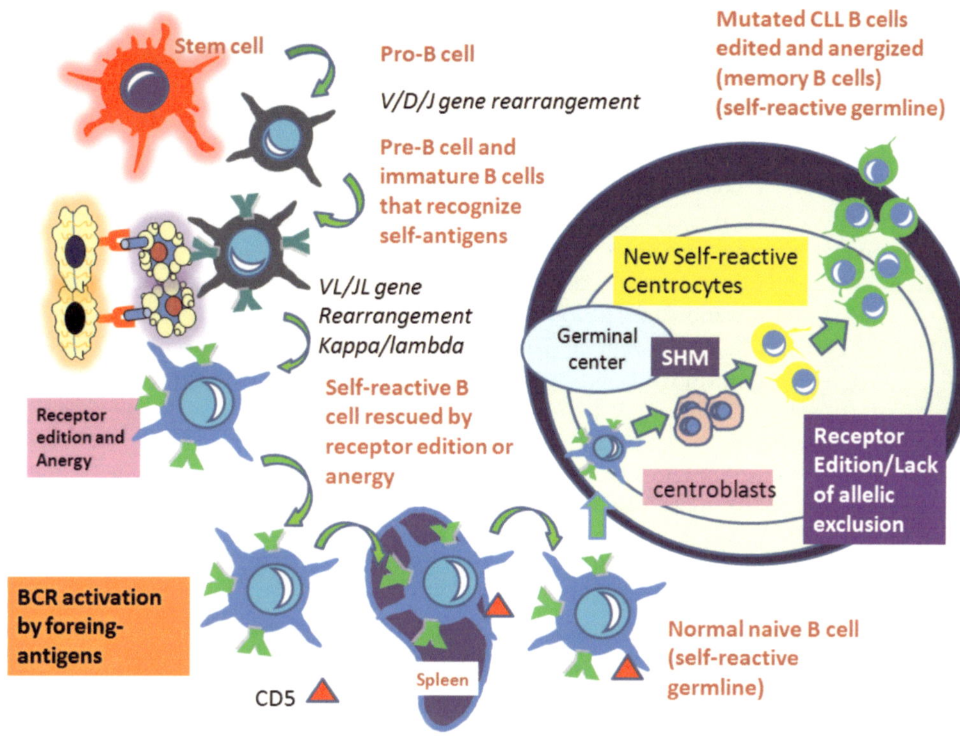

Mutated CLL B-cell development occurs initially in the bone marrow and subsequently in lymphoid organs. In bone marrow, hematopoietic progenitor cells (HSC) differentiate into the pro-B cell that use IGHV genes related with autoimmunity. The pro-B cell undergoes a rearrangement of its immunoglobulin (Ig) heavy chain genes and is called a pre-B cell. Subsequent rearrangement of the light chain enables the cell to express surface self reactive BCR that succeed to be corrected by several rounds of receptor edition. This ex-self-reactive B cells acquire CD5 or other alterations that induce lesser BCR activation. This is the way in which this ex-self-reactive CLL B cells suffer tolerance mechanisms as receptor edition, anergy and inhibition exerted by CD5. These cells leave the bone marrow as unmutated normal naïve B cells. These naïve ex-self reactive B cells enter in germinal centres and suffer somatic hypermutation (SHM) and acquire a new self-reactive BCR, however, again tolerance mechanisms as receptor edition/revision and CD5 expression make this cells in an anergic memory ex-self-reactive B cells. Importantly, reversion of the IGHV mutated sequences to germline counterparts restored the polyreactivity and self-reactivity.

Fig. 4. Mutated CLL B cells generated by somatic hypermutation (García Muñoz et al. Ann Hematol. Accepted).

4. Acknowledgment

The authors declare that a review paper on immunological aspects in CLL is actually accepted in Ann of Hematology.

5. References

Agematsu K, Nagumo H, Yan FC et al. (1997) B cell subpopulations separated by CD27 and crucial collaboration of CD27+ B cells and helper T cells in immunoglobulin production. Eur J Immunol 1997;27:2073-2079

Aqeilan RI, Calin GA, Croce CM, et al. (2010) miR-15 and miR-16-1 in cancer: discovery, function and future perspectives. Cell Death Differ 2010;17:215-20.

Aue G, Njuguna N, Tian X, Soto S, Huges T, Vire B, et al. (2009) Lenalidomide-induced upregulation of CD80 on tumor cells correlates with T cell activation, the rapid onset of a cytokine release syndrome and leukemic cell clearance in chronic lymphcytic leukemia. Haematologica. 2009;94:1266-73.

Bernal A, Pastore RD, Asgary Z, et al.(2001) Survival of leukemic B cells promoted by engagement of the antigen receptor. Blood 2001;98:3050-7

Berland R, Wortis HH.(2002) Origins and functions of B-1 cells with notes on the role of CD5 Annu Rev Immunol 2002;20:253-300

Benschop RJ, Aviszus K, Zhang X et al. (2001) Activation and anergy in bone marrow B cells of a novel immunoglobulin transgenic mouse that is both hapten specific and autorreactive. Immunity 2001;14:33-43.

Binder M, Le´chenne B, Ummanni R, Scharf C, Balabanov S, et al. (2010) Stereotypical Chronic Lymphocytic Leukemia B-Cell Receptors Recognize Survival Promoting Antigens on Stromal Cells. PLoS ONE 2010;5: e15992. doi:10.1371

Binder M, Muller F, Jackst A, Léchenne B, Pantic M, Bacher U, et al. B-cell receptor epitope recognition correlates with the clinical course of chronic lymphocytic leukemia Cancer 2011;117:1891-1900

Broker BM, Klajman A, Youinou P, et al. (1988) Chronic lymphocytic leukemia (CLL) cells secrete multispecific autoantibodies. J Autoinmune 1988;1:469-481Burnet M. (1972) Pathogenesis of auto-immune disease. In Auto-immunity and auto-immune disease (1972). Medical and Technical Publishing CO LTD. 173-290

Caligaris-Cappio F. B chronic lymphocytic leukemia: a malignancy of anti-self B cells. Blood 1996;87:2615-2620

Callin GA,Liu CG, Shimizu M, et al (2004) MicroRNA profiling reveals distinct signatures in B cell chronic lymphocytic leukemia. Proc Natl Acad Sci USA 2004;101:11755-60

Cappione A 3rd, Anolik JH, Pugh-Bernard A, Barnard J, Dutcher P, Silverman G, Sanz I. Germinal center exclusion of autoreactive B cells is defective in human systemic lupus erythematosus. J Clin Invest. 2005;115:3205-3216

Cerutti A, Zan H, Shan S, Schattner E, et al. Ongoing in vivo class switch DNA recombination in chronic lymphocytic leukemia B cells. J Immunol 2002;169:6594-603

Chanan-Khan A, Miller KC, Musial L, Lawrence D, Padmanabhan S, Tajeshita K, et al. (2006) Clinical efficacy of lenalidomide in patients with relapsed or refractory chronic lymphocytic leukemia: results of a phase II stody. J Clin Oncol. 2006;24:5343-9

Chapal N, Peraldi-Roux S, Bresson D, et al. (2000) Human anti-thyroid peroxidase single-chain fragment variable of Ig isolated from a combinatorial library assembled in cell: insights into the In Vivo Situation. J Immunol 2000;114:4162-4169.

Chen L, Apgar J, Huynh L, et al. (2005) Zap-70 directly enhances IgM signaling in chronic lymphocytic leukemia. Blood 2005;105:2036-41.

Chen L, Withopf G, Huynh L, et al. (2002) Expression of ZAP-70 is associated with increased B-cell receptor signaling in chronic lymphocytic leukemia. Blood. 2002;100:4609-46-14

Chiorazzi N, Ferrarini M. (2003) B cell CLL: lessons learned from studies of the B-cell antigen receptor. Ann Rev Immunol. 2003;21:841-94.

Chiorzzi N, Ferrarini M.(2011) Cellular origin(s) of chronic lymphocytic leukemia: cautionary notes and additional considerations and possibilities. Blood.2011;117:1781-1791.

Chiorazzi N, Hatzi K, Albesiano E (2005) B-cell chronic lymphocytic leukemia, a clonal disease of B lymphocytes with receptors that vary in specificity for (auto)antigens. Ann N Y Acad Sci 2005;1062: 1-12.

Chiorazzi N, Rai KR, Ferrarini M. (2005) Chronic lymphocytic leukemia. N Engl J Med 2005;352:804-815

Chu CC, Catera R, Zhang L, Didier S, Agagnina BM, Damle RN, et al. (2010) Many chronic lymphocytic leukemia antibodies recognize apoptotic cells with exposed nonmuscle myosin heavy chain IIA: implications for patient outcome and cell of origin. Blood. 2010;115:3907-3915.

Cimmino A, Callin GA, Fabbri M, et al. (2005) miR-15 and miR-16 induce apoptosis by targeting BCL2. Proc Natl Acad Sci 2005;102:13944-9

Crespo M, Bosch F, Villamor N, et al. (2003) Zap-70 expression as a surrogate for IgV-region mutations in CLL. N Engl J Med 2003;348:1764-1775.

Cyster JG, Hartley SB, Goodnow CC.(1994) Competition for follicular niches excludes self-reactive cells from the recirculating B cell repertoire. Nature 1994;371:389-395.

Dallou A. (2008) CD5: a safeguard against autoimmunity and a shield for cancer cells. Autoimmun Rev 2008;8:349-353

Damle RN, Wasil T, Fais et al,(1999) IGVH gene mutation status and CD38 expression as novel prognostic indicators in CLL. Blood 1999:94:1840-1847.

Diehl LE, Ketchum LH (1998): Autoimmune disease and chronic lymphocytic leukemia: Autoimmune haemolytic anemia, pure red cell aplasia and autoimmune thrombocytopenia. Semin Hematol 25:80-97,1998

Dighiero G, Hart S, Lim A, Borche L, Levy R, et al. (1991) Autoantibody activity of immunoglobulins isolated from B-cell follicular lymphomas. Blood 1991; 78:581-585.

Döhner H, Fischer K, Bentz M, et al.(1995) P53 gene deletion predicts for poor survival and non response to therapy with purine analogs in chronic B-cell leukaemias. Blood 1995;85:1580-9

Döhner H, Stilgenbauer S, Benner A, et al.(2000) Genomic aberrations and survival in CLL. N Engl J Med. 2000:343:1910-1916.

Döhner H, Stilgenbauer S, James MR, et al. (1997) 11q deletions identify a new subset of B-cell chronic lymphocytic leukemia characterized by extensive nodal involvement and inferior prognosis. Blood 1997;89:2516-22.

Dolmetsh RE, Lewis RS, Goodnow CC, et al. (1997) Differential activation of transcription factors induced by Ca2+ response amplitude and duration. Nature 1997;386:855-858

Fais F, et al (1998) Chronic lymphocytic leukemia B cells express restricted sets of mutated and unmutated antigen receptors. J Clin Invest 1998;102:1515-1525.

Forni L, Coutinho A, Köhler G, Jerne NK.(1980) IgM antibodies induce the production of antibodies of the same specificity. Proc Natl Acad Sci USA 1980;77:1125-8

Foreman AL, van de Water J, Gougeon ML, Gershwin ME. (2007) B cells in autoimmune diseases: insights from analyses of immunoglobulin variable (Ig V) gene usage. Autoimmun Rev.2007;6:387-401

Fuda FS, Karandikar NJ, Chen W. (2009) Significant CD5 expression on normal stage 3 hematogones and mature B lymphocytes in bone marrow. Am J Clin Pathol 2009; 132: 733-737

García-Muñoz R. (2009a) Overrall reduction in antibody production could contribute to generate pathogenic autoantibodies and autoimmune manifestations. Clin Rheumatol 2009;28:361-3.

García-Muñoz R, Panizo C, Bendandi M, Llorente L. (2009b). Autoimmunity and lymphoma: is mantle cell lymphoma a mistake of receptor editing mechanism? Leuk Res 2009;11:1437-1439.

García-Muñoz R, Galiacho VR, Llorente L. (2012). Immunological aspects in chronic lymphocytic leukemia (CLL) development. Ann Hematol. (in press)

Gary-Gouy H, Sainz-Perez A, et al. (2007) Natural Phosporylation of CD5 in chronic lymphocytic leukemia B cells and Analysis of CD5 regulated genes in a B cell line suggest a role of CD5 in malignant phenotype. J Immunol 2007;179:4335-4344

Gary-Gouy H, Harriague J, Bismuth G, Platzer C, Schmitt C, Dallou AH. (2002a)Human CD5+ promotes B cell survival through stimulation of autocrine IL-10 production. Blood 2002;100:4537-4543

Gary-Gouy H, Harriague J, Dallou A, Donnadieu E, Bismuth G. (2002b) CD5-negative regulation of B cell receptor signalling pathways originates from tyrosine residue Y429 outside an immunoreceptor tyrosine-based inhibitory motif. J Immunol 2002;168:232-239

Gauld SB, Benschop RJ, Merrel KT, et al. (2005) Maintenance of B cell anergy requires constant antigen receptor occupancy and signaling. Nature Immunol 2005;6:1160-1167).

Gauld SB, Merrell KT, Cambier JC. (2006) Silencing of autoreactive B cells by anergy; a fresh prerspective. Curr Opin Immunol 2006;18:292-297.

Getahun A, O´Neil SK, Cambier JC. (2009) Establishing anergy as a Bona Fide in vivo mechanisms of B cell tolerance. J Immunol 2009;5430-5441

Ghia EM, Jain F, Widhopf II GF, et al.(2008b) Use of IGHV3-21 in chronic lymphocytic leukemia is associated with high risk disease and reflects antigen-driven, post-germinal center leukemogenic selection. Blood 2008;111:5101-5108.

Ghia P, Chiorazzi N, Stomatopoulos K. (2008a) Microenvironmental influences in chronic lymphocytic leukemia: the role of antigen stimulation. J Internal Med. 2008;264:549-62.

Ghia P, Stamatopoulos K, Belessi C, et al. (2005) Geographic patterns and pathogenetic implications of IGHV gene usage in chronic lymphocytic leukemia: the lesson of IGHV3-21 gene. Blood 2005;105:1678-1685.

Ghiotto F, Fais F, Valleto A, et all. (2004) Remarkably similar antigen receptors among a subset of patients with chronic lymphocytic leukemia, J Clin Invest 2004;113:1008-1016.

Goodnow CC. et al. (2005) Self tolerance checkpoints in B cell lymphocyte development. Adv. Immunol 2005;58:279-368.

Goodnow CC, Crosbie J, Adelstein S, et al. (1998) Altered immunoglobulin expression and functional silencing of self reactive B lymphocytes in transgenic mice. Nature 1998;334:676-682.

Goodnow CC, Crosbie J, Jorgensen H, et al. (1989) Induction of self tolerance in mature peripheral B lymphocytes Nature 1989;342:385-391

Griffin DO, Holodick NE, Rothstein TL.(2011) Human B1 cells in umbilical cord and adult peripheral blood express the novel phenotype CD20+CD27+CD43+CD70-. J Exp Med 2011:208:67-80.

Guarini A, Chiaretti S, Tavolaro S, et al. BCR ligation induced by IgM stimulation results in gene expression and functional changes in only in IgVH unmutated chronic lymphocytic leukemia (CLL) cells. Blood 2008;112:782-792.

Hallek M, Cheson D, Catovsky D, Caligaris-Cappio F, Dighiero G, Döner H, Hillmen P, Keating MJ, Montserrat E, Rai KR, Kipps TJ. (2008) Guidelines for the diagnosis and treatment of chronic lymphocytic leukemia: a report from the international Workshop on Chronic Lymphocytic Leukemia updating the National Cancer Institute-Working Group 1996 guidelines. Blood. 2008;111:5446-5456.

Hadzidimitriou A, Darzentas N, Murray F, et al. (2009) Evidence for the significant role of immunoglobulin light chains in antigen recognition and selection in chronic lymphocytic leukemia. Blood 2009;113:403-411.

Hamblin TJ, Davis Z, Gardiner A et al. (1999) Unmutated IGVH genes are associated with a more aggressive form of CLL. Blood 1999;94:1848-1854.

Hamblin TJ, Orchard Ja, Ibbotson RE et al. (2002) CD38 expression and immunoglobulin variable region mutations are independent prognostic variables in chronic lymphocytic leukemias, but CD38 may vary during the course of the disease. Blood 2002;99:1023-1029.

Herve M, Xu K, Ng YS, et al. (2005) Unmutated and mutated chronic lymphocytic leukemias derive from self reactive B cell precursors despite expressing different antibody reactivity. J Clin Invest 2005;115:1636-1643

Hillion S, Saraux A, Youinou P, Jamin C. Expression of RAGs in peripheral B cells outside germinal centers is associated with the expression of CD5. J Immunol 2005;174:5553-61

Hippen KL, Tze LE, Behrens T. (2000) CD5 maintains tolerance in anergic B cells. J Exp Med 2000;191:883-889

Isnardi I, Ng YS, Srdanovic I, Motaghedi R, Rudchenko S, von Bernut H, et al. (2008) IRAK-4/MyD88 dependent pathways are essential for the removal of developing of autoreactive B cells in humans. Immunity 2008;29:746 757

Jerne NK. Idiotipyc networks and other preconceived ideas. (1984) Immunol Rev. 1984:79:5-24

Jerne NK. (1974) Towards a network theory of the immune system. Ann Immunol (Paris) 1974;125C:373-89

Johnson TA, Rassenti LZ, Kipps TJ (1997) Ig VH1 genes expressed in B cell chronic lymphocytic leukemia exhibit distinctive molecular features. J Immunol 1997;158:235-246.

Kalinina O, Doyle-Cooper, Miksanek J et al. Alternative mechanisms of receptor editing in autoreactive B cells. PNAS 2011;108:7125-7130

Kearney ER, Pape KA, Loh DY, et al. Visualization of peptide-specific T cell immunity and peripheral tolerance induction in vivo. Immunity. 1994;1:327-339

Kikushige Y, Ishikawa F, Miyamoto T, et al (2011) Self-renewing hematopoietic stem cell is the primary target in pathogenesis of human chronic lymphocytic leukemia. Cancer Cell. 2011;20:246-59

Klein U, Dalla-Favera R. (2005) New insights into the phenotype cell derivation of B cells in chronic lymphocytic leukemia. Curr Top Microbiol Immunol 2005;294:31-49

Klein U, Rajewsky K, Kuppers R. (1998) Human immunoglobulin (Ig)M+IgD+ peripheral blood expressing CD27 cell surface antigen carry somatically mutated variable region genes: CD27 as a general marker for somatically mutated (memory) B cells. J Exp Med 1998;188:1679-1689

Klein U, Tu Y, Stolovitzky GA, et al. (2001) Gene expression profiling of B cell chronic lymphocytic leukemia reveals a homogeneous phenotype related to memory B cells. J Exp Med 2001;194:1625-1638.

Krober A, Seiler T, Benner A et al. (2002) V(H) mutation status, CD38 expression level, genomic aberrations and prognosis in CLL. Blood 2002;100:1410-1416.

Krober A, Bloehdom J, Hafner S, et al. (2006) Additional genetic high risk features such as 11q deletion, 17p deletion and V3-21 usage characterize discordance of ZAP-70 and VH mutation status in CLL. J Clin Oncol. 2006;24:969-975.

Lanemo Myhrinder A, Hellqvist E, Sidorova E, et al. A new perspective: molecular motifs on oxidized LDL, apoptotic cells, and bacteria are targets for CLL antibodies. Blood. 2008;111:3838-3848

Lanham S, Hamblin T, Oscier D, et al. Differential signaling via surface IgM is associated with VH gene mutational status and CD38 expression in chronic lymphocytic leukemia. Blood 2003;101:1087-1093

Lee J, Kuchen S, Ficher R, et al. (2009) Identification and characterization of circulating human CD5+ pre-naïve B cell population. J Immunol 2009;182:4116-4126.

Luning Prak E, Monestier M, Eisenberg RA. (2011) B cell receptor editing in tolerance and autoimmunity. Ann NY Acad Sci 2011;1217:96-121.

Matutes E, Wrotherspoon A, Catovsky D. (2007) Differential diagnosis in chronic lymphocytic leukemia. Best Pract Res Clin Haematol 2007;20:367-84

Mertens D, Wolf S, Tschuch C et al. (2006) Allelic silencing at the tumor-suppressor locus 13q14.3 suggest an epigenetic tumor-suppressor mechanism. Proc Natl Acad Sci USA 2006;103:7741-6

Mertens D, Bullinger L, Stilgenbauer S. (2011). Chronic lymphocytic leukemia -genomics lead the way. Haematologica 2011;96:1402-1405

Mockridge CI, Potter KN, Wheatley I, Neville LA, Packham G, Stevenson FK. (2007) Reversible anergy of sIgM-mediated signalling in the two subsets of CLL defined by VH-gene mutational status. Blood 2007;109:4424-4431.

Morbach H, Singh S K, Faber C, Lipsky P E, Girschick H J. (2006) Analysis of RAG expression by peripheral blood CD5+ and CD5- B cells in patients with childhood systemic lupus erythematosus Annals of the Rheumatic Diseases 2006;65:482-487

Morikawa K, Oseko F, Morikawa S. (1993) Induction of CD5 antigen on human CD5- B cells by stimulation with staphylococcus Aureus Cowan strain. Int. Immunol 1993;5:809-816.

Murray F, Darzentas N, Hadzidimitriou A, et al.(2008) Stereotyped patterns of somatic hypermutation in subsets of patients with chronic lymphocytic leukemia: implications for the role of antigen selection in leukemogenesis. Blood 2008;111:1524-1533

Muzio M, Apollino B, Scielzo C, et al.(2008) Constitutive activation of distinct BCR-signaling pathways in a subset of CLL patients: a molecular signature of anergy. Blood 2008;112:188-195.

Nakajima PB, Kieffer K, Price A et al. (2009) Two distinct populations of H chain edited B cells show differential surrogate L chain dependence J Immunol. 2009;182:3583-3596.

Nemazee DA, Weigert MG.(2000) Revising B cell receptors. J Exp Med 2000;191:1813-1818.

Oscier DG, Thompsett A, Zhu D, Stevenson FK. (1987) Differential rates of somatic hypermutation in V(H) genes among subsets of chronic lymphocytic leukemia defined by chromosomal abnormalities. Blood 1987;89:4153-4160

Perez-Chacon G, Vargas JA, Jorda J, et al.(2007a) CD5 does not regulate the signalling triggered through BCR in B cells from a subset of B-CLL patients. Leuk Lymphoma 2007;48:147-157.

Perez-Chacon G, Vargas JA, Jorda J, et al.(2007b) CD5 provides viability signals to B cells from a subset of B-CLL patients by a mechanism that involves PKC. Leuk Res 2007;31:183-193

Petlickovski A, Laurenti L, Li X, et al. Sustained signaling through the B-cell receptor induce Mcl-1 and promotes survival of chronic lymphocytic leukemia B cells. Blood. 2005;105:4820-4827.

Puente XS, Pinyol M, Quesada V, Conde L, Ordoñez GR, Villamor N, et al. (2011) Whole genome sequencing identifies recurrent mutations in Chronic lymphocytic leukemia. Nature 2011

Pugh-Bernard, A.E. et al. (2001) Regulation of inherently autoreactive VH4-34 B cells in the maintenance of human B cell tolerance. J Clin Invest. 2001;108:1061-1070.

Rassenti LZ, Kipps TJ. (1997) Lack of allelic exclusion in B cell Chronic lymphocytic leukemia. J Exp Med 1997;185:1435-1445

Radic MZ, Erickson J, Litwin S, et al. (1993) Lymphocytes may scape tolerance by revising their antigen receptor. J Exp Med. 1993;177:1165-1163.

Radic MZ, Wigert M.(1994) Genetic and structural evidence for antigen selection of anti-DNA antibodies. Ann Rev Immunol 1994;12:487-520

Ramsay AG,Johnson AJ, Lee M, Gorgun G, Le Dieur R, Blum W, et al. (2008) Chronic lymphocytic leukemia T cells show impaired immunological synapse formation that can be reversed with an immunomodulating drug. J Clin Invest 2008;118:2427-37

Ravetch JV, Bolland S. IgG Fc Receptors. Annu Rev Immunol. 2001;19:275-290

Ray SK, Putterman C, Diamond B. Pathogenic autoantibodies are routinely generated during response to foreing antigen: a paradigm for autoimmune disease. Proc Natl Acad Sci. USA 1996;93:2019-2024.

Rochas C, Hillion S, Youinou P et al. (2007) RAG mediated secondary rearrangements of B cell antigen receptors in rheumatoid synovial tissue. Autoimmun Rev 2007;7:155-9

Rosenwald A, Alizadeh AA, Widhopf G, et al. (2001) Relation of gene expression phenotype to immunoglobulin mutation genotype in B cell chronic lymphocytic leukemia. J Exp Med 2001;194:1639-1647

Roudier J, Solverman GJ, Chenn PP et al.(1990) Intraclonal diversity in the VH genes expressed by CD5-chronic lymphocytic leukemia producing pathologic IgM rheumatoid factor. J Immunol 1990:144:1526-1530

Rozkova D, Novodna L, Pytlic R, e tal. (2010) Toll like receptors on B cells: Expression and functional consequences of their stimulation. Int J Cancer 2010;126:1132-43

Ruzickova S, Pruss A, Odendahl M, et al. Chronic lymphocytic leukemia preceded by cold agglutinin disease: intraclonal immunoglobulin light chain diversity in VH4-34 expressing single leukemic B cells. Blood 2002;100:3419-3422.

Sandel PC, Monroe JG. (1999) Negative selection of immature B cells by receptor editing or deletion is determined by site of antigen encounter, Immunity. 1999;10:289-299

Shiono H, et al. (2003) Scenarios of autoimmunization of T and B cells in myasthenia gravis. Ann NY Acad Sci 2003;998:237-256.

Shokat KM, Goodnow CC. Antigen induced B cell death and elimination during germinal centre immune responses. Nature 1995;375:334-338.

Stamatopoulos K, Kosmas C, Stavroyianni N, et al (1996) Evidence of immunoglobulin heavy chain variable region gene replacement in a patient with B cell chronic lymphocytic leukemia. Leukemia 1996;10:1551-1556.

Stevenson FK and Caligaris-Cappio F. Chronic lymphocytic leukemia: revelations from the B cell receptor. Blood 2004;103:4389-4395.

Sthoeger ZM, Wakai M, Tse DB, Vinciguerra VP, Allen SL, et al. (1989) Production of autoantibodies by CD5-expressing B lymphocytes from patients with chronic lymphocytic leukemia. J Exp Med 1989;169: 255–268.

Tangye SG, Liu YJ, Aversa G, et al. (1998) Identification of functional human splenic memory B cells by expression of CD148 and CD27. J Exp Med 1998;1691-1703

Thumberg U, Johonson A, Roos G et al.(2001) CD38 is a poor predictor for VH gene mutational status and prognosis in chronic lymphocytic leukemia. Blood 2001;97:1892-1894

Tiegs SL, Russel DM, Nemazee D.(1993) Receptor editing in self-reactive bone marrow B cells. J Exp Med 1993;177:1009-1020.

Tobbin G, Thunberg U, Johnson A, et al. (2002) Somatically mutated Ig V(H)3-21 genes characterize a new subset of chronic lymphocytic leukemia. Blood 2002:99:2262-4.

Tiller T, Tsuiji M, Yurasov S, et al. (2007) Autoreactivity in Human IgG+ Memory B cells. Immunity 2007;26:205-213

Tsuiji M, Yurasov S, Velinzon K, Thomas S, Nussenzweig MC, Wardemann H.(2006) A check point for autoreactivity in human IgM memory B cell development. J Exp Med 2006;203:393-400.

Van Lochem EG, van der Valden VHJ, Wind HK, et al. (2004) Immunophenotypic differentiation patterns of normal hematopoiesis in human bone marrow: Reference patterns for age-related changes and disease induced shifts. Cytometry B Clin Cytom 2004;60:1-13

Vanura K, Le T, Esterbauer H, et al. (2008) Autoimmune conditions and chronic infections in chronic lymphocytic leukemia patients at diagnosis are associated with unmutated IgVH genes. Haematologica 2008;93:1912-16.

Wiestner A, Rosengwald A, Barry TS, et al.(2003) Zap-70 expression identifies a chronic lymphocytic leukemia subtype with unmutated immunoglobulin genes, inferior clinical outcome, and distinct gene expression profile. Blood 2003;101:4944-4951

Yurasov S, Hammersen J, Tiller T, et al. (2005) B cell tolerance check points in healthy humans and patients with systemic lupus erythematosus. Ann N Y Acad Sci. 2005;1062:165-174.

Pattern Recognition Receptors and Cancer: Is There Any Role of Inherited Variation?

Anton G. Kutikhin
Kemerovo State Medical Academy
Russian Federation

1. Introduction

1.1 What are pattern recognition receptors?

The group of the pattern recognition receptors (PRRs) includes families of Toll-like receptors (TLRs), NOD-like receptors (NLRs), C-type lectin receptors (CLRs) and RIG-I-like receptors (RLRs). The summary of the most modern conceptual data about members of these families and about their structure and functions can be obtained from the recent comprehensive reviews (Elinav et al., 2011; Kawai and Akira, 2011; Osorio and Reis E Sousa, 2011; Loo and Gale, 2011), and the schemes of their signaling are presented in Figures 1-2.

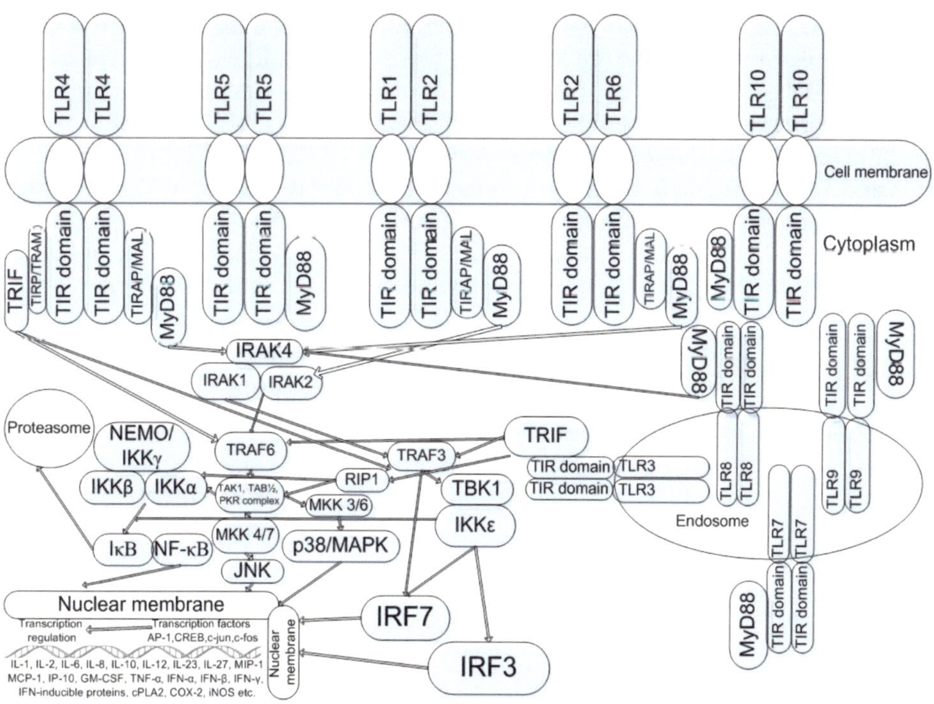

Fig. 1. The signaling of the Toll-like receptor pathway. TLR1, TLR2, TLR4, TLR5, TLR6, and TLR10 are usually located on the cell surface whilst TLR3, TLR7, TLR8 and TLR9 are settled

on the ER membrane (in the resting state) or on the endosomal/lysosomal membrane (after ligand stimulation and trafficking). According to the known data about their structure (Hashimoto et al., 1988), TLRs belong to type I transmembrane glycoproteins and contain three major domains (Matsushima et al., 2007). The ectodomain is oriented towards the extracellular space or cytoplasm (depending on receptor localization) and contains multiple (16-28) leucine-rich repeats (LRRs) that harbor 24–29 amino acids and may contain two types of motifs: typical (T) motifs (LxxLxLxxNxLxxLxxxxF/LxxLxx) and bacterial (S) motifs (LxxLxLxxNxLxxLPx(x)LPxx) (Bell et al., 2003; Matsushima et al., 2007). LRR modules fold into the parallel β-sheets that bend into a concave surface, forming one or two distinct horseshoe structures determining the unique horseshoe shape of TLRs (Matsushima et al., 2007). LRR hydrophobic residues are packed within the interior of ectodomain structure, forming a ligand-binding hydrophobic pocket (Bell et al., 2003, 2006; Kim et al., 2007; Liu et al., 2008). In addition, C-terminal LRRs may control the receptor dimerization and the signal transmission (Takada et al., 2008). The single-spanning transmembrane domain is homologous to IL-1R analog and anchors the receptor in the correct orientation on cell membrane (Huyton et al., 2007; Medzhitov et al., 1997). Third, the cytoplasmic TLR domain (toll/interleukin-1 receptor domain, TIR domain) is usually composed of approximately 150 amino acid residues (Jin and Lee, 2008) and dimerizes after the ligand-ectodomain interaction (TLR ligands are presented in Table 1) and respective alterations in the receptor conformation, triggering the recruitment of the adaptor proteins (MyD88, TIRAP/MAL, TRIF, TRAM, SARM) to initiate the specific signaling pathway of the immune response stimulation (Jin and Lee, 2008; O'Neill and Bowie, 2007). It is important that all TLRs form hetero- or homodimers, and this feature may facilitate the dimerization of the cytoplasmic domain. All adaptors indicated above contain TIR domains, and interactions between such domains of receptor and adaptor are key for the successful signaling (Palsson-McDermott and O'Neill, 2007). The process of TLR signaling is mediated by a number of other adaptor proteins and, finally, leads to activation of NF-κB (Yamamoto et al., 2004), MAPK (Yamamoto et al., 2004), JNK (Takeuchi and Akira, 2001), IRF1, IRF3, IRF5, IRF7 and IRF8 (Honda and Taniguchi, 2006) that move into the nucleus and directly or indirectly control the transcriptional activity of the genes encoding various proinflammatory cytokines (IL-1, IL-2, IL-6, IL-8, IL-10, IL-12, IL-13, IL-23, IL-27, MIP-1, MCP-1, RANTES, SOCS, IP-10, GM-CSF, TNF-α, IFN-α, IFN-β, IFN-γ and IFN-inducible proteins (Chang, 2010; Wong et al., 2011; Zhu and Mohan, 2010).

Member of TLR family	Exogenous ligand	Endogenous ligand
TLR1 (form heterodimers with TLR2)	Triacylated lipopeptides	β-defensin 3
	Lipoarabinomannan	
	Soluble factors of *Neisseria meningitidis* cell wall	
	OspA protein of *Borrelia burgdorferi*	
TLR2	Lipoprotein	HSP22
	Peptidoglycan	HSP60
	Di- and triacylated lipopeptides	HSP70
	Lipoteichoic acid	HSP72
	Zymosan	gp96
	Lipoarabinomannan	HMGB1
	Outer-membrane porins of N.gonorrhoeae and S.dysenteriae	β-defensin 3

	OspA protein of *Borrelia burgdorferi*	Surfactant proteins A and D
	Phenol-soluble modulin of Staphylococcus epidermidis	Eosinophil-derived neurotoxin
	Cell membrane glycolipids of *Trypanosoma cruzi*	Antiphospholipid antibodies
	Hemagglutinin protein of wild-type measles virus	Serum amyloid A
	Envelope proteins of HSV-1 and CMV	Biglycan
	Atypical LPS of *L.interrogans* and *P.gingivalis*	Versican
		Hyaluronic acid fragments
TLR3	dsRNA	mRNA
	Polyinosine-polycytidylic acid	
TLR4	Lipopolysaccharide	HMGB1
	Glucuronoxylomannan	Tenascin-C
	RSV fusion protein	HSP60
	MMTV and MMLV	HSP70
	Taxol	gp96
		Mrp8 and Mrp14
		Neutrophil elastase
		Antiphospholipid antibodies
		Lactoferrin
		Surfactant proteins A and D
		β-defensin-2
		Biglycan
		Low-molecular-weight oligosaccharide fragments of hyaluronan
		Fibrinogen
		Fibronectin
		Heparansulfate
		Oxidized LDL
		Saturated fatty acids
TLR5	Flagellin	
TLR6 (form heterodimers with TLR2)	Diacylated lipoprotein	
	Peptidoglycan	
	Zymosan	
TLR7	Imidazoquinolines	Antiphospholipid antibodies
	ssRNA	ssRNA
TLR8	ssRNA	ssRNA
		Antiphospholipid antibodies
TLR9	Bacterial and viral CpG DNA	IgG-chromatin complexes
	Hemozoin	
TLR10 (may form heterodimers with TLR1 and TLR2)	Unknown	Unknown

Table 1. Ligands of TLRs. Abbreviations: TLR - Toll-like receptor, HSP - heat shock protein, gp - glycoprotein, HSV - herpes simplex virus, CMV - cytomegalovirus, LPS - lipopolysaccharide, dsRNA - double-stranded RNA, HMGB1 - high mobility group box 1, RSV - respiratory syncytial virus, MMTV - mouse mammary tumor virus, MMLV - Moloney murine leukemia virus, Mrp - myeloid related protein.

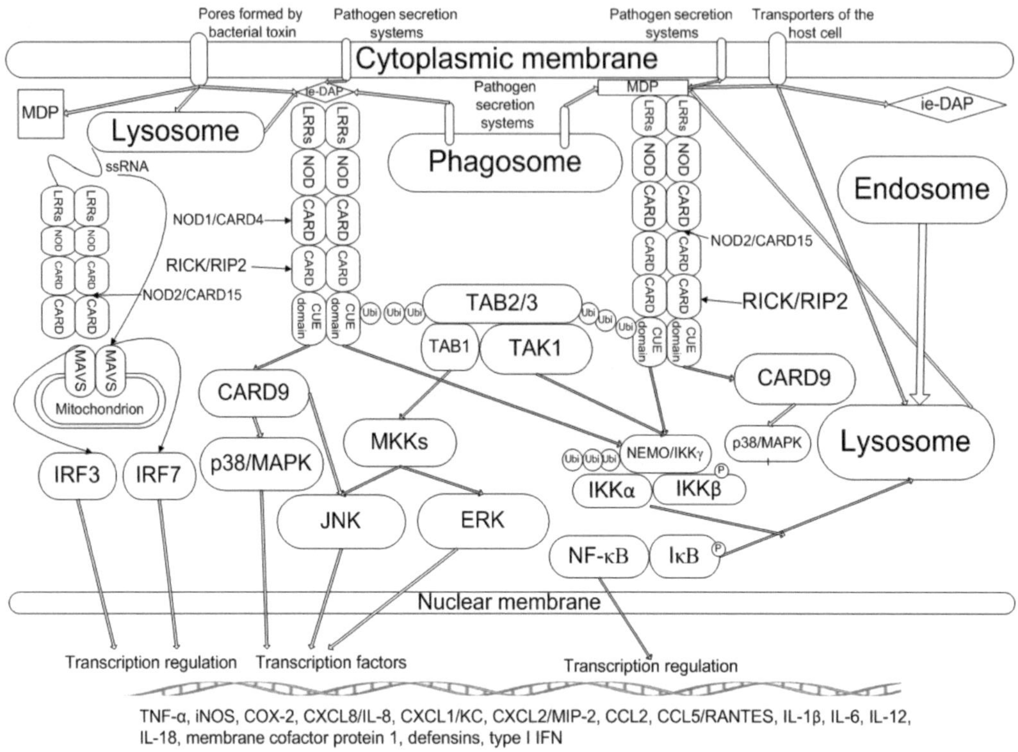

Fig. 2. The signaling of the NOD-like receptor pathway. NLRs usually have three-domain structure (Chen et al., 2009). First, the C-terminal domain, contains multiple leucine-rich repeats (LRRs), directly recognizing exogenous and endogenous ligands (Kumar et al., 2009). The second, central, nucleotide-binding oligomerization domain (NOD) has intrinsic ATPase activity and is responsible for the self-oligomerization and the formation of a complex after the ligand binding for the activation and recruitment of downstream signaling proteins (Kumar et al., 2009). These two domains are common for all known NLRs (Chen et al., 2009). Third, variable, the N-terminal protein-protein interaction domain, may represent a caspase recruitment domain (CARD), death effector domain (DED), pyrin domain (PYD), acidic transactivating domain, or baculovirus inhibitor of apoptosis protein repeat domain (BIR domain) (Kanneganti et al., 2007). The most investigated of NLRs are NOD1/CARD4 and NOD2/CARD15. Both NOD1/CARD4 and NOD2/CARD15 recognize the components of bacteria cell wall: ligands of NOD1/CARD4 are γ-D-glutamyl-m-diaminopimelic acid (iE-DAP) and its synthetic derivatives (particularly having hydrophobic acyl residues) (Chamaillard et al., 2003; Girardin et al., 2003), and the ligand of NOD2/CARD15 is muramyl dipeptide (MDP) (Girardin et al., 2003). These compounds are the components of peptidoglycan (PGN). They can enter the cytosol through the pores formed as a result of bacterial toxin exposure (Ratner et al., 2007), via action of the pathogen secretion systems (Ratner et al., 2007), by endocytosis (Marina-Garcia et al., 2008) or by work of transporters (Ismair et al., 2006), and they can be released in the cytosol of infected cells during a bacterial cell division or from lysosomes where PGN of phagocytosed bacteria is degraded (Shaw et al., 2010). Until the ligand binding, LRR-containing C-terminal domain of NOD1/CARD4 and NOD2/CARD15 prevents the activation of the central domain (NOD)

and its further oligomerization (Faustin et al., 2007); ligand binding causes the conformational alterations in the C-terminal region that, in turn, lead to self-oligomerization of the central domain and to the further activation of N-terminal domain (CARD) that recruits and activates specific adaptor proteins, initiating NOD signaling pathways. Such initiation results in the activation of various transcription factors and, consequently, in the production of proinflammatory mediators (Inohara et al., 1999; Ogura et al., 2001).

Although CLRs and RLRs are investigated relatively less than TLRs and NLRs, it is known that they recognize bacterial, viral, fungal, protozoan, and helminth PAMPs as TLRs and NLRs (Table 2), initiating an immune response against them through their specific signaling pathways (as their structure is not so clear as in the case with signaling pathways of TLRs and NLRs, it will be precisely depicted only in the following years). It is crucially important to note that in many steps signaling pathways of all classes of PRRs may intersect, making possible the crosstalk between them.

Receptor	Ligand
MRC1 (CD206, CLEC13D, mannose receptor)	High mannose, fucose
CD207 (CLEC4K, langerin)	Mannose, fucose, N-acetyl-glucosamine, β-glucan
CD209 (CLEC4L, DC-SIGN)	High mannose, fucose
CLEC7A (Dectin-1)	β-1, 3 glucans
CLEC6A (CLEC4N, Dectin-2)	High mannose, α-mannans
CLEC4E (Mincle)	α-mannose, glycolipids, SAP130
CLEC4A (DCIR)	Mannose, fucose
CLEC4C (BDCA-2, CD303)	Mannose, fucose
RIG-I	Nucleic acids of many viruses
MDA5	Nucleic acids of many viruses

Table 2. The ligands of CLRs and RLRs.

The receptors constituting families of PRRs are united by two general features. Firstly, they directly recognize common antigen determinants of virtually all classes of pathogens (so-called pathogen-associated molecular patterns, or simply PAMPs) and initiate immune response against them via specific intracellular signaling pathways. Secondly, they recognize endogenous ligands (since they are usually released during cell stress, they are called damage-associated molecular patterns, DAMPs), and, consequently, PRR-mediated immune response can be activated without influence of infectious agents. Therefore, PRRs may also initiate the development of aseptic inflammation caused by physical factors such as mechanical pressure, thermal damage, ionizing and non-ionizing radiation, or chemical factors (for instance, acidic damage, alkaline damage, exposure to chemical war gases, croton oil or turpentine, exposure to allergens, liberation of toxic substances during tumor disintegration, aseptic necrosis, internal bleeding, haemolysis, autoimmune processes etc.). It may promote the further progression of inflammation or, on the contrary, prevent the hazardous infectious complications (the combination of these two effects may also be true). The final outcome of PRR working is an enhanced production of the many proinflammatory cytokines participating in a plenty of immune system processes. Expression of PRRs on different levels (transcriptomic or proteomic) was detected in a lot of cells and organs, so it gave an evidence that these receptors control many elements of the complex machinery of human immune system: they allow epithelium and endothelium to defend against infectious agents on their own, they mediate the activation of adaptive immune response by antigen-presenting cells and T-helpers, they stimulate expression of cell adhesion molecules for leukocyte rolling and for other processes of inflammation development, and, finally, they contribute to phagocytosis efficacy (Chang, 2010). As a consequence of all written above, pattern recognition receptors play the key role in realization of innate and adaptive immune response. In addition, many PRRs have a number of other vital functions apart from participation in the immune response realization: they may regulate various aspects of cell proliferation, survival, apoptosis, autophagy, reactive oxygen species generation, pyroptosis, angiogenesis and, consequently, of tissue remodeling and repair (Brown et al., 2007; Fukata et al., 2006; Kim et al., 2007; Rakoff-Nahoum and Medzhitov, 2008).

The fundamental character and diversity of PRR functions have led to amazingly rapid research in this field, and such investigations are very perspective for medicine as immune system plays a key role in vast majority if not all human diseases, and the process of discovering new aspects of the immune system functioning is rapidly ongoing. There is a plethora of papers analyzing the significance of PRRs in various diseases. One of the most actively exploring fields in PRR biology is their role in cancer aetiopathogenesis. Not surprisingly, it is (as well as tumor immunology in general) a hot spot in cancer biology as well.

1.2 The position of pattern recognition receptors in cancer biology

Since PRRs mediate immune response inducing by many immunoadjuvants (Okamoto and Sato, 2003; Seya, 2003), and many of them regulate immune response against potentially carcinogenic infectious agents (*Helicobacter pylori*, EBV, HPV, HHV-8/KSHV, CMV, *Mycobacterium tuberculosis*, *Streptococcus pneumoniae*, enteropathogenic *Escherichia coli*, *Shigella flexneri*, *Salmonella typhimurium*, *Borrelia burgdorferi*, *Chlamydia pneumoniae*, *Chlamydia trachomatis*, *Chlamydia psittaci*, *Campylobacter jejuni*, *Candida spp.*, *Schistosoma mansoni*, *Paracoccidioides brasiliensis*, *Histoplasma capsulatum* etc.), it seems to be possible to stimulate anti-tumor immunity through their enhanced activation. This hypothesis, originally developed for the TLRs, should be also true for the all PRRs as well (Killeen and Wang, 2006; Tsan, 2006). According to this suggestion, a reinforced PRR activation may protect from infectious agents and prevent, inhibit, or block carcinogenesis whilst disrupted functioning of these PRRs may allow infectious agents or tumor cells to avoid recognition by immune system and, consequently, not to be eliminated. At the same time, such PRR activation may promote carcinogenesis, creating a proinflammatory microenvironment (via action of respective cytokines) that is favorable for the tumor progression and chemoresistance development (Chen, 2007). It may also result in immunosuppression caused by chronic inflammation (Tsan, 2006). Chronic inflammation may promote the development of cervical, endometrial, ovarian, breast, prostate, testicular, nasopharyngeal, lung, esophageal, gastric, colorectal, liver, pancreatic, gallbladder, kidney, bladder, lymphatic malignancies, and feasibly several other cancer types (Kinlen, 2004; Okamoto and Sato, 2003). In this case, on the contrary, lower PRR activity should minimize the effects of chronic inflammation such as enhancement of cancer initiation and promotion/progression and, consequently, decrease the probability of tumor development. So, the situation resembles a double-edged sword. The ideal variant, possibly, is the «golden mean» - the balance between low and high PRR activity. This hypothesis, developed for PRRs, may also be successfully projected on PRR intracellular signaling pathways – if their elements are overexpressed/constantly activated, it may lead to similar consequences as enhanced PRR activation. On the other hand, if the members of PRR pathways are underexpressed/inactivated/unable to do their work at the right time in the right place, it may result in the same effects that arise after decreased PRR activity, and the analogical «golden mean» in functioning of all genes encoding proteins constituting PRR signaling pathways will be the optimal variant.

1.3 Structural genomic variation and its relevance to cancer

The novel approaches in healthcare move towards the model of "personalized medicine". Advances in the healthcare service grow annually as well as their social relevance. Diagnostic tests and target therapy have become a part of our life. However, in spite of the neoteric improvements of the screening and treatment modalities, the prognosis of patients with many diseases including cancer remains poor. Thus, modern molecular biology and medicine are concerned on the developing of more and more new genomic markers that possess predictive, therapeutic, or prognostic significance. Several markers may evaluate predisposition of any person to one or another disease with a certain degree of accuracy based on the results of a simple blood test. The widespread application of these tests can reveal the risk groups in populations, and thereafter, the complex of preventive measures among the risk group subjects may be conducted. Moreover, above-mentioned genomic markers can be identified in the perinatal period, so the choice between "include" or "not to include" in the risk group on their basis can be made maximally early, and, consequently, the preventive measures can have the greatest efficacy. As a result, the integrative systems of predictive genomic markers, defined once, will allow to create the programs of cancer prevention based on them and will permit next generations to be informed and forewarned about their risks and predispositions to certain diseases.

Thereby, the discovery and development of predictive, therapeutic, or prognostic markers is the primary problem of biomedicine at the present time. However, the critical barrier for progress in this field is that it is not always easy to find an effective genomic marker that is exactly associated with a particular disease. One of the most widespread and important markers is the type of genomic markers called single nucleotide polymorphisms (SNPs). They represent a variation in the DNA sequence, when a single nucleotide differs between members of a biological species or paired chromosomes in an individual. The finishing of Human Genome Project and the widespread distribution of genotyping technologies have led to the enormous number of studies devoted to the association of the inherited gene polymorphisms with various diseases. The SNPs may result in amino acid substitutions altering protein function or splicing, and they can also change structure of enhancer sequences during splicing (Lamba et al., 2003) or affect mRNA stability (Tierney and Medcalf, 2001). SNPs may also alter transcription factor binding motifs, changing the efficacy of enhancer or repressor elements (Thomas et al., 2006), and they can alter the structure of translation initiation codons that may lead to the downregulation of wild-type transcript (Zysow et al., 1995). Gene polymorphisms located in the leucine-rich repeats constituting ectodomain of PRRs may affect the ability of receptor to bind pathogens they normally recognize (Bell et al., 2003), SNPs in the transmembrane domain can lead to the defects of the intracellular receptor transport that do not allow to locate a receptor on the membrane (Johnson et al., 2007), and, finally, the polymorphisms in the internal domain may result in the altered interaction with the adaptor proteins or in the disrupted dimerization. So, inherited SNPs of the genes encoding PRRs may alter PRR expression and activity, modulating cancer risk and, possibly, influencing on various features of the cancer progression. The same statement should be true for the genes encoding proteins of PRR signaling pathways.

On the basis of the fundamental and epidemiological studies, it is possible to specify the two fundamental mechanisms for the modulation of cancer risk by the polymorphisms of the genes encoding PRRs and proteins of PRR pathways. The first of them is the impairment of the immune response to the certain pathogens (it can be bacteria, viruses, fungi, protozoan, and helminths) that increase the risk of the potentially carcinogenic infection and promote its development along with further chronic persistence. The second mechanism is an increase of production of proinflammatory cytokines after the binding of the ligand (exogenous or endogenous) that create a condition of carcinogenic chronic inflammation.

2. How to connect structural genomic variation in pattern recognition receptors and cancer?

2.1 Relevant malignancies: the first dimension of investigation

There is a variety of cancer types that can be associated with the inherited alterations in the genes encoding PRRs and proteins of PRR signaling pathways:

- Oral cancer (the alteration of the immune response to *Candida spp.* and other infectious agents colonizing oral cavity);
- Esophageal cancer (the variation of immune response to pathogens infecting esophagus);
- Gastric cancer (on the basis of modulation of the immune response to *Helicobacter pylori*, EBV and other infectious agents potentially causing this disease);
- Cancer of the small bowel (the modulation of the immune response to *Campylobacter jejuni*);
- Colorectal cancer (the alteration of the immune response to many infectious agents inhabiting colon and rectum);
- Liver cancer (the variation of the immune response to HBV, HCV, *Helicobacter hepaticus*, or liver flukes);
- Gallbladder cancer (the modulation of the immune response to infectious agents finding in bile);
- Pancreatic cancer (the alteration of the immune response to the pathogens inhabiting the pancreas);
- Endometrial cancer (the modification of the immune response to several kinds of infectious agents colonizing endometrium);

- Cervical cancer (the alteration of the immune response to HPV and some infectious agents colonizing cervix);
- Ovarian cancer (the variation of immune response to *Chlamydia trachomatis*);
- breast cancer (the modulation of the immune response to some viruses infecting breast including HPV and EBV)
- Prostate cancer (the variation of the immune response to *Propionibacterium acnes* and other uncertain pathogens finding in prostate tissue);
- Testicular cancer (the modification of the immune response to EBV);
- Kidney cancer (the variation of the immune response to bacteria and viruses infecting kidneys);
- Bladder cancer (the modulation of the immune response to certain viruses or *Schistosoma spp.*);
- Nasopharyngeal carcinoma (the alteration of the immune response to EBV);
- Lung cancer (the variation of the immune response to *Mycobacterium tuberculosis, Streptococcus pneumoniae, Chlamydia pneumoniae,* and, possibly, to other infectious agents causing chronic inflammatory lung diseases);
- Lymphoma (the modification of the immune response to EBV and many other infectious agents such as *Borrelia burgdorferi* or *Helicobacter pylori*);
- Kaposi sarcoma (the variation of the immune response to HHV-8/KSHV-infection);
- Brain tumors (the alteration of the immune response to CMV and other viruses).

2.2 Selection of valuable polymorphisms: the second dimension of investigation

It is important to remember that there are two main components determining the importance of the SNP in the programs of cancer prevention based on genomic risk markers: the value of odds ratio (OR) between cases and controls (as in the whole population as in subgroups) and the prevalence of the polymorphism in population, and they both may vary in different geographic regions. It is desirable to develop not the one general program, but a number of the individual programs for the different countries/populations/environmental conditions. At the moment, it is possible only to recommend a list of polymorphisms for the further investigation since only small number of studies with perfect design was carried out. The list of relevant polymorphisms that can be admitted as the most perspective for the further oncogenomic investigations may be created according to the following rules:

Gene polymorphism may be included into the short list for the further oncogenomic studies if:

- The SNP leads to the substantial functional consequences on the molecular level (for instance, it strongly affects transcription, splicing, translation, stability and transport of pre-mRNA, mRNA, non-coding RNA or protein encoding by the gene, or it noticeably influences signaling of synthesized protein);
- It is associated with risk of cancer in the population studies;
- It has any functional consequences on the molecular level and it is strongly (threshold OR value may be individual for each cancer type) associated with condition that significantly increases risk of cancer.
- The gene polymorphism can be also included into the extended list if:
- It is characterized by more subtle functional alterations in the gene that, however, still result in qualitative or quantitative alterations of the encoding protein (or non-coding RNA);

- It is associated only with condition that substantially increases risk of cancer but not with risk of cancer.

One question may immediately arise: how to distinguish «substantial» and «more subtle» functional changes on the molecular level? It seems to be difficult to answer only on the basis of general principles of molecular biology since for one gene even the smallest alteration in its structure may lead to critical consequences, for another one converse statement can be true, and the effect also greatly depends on the position of the polymorphism. Therefore, an assessment of power of functional alteration should be individual for each gene, and although conclusions obtained in various investigations may differ, these discrepancies would not distort the general picture: if the polymorphism has «serious» functional consequences according to the results of one research, it definitely should be added into the short list until these conclusions will not be subverted. In any case, the general value of creation of such short and extended lists of the prescriptive polymorphisms seems to overcome difficulties related to these complications. It is important that many polymorphisms can be simply in the linkage disequilibrium with truly functional variants, and fundamental investigations are needed to determine are they only markers of association or indeed causal variants. All polymorphisms that are only in the linkage disequilibrium with functional ones should be excluded from both lists.

In concordance with this conception, the following SNPs of the genes encoding PRRs and proteins of PRR signaling pathways may be accepted as the most valuable for the further oncogenomic investigations on the basis of the analysis of relevant published literature (Table 3):

Gene	Polymorphism
TLR1-TLR6-TLR10 gene cluster:	rs10008492, rs4833103, rs5743815, rs11466657
TLR2	rs3804100, rs4696480, -196 - -174 del (Delta22), GT-microsatellite polymorphism
TLR4	rs4986790, rs4986791, rs16906079, rs11536891, rs7873784, rs1927911, rs10759932, rs10116253, rs11536889, rs11536858
TLR9	rs5743836, rs352140
TIRAP/MAL	rs8177400, rs8177399, rs8177374, rs7932766
MyD88	rs1319438, rs199396
IRAK1	rs1059703, rs3027898, rs10127175
TRAF3	rs7143468, rs12147254, rs11160707
TRAF6	rs331455, rs331457
TOLLIP	rs5743867
IRF3	rs7251
IRF5	rs2004640, rs2280714, rs10954213, 5 bp indel (CGGGG) polymorphism
NOD1	rs2075820, ND(1)+32656
NOD2	rs2066842, rs2066844, rs2066845, rs2006847
MRC1	rs1926736, rs2478577, rs2437257, rs691005
CD209	rs2287886, rs735239, rs735240, rs4804803
CLEC7A	rs16910526
RIG-I	rs36055726, rs11795404, rs10813831

Table 3. The short list of polymorphisms of the genes encoding PRRs and proteins of their signaling pathways promising for the further oncogenomic studies.

The following polymorphisms of the genes encoding PRRs and proteins of PRR signaling pathways may be added into the extended list for the further oncogenomic investigations (Table 4):

Gene	Polymorphism
TLR1-TLR6-TLR10 gene cluster:	rs4833095, rs5743551, rs5743618, rs4129009
TLR2	rs5743704, rs62323857, rs1219178642
TLR3	rs5743305, rs3775291, rs121434431, rs5743316
TLR4	rs1927914, rs2149356
TLR5	rs5744168
TLR7	rs179008
TLR8	rs3764880, rs2407992
TLR9	rs352139, rs187084, rs41308230, rs5743844
TIRAP/MAL	rs7932976, rs595209, rs8177375
MyD88	rs156265, rs7744
IRAK1	rs1059702, rs7061789, rs2239673, rs763737, rs3027907, rs5945174
IRAK3	rs1732886, rs1732888, rs10506481, rs1624395, rs1370128
IRAK4	rs1461567, rs4251513, rs425155
TRAF1	rs6920220, rs10818488, rs3761847, rs7021206
TRAF2	rs7852970
TRAF6	rs540386
TOLLIP	rs5743854
IRF1	rs11242115, rs839, rs9282763
IRF3	rs2304204, rs2304206
IRF5	rs4728142, rs41298401, rs13242262, rs10488631, rs729302, rs3807306
IRF7	rs1131665
IRF8	rs17824933
NOD1	rs72551113, rs72551107, rs6958571, rs2907749, rs2907748, rs2075822, rs2075819, rs2075818
NOD2	rs104895493, rs104895476, rs104895475, rs104895474, rs104895473, rs104895472, rs104895462, rs104895461, rs104895460, rs104895438, rs5743291, rs5743260, rs2076756, rs2066843, Pro371Thr, Ala794Pro, Gln908His
MRC1	rs692527, rs2477664, rs691005, rs2253120, rs2477637
CD209	rs735240
RIG-I	rs3824456, rs669260
MAVS/VISA/IPS-1	rs11905552, rs17857295, rs2326369, rs7269320

Table 4. The extended list of the polymorphisms of the genes encoding PRRs and proteins of their signaling pathways promising for the further oncogenomic studies.

2.3 How to organize the study: the third dimension of investigation

The drawing-up of a rigorous study protocol is the crucial moment in the molecular epidemiology, and in some cases the complexity of the research is considerable. Even if the investigation has a valuable aim, sufficient funding and is carried out in an excellent laboratory, errors in the study design may lead to the misrepresentation of the research results and, hence, to the reduction of their usefulness. All moments that can distort the study accuracy should be taken into account, and certain, the most relevant of them, are discussed below. Obviously, the methods of the sample collection, DNA extraction, and PCR conduction should be reliable enough. Modern methods such as automated DNA extraction, real-time PCR, and pyrosequencing should be used, although traditional methods such as allele-specific PCR with visualization in the agarose gel can be exploited as well, and their application definitely will be continued for the next decade. Anyway, automated methods should be of choice compared to methods where a subjective factor is substantial and can influence the results. The improvement of existing technologies and the development of new ones may elevate the accuracy of DNA extraction and PCR, leading to increase of validity of the results and, consequently, to the further progress in the field.

Other important aspects of the study design also should be considered. To differentiate the impact of the chronic inflammatory conditions from the contribution of the other mechanisms in the association of the polymorphisms of the genes encoding PRRs and proteins of PRR signaling pathways with cancer risk, the stratification of cases and controls by infectious agent status and chronic inflammation status should be mandatory in the further studies devoted to this problem. The sample size should be sufficient, and it depends on the frequency of target polymorphism - if it is high, sample size can be less than in the studies where target SNP frequency is low. There is also a lack of studies investigating functional consequences of the polymorphisms of the genes encoding PRRs and proteins of PRR pathways on molecular level (for instance, alterations in the promoter activity, in the gene expression on the transcriptomic and proteomic levels, in stability or/and localization of the non-coding RNA, pre-mRNA, mRNA and protein inside the cell, in protein structure and functions, etc.). It is important since many polymorphisms can be simply in linkage disequilibrium with the other, truly functional variants, and thus such fundamental studies are necessary to clarify their role (are they only markers of association or indeed causal variants?). In addition, in certain populations replication studies should be conducted to prove results that were obtained in prime investigations, particularly if the sample size was not large.

There are certain disparities in different population studies investigating the association of the polymorphisms of the genes encoding PRRs and proteins of their signaling pathways with various aspects of cancer development. General reasons for these discrepancies may include confounding host, bacterial, or environmental factors in different ethnicities modulating the penetrance of the variant allele and affecting risk of condition increasing cancer risk (such as autoimmune diseases, precancerous gastric lesions, tuberculosis, recurrent pneumonia etc.), different bacterial impact in aetiology of such conditions in different populations (that will be reflected in different features of PRR-mediated immune response because of specific PRR-ligand interaction), differences in the sample size, in age/gender/BMI/ethnicity/TNM stage/other clinicopathological characteristics between the study samples, in the prevalence of infectious agent (e.g. HP or EBV) in case and control groups, differences in diagnostics, stratification, genotyping methods, and chance. In addition, certain studies in which negative results were obtained could never been published (so-called file drawer effect) that may create a significant bias and distort a picture that we can observe at the moment. Unfortunately, although some genome-wide association studies (GWAS) relevant to the discussing problem were performed, it is usually not possible to compare them with the non-GWAS on the same cancer type since there are no non-GWAS investigating association of the same SNPs with similar malignancies. It may be feasible in future when the number of studies devoted to this issue will be enough for correct comparative analysis.

3. Hot spots in the field

The most intriguing moments in the problem of the association of inherited structural variation in the genes encoding PRRs and proteins of PRR signaling pathways with features of cancer development are:

- Are SNPs in the genes encoding PRRs or proteins of PRR signaling pathways associated with the features of cancer progression or only with cancer risk? Existing studies have shown controversial results, and the results of most of them allow to suggest that there is no or weak correlation between such polymorphisms and peculiarities of cancer progression.
- Are the polymorphisms of the genes encoding CLRs, RLRs, or specific proteins of their signaling pathways associated with risk or progression of cancer? If yes, would be appropriate to include them in the list of polymorphisms using in programs of cancer risk determination and further cancer prevention? As it was shown above, there are some premises to think that these SNPs may be associated with cancer risk. Further fundamental and population studies are necessary to answer this question.
- Do the polymorphisms of genes encoding PRRs or proteins of PRR signaling pathways (particularly TLRs and TLR pathway) correlate with altered prostate cancer risk or progression? Despite there are some fundamental mechanisms allowing to hypothesize that *TLR* gene polymorphisms may play a role in prostate cancer aetiology, and a number of comprehensive projects on large samples in various countries was conducted, the reliable associations of these SNPs with prostate cancer risk or with features of prostate cancer progression were not detected, and results vary in different populations.
- Are the polymorphisms of the genes of PRR signaling pathways associated with cancer risk or progression to the same extent as polymorphisms of the genes encoding PRRs? It is logical that if SNP of gene encoding specific PRR is associated with risk or progression features of certain malignancies, polymorphisms in the genes encoding specific signaling molecules constituting pathways of this receptor should correlate with similar neoplasms, if they have substantial functional consequences on the molecular level. In contrast to the polymorphisms of the genes encoding TLRs, whose association with solid tumors is a subject of investigation in a lot of genetic association studies, the polymorphisms of the genes encoding proteins of TLR pathway are investigated mostly in relation to leukemia and lymphoma, and their association with epithelial tumors is discovered very poorly. SNPs affecting functional parts of TLR pathway central elements (MyD88, TRIF/TICAM1, TIRP/TRAM/TICAM2, TIRAP/MAL, IRAKs, TRAF3, TRAF6, TAK1, TAB1, TAB2, PKR, IRF3, IRF7) should be the most significant for the oncogenomic studies analyzing this problem.

- How the polymorphisms of the genes encoding PRRs and proteins of PRR signaling pathways interact with each other in relation to determination of cancer risk and progression? Particularly, how SNPs of positive and negative regulators of PRR activity (especially, miRNA) influence on cancer risk or progression if they are inherited together? Answers to these questions remain elusive at present time, and should be obtained from the fundamental and population studies in the future.
- Which the SNPs of the genes encoding PRRs and proteins of PRR pathways have independent significance, and which are just in the linkage disequilibrium? Knowledge of it may help in listing of the polymorphisms useful in the programs of cancer risk determination and further prevention.
- Which SNPs of the genes encoding PRRs and proteins of PRR pathways should be included in such list? Which of them have universal effect for each cancer type, and which influence on risk or/and progression of one cancer type but have no effect in relation to another malignancy? Differences in the association of the same SNP with different malignancies should be explained by features of specific PAMP-PRR interaction (probably, certain characteristics of ligand binding), or, possibly, on peculiarities of DAMP-PRR interaction. List of SNPs prescriptive for the further oncogenomic investigations may be created according to the conception suggested above.
- How SNPs of the genes encoding PRRs and proteins of PRR pathways affect cancer risk or progression in different populations and their subgroups? How this information may be adjusted for application in the creation of the programs of cancer risk determination and further prevention? Only large, comprehensive, well-designed population studies may give answer to these questions.
- Do the polymorphisms of the genes encoding PRRs and proteins of PRR pathways influence on cancer risk only through increase of risk of chronic inflammatory conditions, or they can affect it also through other mechanisms? How this information may be used in the programs of cancer risk determination and further prevention? To answer these questions, control group in population studies should include not only healthy controls, but also controls with the chronic inflammatory conditions predisposing to investigating cancer type.
- Which infectious agents recognizing by various PRRs are carcinogenic, and which are not? It may help to define the cancer types associated with the SNPs of the genes encoding specific PRRs and proteins constituting PRR signaling pathways. Fundamental studies devoted to the investigation of infectious agent-PRR interactions, to the investigation of carcinogenicity of known infectious agents and to the discovery of new, possibly carcinogenic, infectious agents, should answer this question.

No doubt, the determination of the role of SNPs in genes encoding PRRs and proteins of PRR signaling pathways in fields of tumor immunology and molecular epidemiology of cancer may open new pages in the cancer biology and cancer prevention.

4. Acknowledgements

I would like to thank Prof. Elena B. Brusina and Arseniy Yuzhalin for their support during the writing of this chapter.

5. References

Bell, J.K.; Mullen, G.E.; Leifer, C.A.; Mazzoni, A.; Davies, D.R. & Segal, D.M. (2003). Leucine-rich repeats and pathogen recognition in toll-like receptors. *Trends in Immunology*, Vol.24, No.10, (October 2003), pp. 528–533, ISSN 1471-4906

Bell, J.K.; Botos, I.; Hall, P.R.; Askins, J.; Shiloach, J.; Davies, D.R. & Segal, D.M. (2006). The molecular structure of the TLR3 extracellular domain. *Journal of Endotoxin Research*, Vol.12, No.6, (December 2006), pp. 375-378, ISSN 0968-0519

Brown, S.L.; Riehl, T.E.; Walker, M.R.; Geske, M.J.; Doherty, J.M.; Stenson, W.F.; Stappenbeck, T.S. (2007). Myd88-dependent positioning of Ptgs2-expressing stromal cells maintains colonic epithelial proliferation during injury. *The Journal of Clinical Investigation*, Vol.117, No.1, (January 2007), pp. 258–269, ISSN 0021-9738

Chamaillard, M.; Hashimoto, M.; Horie, Y.; Masumoto, J.; Qiu, S.; Saab, L.; Ogura, Y.; Kawasaki, A.; Fukase, K.; Kusumoto, S.; Valvano, M.A.; Foster, S.J.; Mak, T.W.; Nuñez, G. & Inohara, N. (2003). An essential role for NOD1 in host recognition of bacterial peptidoglycan containing diaminopimelic acid. *Nature Immunology*, Vol.4, No.7, (July 2003), pp. 702-707, ISSN 1529-2908

Chang, Z.L. (2010). Important aspects of Toll-like receptors, ligands and their signaling pathways. *Inflammation Research*, Vol.59, No.10, (October 2010), pp. 791-808, ISSN 1023-3830

Chen, G.; Shaw, M.H.; Kim, Y.G. & Nuñez, G. (2009). NOD-like receptors: role in innate immunity and inflammatory disease. *Annual Review of Pathology*, Vol.4, pp. 365-398, ISSN 1553-4006

Chen, R.; Alvero, A.B.; Silasi, D.A. & Mor, G. (2007). Inflammation, cancer and chemoresistance: taking advantage of the toll-like receptor signaling pathway. *Americam Journal of Reproductive Immunology*, Vol.57, No.2, (February 2007), pp. 93–107, ISSN 1046-7408

Elinav, E.; Strowig, T.; Henao-Mejia, J. & Flavell, R.A. (2011). Regulation of the antimicrobial response by NLR proteins. *Immunity*, Vol.34, No.5, (May 2011), pp.665–679, ISSN 1074-7613

Faustin, B.; Lartigue, L.; Brucy, J.M.; Luciano, F.; Sergienko, E.; Bailly-Maitre, B.; Volkmann, N.; Hanein, D.; Rouiller, I. & Reed, J.C. (2007). Reconstituted NALP1 inflammasome reveals two-step mechanism of caspase-1 activation. *Molecular Cell*, Vol.25, No.5, (March 2007), pp. 713-724, ISSN 1097-2765

Fukata, M.; Chen, A.; Klepper, A.; Krishnareddy, S.; Vamadevan, A.S.; Thomas, L.S.; Xu, R.; Inoue, H.; Arditi, M.; Dannenberg, A.J. & Abreu, M.T. (2006). Cox-2 is regulated by Toll-like receptor-4 (TLR4) signaling: role in proliferation and apoptosis in the intestine. *Gastroenterology*, Vol.131, No.3, (September 2006), pp. 862–877, ISSN 0016-5085

Girardin, S.E.; Boneca, I.G.; Viala, J.; Chamaillard, M.; Labigne, A.; Thomas, G.; Philpott, D.J. & Sansonetti, P.J. (2003). Nod2 is a general sensor of peptidoglycan through muramyl dipeptide (MDP) detection. *Journal of Biological Chemistry*, Vol.278, No.11, (March 2003), pp. 8869-8872, ISSN 0021-9258

Girardin, S.E.; Travassos, L.H.; Hervé, M.; Blanot, D.; Boneca, I.G.; Philpott, D.J.; Sansonetti, P.J. & Mengin-Lecreulx, D. (2003). Nod1 detects a unique muropeptide from gram-negative bacterial peptidoglycan. *Science*, Vol.300, No.5625, (June 2003), pp. 1584-1587, ISSN 0036-8075

Hashimoto, C.; Hudson, K.L. & Anderson, K.V. (1988). The Toll gene of Drosophila, required for dorsal-ventral embryonic polarity, appears to encode a transmembrane protein. *Cell*, Vol.52, No.2, (January 1988), pp. 269-279, ISSN 0092-8674

Honda, K. & Taniguchi, T. (2006). IRFs: master regulators of signalling by Toll-like receptors and cytosolic pattern-recognition receptors. *Nature Reviews. Immunology*, Vol.6, No.9, (September 2006), pp. 644-658, ISSN 1474-1733

Huyton, T.; Rossjohn, J. & Wilce, M. (2007). Toll-like receptors: structural pieces of a curve-shaped puzzle. *Immunology and Cell Biology*, Vol.85, No.6, (August-September 2007), pp. 406–410, ISSN 0818-9641

Inohara, N.; Koseki, T.; del Peso, L.; Hu, Y.; Yee, C.; Chen, S.; Carrio, R.; Merino, J.; Liu, D.; Ni, J. & Núñez, G. (1999). Nod1, an Apaf-1-like activator of caspase-9 and nuclear factor-kappaB. *Journal of Biological Chemistry*, Vol.274, No.21, (May 1999), pp. 14560-14567, ISSN 0021-9258

Ismair, M.G.; Vavricka, S.R.; Kullak-Ublick, G.A.; Fried, M.; Mengin-Lecreulx, D. & Girardin, S.E. (2006). hPepT1 selectively transports muramyl dipeptide but not Nod1-activating muramyl peptides. *Canadian Journal of Physiology and Pharmacology*, Vol.84, No.12, (December 2006), pp. 1313–1319, ISSN 0008-4212

Jin, M.S. & Lee, J.O. (2008). Structures of the toll-like receptor family and its ligand complexes. *Immunity*, Vol.29, No.2, (August 2008), pp. 182-191, ISSN 1074-7613

Johnson, C.M.; Lyle, E.A.; Omueti, K.O.; Stepensky, V.A.; Yegin, O.; Alpsoy, E.; Hamann, L.; Schumann, R.R. & Tapping, R.I. (2007). Cutting edge: a common polymorphism impairs cell surface trafficking and functional responses of TLR1 but protects against leprosy. *Journal of Immunology*, Vol.178, No.12, (June 2007), pp. 7520–7524, ISSN 0022-1767

Kanneganti, T.D.; Lamkanfi, M. & Núñez, G. (2007). Intracellular NOD-like receptors in host defense and disease. *Immunity*, Vol.27, No.4, (October 2007), pp. 549-559, ISSN 1074-7613

Kawai, T. & Akira, S. (2011). Toll-like receptors and their crosstalk with other innate receptors in infection and immunity. *Immunity*, Vol.34, No.5, (May 2011), pp. 637–650, ISSN 1074-7613

Killeen, S.D.; Wang, J.H.; Andrews, E.J. & Redmond, H.P. (2006). Exploitation of the toll-like receptor system in cancer: a doubled-edged sword? *British Journal of Cancer*, Vol.95, No.3, (August 2006), pp. 247–252, ISSN 0007-0920

Kim, D.; Kim, M.A.; Cho, I.H.; Kim, M.S.; Lee, S.; Jo, E.K.; Choi, S.Y.; Park, K.; Kim, J.S.; Akira, S.; Na, H.S.; Oh, S.B. & Lee, S.J. (2007). A critical role of toll-like receptor 2 in nerve injury-induced spinal cord glial cell activation and pain hypersensitivity. *Journal of Biological Chemistry*, Vol.282, No.20, (May 2007), pp. 14975–14983, ISSN 0021-9258

Kim, H.M.; Park, B.S.; Kim, J.I.; Kim, S.E.; Lee, J.; Oh, S.C.; Enkhbayar, P.; Matsushima, N.; Lee, H.; Yoo, O.J. & Lee JO. (2007). Crystal structure of the TLR4-MD-2 complex with bound endotoxin antagonist eritoran. *Cell*, Vol.130, No.5, (September 2007), pp. 906–917, ISSN 0092-8674

Kinlen, L. (2004). Infections and immune factors in cancer: the role of epidemiology. *Oncogene*, Vol.23, No.38, (August 2004), pp. 6341–6348, ISSN 0950-9232

Kumar, H.; Kawai, T. & Akira, S. (2009). Pathogen recognition in the innate immune response. *The Biochemical Journal*, Vol.420, No.1, (April 2009), pp. 1-16, ISSN 0264-6021

Lamba, V.; Lamba, J.; Yasuda, K.; Strom, S.; Davila, J.; Hancock, M.L.; Fackenthal, J.D.; Rogan, P.K.; Ring, B.; Wrighton, S.A. & Schuetz, E.G. (2003). Hepatic CYP2B6 expression: gender and ethnic differences and relationship to CYP2B6 genotype and CAR (constitutive androstane receptor) expression. *The Journal of Pharmacology and Experimental Therapeutics*, Vol.307, No.3, (December 2003), pp. 906–922, ISSN 0022-3565

Liu, L.; Botos, I.; Wang, Y.; Leonard, J.N.; Shiloach, J.; Segal, D.M. & Davies, D.R. (2008). Structural basis of toll-like receptor 3 signaling with double-stranded RNA. *Science*, Vol.320, No.5874, (April 2008), pp. 379–381, ISSN 0036-8075

Loo, Y.M. & Gale, M. Jr. (2011). Immune signaling by RIG-I-like receptors. *Immunity*, Vol.34, No.5, (May 2011), pp. 680-692, ISSN 1074-7613

Marina-García, N.; Franchi, L.; Kim, Y.G.; Miller, D.; McDonald, C.; Boons, G.J. & Núñez, G. (2008). Pannexin-1-mediated intracellular delivery of muramyl dipeptide induces caspase-1 activation via cryopyrin/NLRP3 independently of Nod2. *Journal of Immunology*, Vol.180, No.6, (March 2008), pp. 4050-4057, ISSN 0022-1767

Matsushima, N.; Tanaka, T.; Enkhbayar, P.; Mikami, T.; Taga, M.; Yamada, K. & Kuroki, Y. (2007). Comparative sequence analysis of leucine-rich repeats (LRRs) within vertebrate toll-like receptors. *BMC Genomics*, Vol.8, (May 2007), p. 124, ISSN 1471-2164

Medzhitov, R.; Preston-Hurlburt, P. & Janeway, C.A. Jr. (1997). A human homologue of the Drosophila Toll protein signals activation of adaptive immunity. *Nature*, Vol. 388, No. 6640, (July 1997), pp. 394-397, ISSN 0028-0836

Ogura, Y.; Inohara, N.; Benito, A.; Chen, F.F.; Yamaoka, S. & Nunez, G. (2001). Nod2, a Nod1/Apaf-1 family member that is restricted to monocytes and activates NF-kappaB. J *Journal of Biological Chemistry* , Vol. 276, No.7, (February 2001), pp. 4812-4818, ISSN 0021-9258

O'Neill, L.A. & Bowie, A.G. (2007). The family of five: TIR-domain-containing adaptors in Toll-like receptor signalling. *Nature Reviews. Immunology*, Vol. 7, No.5, (May 2007), pp. 353-364, ISSN 1474-1733

Okamoto, M. & Sato, M. (2003). Toll-like receptor signaling in anti-cancer immunity. *The Journal of Medical Investigation*, Vol. 50, No.1-2, (February 2003), pp. 9–24, ISSN 1343-1420

Osorio, F. & Reis E Sousa, C. (2011). Myeloid C-type lectin receptors in pathogen recognition and host defense. *Immunity*, Vol. 34, No.5, (May 2011), pp. 651–664, ISSN 1074-7613

Pålsson-McDermott, E.M. & O'Neill, L.A. (2007). Building an immune system from nine domains. *Biochemical Society Transactions*, Vol. 35, No.6, (December 2007), pp. 1437-1444, ISSN 0300-5127

Rakoff-Nahoum, S. & Medzhitov, R. (2008). Role of toll-like receptors in tissue repair and tumorigenesis. *Biochemistry (Moscow)*, Vol.73, No.5, (May 2008), pp. 555–561, ISSN 0006-2979

Ratner, A.J.; Aguilar, J.L.; Shchepetov, M.; Lysenko, E.S. & Weiser, J.N. (2007). Nod1 mediates cytoplasmic sensing of combinations of extracellular bacteria. *Cellular Microbiology*, Vol. 9, No.5, (May 2007), pp. 1343-1351, ISSN 1462-5814

Seya, T.; Akazawa, T.; Uehori, J.; Matsumoto, M.; Azuma, I. & Toyoshima, K. (2003). Role of toll-like receptor and their adaptors in adjuvant immunotherapy for cancer. *Anticancer Research*, Vol.23, No.6a, (November-December 2003), pp. 4369–4376, ISSN 0250-7005

Shaw, P.J.; Lamkanfi, M. & Kanneganti, T.D. (2010). NOD-like receptor (NLR) signaling beyond the inflammasome. *European Journal of Immunology*, Vol.40, No.3, (March 2010), pp. 624-627, ISSN 0014-2980

Takada, E.; Okahira, S.; Sasai, M.; Funami, K.;, Seya, T. & Matsumoto, M. (2007). C-terminal LRRs of human Toll-like receptor 3 control receptor dimerization and signal transmission. *Molecular Immunology*, Vol. 44, No.15, (July 2007), pp. 3633-3640, ISSN 0161-5890

Takeuchi, O. & Akira, S. (2001). Toll-like receptors; their physiological role and signal transduction system. *International Immunopharmacology*, Vol.1, No.4, (April 2001), pp. 625-635, ISSN 1567-5769

Thomas, K.H.; Meyn, P. & Suttorp, N. (2006). Single nucleotide polymorphism in 5'-flanking region reduces transcription of surfactant protein B gene in H441 cells. *American Journal of Physiology. Lung Cellular and Molecular Physiology,* Vol.291, No.3, (September 2006), pp. 386–390, ISSN 1040-0605

Tierney, M.J. & Medcalf, R.L. (2001). Plasminogen activator inhibitor type 2 contains mRNA instability elements within exon 4 of the coding region. Sequence homology to coding region instability determinants in other mRNAs. *Journal of Biological Chemistry*, Vol.276, No.17, (April 2001), pp. 13675–13684, ISSN 0021-9258

Tsan, M.F. (2006). Toll-like receptors, inflammation, and cancer. *Seminars in Cancer Biology*, Vol.16, No.1, (February 2006), pp. 32-37, ISSN 1044579X

Wong, Y.; Sethu, C.; Louafi, F. & Hossain, P. (2011). Lipopolysaccharide Regulation of Toll-Like Receptor-4 and Matrix Metalloprotease-9 in Human Primary Corneal Fibroblast Cells. *Investigative Ophthalmology and Visual Science*, Vol.52, No.5, (April 2011), pp. 2796-2803, ISSN 0146-0404

Yamamoto, M.; Takeda, K. & Akira, S. (2004). TIR domain-containing adaptors define the specificity of TLR signaling. *Molecular Immunology*, Vol.40, No.12, (February 2004), pp. 861–868, ISSN 0161-5890

Zhu, J. & Mohan, C. (2010). Toll-like receptor signaling pathways--therapeutic opportunities. *Mediators of Inflammation*, Vol.2010, p. 781235, ISSN 0962-9351

Zysow, B.R.; Lindahl, G.E.; Wade, D.P.; Knight, B.L. & Lawn, R.M. (1995). C/T polymorphism in the 5'untranslated region of the apolipoprotein(a) gene introduces an upstream ATG and reduces in vitro translation. *Arteriosclerosis, Thrombosis and Vascular Biology*, Vol.15, No.1, (January 1995), pp. 58–64, ISSN 1049-8834

Section 2

Basics of Autoimmunity and Multiple Sclerosis

6

Glial and Axonal Pathology in Multiple Sclerosis

Maria de los Angeles Robinson-Agramonte[1], Alina González-Quevedo[2] and Carlos Alberto Goncalves[3]
[1]*International Center for Neurological Restoration,*
[2]*Institute of Neurology and Neurosurgery,*
[3]*Federal University of Rio Grande del Sur. Porto Alegre,*
[1,2]*Cuba*
[3]*Brazil*

1. Introduction

The central nervous system (CNS) consists of a series of complex structures which comprise cellular elements with basic communication functions and elaboration of information as part of their role in the process of biological adaptation and maintenance of homeostasis [Hickey WF, 2001].

1.1 Mayor components of the CNS

The major components of the CNS; neurons and neurites, microglias, astrocytes, ependymal cells and oligodendrocytes, establish all an important interrelationship, vital to the brain maintenance homeostasis. Ependymal cells lay around layers of astrocytes, which in turn envelop neurons, neurites and vascular elements. In addition, the normal CNS parenchyma contains blood vessels and resident macrophages. Glial cells, as they possess no conventional synaptic contacts, differ from neurons mainly establishing a rich interrelationship with other CNS components. The neuroglia, brain interstitial element, is recognized as including three groups of glial cells: 1) macroglias, such as astrocytes and oligodendrocytes,2) microglia and 3) ependymal cells.

Regarding glial function, the astrocytes are involved in glutamate uptake, repair and transport, and are part of the blood brain barrier (BBB). Studies conducted by Reese and Karnowosky [1967] indicate that the astrocyte end-feet provide little resistance to molecule movement, and that the blockage of their passage into the brain occurs at the endothelial-cell-lining blood vessels. In this case, endothelial cells forming for brain vascular endothelium, play an important role in the communication between the CNS and the periphery, this latter understood as intravascular space.

Oligodendrocytes are the myelin producing cells within the CNS and are potentially highly vulnerable to immune mediated damage, since they share together with the myelin sheath many molecules with affinities to elicit specific T and B cell responses, which lead to their destruction. Oligodendrocytes do not express class I or II MHC molecules, but a wide profile of cytokine receptors, both pro-inflammatory and regulatory which have been found on this cell-type, suggesting their innate and adaptative ability to participate in immune response.

Microglial cells, the most interesting and enigmatic CNS type cells, play a role in phagocytosis and inflammatory response in the CNS. Under normal conditions these cells seem to be in a resting state, becoming a very active macrophage during the disease, and constituting the major effector cell in immune-mediated damage in the CNS. An explosive activity in the field of microglia cell-research conducted in the past 15 to 20 years has led to the identification of microglia as a highly efficient accessory and effector cell of the immune system. Microglia expresses class II MHC antigen upon activation [Perry & Gordon, 1997] in the absence of a T cell response, which suggests that major histocompatibility complex (MHC) antigen expression may represent a marker of activation and/or a state of immunological competence. Microglia are also major producers of a large number of proinflammatory cytokines with well-known effects on T cells [Perry & Gordon, 1997]. All the previous information supports a wide glial involvement in brain internal homeostasis maintenance that plays a major role in the regulatory function of barrier systems.

1.2 Brain neurovascular unit

The blood-brain barrier (BBB) system, located between the intravascular space and the brain tissue, constitutes a phenomenon of selective permeability and reduced exchange of products between the blood and the nervous system. It is a characteristic of brain capillaries and is regulated by the cells that form the neurovascular unit (NVU) [Becher et al, 2006; Nathanson & Chun, 1990; Seyfert & Faultish, 2003] and the dynamics of cerebrospinal fluid (CSF) flow [Becher et al, 2006; Seyfert & Faultish, 2003]. NVU refers to the dynamic exchange among the cellular elements forming these barriers in the brain; there is a regional specialized interface between the neural tissue and the blood [Neutwelt et al, 2008].

The NVU is formed by: 1) The CSF-blood barrier, site of immunological communication between the CSF and intravascular space, which favours antigenic recognition and lymphocyte activation at this level [Bigio, 1995; Nathanson & Chun, 1990a; Redzic et al, 2005]; 2) The meningeal barrier, that is, the aracnoid membrane, bordering the duramater, where the CSF drains to the dural venous sinuses, the olfactory nerve and the carotid sheaths[Nag S. 2003]; 3) the BBB, constituted by the brain vascular endothelium, regulates the entrance of molecules and supply of nutrients to the brain, as well as preserving the ionic homeostasis in the brain environment [Petty & Lo, 2002]; 4) the blood-nerve barrier, which surrounds the axon tangles and includes the endothelial membrane of the endoneural capillary and the perinerium [Hemmer, 2004]; 5) the blood–retinal barrier, formed by the retinal endothelial capillary and the retinal tissue, like BBB; 6) the blood-labyrinth barrier, which has as anatomical reference the endolymph-blood and endolymph-perilymph barriers.These capillaries are lined with endothelial cells that are joined by tight junctions and physiologically form the blood–labyrinth barrier that is essential for sensitive auditory function; and 7) the blood-spinal cord barrier - with a greater permeability than the BBB - which communicates with the periphery through the nerve roots plexus [Haukins & Davis , 2005].

For centuries, the BBB, the lack of conventional lymphatic drainage and low response to aloantigens inoculated in the CNS, were arguments to consider this compartment as a privileged site. Nevertheless, today it is well known, that there is no such privilege, but rather the main differences of the immune response in the brain, regarding the periphery, are in the kinetics and the degree of regulation of the different stages of the immune response at this level, which will take place under the functional control of the immune response and influence of cellular mediators acting in a regulated quantitative and temporally balanced sequence[Fisher & Gage, 1993].

In normal conditions, neurons are unable to interact with T-cells, via MHC expression antigens, however, neurons possess unique antigenic proteins, which are normally sequestered by the BBB from the circulating immune system, making the CNS vulnerable to immune-mediated damage. On the other hand, there is increasing evidence on the ability of astrocytes to act as accessory cells of the immune system, as a facultative phagocyte able to interact with lymphocytes, since astrocytes express class II MHC antigens, essential molecules for antigen presentation to T helper cells. Astrocytes are also able to synthesize cytokines like interleukin 1, interferon γ and tumor necrosis factor, among others. During inflammation, the mechanism of selective transport displayed by endothelial cells (EC) is disrupted and endothelial tight junctions display altered permeability with subsequent edema within and around neighboring astrocytes. Evidence of the immunological role of microglia in demyelinating diseases like Multiple Sclerosis, as well as evidences of their putative role as a major effector-cell of immune mediated cell damage at this level has been well established.

1.3 Astrocytes as dynamic regulators of neuronal functional activity

One of the main functions of astrocytes is the uptake of neurotransmitters released from nerve terminals. But astrocytes can also release neuroactive agents, including transmitters, eicosanoids, steroids, neuropeptides and growth factors [Anderson & Swanson, 2000]. The regulation and mechanism (or mechanisms) of astrocyte-mediated release of neuroactive compounds are for most agents poorly defined. Release of glutamate appears to be the primary mechanism by which astrocytes modulate synaptic transmission [Kang, 1998].

In addition, astrocytes might serve neurons not so much as servants but as parents - both literally, as a developmental source of new neurons, and figuratively, as the regulators and judges of neuronal behaviour and activities. Simply stated, astrocytes command neurons what to do, besides keeping their environment clean. Interactions among astrocytes, neurons and endothelial cells define the gliovascular unit.

BBB is a diffusion barrier that regulates the exchange of molecules between the two tissues. The primary seal of the blood-brain barrier is formed by endothelial tight junctions. Astrocytes enwrap the vasculature with a large number of endfeet covering the vessel wall, although their role in BBB is poorly defined, they do not have a barrier function in the mammalian brain [del Zoppo & Hallenbeck, 2000]. Several factors released by astrocytes might be important for the induction and maintenance of the blood-brain barrier, as manifested by the appearance of endothelial tight junctions in cells ensheathed by astrocytic endfeet. Several investigators have studied this issue and have identified agents released by astrocytes, including transforming growth factor-a (TGFa) and glial-derived neurotrophic factor (GDNF), that support the formation of tight junctions in cultured endothelial cells [Abbott, 2002].

In general, the interactions between the barriers conforming the neurovascular unit, constitute the base of pathological events involved in neurological diseases, with inflammatory, neurodegenerative or autoimmune components as in MS, neuromyelitis optica (NMO), posterior uveitis, CNS vasculitis, cerebral ischemia, Alzheimer´s disease, among others [Brown, 2001] and at the same time they derive from transduction signals, disruption and assembling of the BBB in pathological conditions [Friese & Fugger, 2005]. As an extension of surveys on neuroaxonal loss and inflammatory demyelination in MS, this chapter focuses on the involvement of immune factors in axonal and neuronal neurodegeneration and summarizes concepts on immune-mediated axoneuronal dysfunction and highlights the potential pathways amenable to therapeutic interventions.

This chapter will focus on the physiopathology of Multiple Sclerosis with special emphasis on glial pathology, information on viral diseases and their relationship in its physiopathology, as well as on current therapeutic aspects.

2. Multiple Sclerosis

2.1 Heterogeneity in Multiple Sclerosis

Multiple Sclerosis (MS) is a primary inflammatory demyelinating autoimmune disease affecting the CNS and the peripheral nervous system (PNS). Recent results suggest a degenerative and hemodynamic profile in this disease, which arises from the evidence of early axonal damage [Kira, 2007; Porras-Betancourt et al, 2007] and stenotic changes in the extracranial vessels that modify the NVU [Rose & Carlson, 2007].

MS is included among the 50 neurological autoimmune diseases that affect approximately 75 $x10^6$ persons in the world [Lucchinetti et al, 2000], it is more frequent in women between 20 and 40 years of age and it constitutes the major cause of neurological disability in young adults [Martinez et al, 2005; Martinez-Yélamo et al, 1998].

Neuropathology of MS shows periventricular vascular impairment and leukocyte infiltration directed toward the myelin sheath and axon [Babbe et al, 2000; Forman et al, 2006; Jiang & Chess, 2006; Komek, 2003; Neumann et al, 2002]. Inflammation leading to progressive focal tissue damage and early axonal damage in MS could explain the current paradox concerning the temporal sequence of events that mediate axoneuronal damage in this disease, as well as the influence of immunomodulating therapy on the rate of relapses [Coles et al, 2006; Pittock et al, 2004], the persistence of oligoclonal response in the CSF and response against neurofilament proteins observed previous to demyelination. These are features that support the primary degenerating character of the disease.

MS is a prototype of neurodegenerative disease affecting primarily the axons and myelin in the CNS and the PNS. In spite of the fact that it is a disease which was described more than a century ago, the mechanism triggering the immunological reaction against myelin antigens remains unknown. Loss of myelin is accompanied by an impairment of nerve conduction leading to varied symptoms observed in this disease, that follow the formation of demyelinating plaques present in different parts of the brain and spinal cord.

It has been suggested that MS occurs as a consequence of an inflammatory response induced by the interaction of immune, environmental and genetic factors, which lead to demyelination, oligodendrocyte death, gliosis, axonal damage and neurodegeneration. In this sense, three aspects are of interest in the neuropathological approach of the disease: heterogeneity, viral or immune-environmental hypothesis and the axoneuronal degeneration that occurs in early stages of the disease.

MS displays a great heterogeneity that manifests itself not only in the immunogenetic pattern and the clinical forms of presentation, but also in the neuropathology, diagnosis and therapeutic response. Different authors have referred to these aspects [Bielekova et al, 2005; Lim et al, 2005] that could be defined as a) clinical neuropathological heterogeneity and b) heterogeneity related to the interpretation of neurobiological findings with respect to the diagnosis and clinical course of the disease.

Heterogeneity due to the influence of genetic and immuno-environmental factors in MS

The influence of genetic and immune-environmental factors in MS ranges from the geographic north-south distribution gradient of the disease, with a higher prevalence in developed countries, to the hygienic hypothesis [Cabre et al, 2005].

From a genetical point of view, MS displays a dominant poligenic character, with an incidence 20 to 50 times higher in first-degree relatives as compared with the general population and more than 100 genes reported. [Mirsattari et al, 2001]. Nevertheless, the highest individual genetic susceptibility is linked to MHC genes, with a distinctiveness for HLA DR 15* aplotypes in those exhibiting a more benign course, and HLA DR4 for those with a progressive form of the disease. Also, studies in monozygotic twins show a concordance of 25% and for dizygotic twins of less than 5%[Hillert, 2006; Lisak, 2006; Wingerchuck & Kantarci, 2007].

Other genes reported in MS include transcription genes of MHC class II, complement system, cytokines such as IL 17 e IL 17R, IL 1R, TNFp75R, GFAP, TNFα, TNFβ, TNFαR, beta linfotoxin, adhesion molecules (CD11a, CD18, CD49, β7-Integrin, transcripts for T-cells (TCR α), NK cells, B cells and proteases involved in antigen processing [Camerona, 2009; Gandhi , 2008]. The other hypothesis has strong supporters, due to the autoimmune character of the disease and the inflammatory and excitotoxic axonal degenerative reaction underlying the demyelinating process.

Clinical heterogeneity and neuropathology in MS

Clinical heterogeneity of MS is a consequence of the brain and spinal cord regions where plaques are located and the relapse rate - the latter is a very important element in the progression of the disease. From a clinical point of view, MS displays 4 clinical forms of presentation:1) relapsing-remitting MS, characterized by episodic exacerbations (relapses)followed by partial or complete recovery in approximately one month, and periods of clinical stability (remission); 2) primary progressive MS that displays a chronic progressive course, with no relapses; 3) secondary progressive MS characterized by relapses that progress in time, with less exacerbations, more incomplete recovery and irreversible disability; and 4) benign MS, which does not display a secondary progressive phase, or does not accumulate a significant disability until several decades after the onset of the disease [Fox et al, 2006; Lee et al, 2007; McDonald et al, 2001].

In all cases, MS clinical forms overlap, along with the neuropathological patterns described for the disease [Luchinetti, 2007]. In RR-MS an inflammatory pattern prevails, while in the progressive form a degenerative pattern prevails.Changes in the disability scale also correspond to clinical findings and imaginological changes in MRI studies. Although other factors are involved in the heterogeneous and multiorgan character of MS, all converge with the clinical picture to characterize the disease´s behavior individually.

Clinical and diagnostic heterogeneity

This aspect refers to the heterogeneity the disease management introduces in the interpretation of neurobiological variables, that allow the establishment of criteria from a prognostic point of view of the clinical course of MS, specifically for the immunological evaluation of CSF and MRI studies [Chabas, 2010; Villar, 2005].

The persistence of an oligoclonal response in the CSF of MS patients indicates the presence of a chronic inflammatory process with confirmatory value in this disease. CSF oligoclonal banding is an immunological feature not only of MS, but also of other neuroinflammatory diseases, including neuromyelitis optica.

The oligoclonal pattern that prevails in the CSF of MS patients is the presence of oligoclonal bands in CSF, but not in serum [Andersson, 1994, Correales, 2004, Falip, 2001]. It is suspected that autoantibodies can exacerbate inflammation and neurodegeneration in patients with MS, but which antigens intrathecal oligoclonal IgG recognize and how the autoimmune response is induced are still unknown [Meinl, 2008].

Heterogeneity is also associated with specific oligoclonal patterns in specific clinical forms. Thus, in the majority of cases, with primary progressive MS, a pattern of CSF and serum oligoclonal bands with additional bands in CSF is also found. On the other hand, oligoclonal bands directed to myelin lipids have been detected in RR-MS, secondarily progressive MS, but not in primary progressive MS [Camerona, 2009, Villar, 2005].

The presence of oligoclonal bands in the CSF has been considered a prognostic tool for the clinical management of these patients. Heterogeneity has also been introduced in the concordance of CSF analysis and the results of the MRI studies. According to Barkhof's criteria, different lesión patterns have been reported in patients positive or negative for CSF oligoclonal bands [Sospedra, 2009]. A lower frequency of infratentorial lesions have been reported in the MRIs of MS patients who are negative for oligoclonal bands and a higher frequency of juxtacortical lesions in patients with CSF oligoclonal bands. These associations are important in order to acquire a better comprehension and management of these patients based on the topography of the MRI lesions and their relation with the immunological response in the CSF [Sospedra & Martin, 2009].

2.2 Multiple Sclerosis pathology

2.2.1 Pathogenic mechanisms inducing Multiple Sclerosis

The oligoclonality and specificity of autoreactive T-cells suggest that myelin protein peptides are the activating antigens predominating in MS, whose essential attributes allow them to bind the T-cell receptor related with the structure of the lateral chain of the variable region of MHC Ag. Actually, it has been stated that the degeneration of the T-cell receptor´s ligand specificity is a main mechanism through which infectious agents can cause MS [Lee et al, 2007; Levin et al, 2010].

Among the pathogenic viruses in humans, those which induce persistent infection are relevant in MS as the triggering element of the autoimmune process that damages myelin. Herpes virus is of particular interest due to its neurotrophism, ubiquitous nature and tendency to produce latent recurrent infection. In general, there are 3 mechanisms through which viral agents can induce MS: a) molecular mimicry, b) "bystander" activation, and c) recognition of cryptic antigens [Lu et al, 2011; Levin et al, 2010].

a. Molecular mimicry

Considering the viral agents involved in the pathogenesis of MS, 83% of the patients show high titers of IgG antibodies for Epstein Barr´s virus [Barnett, 2006; Wingerchuck, 2006]. The molecular mimicry hypothesis is based on the structural similarity between myelin basic protein (MBP) peptide and Epstein Barr virus peptide, followed by the activation of autoreactive T-cells for myelin and the subsequent loss of the axon´s myelin [Haahr & Hollsberg, 2006; Maghzi et al, 2010].

b. Bystander activation

Autoreactive T-cells are also activated by unspecific inflammatory events. These events can depend on the specific recognition of exposed self-antigens due to tissue damage induced by viruses, by the autoreactive immunocompetent cell´s receptor or by independent recognition of viral antigens via autoreactive T/B cell´s receptor. In this case, 3 mechanisms have been proposed: activation by superantigens, action of pro-inflammatory cytokines derived from viral persistence and activation by Toll- like receptors [Fujinami et al, 2006; McCoy et al, 2006].

Activation by superantigens

This mechanism involves the exposure to superantigens (superAgs), toxins derived from viral agent induced relapses. This was demonstrated in the EAE model by interaction with specific T-cell clones for MBP expressing the βV TCR chain [Torkildsen et al, 2006].

Superantigens, are active mitogens, mostly all small basic proteins (20-30 kD), that induce a response by binding to the MHC Ags´ lateral part, which is not the usual location. Binding does not take place through the polymorphic trimolecular complex or binding Ag site, but laterally, at a specific sequence coded by genes of the βV TCR chain. After MHC-II and TCR bind, aggregation of the receptor and cellular activation follows. Contrary to what conventionally occurs, superAgs are not processed by the antigen-presenting cells, nor are they presented in the restricted MHC self-antigens context [Fujinami et al, 2006; McCoy et al, 2006].

Viral persistence and activation mediated by inflammatory cytokines

As a consequence of persistent viral infection, virus infected antigen-presenting cells (APC), present viral peptides to T $CD4^+$and $CD8^+$ cells together in the context of MHC class antigens. The activation of these cells induces the production of INFγ and the differentiation of T-cells via IL-12. T CD4 effector - cells secrete more INFγ and IL-12 that stimulates the T-cells differentiation to effectors, secreting more mediators like INFγ and TNFα. Activated macrophages also, secrete TNFα, nitric oxide and other reactive oxygen species that damage the infected cells and other bystander non-infected cells, to be phagocytized by macrophages and dendritic cells who process and present self-antigens to T CD4 and CD8 autoreactive cells, destroying the tissue´s infected self-cells via perforins, among other mechanisms [Lassmann, 2011]. The resulting cellular detritus are captured and processed by APC and presented to autoreactive CD8-T lymphocytes who display an autoimmune reaction. In this manner, the pro-inflammatory cytokines and chemokines secreted during the infection mediate the damage, becoming activators of the T CD8 cells specific for viral antigen and autoreactive inductors of the autoimmune process [Pender: 2011]. In this case the activation and differentiation of T CD8 cells occurs in an unspecific way [Becher et al , 2007; Haahr & Hollsberg, 2006].

On the other hand, the CNS antiviral polyspecific immune response in MS, has become a potential tool to evidence chronic autoimmune response in these patients [Cohrs, 2007]. This hypothesis has been supported by the reports showing that more than 80% of people with MS display humoral intrathecal response against neurotrophic viruses (herpes simplex, measles, rubella and varicela zoster, among others). The combined response against these neurotrophic viruses in the CNS of MS patients, was coined by Reiber et al as MRZ reaction, and many others groups have disagreed on the diagnostic value of this detection from CSF analysis in more than 90% of MS patients [Colleen et al, 2006; Correales, 2004; Jarius, 2008, Jarius et al, 2009; Luchinetti, 2007], since a similar frequency of this autoimmune chronic reaction was observed in other neurological diseases [Jarius, 2008; Jarius et al, 2009]. The MRZ reaction has also been reported in NMO patients, although in a lower frequency than in MS, and it has been useful to establish a differential diagnosis between both demyelinating diseases [Jarius, 2008]. Other MRZ reaction results were reported in tropical regions with variations regarding the previous reports [Robinson et al, 2001; Robinson et al, 2007]. In this case, a lower response to rubella virus was observed in the CNS in a smaller series of patients regarding varicela zoster and measles virus. The later showed a neurotrophic virus response similar to those reported by Reiber et al in German MS persons [Reiber et al, 1998].

We could think that a reliable interpretation of these last findings probably comes from different epidemiological factors in the two countries, or that a previous contact with this neurotrophic virus could be necessary for a detectable intrathecal polyspecific MRZ antibody response, either by immunization or native infection. In this case, as rubella is a mild disease, it may be under-reported, even in areas where reporting has been mandatory for years. As it has been previously stated [Cooper & Alford, 2001], antibodies to rubella in people under 35 years of age is as low as 30% in tropical countries like Trinidad or Panama, compared with more than 80% in Europe or the USA [Cooper & Alford, 2001]; thus, the results found in Cuban patients could be comparable for our region without the influence of any additional factor.

Activation by Toll- like receptors

Although the role of innate - immunity involves native protection and maintenance of homeostasis, in some cirscumstances, it could result in a destructive autoimmunity via toll - like receptor (TLR), or unspecific mechanisms due to the action of lysozime, lactoferrin, oxidative stress or the recognition of molecular structures expressed in non - infected cells with an inhibitory effect on the immune response (NK cells, complement proteins and family receptors of type C lectins, among others [Frischer; 2009]. The TLR is expressed in a wide range of immune and non-immune cells like microglias, oligodendrocytes and astrocytes, which act as centinels, a) by recognition of a conserved molecular pattern associated with pathogens or b) generating pro-inflammatory signals that influence the adaptative immune response [Chauhan & Marriott, 2007].

It is believed that this mechanism initiates the lesion, previously preceded by peripheral activation. The LPS binding TLR4 increase cytokine expression and oxygen reactive species inducing peripheral autoreactive T cell activation and where an inappropriate TLR signal can contribute to MS development [Kielian; 2005]. In this way, the increased expresion of TLR on dendritic cells inhibit the immunosupresor effect of regulatory T cells CD4+/CD25+ on autoreactive T cells vía IL 6, causing loss of peripheral tolerance. The increase of exacerbations around viral infections in MS supports this hypothesis.

Cryptic Antigens

Cryptic or sequestered antigens are exposed as a consequence of myelin loss, induce an antibody response against them, causing reactive changes within the neuron cellular body and axon, blocking the interaction of oligodendrocyte precursors with the axon and consequently promoting remyelination and axonal repair [Devries, 2006; Magliozzi et al, 2010].

2.2.2 Mechanism involving the axoneuronal degeneration in MS

The investigation of neurodegeneration in MS has received the highest priority in the last few years, establishing a multifactorial process involving myelin loss, immune-mediated histotoxicity, decreased trophic support, mitochondrial damage, metabolic-energetic changes, and altered signalling [Ghafourifar, 2008; Klawiter & Cross, 2007; Lindberg et al, 2008; Sobel, 1998].

It is commonly accepted that the initial activation of the T cell system takes place in the systemic immune compartment outside the CNS, where T lymphocytes encounter a specific autoantigen presented in the context of MHC class II molecules [Neumann et al, 2002] and the simultaneous delivery of additional co-stimulatory signals, such as B7-1 (CD80) and B7-2 (CD86), on the cell surface of antigen presenting cells. Such autoreactive T cells may reside quiescently at this level, until an external trigger - most likely a viral infection- renders these cells active to develop their auto aggressive potential.

The degree of neurological impairment seems to be determined by the extent of axonal loss, which is proposed to be the final step in the pathogenesis of the MS lesions. However, so far it remains unclear: (a) whether axonal injury is the result of an active destructive process targeting the axon; (b) if it occurs as a result of increased vulnerability of demyelinated axons or as part of a bystander effect; or (c) if axonal degeneration takes place as a physiological response to permanent demyelination inhibiting the extrinsic trophic signal to axons [Luchinetti. 2007].

Pathogenic events involved in axoneuronal degeneration

Two main pathogenic events must be considered as the cause of axoneuronal damage leading to irreversible discapacity in MS: a) damage of the myelin oligodendrocytic unit and b) the axoneuronal neurodegeneration process.

Damage of the myelin oligodendrocytic unit

Indirect effect of T cells can also mediate damage to the myelin-oligodendrocytic unit. Autoreactive T lymphocytes activated from the periphery get into the CNS by degradation of the brain vascular endothelial cells. Th1 lymphocytes expressing adhesion molecules such as VLA-4 y LFA-1, release cytokines and metalloproteinases MMP2/9 that acting at the BBB level, induce an increase of its permeability. The later, linked with a higher integrin expression (V-CAM /I-CAM) induced by INFγ and TNFα, facilitate the migration of activated T cells into the CNS. Once in the CNS, these activated T-cells release cytokines - such as INFγ- which induces activation and differentiation of others autoreactive T cells resting in the Tho state, to transform into effector cells, activating microglias, resident macrophages in the CNS and Tγδ cells, thus contributing to the damage. Recently it has also been postulated that T cell regulators can transform into Th-17 effector cells, contributing to a major lesional effect on the myelin-oligodendrocytic unit [Ishizu , 2010]. Figure 2 shows the mechanisms related with the indirect effect of T lymphocytes and microglia in the damage of the myelin-oligodendrocyte unit.

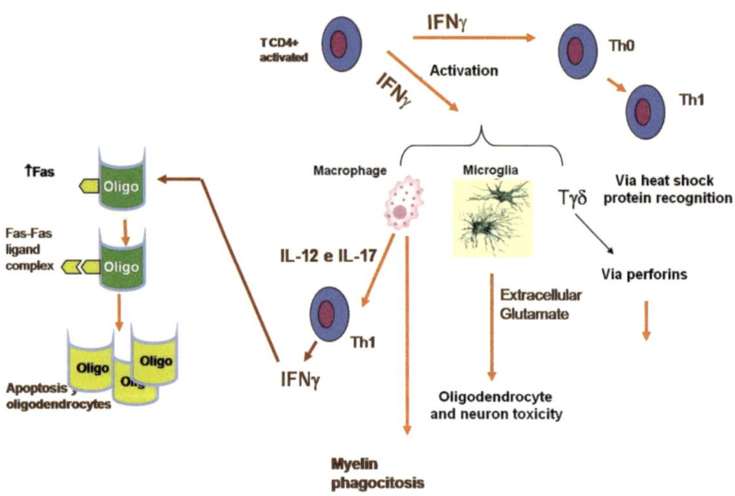

Fig. 1. Pathogenic mechanism, involving damage of the myelin oligodendrocytic unit. Microglia interfere the oligodendrocyte repopulation and mediate their toxicity and death with the main intervention of cytokine like IFNγ and TNFα.

Microglia also cause a toxic effect on oligodendrocytes and neurons via extracellular glutamate and nitric oxide secretion, while Tγδ cells induce direct oligodendrocyte damage, via perforine. INFγ- activated macrophages are also induced to secrete cytokines such as IL-12 and IL 17 that induce Th1 cells to secrete more INFγ. INFγ then induces the expression of Fas molecules on the oligodendrocyte surface promoting a Fas-Fas ligand interaction, followed by oligodendrocyte apoptotic death, Fig 1. Thus, the microglia, main mediator of glial -neuron interaction becomes a binding point between the innate and adaptative immune systems. In acute inflammation, microglia act as antigen presenting cells (APC), and contribute to antibody clearance and elimination of myelin detritus after clinical relapse. However, during the chronic phase of a pathological condition like MS, this cell type contributes to irreversible damage. Glial-derived INFγ, also interferes with the vitality, recruitment and function of OPC, interfering with complete remyelination at lesion sites.

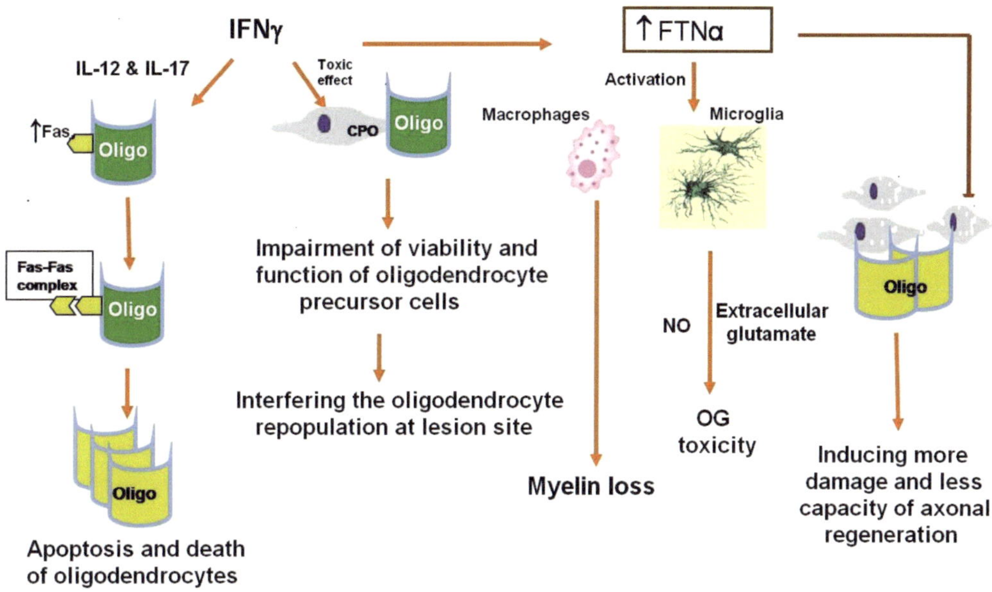

Fig. 2. Indirect T cell effect, on the myelin-oligodendrocytic unit in MS. Microglia also, causes a toxic effect on oligodendrocytes and neurons via extracellular glutamate and nitric oxide secretion. Th1: T-helper-1 cells.

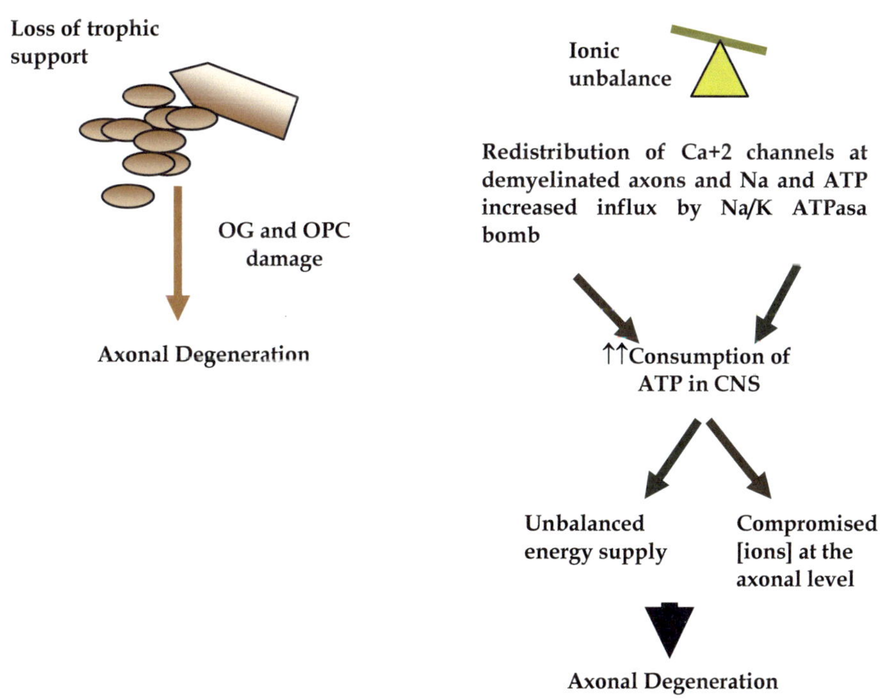

Fig. 3.Axonal damage mediated by mechanisms independent of active inflammation in MS. OG; oligodendrocyte, OPC: oligodendrocyte precursor cells.

On the other hand, damage to the myelin-oligodendrocytic unit occurs as a consecuence of an increased vulnerability of demyelinated axons to immune attack, a reduced trophic support, since myelination provides an extrinsic trophic signal to axons. Fig 3 shows the mechanisms leading to axonal damage independent from active inflammation: loss of trophic factors and ionic and energetic unbalance, Fig 3.

Neuronal damage in MS results from two insults: on one side mediated by microglia, via IL 1beta, TNFα, IL 6 and NO, all neurotoxic to neurons which are functionally compromised by hypoxic damage, and on the other side due to an excess of extracellular glutamate, oligodendrocyte toxicity, and axonal loss. Gene transcripts for TNF and IL 6 with an impact on the pathophysiology of MS have been identified in the margins and center of the active lesions, but not in the inactive lesions [Jack et al, 2007].

Axoneuronal degeneration in MS

Loss of trophic support in MS pathophysiology: Reduced inflammation occurring during the course of chronic demyelination suggests the existence of mechanisms not related to active inflammation as being responsible of continuous axonal loss and progressive and irreversible inability. It has been acknowledged that this is due to the loss of trophic support derived from oligodendrocyte damage, which is necessary for axonal survival independent from compact myelin (Fig 4).

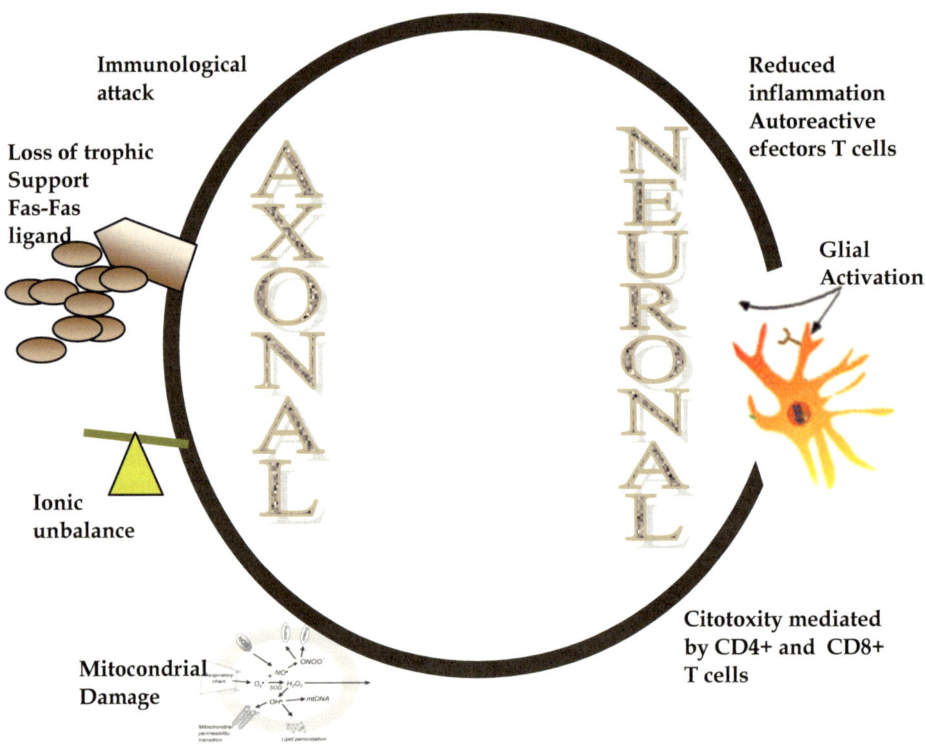

Fig. 4. Mechanism involved in the axoneuronal degeneration process. Neuroaxonal loss represents the major pathophysiological element correlating with clinical disability. The figure summarizes the mechanisms causing demyelination and axoneuronal degeneration in MS and their combined contribution to disease progression and irreversible inability.

Ionic unbalance in MS pathophysiology: Ionic unbalance -as a result of compensatory changes to restore nervous conduction following demyelination- can induce long term axonal degeneration. Therefore, the redistribution of Na channels on demyelinated axons restores the action potential, neuronal function and increases Na and ATP influx, via the Na/K ATPase pump to maintain the ionic gradient, which is necessary for neurotransmission. Both processes are highly energy consuming, leading to energetic unbalance, altered axonal ion concentrations and subsequent neurodegeneration (Fig4).

Antibodies to Cytoskeletal Proteins: Neurofilaments are a group of cytoskeletal proteins expressed in neuronal cells and axons. Neurodegenerative disorders like Alzheimer's disease and Parkinson's disease are characterized by accumulation of NF proteins leading to abnormalities in axonal transport and an impending neuronal loss [Amor et al, 2010; Arumugam et al, 2008]. Antibodies to axonal cytoskeletal proteins may be markers of axonal damage, as well as important contributors to neurodegeneration and clinical disability in MS. CSF levels of antibodies against the NFL correlate with disease duration, clinical disability, IgG index, and the degree of cerebral atrophy measured by MRI [Bartos et al, 2007; Eikelenbom, 2003]. Although elevated levels of NFL-specific antibodies are present in sera of patients with PP-MS, these antibodies are also increased in sera of patients with other neurological diseases [Bartos et al, 2007; Huizinga, 2008].

Although there is no confirmed evidence to establish that antineurofilament antibodies themselves contribute to mayor neuroaxonal damage, experimental models provide supportive evidence [Amor et al, 2010]. Immunization of mice with NFL triggers the development of a CNS disease characterized by axonal damage, paralysis, and spasticity [Huizinga et al, 2008]. Furthermore, microinjections of anti-kinesin or anti-dynein antibodies cause impairment of the anterograde and retrograde NF transport in cultured neurons [Theiss et al, 2005] and induce the formation of long and branched mitochondrial structures redistributed to the nuclear periphery. These intracellular changes are associated with altered calcium homeostasis, apoptosis, and neurodegeneration [Arumugam et al, 2009]. Antibodies to neurofilaments and possibly to other cytoskeletal proteins are produced during tissue damage in MS. Experimental data support that these antibodies may gain access to their intracellular target and cause changes in axonal transport, mitochondrial distribution and calcium homeostasis, and thus contribute to apoptosis and neurodegeneration [Vishkina & Kalman, 2008].

Criteria based on evidence regarding the role of Ab-mediated autoreactivity to neurofilament proteins in MS has been controversial [Silber et al, 2002; Bartos et al, 2007; Bartos el al, 2007a; Bejartmar & Trapp, 2003; Semra et al, 2002; Eikelenboom et al, 2003]. Bartos et al for example, detected increased intrathecal IgG and IgM antibodies against the medium subunit of neurofilaments (NFM) in patients with all subtypes of MS [Bartos et al, 2007; Bartos et al, 2007a] while Silber et al [2002] maintained the relevance of autoantibody to NFL in CSF as progression markers in MS. Unexpectedly, anti-NFM antibody levels appeared to be higher in the serum than in CSF, possibly related to NF antigen leakage from the CNS to the peripheral blood, or to the higher concentration of plasma cells in the blood. Alternatively, anti-NFM antibodies may be triggered by exogenous antigens and molecular mimicry in the peripheral blood [Bartos et al, 2007; Bartos et al, 2007a; Bejartmar et al, 2003; Eikelenboom et al, 2003; Semra et al, 2002; Silber et al, 2002].

Besides these considerations, the evaluation of axonal markers from CSF analysis, have shown different results; some experiences considering these biomarkers promissory for monitoring progression and/or relapsing rate in MS. So, a study in patients published by Eikelenboom et al, reported a significant correlation between intrathecal production of NFLP antibody in CSF and cortical atrophy and more recently a significant relationship between NFLP antibody index and relapsing rate was observed in patients bearing MS [Eikelenboom et al 2003; Robinson, 2010]. Fig 5 shows a study conducted in a group of 26 Cuban MS patients with different clinical forms of the disease. The evaluation of Ab reactivity to NFLP in CSF was significantly correlated with the relapsing rate, denoting an association between both clinical and biological parameters. These results are interesting since they show another aspect of the idiotipic response in MS, and its possible insertion not only from the view point of the pathogenic mechanism of the disease, but also as a useful clinical tool, at least to predict or monitor treatment response.

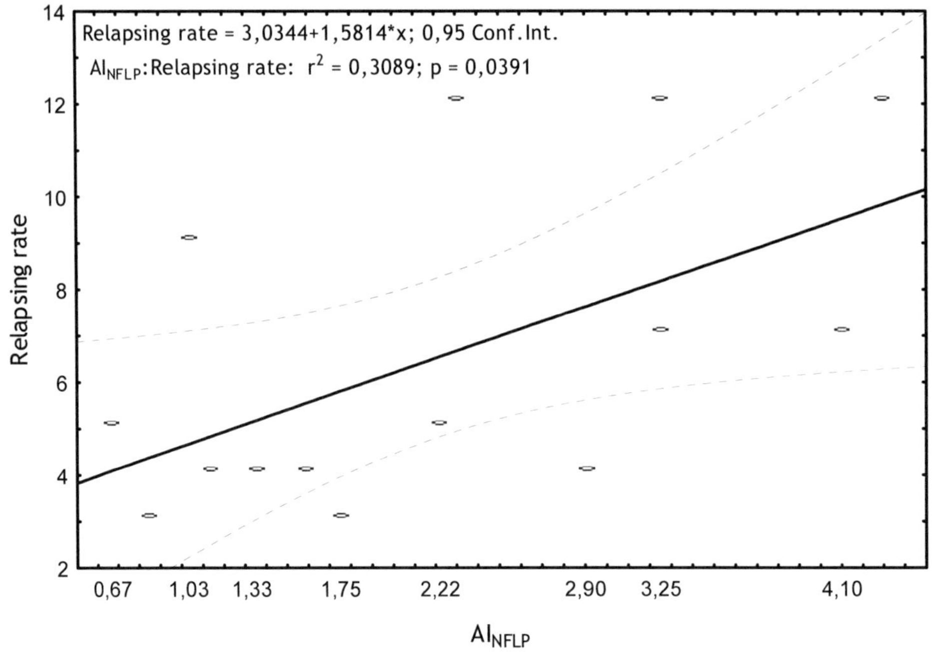

Fig. 5. Statistical analysis between AI_{NFLP} and relapsing rate in MS patients showed a significant correlationship between both parameters. * Spearman´s correlation test, $p<0.05$. AI_{NFLP}: Antibody index to neurofilament light protein. AI_{NFLP}: NFLP CSF/NFLP Serum / IgG CSF/IgG serum.

2.3 Autoimmunity contributing to glial pathology in MS

Neurodegeneration in MS occurs in response to a multifactorial process involving loss of myelin protection by immune-mediated histotoxicity, decreased trophic support, mitochondrial damage, metabolic changes and altered signaling [Ghafourifar et al, 2008; Lindberg et al, 2008]. Nevertheless, different neuronal targets have been identified as causing neuronal dysfunction, following a humoral immune mechanism in MS which can be classified as neuronal surface molecules, intracellular enzymes, signaling molecules and chaperones, nuclear antigens and cytoskeletal protein among others (Vyshkina & Kalman, 2008|. On the other hand, it has been suggested that microglial responses are tailored in regional and insult-specific manners [Carson et al, 2007]. The most recognizable role of microglia in brain defense is as a scavenger of cellular debris by phagocytosis, as occurs in the event of infection, inflammation, trauma, ischemia, and neuronal death [Kraft & Harry, 2011]. However, it is well known that, not only do microglia dynamically survey the CNS to clear damaged cellular debris, but they are also capable of initiating a rapid and specific response to subtle changes in the microenvironment. Different types of neuronal pathology and other activating stimuli clearly elicit differing responses from brain-resident microglia [Colton & Wilcock, 2010; Rivest, 2009], evidencing the autoimmune process that leads to brain damage as occurs in MS.

B cells and autoimmunity in MS

B cells are involved in multiple immune pathways including the presentation of antigenic determinants and the expression of costimulatory signals for T lymphocytes, immunoglobulin production, secretion of cytokines, and recruitment of T cells into the CNS. The B-cell lineage is represented by B lymphocytes (CD19þ, CD138), plasma blasts (CD19þ, D138þ), and plasma cells (CD19_, CD138þ; all detectable in CNS and CSF. In MS most of these cells express memory phenotypes, CD27þ positive. A relevant contribution of humoral autoimmunity in myelin loss has been proposed in demyelinating diseases with a prominent intervention of complement molecules and Ab itself [Lucchinetti et al, 2000; Serafini et al, 2010]. Thus, immunological and molecular results have repeatedly been reported by differents groups in this field, all of them directed towards the characterization of the cellular arm of autoimmunity.

Mechanisms leading to autoimmune B-cell activation may be initiated by CD4 T helper type 2 (TH2) lymphocytes and their soluble inflammatory products (eg. interleukins 4, 5 and 13) followed by an antigen-specific expansion of clones either in the peripheral circulation or in the damaged CNS tissue, where intracellular proteins are released. As it was expressed earlier in this chapter, bystander activation describes a non-antigen-specific activation of T or B cells usually mediated by soluble inflammatory products of nearby immune cells, while the humoral immune system appears to be more successful in breaking anti-neuronal tolerance than the cellular system, and has greater pathogenic significance supporting the involvement of the humoral immune response in MS-related neurodegeneration [Huizinga et al, 2008].

From a molecular view point, data also support the involvement of B lymphocytes and their products in MS. Intrathecal production of immunoglobulins with an oligoclonal electrophoretic distribution pattern is a hallmark of the disease. Clonally expanded autoreactive B cells in the CSF and CNS have increased VH mutation rates concentrated in the complementarity determining regions. VH sequences expressed in plaques are absent in the peripheral blood [Owens et al, 2001]. B-cell heavy and light chain editing, a mechanism to prevent autoimmunity by the replacement of elements in rearranged immunoglobulin genes after the re-expression of recombination activating genes —RAG1/RAG2, is inefficient in MS, a fact which is suggested by the detection of autoreactive B cells with unsuccessfully edited receptors in the CSF [Lambracht-Washington et al, 2007; O'Connor et al, 2007] These observations suggest that CNS antigen-specific and clonally expanded B cells present in CNS and CSF of MS patients exhibit complex molecular characteristics and intraclonal diversity.

Neuroaxonal targets of humoral autoimmunity in MS and EAE have been identified in the CNS during the process of demyelination. Immunoglobulins produced by activated B cells in the CNS and CSF target numerous self-antigens including components of CNS myelin such as myelin basic protein, proteolipid protein, myelin-associated glycoprotein, and myelin oligodendrocyte glycoprotein [Dutta & Trapp, 2007]. A great number of papers discuss the involvement of myelin-specific antibodies in the development of demyelination and disease progression and although not uniformly, the use of some of these antibodies as biomarkers is accepted as a support to the diagnosis or to monitor disease activity and course [Amor et al, 2007; Lutterotti et al, 2007]

Anti-Neuronal Antibodies in MS

Antibodies to a variety of intracellular molecules including enzymes, signaling molecules, HSPs, and nuclear proteins are detected in MS and other inflammatory and neurological disorders. The production of these antibodies may be related to bystander immune activation and epitope spreading during tissue injury, as was referred before, although their pathogenic significance remains uncertain in some cases.

Antibodies Targeting Neuronal Cell-Surface Molecules: Neuronal cell-surface antigen molecules in the surface membrane of myelinated axons are normally hidden from the immune system, and only become exposed after demyelination becoming antigenic and inducing the production of neuron-specific antibodies. IgG and IgM antibodies binding to the surface of a neuronal cell line were found in 70% of sera from patients with secondary progressive (SP)-MS and in 25% of sera from patients with relapsing-remitting (RR)-MS [Kraft & Harry, 2011] . This finding may indicate the spreading of autoimmunity to neuronal antigens as a consequence of CNS expansion and tissue damage.

Axolemma-enriched fractions: Antibodies to axolemma-enriched fractions (AEF) of the CNS are also present in CSF and sera of MS patients, [Zaffaroni, 2003].From in vitro assays, there is evidences that these antibodies damage neurites and prevent neuronal outgrowth. The production of anti-axolemma and anti-myelin IgGs appears to be independent. Criteria to consider antiaxolemmal IgG antibodies as markers of axonal damage are based on these observations [Zaffaroni, 2003].

Neurofascin: One of the targets in antibody-mediated axonal injury is the cell-adhesion molecule neurofascin. The 186 kDa neuronspecific isoform of neurofascin (NF186) is involved in the clustering of voltage gated Na channels at Ranvier´s nodes, while the 155 kDa glial-specific isoform (NF155) is required for the proper assembly of paranodal junction, targeting the interaction sites between myelin and axon. Early in the disease course and preceding demyelination, changes in the distribution of NF155 have been observed in MS lesions [Vyshkina1 & Kalman, 2008]. Maier et al [2007] showed that the NF155-levels were reduced, suggesting that NF155 is subject to protein degradation in the lesions. On the other hand, studies in sera showed levels significantly higher in patients with chronic progressive forms of MS compared to other inflammatory neurological diseases. At the same time, studies in vitro showed that antibodies to neurofascin inhibit axonal conduction and that NF155-specific antibodies cross-react with NF186-transfected cells at the nodes of Ranvier possibly initiating axonal injury and accelerating disease progression [Mathey et al, 2007]. Neurofascin-specific antibodies can also inhibit remyelination by binding to NF155 expressed on the surface of oligodendrocytes. In vivo experiments revealed that antibodies to neurofascin and complement can selectively target nodes of Ranvier, cause axonal injury, and trigger disease exacerbation in EAE [Mathey et al, 2007].

Anti ganglioside antibodies: It is well known that gangliosides are glycolipids with sialic residues in the outer layer of cell membranes, particularly enriched in the membranes of neurons. Experimental data reveal that antiganglioside antibodies can disrupt the BBB, create neuromuscular block by binding to neuronal gangliosides at the neuromuscular junction and inhibit axonal regeneration after peripheral nerve injury in mice [Amor et al, 2010],. Increased levels of anti-GM3 (monosialoganglioside) antibodies can be found in sera of a great proportion of patients with progressive forms of MS (56.3%) in primary progressive (PP)-MS and in 42.9% of SP-MS vs 2.9% in RR-MS and 14.6% in OND. Anti-GD2 (disialo-ganglioside)-like IgM autoantibodies were detected in sera of 30% of MS patients, and a positive correlation of anti-GD2-like IgM reactivity with neurological disability was observed [*Kanda et al, 2000*]. The increased prevalence of GD2-specific IgM antibodies in SP-MS (47.8%) compared to RR-MS (24.2%) and PP-MS (26.7%), also suggests the involvement of these antibodies in inflammation-induced neurodegeneration [Marconi et al, 2006]. It should be emphasized; that it is not clear whether anti-ganglioside antibodies can cause or result from axonal damage, and whether they may definitely function as putative markers of neurodegeneration in MS.

In general, these data suggest that antibodies specific to neuronal cell-surface molecules are produced during demyelination, and that they may themselves contribute to glial pathology or axonal injury in MS. These antibodies can activate complement and exert cytotoxicity, provide binding sites for the Fc receptors on macrophages and microglial cells, interrupt axon–myelin interaction, inhibit axonal conduction and outgrowth, disrupt the BBB, and alter oligodendrocyte functioning. Correlation of the antibody titers with the severity of disability offers an opportunity of using these neuronal cell-surface antibodies as biomarkers.

Antibodies to Intracellular Molecules: Arrestins, glutamate decarboxylase and nuclear antigens

MS patients show a high prevalence of autoreactivity to intracellular antigens such as neuron-specific enolase (metabolic enzyme), b-arrestin and retinal arrestin among others. So, antibody reaction to arrestins, a family of multifunctional, intracellular proteins that regulate signal transduction and the activity of G-protein-coupled receptors, has been reported in MS; while b-arrestin-1 enhances the expression of antiapoptotic Bcl2 that may control the development of both MS and EAE. Anti-b-arrestin-specific antibodies and antibodies to retinal arrestin can be found in sera of patients with MS. [Gorczyca et al, 2004]. B-Arrestin-1-knockout mice are more resistant, and b-arrestin-1 transgenic mice are more susceptible to EAE [Frederick & Miller, 2007; Shi et al, 2007].

Immunity to glutamate decarboxylase (GAD), an enzyme that converts glutamate into the inhibitory neurotransmitter aminobutyric acid (GABA), can also be detected in MS. GAD is expressed in various cell types including neurons, and its activity is reduced in sera of MS patients. Serum anti- GAD65 antibodies are present in 10% of MS patients [Hermitte et al,

2000]. Anti-GAD antibodies have also been associated with systemic autoimmune disorders, such as type 1 diabetes, although without a clear understanding of the pathogenic significance [Taplin & Barker, 2008]. Elevated antinuclear antibodies (ANA) in sera of MS patients have been reported at varying frequencies (2.5–81%) depending on the methodological approaches [Ferreira et al, 2005; Roussel et al, 2000]. In contrast, the ANA titers are low (between 1:40 and 1:100) in sera of MS patients, who also often have low-affinity IgG antibodies to multiple other nuclear and cytoplasmic epitopes. [Ferreira et al, 2005; Roussel et al, 2000; Lu & Kalman, 1999]. These data suggest that detection of ANA and related antibodies in MS may result from a nonspecific immune activation.

Furthermore, these observations support that B cells may contribute directly or indirectly to MS development. Removal of immunoglobulins from the peripheral blood by plasmapheresis appears to be beneficial in the subgroup of patients with type II lesions [Keegan et al, 2005] and depletion of CD20 B cells by rituximab results in a significant reduction in the number of enhancing MRI lesions. The latter intervention, however,does not exert its beneficial effects by directly affecting the immunoglobulin pool, but by depleting memory B cells and altering antigen presentation, T-cell activation, or T-cell recruitment into the CNS [Hauser et al, 2008].

Autoimmunity and Glutamate-Mediated Neurotoxicity

Glutamate is a neurotransmitter released by neurons into the synaptic space where it binds to its postsynaptic receptors. Elevated levels of extracellular glutamate can lead to the death of neurons, astrocytes and oligodendrocytes [Matute et al, 2006]. Excitotoxic tissue damage mediated by glutamate has been described in a number of neurologic diseases (eg stroke, traumatic injury, neurodegeneration) including MS [Vercellino et al, 2007].

Glial cells and neurons express various types of glutamate excitatory amino-acid transporters (EAAT1–EAAT5). The reuptake of glutamate appears to be impaired in MS due to the downregulation of EAAT1 and EAAT2 molecules in white matter and cortical lesions[Vercellino et al, 2007]. Glutamate levels in the CSF are higher during relapses than remissions, and correlate with disease severity [Sarchielli et al, 2003.) These observations suggest that inflammation upsets the balance of glutamate release and re-uptake, and the excessive glutamate may escalate tissue injury in MS.

Glutamate toxicity may be further enhanced by altered receptor expression and signaling.Two main subtypes of glutamate receptors have been identified: ionotropic, coupled directly to membrane ion channels; and metabotropic, coupled to G proteins. The ionotropic receptors are divided into three subtypes based on their selective agonists: N-methyl-D-aspartate (NMDA), a-amino-3-hydroxy-5-methyl-4-isoxazolepropionate (AMPA), and kainate [Lipton & Rosenberg, 1994]. An elevated expression of subunit 1 of AMPA receptor (GluR1) on oligodendrocytes at the borders of active plaques, and subunit 3 of AMPA receptor (GluR3) and metabotropic glutamate receptors (mGluR) on reactive astrocytes in MS lesions have also been reported. Activated microglia and macrophages are immunopositive for NMDA receptor subunit 1 (NR1) in plaques and may also play a role in Ca-dependent injury of oligodendrocytes and neurons. NMDA receptor antagonists, memantine, amantadine, and MK-801 reduce neurological deficits in EAE, and the blockade of AMPA receptors by antagonists, also ameliorate clinical signs of EAE. [Bolton & Paul, 1997; Smith et al, 2000; Stys & Lipton, 2007; Wallstrom 1996].

Antibodies targeting glutamate receptors may have agonist or antagonist effects. Agonists usually cause excitotoxicity and complement-mediated cell death [Groom et al, 2003]. Anti-GluR3 antibodies are implicated in epilepsy syndromes but not in MS. In summary, these observations suggest that glutamate homeostasis is being upset in inflammatory lesions of MS, where the concentration of glutamate is increased, at least in part, due to a decreased re-uptake. In addition, anti-glutamate receptor antibodies are associated with inflammatory and neurodegenerative disorders, like MS, often correlating with clinical improvement.

Induction of Central Nervous System Autoimmunity by Th17 lymphocyte in MS

T-helper cells classically divide into two functional subsets including: Th1 and T-helper-2 (Th2); each one with a distinct activity of transcription factor and pattern of cytokine-secretion phenotype [Mosmann et al, 1986.]. Th1 cells produce IFN-γ, TNF-β and interleukin-10 (IL-10), and mediate cellular immune responses against tumor cells, intracellular viruses and bacteria via macrophages and cytotoxic T-cell activation. In addition, Th1 cells drive cell-mediated response leading to tissue damage and drive humoral immune responses to Ig2a subclasses. Innate immune cells, through STAT6 signals, secrete IL-4 that induces the transformation of naıve CD4+ T cells into Th2 cells, leading to the expression of transcription factor GATA3. This cascade of events in turn results in the production of IL-4, IL-5, IL-13, IL-21 and IL-31, important for host defense against helminths and contribute to the pathogenesis of asthma and allergy [Monteleone et al, 2008; Steinman, 2007; Wilson et al, 2009]. Other T-cell subsets that co-express CD4 and CD25 are Th3 cells, or regulatory T (TREG) cells, which regulate both Th1 and Th2 cell function, and maintain homeostasis of the immune system [Vojdani & Lambert, 2011]. TREG cells can develop from thymic CD4+ T-cell precursors in the presence of IL-2 and TGF- β, which are termed natural TREG cells. TREG cells produce low levels of IL-2 and IFN-γ, but produce high levels of IL-10, IL-35 and TGF-β, suppressing immune responses to self-antigens and preventing autoimmune disease by two different immunoregulatory immunosuppressive or antiinflammatory cytokines, IL-10 and TGF-β , Fig 6.

More recently, a specific T-cell subset, termed Th17 cell, that secretes a cytokine called IL-17, has been identified. This cell develops from naıve CD4+ T cells in response to IL-6, IL-23, TGF-β and IL-1β. IL-6 and IL-23 activate STAT3, which increases the expression of RORγt and RORγ transcription factors, promoting the expression of IL-17A, IL-17F, IL-21 and IL-22. These cells, important for host defense against extracellular bacteria, are also involved in mediating autoimmune diseases [Chung & Dong, 2009; Stockinger & Veldhoen, 2007]. The immunopathogenic activities of Th17 cell in inflammation and autoimmunity has been linked to a growing list of cancers, autoimmune and inflammatory diseases such as rheumatoid arthritis, systemic lupus erythematosus, multiple sclerosis, asthma, psoriasis, systemic sclerosis, chronic inflammatory bowel disease and allograft rejection [Chung & Dong, 2009; McGeachy et al, 2009; Steinman, 2007].

Th1 and Th2 effector molecules antagonize the development of Th17 cells, which are responsible for destructive tissue pathology in autoimmune diseases including neuroinflammation; whereas, naıve CD4 cells in the presence of IL-12 and transcription factors, such as T-bet and STAT4, become Th1 cells, which express IL-12R and produce IFN-γ. Naıve CD4 cells in the presence of IL-4, GATA-3 and STAT6 become Th2 cells, which produce IL-4. Finally, naive CD4 cells in the presence of TGF-β, IL-23 and transcription factor RORγt become IL-17-producing Th17 cells [Batten et al, 2006; Cheung et al, 2008].

As it was previously mentioned, the pathogenic contribution of Th1, Th2 and Th17 lymphocytes to autoimmune disorders has been reported both in systemic and in neurological diseases [Zheng et al; 2007]. IL-17-producing T-helper cells play an important role in the induction of neuroimmune diseases, like MS and its animal model called experimental autoimmune encephalomyelitis (EAE) [Iwakura & Ishigame, 2006.]. This observation is based on the detection of IL-17 levels in both the plaques and cerebrospinal fluid of MS patients [Ishizu et al, 2005].

It has been established that IL-17 is a proinflammatory cytokine that stimulates epithelial, fibroblast and endothelial cells to produce other inflammatory chemokines and cytokines, including macrophage inflammatory protein (MIP)-2, monocyte chemoattractant protein (MCP-1), granulocyte-colony stimulating factor (G-CSF) and IL-6 and synergizes with IL-1β and TNF-α, to induce more chemokine expression [Vojdani & Lambert, 2011].

Also, microglia is known either as antigen presenting cells and effector cells and is involved in inflammatory demyelination of the CNS. It was shown that treatment of microglia with IL-17 upregulated microglia production of IL-6, MIP-2, nitric oxide, neurotrophic factors and adhesion molecules. In a similar way IL-1β and IL-23 may induce microglial IL-17 production, contributing to neuroimmune pathology in MS [Kawanokuchi et al, 2008]. An additional support to this hypothesis came from the experience in mice injected with specific antibodies against IL-17, which resulted in inhibition of chemokine expression, whereas overexpression of IL-17 in lung epithelia resulted in chemokine production and leukocyte infiltration [Vojdani & Lambert, 2011].

In MS, the location and distribution of CNS lesions under the influence of genetic susceptibility is determinant for clinical outcome and disease course and suggests that T-cell immune response specificity influences the sites of inflammation. A recent study published by Stromnes et al in 2008, demonstrated that T-cells specific to MBP epitopes generate two different populations of helper cells, Th17 and Th1 [Stromnes et al, 2008]. Notably, the Th17 to Th1 ratio of infiltrating T-cells determines that inflammation in the brain parenchyma occurs when the ratio of Th17 to Th1 cells is much greater than one, triggering a disproportionate increase of IL-17 in the brain that results in inflammation, Fig.6. At the same time, these results indicate that Th17, Th1 and their ratio, are main mechanisms regulating cell infiltration into the brain parenchyma.

Stromnes´ group also considered that a differential regulation of inflammation in the brain with a Th17:Th1 ratio >1, and in the spinal cord with a Th17: Th1 ratio <1, indicates that Th1 cells play a significant pathologic role in spinal cord autoimmunity [Stromnes et al, 2008]. It was concluded that IL-17 produced by Th17 cells is the major regulator of CNS autoimmunity. So, IL-17, deemed as the most pathogenic cytokine in inflammatory neuroimmune and autoimmune disorders, induces the activation of matrix metalloproteinase-3 (MMP-3) and recruits neutrophils to the site of inflammation, which also activates MMPs, proteases and gelatinases, contributing to BBB breakdown and a further enhancement of neutrophil recruitment. This increase in protease activity, which attracts a significant number of monocytes and macrophages to the inflammatory sites, with a subsequent citokine secretion and glial activation, reinforces the eventual myelin and axonal damage [Tester et al, 2007]. Thus, it is possible to consider that under CNS inflammatory conditions, microglia, which act as antigen presenting cells, produce IL-1β

and IL-23 and act in an autocrine manner, via IL-17 expression in microglia and IL-17-induced activation of MMP-3, contributing to neuroimmune pathology in MS.

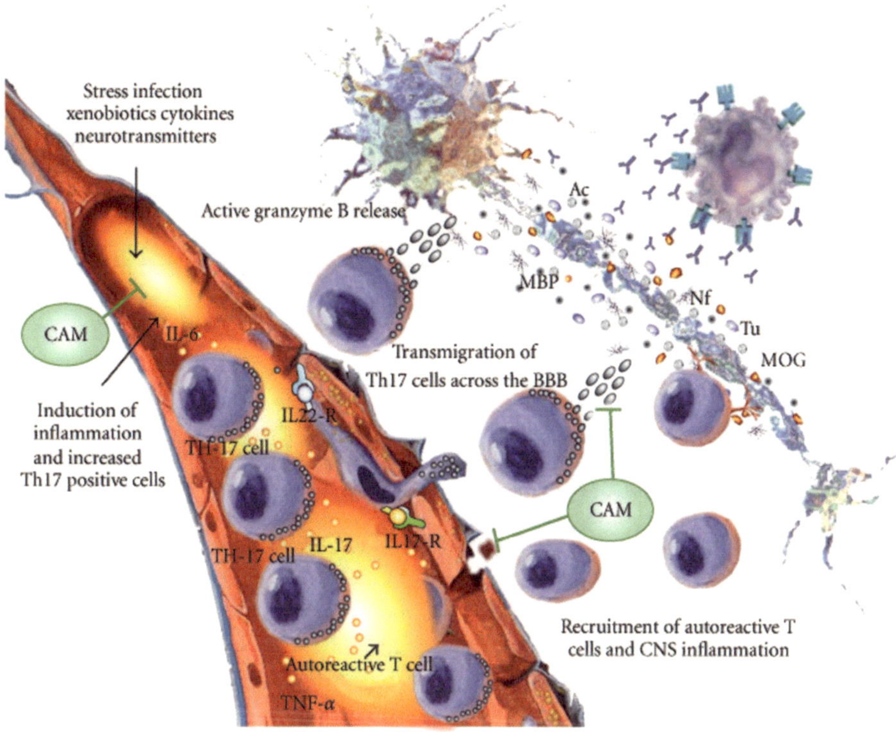

Fig. 6. The role of Th17 lymphocytes in the pathogenesis of inflammatory and neuroimmunological disorders. Environmental factors' induction of inflammatory response, production of cytokines and increase in the number of Th17 positive cells in circulation. Expression of IL-17 and IL-22 receptors on blood-brain barrier endothelial cells result in the binding of Th17 cells to BBB tight junctions. This disrupts the tight junctions, and the Th17 cells then transmigrate across the BBB, setting the stage for the killing of neurons by the release of granzyme B. CAM protocols may be used to block the inflammatory cascade induced by infection. CAM: Complementary alternative medicine, BBB; blood brain barrier. Taken from: The Role of Th17 in Neuroimmune Disorders: Target for CAM Therapy. Part II. In Hindawi Publishing Corporation Evidence-Based Complementary and Alternative Medicine, Volume 1-7, 2011.

Induction of BBB Disruption and Neuroinflammation mediated by IL 17 in MS

The BBB is composed of two layers: the microvascular endothelial cells and the glia limitans formed by glial foot processes [Maes et al 2007]. The perivascular space between the endothelial cells and astrocytes is populated by macrophages, which behave like immature dendritic cells [Vojdani & Lambert, 2011]; thus factors able to open the epithelial barrier will destroy both the BBB and neural tissue [Maes et al 2007; Maes et al, 2008].

Since microglia play a significant role in MS, to further strengthen the role of IL-17 in CNS inflammation, microglia were treated with IL-17. Treatment with IL-17 upregulated the microglial production of IL-6, MIP-2, nitric oxide, adhesion molecules and neurotrophic factors [Kawanokuchi et al, 2008]. Since it is known that IL-17 can be secreted by microglia in response to IL-1β or IL-23, these results strongly suggest that the cells co-expressing IL-17, IL-22 and granzyme B through the action of IL-17 and IL-22, play a significant role in the induction and breach in the BBB and its permeabilization to circulating CD4+ lymphocytes and soluble molecules resulting in CNS inflammation [Vojdani & Lambert, 2011]. The role of Th17 lymphocytes in the pathogenesis of inflammatory and neuroimmunological disorders is shown in Figure 6. This role of Th17 cells and the IL-17 produced by them in neuroinflammation could make these novel CD4 cells a suitable target for treatment in demyelinating diseases like MS.

Therapies towards BBB repair and the inhibition of lymphocyte transmigration can reduce neuro-inflammation, and at the same time, could be relevant since resident microglia and astrocytes, play an important role in the initiation and progression of immune responses induced by pathogen invasion or their antigens [Chauhan and Marriott ; 2007]. So, infections associated with high levels of inflammatory cytokines including IL-1β, IL-6, TNF-α and IL-17 in the CNS may result in neurological dysfunction. In this case, microglia and astrocytes via TLR and nucleotide-binding domain promote the recruitment and antigen-specific activation of infiltrating leukocytes [Rock et al.; 2004; Kielian; 2005].

Accumulated evidence has shown that substance P (SP), the most abundant tachykinin in the brain, also plays an important role in the inflammatory immune responses at peripheral sites [Vojdani & Lambert, 2011]. Neuropeptide SP, with its high affinity receptor NK-1R is expressed on microglia and can also modulate the function of myeloid cells, such as dendritic cells and macrophages via a high affinity receptor called neurokinin-1 (NK-1). SP with NK- 1R activate the transcription factor NF-κB, which facilitates the production of key proinflammatory cytokines such as TNF-α, IL-6 and IL-17, and also reduce the production of immunoregulatory cytokines (TGF-β, IL-10) by macrophages; thereby further exacerbating inflammation [Vojdani & Lambert, 2011]. The mechanism of bacterial antigens inducing the neuronal SP production and it´s binding to SP receptors, result in cytokine production and brain inflammation. Furthermore, products, such as SP receptor antagonists for the inhibition of NF-κB, or minocycline, α-Lipoic acid, resveratrol [Aebischer & Kato; 2007; Lampl et al, 2007] or quercetin [Sternberg et al, 2008], which are known to be effective in the repair of BBB damaged by infections, may represent important new therapeutic strategies to combat potentially disabling consequences of inflammation within the brain.

2.4 Current perspective on treatment in MS

Further evidence to support the importance of neurodegeneration in MS is obtained from clinical data showing only a partial success of the available disease-modifying drugs (interferons, Glatiramer Acetate, monoclonal antibodies to antigenic determinants expressed on T lymphocytes, among others), which impede activation and migration of inflammatory cells via the BBB, but have no direct effect on the degenerative processes in the CNS. [Antel & Miron, 2008; Bergamaschi et al, 2006; De Jager , 2007; Miron et al, 2008; Weinstock-Guttman, 2006].

The research community has clarified the underlying biology of MS and shown great promises for developing an improved therapy. Areas of research that hold promise in the near future include: 1) the development of drugs that block the movement of myelin-attacking T cells from the bloodstream into the brain, 2) engineering drugs that specifically inhibit the damaging T cells or antibodies, 3) finding approaches that promote remyelination (myelin ro treatment in MS repair), which may allow individuals to regain function and 4) studies of MRI, immune, and genetic variables that improve our ability to predict the disease course, and tailor or engineer therapy to individuals with MS.

Trials of stem cell transplantation, with the goal of repopulating oligodendrocytes, are underway in people with MS. Remyelination may also be promoted by blocking leucine rich repeat and Ig domain-containing, Nogo Receptor-interacting protein 1 (LINGO-1), a protein on the surface of neurons that inhibits differentiation of precursor oligodendrocytes into mature cells. Antibody blockade of LINGO-1 has shown promise in an animal model of MS [Loeb, 2007]. Neurotrophins are protein factors produced by CNS cells that support neuronal growth, survival and differentiation [Azoulayet al, 2008]. In MS, secretion of the neurotrophin brain-derived neurotrophic factor is low and dysregulated [Mi et al, 2009] and BDNF is therefore also being considered as a therapeutic target. Current MS therapeutics are moderately effective for modifying disease during its relapsing-remitting phase. There are a number of oral and parenteral agents that target developing inflammation, and several are likely to be approved for treatment of RRMS within the next few years. These therapies will likely more effectively control RRMS but will also carry greater known and, as yet, unknown safety risks. These risks and benefits will have to be weighed carefully against the efficacy and proven safety of the IFNs and Glatiramer acetate. Furthermore, none of the anti-inflammatory therapies currently in late stage of development are likely to benefit patients with SPMS and PPMS. Development of effective neuroprotective and neurorestorative therapies are needed in order to benefit patients with progressive MS.

3. Conclusion

Since MS shows a great heterogeneity, the influence of multiple etiopathogenic factors could be considered as the main cause of this behavioral pattern. Nevertheless the well established hypothesis on the aetiology and pathogenic mechanisms described for this disease are not enough, at least to explain the wide clinical variations in response to treatment. From this view point, it is true that serious contributions have been achieved, but more protocols must be conducted for a major understanding of MS pathology, as well as for a more effective response to treatment.

4. References

Abbott NJ 2002 .Astrocyte-endothelial interactions and blood-brain barrier permeability. J. Anat. 2009, 629-638.

Aebischer P and. Kato A C. 2007. Playing defense against Lou Gehrig's disease. *Scientific American*, 297: 86- 93.

Amor S, Giovannoni G. 2007 Antibodies to myelin oligodendrocyte glycoprotein as a biomarker in multiple sclerosis—are we there yet? Mult Scler, 13:1083-1085.

Amor S, Puentes F, Baker D & van der Valk P. 2010. Inflammation in neurodegenerative diseases. Immunology, 129: 154-169.

Anderson, C.M. and Swanson, R.A. 2000 Astrocyte glutamate transport: review of properties, regulation, and physiological functions. Glia 32: 1-14.

Anderson, M, Alvarez-Cermeño, J, Bernardi, G & Cogato, I. 1994. Cerebro Spinal fluid in the diagnosis of multiple sclerosis: a consensus report. J Neurol Neurosurg Psych, 57: 897-902.

Antel JP & Miron VE. 2008. Central nervous system effects of current and emerging multiple sclerosis-directed immuno-therapies. Clinical Neurology and Neurosurgery 110: 951–957 .

Arumugam TV, Woodruff TM, Lathia JD, Selvaraj PK, Mattson MP, Taylor SM. 2009 Neuroprotection in stroke by complement inhibition and immunoglobulin therapy. Neuroscience.

Azoulay D, Urshansky N, Karni A. 2008Low and dysregulated BDNF secretion from immune cells of MS patients is related to reduced neuroprotection. *J Neuroimmunol,* 195:186–193.

Babbe, H, Roers, A & Waisman, A. 2000. Clonal expansion CD8+ T cells dominate the T cell infiltrate in active multiple sclerosis lesions as shown by micromanipulation and single cell polymerasa chain reaction. J Exp Med, 192: 393-404.

Barnett M.H. &, Sutton I. 2006. The pathology of multiple sclerosis: a paradigm shift. Curr Opin Neurol , 19: 242-47.

Bartos A, Fialova L, Soukupova J, Kukal J, Malbohan I & Pitha J. 2007 Antibodies against light neurofilaments in multiple sclerosis patients. Acta Neurol Scand,116: 100-7.

Bartos A, Fialova L, SoukupovÃ¡ J, Kukal J, Malbohan I & Pitha J. 2007a. Elevated intrathecal antibodies against the medium neurofilament subunit in multiple sclerosis. J Neurol, 254: 20-25.

Batten M., Li J., Yi S et al. 2006. Interleukin 27 limits autoimmune encephalomyelitis by suppressing the development of interleukin 17-producing T cells. Nature Immunology, 7: 929–936.

Becher B, Bechmann, I & Greter, M. 2006. Antigen presentation in autoimmunity and CNS inflammation: how T lymphocytes recognize the brain. J Mol Med; 84: 532-43.

Bejartmar C, Trapp B.D. 2003. Axonal degeneration and progressive neurologic disability in multiple sclerosis. Neurotox Res , 5: 157-64.

Bergamaschi R, Kappos L, Antel J, Comi G, Montalban X, O'Connor P, et al. 2006. Oral Fingolimod (FTY720) for Relapsing Multiple Sclerosis. N Engl J Med; 355: 1124-40.

Bielekova, B, Kadom, M & Fisher, E. 2005 MRI as a marker for disease heterogeneity in Multiple sclerosis. Neurology, 65: 1071-76.

Bigio, MR. 1995. The ependyma. A protective barrier between brain and cerebrospinal fluid. Glia; 14:1-13.

Bolton C, Paul C. MK-801 limits neurovascular dysfunction during experimental allergic encephalomyelitis. J Pharmacol Exp Ther 1997; 282: 397–402.

Brown K.A. 2001. Factors modifying the migration of lymphocytes across the blood-brain barrier. Int Immunopharmacol, 1: 2043-62.

Cabre P, Signate,A, Olindo, S; Merle,H ; Caparros-Lefebvre, D, et al. 2005. Role of return migration in the emergence of multiple sclerosis in the French West Indies. Brain, 128: 2899–2910.

Camerona EM; Spencera S; Lazarinia, J; Harpa, CT; Wardb,ES; et al.2009. Potential of a unique antibody gene signature to predict conversion to clinically definite Multiple Sclerosis. J Neuroimmunol, 213: 123–130.

Carson, M.J.; Bilousova, T.V.; Puntambekar, S.S.; Melchior, B.; Doose, J.M.; Ethell, I.M. 2007. A rose by any othername? The potential consequences of microglial heterogeneity during CNS health and disease. Neurotherapeutics, 4: 571-579

Chabas, D; Ness, J; Belman, A; Yeh, EA; Kuntz, N; Gorman, MP; et al. 2010. Younger children with MS have a distinct CSF inflammatory profile at disease onset. Neurology, 74: 399–405.

Chauhan V S & Marriott I. 2007. Bacterial infections of the central nervous system: a critical role for resident glial cells in the initiation and progression of inflammation. Curr Immunol Rev, 3: 133–143.

Cheung P.F.Y., Wong C.K., and Lam C.W.K. 2008. Molecular mechanisms of cytokine and chemokine release from eosinophils activated by IL-17a, IL-17f and IL-23: implication for Th17 lymphocyte-mediated allergic inflammation. J Immunol 180: 5625–35.

Chung Y. & Dong C. 2009. Don't leave home without it: the IL- 23 visa to TH-17 cells. Nat Immunol, 10: 236–38.

Cohrs RJ, Gilden DH. 2005. Prevalence and abundance of latently transcribed varicella-zoster virus genes 17. Nature Immunol 6: 1133–41.

Coles AJ, Cox, A, Le Page, E. 2006. The window of therapeutic opportunity in multiple sclerosis: Evidence for monoclonal antibody therapy. J Neurol, 253: 98-108.

Colleen MK, Burns BA, and KevinAA. 2006. Does rubella immunity predict méasles immunity? A serosurvey of pregnant women.Infectious Disease Obstetrics and Gynecology. Clinical Study. Hindawi Publishing Corporation. pp. 23.

Colton C.A.; Wilcock, D.M. 2010. Assessing activation states in microglia. CNS Neurol. Disord. Drug Targets, 9: 174-191.

Cooper LZ, Alford CA. 2001. Rubella. In: Remington JS, Klein, JO, eds. Infectious diseases of the fetus and newborninfant. London: W.B. Saunders; 347–87.

Correales J. 2004. Oligoclonal bands and antibody response in multiple sclerosis.In: Focus on Multiple sclerosis Research. Frank Columbus (ed): pp. 37-65.

De Jager, PL & Hafler, DA. 2007. New therapeutic approaches for multiple sclerosis. Annu Rev Med, 58:417–432.

Del Zoppo, GJ & Hallenbeck, JM 2000. Advances in the vascularpathophysiology of ischemic stroke. Thromb. Res. 98: 73–81.

Departamento de análisis de datos. 2004. Dirección nacional de estadística y registros médicos. Ministerio de Salud Pública de Cuba, Havana City, Cuba.

Devries HG 2006. Cryptic axonal antigens and axonal loss in multiple sclerosis. Neuroch Res, 29:1999- 2004.

Dutta R, Trapp BD. Pathogenesis of axonal and neuronal damage in multiple sclerosis. Neurology 2007. 68(Suppl 3): S22–S31.

Eikelenboom MJ, Petzold A, Lazeron RHC, Silber E, Sharief M, Thompson EJ; et al. 2003 Neurofilament light chain antibodies are correlated to cerebral atrophy. Neurology, 60: 219-23.

Falip M; Tintore, M; Jardi, R; Duran, I; Link; H & Montalban, X. 2001.Utilidad clínica de las bandas oligoclonales. Rev Neurol, 32: 1120-24.

Ferreira S, D'Cruz DP, Hughes GRV. 2005. Multiple sclerosis, neuropsychiatric lupus and antiphospholipid syndrome: where do we stand? Rheumatology (Oxford); 44: 434–442.

Fisher LJ & Gage, F.H. 1993. Grafting in the mammalian central nervous system. Physiol Rev, 73: 583-16.

Forman, ME; Racke, KM & Raine, SC. 2006. Multiple Sclerosis- the plaque and its pathogenesis. N Eng J Med, 354: 942-55.

Fox RJ, Bethoux F, Goldman MD, Cohen JA. 2006. Multiple sclerosis: advances in understanding, diagnosing, and treating the underlying disease. Cleve Clin J Med, 73: 91-102.

Frederick TJ, Miller SD. 2007. Arresting autoimmunity by blocking beta-arrestin-1. Nat Immunol; 8: 791–792.

Friese, MA & Fugger, L. 2005. Autoreactive CD8+ T cells in multiple sclerosis: a new target for therapy? Brain, 128: 1747–63.

Frischer J M, Bramow S, Dal-Bianco A, Lucchinetti CF,Rauschka H, Schmidbauer M, Laureen H, Sorensen PS & Lassmann H. 2009. The relation between inflammation and neurodegeneration in multiple sclerosis brains. Brain, 132; 1175–1189.

Fujinami RS, von Herrath MG, Christen U, Whitton JL. 2006. Molecular mimicry, bystander activation, or viral persistence: infections and autoimmune disease. Clin Microbiol Rev, 19: 80–94.

Gandhi, KS, McKay FC, Schibeci SD, Arthur JW, Heard RN, StewartGJ & Booth DR. 2008. BAFF is a Biological Response Marker to IFN-β Treatment in Multiple Sclerosis. J Inter & Cytok Res 28: 529–540.

Ghafourifar P, Mousavizadeh K, Parihar MS, et al. Mitochondria in multiple sclerosis. 2008. Front Biosci 13: 3116–3126.

Gorczyca WA, Ejma M, Witkowska D, et al. 2004. Retinal antigens are recognized by antibodies present in sera of patients with multiple sclerosis. Ophthalmic Res; 36: 120–123.

Groom AJ, Smith T, Turski L Xiong ZQ, Qian W, Suzuki K, et al. 2003. Formation of complement membrane attack complex in mammalian cerebral cortex evokes seizures and neurodegeneration. J Neurosci; 23: 955–960.

Haahr S, Hollsberg P. 2006. Multiple sclerosis is linked to Epstein-Barr virus infection. Rev Med Virol, 16: 297-10.

Haukins, BT & Davis, TP. 2005. The blood-brain barrier/neurovascular unit in health and disease. Pharmacol Rev, 57: 173-85.

Hauser SL, Waubant E, Arnold DL, , et al. 2008. Hermes Trial Group. B-cell depletion with rituximab in relapsing-remitting multiple sclerosis. N Engl J Med; 358: 676–688.

Hemmer, B, Cepok, S, Zhou, D & Sommer, N. 2004. Multiple sclerosis – a coordinated immune attack across the blood brain barrier. Current Neurovasc Res; 1: 141-50.

Hermitte L, Martin-Moutot N, Boucraut J, et al. 2000. Humoral immunity against glutamic acid decarboxylase and tyrosine phosphatase IA-2. J Clin Immunol; 20: 287–293.

Hickey, WF. 2001. Basic principles of immunological surveillance of the normal central nervous system. Glia, 36: 118–24.

Hillert J. 2006. Multiple sclerosis: postlinkage genetics. Clin Neurol Neurosurg , 108:220-2.

Huizinga R, Linington C, Amor S. 2008. Resistance is futile: antineuronal autoimmunity in multiple sclerosis. Trends Immunol ; 29: 54–60.

Ishizu T, Osoegawa M., Mei F.-J. et al, 2005. Intrathecal activation of the IL-17/IL-8 axis in opticospinal multiple sclerosis. Brain, 128: 988–1002.

Ishizu, KJ. 2009. Intrathecal activation of the IL-17-IL-8 axis in opticospinal multiple sclerosis. Pharmacol Res, 128: 207-09.

Iwakura Y. & Ishigame. 2006. The IL-23/IL-17 axis in inflammation. J Clin Invest, 116: 1218–22.

Jack, C; Jack, A, Wolfgang B & Tanja K. 2007. Contrasting Potential of Nitric Oxide and Peroxynitrite to Mediate Oligodendrocyte Injury in Multiple Sclerosis. GLIA 55: 926–934.

Jarius S, Eichhorn P, Jacobi C, Wildemann B, Wick M, Voltz R. 2009. The intrathecal, polyspecific antiviral immune response: Specific for MS or a general marker of CNS autoimmunity? J Neurol Sci, 280: 98-100.

Jarius S. 2008. Polyspecific, antiviral immune response distinguishes multiple sclerosis and neuromyelitis optica. Nature Clin Pract Neurol; 4: 524.

Jiang, H & Chess, L. 2006. Regulation of immune response by T cell. New Engl J Med 354: 1166-76.

Kanda T, Iwasaki T, Yamawaki M, et al. 2000. Anti-GM1 antibody facilitates leakage in an in vitro blood-nerve barrier model. Neurology; 55: 585–87.

Kawanokuchi J, Shimizu K., Nitta A. et al. 2008. Production and functions of IL-17 in microglia. J Neuroimmunol, 194: 54–61.

Kang, J. 1998 Astrocyte-mediated potentiation of inhibitory synaptic transmission. Nat. Neurosci, 1: 683–92.

Keegan M, Kónig F, McClelland R, et al. 2005. Relation between humoral pathological changes in multiple sclerosis and response to therapeutic plasma exchange. Lancet; 366: 579–82.

Kielian T, Esen N and Bearden E. D. 2005. Toll-like receptor 2 (TLR2) is pivotal for recognition of S. aureus peptidoglycan but not intact bacteria by microglia. *GLIA*, 49: 567–76.

Kira J. 2007. Etiology of multiple sclerosis. In: Multiple Sclerosis for the Practicing Neurologist. Theodore (ed). pp. 1-6, Demos Medical Publishing LLC, Vol 5, New York.

Klawiter, EC & Cross, AH. 2007. B cells: no longer the nondominant arm of multiple sclerosis. Curr Neurol Neurosci Rep; 7: 231–238.

Komek, BL. 2003. Neuropathology of multiple sclerosis-new concepts. Brain Res Bull, 61: 321-26.

Kraft AD & Harry GJ. 2011. Features of Microglia and Neuroinflammation Relevant to Environmental Exposure and Neurotoxicity Int. J. Environ. Res. Public Health, 8: 2980-3018

Lambracht-Washington D, O'Connor KC, Cameron EM, et al. 2007. Antigen specificity of clonally expanded and receptor edited cerebrospinal fluid B cells from patients with relapsing remitting MS. J Neuroimmunol; 186: 164–76.

Lampl Y, Boaz M, Gilad R, et al. 2007. Minocycline treatment in acute stroke: an open-label, evaluator-blinded study. *Neurology*, 69: 1404–10.

Lassmann H, Niedobitek G,Aloisi F, & Middeldorp JM. 2011. Epstein–Barr virus in the multiple sclerosis brain: a controversial issue—report on a focused workshop held in the Centre for Brain Research of the Medical University of Vienna, Austria. Brain: 134: 2772–86.

Lee, MA, Palace D, Palace J. 2007. The diagnostic and differential diagnostic in multiple sclerosis.In: Multiple Sclerosis for the Practicing Neurologist Theodore E (ed). New York: Demos Medical Publishing, LLC, Vol 5, p. 33-50.

Levin LI, Munger KL, O'Reilly EJ, Falk KI, Ascherio A. 2010, Primary infection with Epstein-Barr virus and risk of multiple sclerosis. Ann Neurol; 67: 824–30.

Lim, ET, Sellebjerg, F, Jensen, CV, Altmann, DR, Grant, D & Keir, G. 2005 .Acute axonal damage predicts clinical outcome in patients with multiple sclerosis. Mult Scler ,11: 532-6.

Lindberg RL, Achtnichts L, Hoffmann F, et al. 2008. Natalizumab alters transcriptional expression profiles of blood cell subpopulations of multiple sclerosis patients. J Neuroimmunol; 194: 153–64.

Lipton SA, Rosenberg PA. 1994. Excitatory amino acids as a final common pathway for neurologic disorders. N Engl J Med; 330: 613–22.

Lisak, PR. 2007.Neurodegeneration in multiple sclerosis.Defining the problem. Neurology 2007; 68: S5-S12.

Loeb JA. 2007. Neuroprotection and repair by neurotrophic and gliotrophic factors in multiple sclerosis. Neurology; 68(Suppl 3): 38–54.

Lovato L, Willis SN, Rodig SJ, Caron T, Almendinger SE, Howell OW, et al. 2011. Related B cell clones populate the meninges and parenchyma of patients with multiple sclerosis. Brain; 134: 534–41.

Lu F, Kalman B. 1999. Autoreactive IgG to intracellular proteins in sera of MS patients. J Neuroimmunol; 99:72–81.

Lu J, Murakami M, Verma SC, Cai Q, Haldar S, Kaul R, et al. 2011. Epstein-Barr virus nuclear antigen 1 (EBNA1) confers resistance to apoptosis in EBV-positive B-lymphoma cells through upregulation of survivin. Virology; 410: 64–75.

Lucchinetti, C, Brück W, Scheithauer B, Rodriguez M Lassman H. 2000, Heterogeneity of multiple sclerosis lesions: implications for the pathogenesis of demyelination. Ann Neurol, 47: 707-17.

Luchinetti CF. 2007. Advances in the neuropathology of multiple sclerosis: evolving pathogenesis insight. Continuum Lifelong Learning. Neurology 13: 86-116.

Lutterotti A, Berger T, Reindl M. 2007. Biological markers for multiple sclerosis. Curr Med Chem; 14:1956–65.

Maes M, Kubera M., and Leunis JC. 2008. The gut-brain barrier in major depression: intestinal mucosal dysfunction with an increased translocation of LPS from gram negative enterobacteria (leaky gut) plays a role in the inflammatory pathophysiology of depression. Neuroendocrinol Letters, 29: 117–24.

Maes M, Coucke F, and Leunis JC. 2007. Normalization of the increased translocation of endotoxin from gram negative enterobacteria (leaky gut) is accompanied by a remission of chronic fatigue syndrome. Neuroendocrinol Letters, 28: 739–44.

Maghzi AH, Marta M, Bosca I, Etemadifar M, Dobson R, Maggiore C, et al. 2010. Viral pathophysiology of multiple sclerosis: a role for Epstein-Barr virus infection? Pathophysiology; 18: 13–20.

Magliozzi R, Howell OW, Reeves C, Roncaroli F, Nicholas R, Serafini B, et al. 2010. A gradient of neuronal loss and meningeal inflammation in multiple sclerosis. Ann Neurol; 68: 477–93.

Maier O, Baron W, Hoekstra D. 2007. Reduced raft-association of NF155 in active MS-lesions is accompanied by the disruption of the paranodal junction. Glia; 55: 885–95.

Marconi S, Acler M, Lovato L, et al. 2006. Anti-GD2-like IgM autoreactivity in multiple sclerosis patients. Mult Scler; 12: 302–08.

Martinez, A; Mas, A; de las Heras, V; Arroyo, R; Fernandez-Arquero, M; de la Concha, EG et al. 2005. Early B-cell Factor gene association with multiple sclerosis in the Spanish population. BMC Neurol, 5: 19-22.

Martinez-Yélamos, S, Ballabriga, J, Martinez-Yélamos, A, Hernandez, JJ & Arbizu, T. 1998. Evolución y pronóstico de la esclerosis múltiple. Medicine; 7: 4333-37.

Mathey EK, Derfuss T, Storch MK, et al. 2007. Neurofascin as a novel target for autoantibody-mediated axonal injury. J Exp Med; 204: 2363–72.

Matute C, Domercq M, Sanchez-Gomez MV. 2006. Glutamate-mediated glial injury: mechanisms and clinical importance. Glia; 53: 212–24.

McCoy, L; Tsunoda, I & Fuginami, RS. 2006. Multiple sclerosis and virus induced immune responses: autoimmunity can be primed by molecular mimicry and augmented by bystander activation. Autoimmunity, 39: 9-19.

McDonald, W, Compston, A, Edan, G, Hangtung, H, Lublin, F, McFarland H et al. 2001. Recommended diagnostic criteria for multiple sclerosis. Ann Neurol , 50: 121-27.

McGeachy M. J., Chen Y, Tato C.M et al. 2009. The interleukin 23 receptor is essential for the terminal differentiation of interleukin 17-producing effector T helper cells in vivo. Nat Immunol, 10: 314–24.

Meinl E, Krumbholz M, Derfuss T, Junker A,Hohlfeld R. 2008. Comparmentalization of inflammaion in the CNS:A major mechanism driving progressive multiple sclerosis. J Neurol Sci; 274: 42-44.

Mi S, Miller RH, Tang W, Lee X, Hu B, Wu W, Zhang Y, Shields CB, Zhang Y, Miklasz S, Shea D, Mason J, Franklin RJ, Ji B, Shao Z, Chédotal A, Bernard F, Roulois A, Xu J, Jung V, Pepinsky B. *2009*. Promotion of central nervous system remyelination by induced differentiation of oligodendrocyte precursor cells. *Ann Neurol*; 65: 304–15.

Miron VE, Jung CG, Kim HJ, Kennedy TE, Soliven B &. Antel JP. 2008. FTY720 Modulates Human. Oligodendrocyte Progenitor Process Extension and Survival Ann Neurol; 63: 61–71.

Mirsattari, SM, Johnston, J, McKenna R, et al. 2001. Aborigenals with multiple sclerosis HLA types and proedominance of neuromyelitis óptica. Neurology, 56: 317-23.

Monteleone G., Pallone F, & MacDonald T.T. 2008. Interleukin- 21: a critical regulator of the balance between effector and regulatory T-cell responses. Trends Immunol, 29: 290–94.

Mosmann T. R.; H. Cherwinski, M.W.; Bond, M.A.; Giedlin, & Coffman R.L. 1986. Two types of murine helper T cell clone. I. Definition according to profiles of lymphokine activities and secreted proteins. J Immunol, 136: 2348–57.

Nag, S. 2003. Pathophysiology of blood brain barrier breakdown. Methods Mol Med, 89: 97-111.

Nathanson, JA & Chun, LYL. 1990. Possible role of the choroid plexus in immunological communication between the brain and periphery. BB Johansson, Ch Owman, H Widner (Eds). In. Pathophysiology of the blood brain barrier, Elsevier Science Publisher, pp. 501 505.New York.

Nathanson, JA, Chun, LYL. 1990a. Immunological function of the blood- cerebrospinal fluid barrier. Proc Natl Acad Sci. USA, 86: 1684-88.

Ness, JM; Chabas, D; Sadovnick, AD; Pohl, D; Banwell, B & Weinstock-Guttman, B. 2007. Clinical features of children and adolescents with multiple sclerosis. Neurology, 68; 37-45.

Neumann, H, Medana, IM, Bawer, J & Lassmann, H. 2002. Cytotoxic T lymphocyte in autoimmune and degenerative CNS diseases. Trends Neurosci, 25: 313-19.

Neutwelt, E, Abbott, NJ , Abrey, L, Banks, W A, Blakley, B, Davis, T, et al. 2008. Strategies to advance translational research into brain barriers. Lancet Neurol; 7: 84-96.

O'Connor KC, Cameron EM, et al. 2007. Antigen specificity of clonally expanded and receptor edited cerebrospinal fluid B cells from patients with relapsing remitting MS. J Neuroimmunol; 186: 164–76.

Owens GP, Burgoon MP, Anthony J, et al. 2001. The immunoglobulin G heavy chain repertoire in multiple sclerosis plaques is distinct from the heavy chain repertoire in peripheral blood lymphocytes. Clin Immunol; 98: 258–263.

Pender MP. 2011. The essential role of Epstein-Barr Virus in the pathogenesisof multiple sclerosis. Neuroscientist, 17: 351–67.

Perry, V H & Gordon, S. 1997. Microglias and macrophages. In: Immunology of the nervous system, R W Keane and WE Hickey (eds), pp (155-172) Oxford University Press,New York.

Petty, MA & Lo, HE. 2002. Junctional complexes of the blood–brain barrier: permeability changes in neuroinflammation. Prog Neurobiol, 68: 311–23.

Pittock, SJ, Mayr, WT, McClelland RL. 2004. Change in MS-related disability in a population- based cohort: a 10- year follow–up study. Neurology; 62: 51-59.

Porras-Betancourt, M; Nuñez-Orozco, L; Plascencia-Alvarez, NI; Quiñones-Aguilar, S & Sauri-Suarez, S. 2007. Esclerosis Multiple. Rev Mex Neurosc; 8: 57-66.

Prat A, Antel J. 2005. Pathogenesis of multiple sclerosis.Curr Opin Neurol , 18: 225-30.

Rauer, S; Euler, B; Reindl,M & Berger TH. 2006. Antimyelin antibodies and the risk of relapse in patients with a primary demyelinating event. J Neurol Neurosurg Psychiatry, 77: 739–42.

Redzic, ZB, Preston, JE, Duncan, JA, Chdobski, A & Szmydynger Chdobsk, J. 2005. The choroid plexus- cerebrospinal fluid system from development to ageing. Curr Top Dev Biol, 71: 1-52.

Reese, TS & Karnowosky, MJ 1967. Fine structural localization of a blood-brain barrier to exogenous peroxidase. J Cell Biol 34: 207-17.

Reiber H, Ungefehr ST, Jacobi CHR. 1998. The intrathecal, polyspecific and oligoclonal immune response in multiple sclerosis. Mult Scler; 4: 111–17.

Rivest S. 2009. Regulation of innate immune responses in the brain. Nat. Rev. Immunol, 9: 429-39.

Robinson-Agramonte MA. 2010. Asimilación del método de focalización isoeléctrica en agarosa y aplicación del ELISA al estudio de la respuesta de anticuerpos en el sistema nervioso central de personas con esclerosis múltiple. Revista CENIC Ciencias Biológicas, 21: 206-07.

Robinson-Agramonte M, Reiber H, Cabrera-Gomez JA, Galvizu R. 2007. Intrathecal polyspecific immune response to neurotropic viruses inmultiple sclerosis: a comparative report from Cuban patients. Acta Neurol Scand, 115: 312–18.

Robinson-Agramonte M, Reiber H, Dorta-Contreras AJ,Herna´ndez-Dıaz E. 2001. Respuesta inmune intratecal oligoclonaly poliespecı´fica en la esclerosis múltiple. Rev Neurol; 33: 809–11.

Rock R. B, Gekker G, Hu S et al. 2004. Role ofmicroglia in central nervous system infections. Clinical Microbiology Reviews, 17: 942–64.

Rose, WJ & Carlson, GN. 2007. Pathogenesis of multiple sclerosis. Continuum Lifelong Learning Neurol , 13: 35-62.

Roussel V, Yi F, Jauberteau MO, et al. 2000. Prevalence and clinical significance of anti-phospholipid antibodies in multiple sclerosis: a study of 89 patients. J Autoimmun; 14: 259–65.

Sarchielli P, Greco L, Floridi A, et al. 2003. Excitatory amino acids and multiple sclerosis: evidence from cerebrospinal fluid. Arch Neurol; 60: 1082–88.

Semra YK, Seidi OA, Sharief MK. 2002. Heightened intrathecal release of axonal cytoskeletal proteins in multiple sclerosis is associated with progressive disease and clinical disability. J Neuroimmunol, 122: 132-39.

Serafini B, Severa M, Columba-Cabezas S, Rosicarelli B, Veroni C, Chiappetta G, et al. 2010. Epstein-Barr virus latent infection and BAFF expression in B-cells in the multiple sclerosis brain: implications for viral persistence and intrathecal B-cell activation. J Neuropath Exp Neurol; 69: 677–93.

Seyfert, S & Faultish, A. 2003. Is the blood-CSF barrier altered in disease? Acta Neurol Scand, 108: 252-56.

Shi Y, Feng Y, Kang J, et al. 2007. Critical regulation of CD4+ T cell survival and autoimmunity by beta-arrestin-1. Nat Immunol; 8: 817–24.

Silber, E; Semra, YK; Gregson, NA & Sharief MK. 2002. Patients with progressive multiple sclerosis have elevated antibodies to neurofilament subunit. Neurology 58: 1372-78.

Smith T, Groom A, Zhu B, et al. 2000. Autoimmune encephalomyelitis ameliorated byAMPA antagonists. Nat Med; 6: 62–66.

Sobel, RA. 1998. The extracellular matrix in multiple sclerosis lesions.J Neuropathol Exp Neurol, 57: 205–17

Sospedra, M &. Martin, R. 2009. MRI criteria in MS patients with negative and positive oligoclonal bands: equal fulfillment of Barkhof's criteria but different lesion patterns. J Neurol, 256: 1121-25.

Steinman L. 2007. A brief history of TH17, the first major revision in the TH1/TH2 hypothesis of T cell-mediated tissue damage. Nature Medicine, 13: 139–45.

Sternberg Z, Chadha K, Lieberman A et al. 2008. Quercetin and interferon-β modulate immune response(s) in peripheral blood mononuclear cells isolated from multiple sclerosis patients. Journal of Neuroimmunology, 205: 142–47.

Stockinger & Veldhoen M. 2007. Differentiation and function of Th17 T cells. Curr Op Immunol,19: 281–86.

Chung Y. & Dong C. 2009. Don't leave home without it: the IL- 23 visa to TH-17 cells. Nat Immunol, 10: 236–38.

Stromnes I. M., Cerretti L.M, Liggitt D., Harris R.A. & Goverman J. M. 2008. Differential regulation of central nervous system autoimmunity by TH1 and TH17 cells. Nature Medicine, 14: 337–42.

Stys PK, Lipton SA. 2007. White matter NMDA receptors: an unexpected new therapeutic target? Trends Pharmacol Sci; 28: 561–66.

Taplin CE, Barker JM. 2008. Autoantibodies in type 1 diabetes. Autoimmunity; 41: 11–18.

Tester A.M., Cox J. H., Connor A. R. et al, 2007. LPS responsiveness and neutrophil chemotaxis in vivo require PMN MMP-8 activity. PLoS ONE, 2: article e312.

Theiss C, Napirei M, Meller K. 2005. Impairment of anterograde and retrograde neurofilament transport after anti-kinesin and anti-dynein antibody microinjection in chicken dorsal root ganglia. Eur J Cell Biol 84: 29–43.

Torkildsen, O; Vedeler, CA; Nyland, HI; Myhr KM. 2006. FcγR and multiple sclerosis: an overview. Acta Neurol Scand ,113: 61–63.

Vercellino M, Merola A, Piacentino C, et al. 2007. Altered glutamate reuptake in relapsing-remitting and secondary progressive multiple sclerosis cortex: correlation with microglia infiltration, demyelination, and neuronal and synaptic damage. J Neuropathol Exp Neurol; 66: 732–39.

Villar, LM; Sádaba,MC;Roldán, E; Masjuan, J; González, P; Villarrubia, N; et al. 2005. Intrathecal synthesis of oligoclonal IgM against myelin lipids predicts an aggressive disease course in MS. J Clin Invest,115 :187-90.

Vojdani A & Lambert J. 2011a The Role of Th17 inNeuroimmuneDisorders: Target for CAM Therapy. Part II Hindawi Publishing Corporation Evidence-Based Complementary and Alternative Medicine Volume 1-7.

Vojdani A & Lambert; J. 2011.The Role of Th17 inNeuroimmuneDisorders: Target for CAM Therapy. Part I Hindawi Publishing Corporation Evidence-Based Complementary and Alternative Medicine Volume 1-8.

Vyshkina T & Kalman B. 2008. Autoantibodies and neurodegeneration in multiple sclerosis. Lab Invest, 1–12.

Wallstrom E, Diener P, Ljungdahl A, et al. 1996. Memantine abrogates neurological deficits, but not CNS inflammation, in Lewis rat experimental autoimmune encephalomyelitis. J Neurol Sci; 137: 89–96.

Weinstock-Guttman B; Ramanathan M; Lincoff N; Napoli SQ; Sharma J; et al. 2006. Study of Mitoxantrone for the Treatment of Recurrent Neuromyelitis Optica Devic Disease. Arch Neurol, 63: 957-63.

Wilson C. B, Rowell E. & Sekimata M. 2009. Epigenetic control of T-helper-cell differentiation. Nat Rev Immunol, 9: 91–105.

Winer JB. 2001. Guillain Barre syndrome. Mol Pathol; 54: 381–85.

Wingerchuck, D & Kantarci O. 2006. Epidemiology and natural history of multiple sclerosis: new insights. Curr Opin Neurol, 19: 248-54.

Zaffaroni M. 2003. Biological indicators of the neurodegenerative phase of multiple sclerosis. Neurol Sci; 24 (Suppl 5): S279–S282.

Zheng et al. 2007. Interleukin-22, a TH17 cytokine, mediates IL-23-induced dermal inflammation and acanthosis. Nature, 445 (7128): 648–51.

Adaptive Immune Response in Epilepsy

Sandra Orozco-Suárez[1,*], Iris Feria-Romero[1], Dario Rayo[2], Jaime Diegopérez[2], Ma.Ines Fraire[2], Justina Sosa[3], Lourdes Arriaga[4], Mario Alonso Vanegas[5], Luisa Rocha[6], Pietro Fagiolino[7] and Israel Grijalva[1]
[1]*Unidad de Investigación Médica en Enfermedades Neurológicas,*
[2]*Hospital de Pediatria, CMN Siglo XXI,*
[3]*Hospital de Especialidades, CM "La Raza",IMSS.México D.F.,*
[4]*Unidad de Investigación en Inmunoquímica,Hospital de Especialidades, CMN Siglo XXI, IMSS México D.F.,*
[5]*Instituto Nacional de Neurología y Neurocirugía,"Manuel Velasco Suárez", México D.F.,*
[6]*Departamento de Farmacobiología, Centro de Investigacion y de Estudios Avanzados, Sede Sur,*
[7]*Centro de Monitoreo de Fármacos, Universidad de la República, Montevideo,*
[1,2,3,4,5,6]*México*
[7]*Uruguay*

1. Introduction

Various brain injuries in humans such as neurotrauma,stroke, infection, febrile convulsions and status epilepticus are associated with the acute occurrence of seizures and an increased risk of developing epilepsy, Experimental studies in rodents have shown that these events induce a chronic decreased seizure threshold or the development of spontaneous seizures, supporting the notion, that central nervous system (CNS) injury can lead to lasting hyperexcitability. These injuries trigger inflammatory processes in the brain, which are rapidly ensuing and long-lasting, raising the possibility that inflammatory mediators may contribute to the development of epileptogenesis, and the consequent precipitation of spontaneous seizures.

On the other hand a pathogenic role of immunity in epilepsies has long been suggested based on observations of the efficacy of immune-modulating treatments and, more recently, by the finding of inflammation markers including autoantibodies in individuals with a number of epileptic disorders. Clinical and experimental data suggest that both innate and adaptive immunity may be involved in epilepsy. Innate immunity represents an immediate, nonspecific host response against pathogens via activation of resident brain immune cells and inflammatory mediators. These are thought to contribute to seizures and epileptogenesis. Adaptive immunity employs activation of antigen specific B and T lymphocytes or antibodies in the context of viral infections and autoimmune disorders.

* Corresponding Author

This review focused first on the description of the interaction between the immune system and CNS peculiar aspects and relevance for the pathogenesis of immune-mediated diseases of the CNS, second, we offer an overview of the experimental evidence in experimental models of seizures to discuss how inflammation modulates epilepsy, and whether inflammation is always detrimental to cell survival. Such research has also sought to determine how inflammatory mechanisms might be harnessed to develop therapies for epilepsy and third we describe causal clinical evidences of various forms of human epilepsy in which CNS inflammation and markers of adaptive immunity have been described, also we describe some of the treatments used in pharmacoresistan epilepsy with probable autoimmune origin.

2. Overview of the immune system

The natural defences presented by an individual to any external agent are included in the immune system; this is generally divided into innate and adaptive immunity. Innate immunity is the first response presented against insult, that is triggered by physical, chemical or bacteriological damage, the latter is the most familiar and easier to reproduce by introducing systemic lipopolysaccharide or LPS, which is the substance that covers the outer membrane of Gram (-)bacteria (Condie, 1955; Rivest , 2000). For its study, innate immunity is divided into the afferent arm, which identifies or perceives to insult, and the efferent arm, which is how the infection is eradicated (Tracey, 2009). Several studies have shown that depending on the agent causing the damage, pathway, organ and even insult cells triggers a series of molecules for defence of the individual and the communication between immune system cells can lead to out both by direct contact between cells or by the involvement of soluble factors known as cytokines. This will differentiate the humoral components of the afferent arm (LBP, CD14, collectins, properdin, C3b, pentraxins) and efferent (cytokines, antimicrobial peptides, lysozyme, BPI, complement, lactoferrin, acute phase reactants) and cellular components of the afferent arm (TLRs, dectina-1, CD14, formyl peptide receptor or FMLP, NOD1, NOD2) and efferent (antimicrobial peptides, proteases, lipases, glycosidases, cell adhesion molecules, H2O2, hydroxyl radical, oxygen halides, nitric oxide, peroxynitrite, etc.) (Beutler, 2004; Vezzani, 2005).

Until recently, adaptive immunity was considered a type of immune response independent of the innate immune response; now it is known that both responses are intertwined, so the participation of dendritic cells, monocytes, macrophages, B lymphocytes and T, specialized molecules of immune histocompatibility, complex class I and II (MHC I and II) that are present during the innate response, are the beginning of the adaptive response (Iwasaki, 2010). In this type of response antigen recognition is carried by the specific antigen-presenting cells (APCs) and antigen receptors. In the adaptive immune response; it is identified two ways: the conventional adaptive immunity in jawed vertebrates and unconventional characteristic of jawless vertebrates.

The first is mediated by immunoglobulins (Ig) and T cell receptors (TCRs) (Fig 1). Low-affinity IgM antibodies circulate in the blood prior to encountering pathogens, however, high-affinity IgG and IgA antibodies are required to inactivate toxins, neutralize viruses, and promote the clearance of microorganisms (Li, 2004). Prior to antigen exposure, the initial generation of a diverse antibody repertoire is achieved early in B-lymphocyte development by the successful rearrangement of the V, D, and J gene. This recombination process depends on the recognition of recombination signal sequences (RSSs), which flank the segmental elements and create extensive variation in the receptor structure at junctional (joining) interfaces. V(D)J rearrangement form of somatic recombination occurs in the progenitors of B and T cells and is mediated by recombination-activating gene 1 (RAG1) and RAG2, which function in a lymphocyte- and site-specific recombinase complex and are supported by ubiquitous DNA repair factors (Fig **1A**)(Gellert, 2002). The Immunoglobulins function first as membrane-bound receptors on B cells and their precursor cells, and they are selected for both antigen-binding specificity and affinity. A change in RNA splicing converts the membrane-bound receptor to a soluble product and is associated with the differentiation from receptor-expressing B cells to immunoglobulin-secreting plasma cells. A second wave of antibody diversification occurs through somatic hypermutation (SHM) (Fig. 1**B**) and/or gene conversion (GC) of the V region to generate high-affinity antigen binding sites (MacLennan, 1994). SHM is the predominant mechanism in mice and humans, whereas GC occurs in chickens and some other species (Weill and Reynaud 1996). In the same centroblast B cell, the heavy-chain V regions encoding the antigen binding sites are rearranged down the chromosome through class switch recombination (CSR) so that they can be expressed with one of the constant (C) region genes to carry out many different effector functions and be distributed throughout the body (Fig. 1**C**). Activation-induced cytidine deaminase (AID) mediates SHM, gene conversion and class-switch recombination (CSR).

The TCR is a clonotypic, membrane-bound receptor that binds peptide-MHC (pMHC). Similar to immunoglobulins, both classes of TCRs (αβ TCRs and γδ TCRs) are heterodimers in which a D segment is a rearranging component of one unit of the receptor heterodimer. The function of αβ TCRs relies on the polymorphic MHC class I and class II molecules expressed by antigen-presenting cells. By contrast, γδ TCRs function independently of MHC class I and class II molecules and it has been proposed that a forerunner of the rearranging antigen-binding receptors might have been a γδ TCR-like receptor (--12--). Genetically, TCRs are rearranged into α and β-chains from a selection of 176 variable (V), diversity (D), joining (J), and constant (C) genes on chromosomes 7 and 14. Random recombination of these genes generates only 5–10% of the potential diversity within the TCR repertoire; exonucleolytic activity, random N nucleotide additions at the V(D)J junctions (Cabaniols, 2001) and αβ chain pairing contribute the remainder (Fig 1). Theoretical TCR diversity in humans has been placed in the region of 10^{15} - 10^{20} unique structures (Davis, 1988; Lieber 1991; Shortman, 1990), with direct *in vivo* estimates greater than $2.5X10^{7}$ unique structures (Arstila, 1999). Structurally, TCR α- and β-chains fold to expose six highly flexible complementary determining region (CDR) loops that can contact the pMHC binding face. The germline-encoded CDR1 and CDR2 loops, from the TRAV and TRBV genes, participate heavily in MHC contacts and occasionally peptide contacts. The variable CDR3 loops, which span the V(D)J joints, are key to TCR diversity and participate heavily in peptide contacts. TCRs dock with pMHC complexes in a roughly diagonal fashion, such that the CDR3α loops are placed over the peptide N-terminus and the CDR3β loops lie over the peptide C-terminus (Miles, 2010).

In unconventional adaptive immunity, the specific response to antigens of bacteria and blood cells is similar to cellular immunity and identified lymphocyte-like cells in organs and tissues (Alder, 2005). On the other hand humoral mediators are somatically derived variants of leucine-rich repeats or LRRs, termed variable lymphocyte receptors (VLRs), which are as efficient as V (D) J process. The mechanism of VLRs assembly seems to be driven by a copy choice mechanism of recombination that is based on sequence similarities of individual LRR segments rather than by specific recombination elements (Han, 2008; Nagawa, 2007).

Although immunoglobulins, TCRs, and VLRs are structurally unrelated and somatic variations generated through unrelated mechanisms, these molecules develop clonal specificity through somatic recombination, show evidence of specific cell lineage compartmentalization in receptor expression and can share common features in the recipient's immune regulation (Litman, 2010).

3. Immunology of the nervous system

The CNS has developed strategies to limit the entry of immune elements as well as to limit the emergence of immune activation with the tissue itself. Immune privilege in the CNS is partially dependent on the blood–brain barrier (BBB), which is designed to limit the entry of solutes and ions into the CNS(Carson et al.,2006). Exclusion from, and selective entry of compounds into the CNS takes place in the capillary venules. In contrast ,cell migration takes place at the post-capillary venules, where cell migration is controlled by adhesion molecules, cytokines and chemokines, and their receptors (Fig.2)(Owens et al., 2008). Not only the physical properties of the BBB, but also potentially damaging immune responses as such are regulated by the suppressive environment within the CNS. Both astrocytes and microglia play a major role in this regulation, while neurons are assumed to play a largely passive role being only the victims of immune responses. Microglia invade the brain early in development and take on a resting 'protective' role as sentinels, scattered uniformly throughout the CNS and forming a network of potential effectors cells. In contrast to peripheral macrophages that are highly effective at inciting pro-inflammatory responses, microglia take on an opposing role, limiting inflammation. This role is extended also to astrocytes, the first cells that CNS-infiltrating immune cells encounter. Astrocytes suppress T helper 1 (Th1) and T helper 2 (Th2) cell activation, the proliferation and effector functions of activated T cells, and possess a wide variety of molecular mechanisms to induce apoptosis in activated T cells. Contrary to the idea that neurons only play a passive role, many of their products (i.e. neuropeptides and transmitters), as well as the neuronal membrane proteins CD22, CD47, CD200, CX3CL1 (fractalkine), intercellular adhesion molecule (ICAM), neural cell adhesion molecule (NCAM), semaphorins and C-type lectins all regulate inflammation (Tian, 2009). In addition, neurons express low levels of major histocompatibility complex (MHC) molecules and actively promote T-cell apoptosis via the Fas–Fas ligand pathway (CD95–CD95L). Neuronal expression of the cannabinoid (CB1) receptor is also implicated in suppressing inflammation. CB1 knockout mice more readily develop experimental autoimmune encephalomyelitis (EAE), the autoimmune model of multiple sclerosis (MS). Neurons also favour the differentiation of T-regulatory cells, by providing a local microenvironment dominated by transforming growth factor-b1 (TGF-b1). Damaged neurons, however, are less able to maintain this protective shield, allowing further insults.

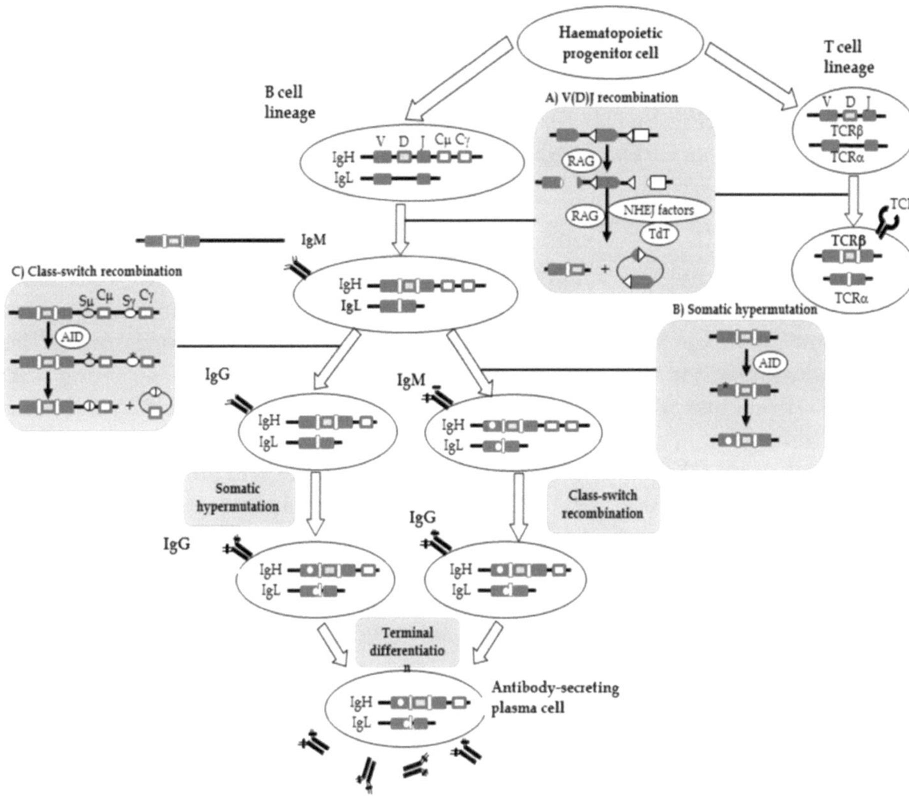

Fig 1. Conventional adaptative immune response in jawed vertebrates. A haematopoietic progenitor cell gives rise to distinct B and T cell lineages. During the development of Ig and TCR different recombination processes are involved. **A) V(D)J recombination.** In this process, RSSs (dark and white triangles) direct the RAG1–RAG2 recombinase complex to individual gene segments (dark and white boxes). The recombinase introduces two double-strand DNA breaks with blunt signal ends and hairpin-sealed coding ends. In the subsequent joining phase, TdT a template-independent DNA polymerase, adds random nucleotides to the junction of the gene elements, thereby increasing repertoire diversity dramatically; the RSSs are joined without further end processing and form excision circles. The key factors that facilitate each diversification step are NHEJ factors. Once functional DNA rearrangements occur, TCR sequences are unaltered. **B) Somatic hypermutation** is initiated by AID, which deaminates individual cytidines within the V(D)J exon of the immunoglobulin gene, leading to U:G mismatches (asterisk). Subsequent error-prone repair results in individual point mutations (white dot in the gene and white bar in the immunoglobulin molecules), and B cells with higher affinity for the original antigen are selected. **C) Class-switch recombination.** The AID creates U:G mismatches in the highly repetitive S regions (dark and white ovals) that are upstream of the exons encoding the constant regions of different isotypes. Error-prone repair leads to the generation of double-strand DNA breaks, excision of the intervening DNA (containing the Cμ exons) and joining of the remains of the S regions. The recombined, somatically mutated V(D)J region is then associated with Cγ, instead of Cμ. (Modified from Litman, 2010). **B and T cell lineages.** Immunoglobulin heavy and light chain: IgH and IgL; T cell receptor α and β chain: TCRα and TCRβ. **A) V(D)J recombination.** Variable, diversity,

joining genes: V(D)J; Recombination signal sequences: RSSs; Recombination activating gene 1 and 2: RAG1 and RAG2; Terminal deoxynucleotidyl transferase: TdT; Non-homologous end-joining: NHEJ. **B) Somatic hypermutation.** Activation-induced cytidine deaminase: AID. **C) Class-switch recombination.** Switch (S); Constant region for the Igμ isotype (Cμ) and a single representative downstream Cγ exon within the IgH locus.

4. Innate and adaptive responses in epilepsy

Despite the immune-privileged environment, it is clear that both innate and adaptive inflammatory responses do occur in the CNS. Activation of the innate immune system is a crucial first line of defense, to opsonize and clear apoptotic cells. Furthermore, innate immune responses recruit cells of the adaptive immune system by secreting various cytokines and chemokines that induce adhesion molecules on the BBB, and by inducing the expression of costimulatory molecules on microglia. Through conserved pattern-recognition receptors (PRRs), local CNS cells may be triggered to develop innate responses. Among these receptors are Toll-like receptors (TLRs), which bind highly conserved structural motifs either from pathogens (pathogen-associated molecular patterns, or PAMPs) or from damaged or stressed tissues (danger-associated molecular patterns, or DAMPs). Thus, not only invading micro-organisms, but also endogenous signals can switch on innate responses in the CNS. Some DAMPs, including heat shock proteins, uric acid, chromatin, adenosine and ATP, high mobility group box chromosomal protein 1 (HMGB-1), galectins and thioredoxin have adjuvant and pro-inflammatory activity. TLRs can be widely up-regulated during neurological disorders in varying patterns on microglia, astrocytes, oligodendrocytes and neurons (Bsibsi, 2002). When activated, TLRs are generally assumed to promote the production of pro-inflammatory cytokines, evoking a damaging environment that may contribute to neuronal damage. In vitro, Ab activates microglia through TLRs (Jackson et al., 2006, Okun et al., 2009;Letiembre et al.,2009). TLRs also aid the uptake of Ab and other aggregated proteins, thereby promoting their clearance from the CNS. Although in this manner, TLRs may seem to play a beneficial role in epilepsy it is currently unclear whether cellular activation by TLRs in another way may also contribute to epileptogenesis (Ravizza et al., 2011) . Therefore, rather than only playing a pathogenic role, several TLRs also play a role in repair during neurodegenerative disorders, under non-infectious conditions, suggesting that activation of at least some TLRs can also be used as a therapeutic strategy in CNS disorders(van Noort, 2007)

4.1 Experimental evidence

Due to advances in both structural and functional neuroimaging, as well as opportunities to perform invasive investigations of the human brain in an epilepsy surgery setting, an increasing amount of research on focal epilepsy is now utilizing patients and tissue obtained from patients. Nevertheless, parallel studies on patients and well validated equivalent animal models remain indispensable to circumvent difficulties in clinical research resulting from ethical limitations, cost, inadequate sampling, and absence of appropriate controls. The reliability of animal models in analysing epileptogenic mechanisms and testing the efficacy of antiepileptic drugs (AEDs) depends on how faithfully the epileptic phenomenology mimics both the clinical and EEG features of human seizures. Moreover, since human epilepsies are defined as pathological conditions characterized by the recurrence of epileptic

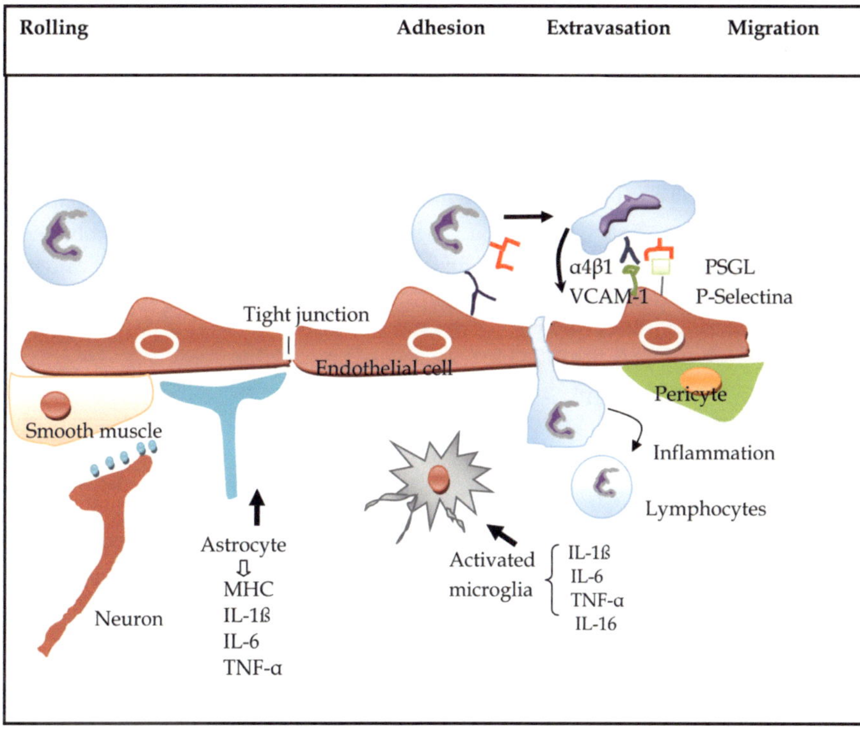

Fig. 2. T cell migration through the BBB in epilepsy. T-cell can enter the brain parenchyma by extravasation across the blood–brain barrier nonfenestrated endothelium and basal lamina. Antigen-presenting cells such as dendritic cells and macrophages are found in the subarachnoid space, in the perivascular space, and in the choroid plexus, whereas microglia are located in brain parenchyma; at these locations, these cells may encounter circulating CNS-borne antigens. The abnormal permeation across the barrier results in further, and perhaps distal, disruption of tight junctions, this time mediated by release of inflammatory mediators by both extravasated blood cells and activated microglia. Frank cellular immunoagression occurs if and when histocompatibility mechanisms are activated and antibody-mediated reactions occur. IL, interleukin; TNF, tumor necrosis factor; IFN, interferon; CSF, colony-stimulating factor; MHC, major histocompatibility complex, modify by Mix et al (2007) and Oby and Janigro (2006).

seizures only animals presenting with recurrent seizures can be defined as animal models of epilepsy. The acute experimental procedures designed to induce seizures, such as the injection of convulsant drugs, maximal electroshock etc., should therefore be referred to as animal models of seizures and not epilepsies unless they also induce a permanent epileptogenic. In this way the models have been described as **acute experimental seizure models**, in which seizures are induced by electrical stimulation, topical convulsants that block inhibition (e.g., penicillin, bicuculline, picrotoxina, pentylenetetrazol, strychnine), or topical convulsants that enhance excitation (e.g., carbachol, kainic acid). **Chronic models** of focal epilepsy can be induced with freeze lesions, partially isolated cortical slabs, metals (e.g., alumina, cobalt, tungstic acid, ferric chloride), kindling, tetanus toxin, anti-GM1 ganglioside antibodies, hippocampal sclerosis (kainic acid, pilocarpine, self-sustained status epilepticus), or focal dysplasia (neonatal freeze, prenatal radiation, MAM) (Engel, 2004).

Some of these epilepsy models in rodents trigger a prominent inflammatory response in brain regions recruited in the onset and propagation of epileptic activity; depending on the severity of the seizures, the inflammatory activity is affected in different ways (Minami, 1990;1991; Gahring, 1991;Jankowsky &Patterson, 2001; Kubera,2001; Oprica,2003; Turrin,2004). In models of temporal lobe epilepsy, the seizures produce changes in the function of the peripheral immune system. The thymus, for example, displays reduced weight, probably due to elevated corticosterone plasma levels during kainate-induced seizure; this steroid is induced during some kinds of stress or after a pathogenic infection. An increase in metabolic activity of splenocytes at the cellular level may be connected to enhanced phagocytic activity of macrophages (Kubera et al., 2001). The inflammatory response occurs during the 3 days following seizures. Although IL-1*β*, TNF-*a*, and IL-6 are expressed at very low levels in normal brain, their messenger RNA (mRNA) and protein levels are rapidly (≤30 min) increased after the induction of seizures, declining to basal levels within 48–72 h from the onset of seizures. However, IL-1β is still up regulated in the brain 60 days after status epilepticus in rats with spontaneous seizures (Plata et al., 2000). The increase in interleukin (IL)-1β, IL-6 and TNF-α in microglia and astrocytes is followed by a cascade of downstream inflammatory events which may recruit cells of the adaptive immune system (Vezzani and Granata, 2005).

The kindled model exhibited a significant up-regulation of IL-1 β, IL-1RI, TNF-*a* and TGF-*β*1 mRNAs in several limbic brain regions. The overall profile of mRNA changes shows specificity of transcriptional modulation induced by amygdala kindling. The data support a role for cytokines and NPY in the adaptive mechanisms associated with generalized seizure activity (Gahring, 1997). Cytokine production is also induced in brain by audiogenic seizures(Lee, 2008). Production of proinflammatory molecules (a cytokine induced portfolio of genes that are established mediators of inflammation (Dinarello, 2000) is typically accompanied by the concomitant synthesis of anti-inflammatory mediators and binding proteins apt to modulate the inflammatory response, thus avoiding the occurrence of deleterious induction of genes that mediate inflammatory effects. In this respect, up regulation of IL-1–receptor antagonist (Ra), a naturally occurring antagonist of IL-1β, has been described after acute seizures, status epilepticus, and in kindling (Gasque ,1997; Gorter, 2006;Avignone ,2008). However, IL-1Ra and IL-1β are induced by seizures and IL-1Ra is produced with a delayed time course, differing from classic inflammatory reactions in which IL-1Ra is produced at 100- to 1,000-fold excess and concomitant with IL-1β production. Thus the brain is less effective than the periphery in inducing a crucial mechanism for rapidly terminating the actions of a sustained increase in endogenous IL-1β. Cytokine receptors in the CNS are expressed by neurons, microglia, and astrocytes. However, it is primarily microglia activation that has morphologic changes related to the seizures and inflammation; this is a complex process that includes changes in pharmacological and electrophysiological properties, migration, proliferation, and release of a variety of mediators. In the context of status epilepticus induced by kainate, microglia are activated within the same time course that is observed for neuronal degeneration (Hosokawa, 2003; Xiong,2003).

The immune response changes during all three phases of epileptogenesis. The genes related to immune response are induced during both acute and latent phases of epileptogenesis but also during the chronic phase (in CA3). Although the immune response was greater one week after status epilepticus, the levels of secreted phosphoprotein 1 (Spp1 or osteopontin), a glycoprotein that promotes macrophage migration, Hg2a (or CD74; H-2 class II histocompatibility antigen), proteasomes (Psmb9, macropain), toll-like receptor 4 (Tlr4), and tumor necrosis factor (Gorter,2006), also, the prostaglandin synthesis, illustrated by Cox-2 induction, was activated in the acute and chronic phases but not in the latent period, indicating that this process is related to the occurrence of seizure activity. Activation of prostaglandin receptors could increase intracellular calcium and subsequent glutamate release, which would increase excitability in the surrounding networks (Bezzi et al., 1998; Rozovsk et al.,1994)

An important component of the immune response is activation of the complement pathway. Although complement factors might invade the brain via a leaky BBB, part of the increased expression is likely to originate from activated glial cells (Ravizza et al., 2006;Vezzani, 2008). The complement system may be useful for eliminating aggregated and toxic proteins. However, overactivation of the complement system can also have damaging effects through the activation of microglia and proinflammatory cytokines. Interestingly, sequential infusion of individual proteins of the membrane attack pathway into the hippocampus of freely moving rats induces seizures as well as cytotoxicity (Ravizza et al., 2006).

The complement cascade is activated by three pathways: the classical, the alternative, and the lectin pathway; the lectin pathway leads to the formation of the C5b-C9 membrane attack protein complex (MAC). Complement activation in the CNS is increasingly recognized to be associated with exacerbation and progression of tissue injury in different degenerative and inflammatory diseases. Interestingly, sequential infusion of individual proteins of the membrane attack pathway (C5b6, C7, C8, and C9) into the hippocampus of awake, freely moving rats induces both behavioral and electrographic seizures as well as cytotoxicity, suggesting a role for the complement system in epileptogenesis. Rozowski and colleagues (1994) showed increased C1q and C4 mRNA in rat pyramidal neurons after systemic injection of convulsant doses of kainic acid in neuronal layers of limbic areas that are vulnerable to kainic acid-induced neurodegeneration (Vezzani, 2008); moreover, clusterin and C1q immunoreactivities were observed in both neurons and astrocytes, while increased immunoreactivities (as observed in vivo after seizures) were demonstrated following prolonged exposure of primary cultures of hippocampal neurons to glutamate. Additionally, with sequential infusion into the rat hippocampus the individual proteins of the MAC induced both behavioral and electrographic seizures as well as cytotoxicity (Ravizza et al, 2006).

In addition, there is prominent activation of the complement cascade during the epileptogenesis phase in the experimental model and in sclerotic hippocampi from a rat model of TLE and human TLE (Aronica et al., 2007). Interestingly, the expression of CD59, a complement inhibitor of the MAC, was increased in microglia, but only modestly in neurons, suggesting that in this cell population complement activation may be poorly controlled (Rozovsky et al., 1994). These findings are corroborated by clinical evidence showing that both IL-1β and IL-1 receptor type I (RI), NFkB and complex are overexpressed in lesional brain tissue of patients with diverse types of pharmacoresistant epilepsy (Sheng et al., 1994, Crespel et al., 2002)

4.2 Clinical evidence

From a clinical standpoint, a role of inflammation in the pathophysiology of human epilepsy is still hypothetical, although this possibility is supported by abundant evidence. The first insight into a role for inflammation in epilepsy originated from the demonstrated antiepileptic activity of select, powerful anti-inflammatory drugs, including steroids. Moreover, several reports showed increased markers of inflammation in serum, CSF, and brain resident cells in patients with epilepsy. For example, epileptic patients who have recently experienced tonic–clonic seizures display a proinflammatory profile of cytokines in plasma and CSF, consisting of higher IL-6 levels and a lower IL-1Ra–to–IL-1α ratio. Because the IL-6 concentration is much higher in CSF than in plasma (Pacifici et al., 1995; Peltola et al., ,1998) and the contribution of peripheral blood mononuclear cells (PBMCs) to increased plasma levels of cytokines is still unclear (Sheng et al., 1994), the most likely origin of CSF cytokines appears to be the brain. In the same way, Sinha et al. (2008) analyzed cytokine levels in patients with partial epilepsy, status epilepticus and some epilepsy syndromes. Compared to controls, the patient group showed detectable levels of the following cytokines in serum: IL-6, TNF-α, IL-2, IL-4, IFN-γ and IL-1β. Serial analysis during the seizure-free period revealed a decrease in cytokine levels: TNF-α (25% to 12.5%), IFN-γ (12.5%to 0%), IL-1 (25% to 0) and IL-2 (6.2% to 6.2%), IL-4 (18.8% to 0%) and IL-6 (18.8% to 6.2%). On the other hand, increased post-ictal serum cytokine levels were found in patients with several epilepsy syndromes. However, data collected using tissue of patients with TLE show that specific inflammatory pathways are chronically activated during epileptogenesis and that they persist in chronic epileptic tissue, suggesting that they may contribute to the etiopathogenesis of some types of epilepsy, such as TLE (Ravizza et al., 2008).

4.3 Temporal lobe epilepsy (TLE)

Temporal lobe epilepsy refers to both lesional and nonlesional epilepsies characterized by focal seizures arising from either the neocortex or the mesial temporal structures. One of these syndromes is TLE, associated with hippocampal sclerosis (HS), a histopathologic condition characterized by neuronal loss and gliosis, predominantly affecting the CA1 region and the dentate gyrus. Increased IL-1*a* expression in microglia-like cells (Aronica et al., 2007), TLE with hippocampal sclerosis, and astroglial, microglial, and neuronal (5/8 cases) expression of C1q, C3c, and C3d were observed, particularly within regions where neuronal cell loss occurs (Crespel et al., 2002). Bauer et al (2009) showed that patients with well-characterized TLE led to immediate and long lasting posictal increase in systemic IL-6 levels; however this rise of IL-6 was lacking in patients with hippocampal sclerosis. The authors in accord with Meador et al.,(2004) suggest the cerebral lateralization of immune functions. On the other hand, there was expression of proinflammatory molecules in neurons and glia in brain tissue obtained from patients surgically treated for drug-resistant epilepsies (Crespel et al., 2002; Maldonado et al., 2003). In particular, the genes involved in the biological process of immunity and host defense are highly overrepresented in HS TLE patients; the functional gene classes most affected are chemokines and neuropeptides (De Simoni et al.,2000; van Gassen et al., 2008). Evaluation of immunological parameters applied to different groups of epileptogenic focus localization has shown that the increase of CD8+ lymphocytes is limited to temporal and lateralized patients. Patients with extratemporal localization of focus, as well as psychogenic cases, show normal levels of immunological lymphocyte markers (Lorigados-Pedre., 2004). Thus, upregulation of these chemokines in the human TLE hippocampus may contribute not only to neuropathology, but also to epileptogenesis. Early up regulation of chemokines, for instance, after viral infection, may represent a common pathway linking the various predisposing factors in the etiology of TLE, such as trauma, febrile seizures, meningitis, encephalitis, and tumors.) These data show that specific inflammatory pathways are chronically activated during epileptogenesis and that they persist in chronic epileptic tissue, suggesting that they may contribute to the etiopathogenesis of TLE (van Gassen et al, 2008)

4.4 Rasmussen's encephalitis

Rasmussen's encephalitis serves as a prototype of inflammatory epilepsy. The autoimmune nature of this condition was suspected after the discovery of autoantibodies against the glutamate receptor GluR3, one of the AMPA (α-amino-3-hydroxy-5-methyl-4-isoxazolepropionic acid) subunits. Subsequently, anti-GluR3 antibodies were detected in other epilepsy syndromes, including early-onset noninflammatory focal epilepsy and catastrophic infantile epilepsy (Mantegazza et al., 2002). There is no effective medical treatment for Rasmussen's encephalitis, except perhaps steroids, which can be useful when given early in the course of the disease (Robitaille, 1991). Functional hemispherectomy has been the main procedure used to stop progression of the disease; in this way, the tissue could be examined and the progression of an inflammatory process confirmed. Pardo et al. (2004) describe the effect of disease duration on the burden of pathology. The greatest intensity of inflammation and microglial proliferation with nodule formation are generally seen in early states (Fig.3), followed by a decrease in the later stages. The intensity of inflammation, as represented by accumulation of T cells and microglial proliferation (Fig.3), has been reported to bear an inverse correlation with disease duration (Bauer et al., 2002; 2007). Different stages of inflammation may coexist in the same patient with a multifocal distribution, which is consistent with an ongoing and progressive immune-mediated process (Gahring et al., 2001;Neumann et al., 2002). CD8+ T cells are located in close opposition to degenerating neurons and may contribute to neuronal cell death via secretion of granzyme B, a strong activator of caspase-mediated apoptosis (He et al., 1998; Bien et al., 2002; 2005). Activated CD4+ T cells may also prime B cells to produce autoantibodies. The resulting autoantibodies may destroy neurons, either directly by excessive stimulation of receptor-mediated ion channels or indirectly by binding complement factors and leading to the formation of the MAC (Bien et al., 2002;2007) which can induce neuronal loss and seizures (Xiong et al., 2003). Epileptic activity may induce inflammatory mediators in microglia, astrocytes, neurons, and endothelial cells and may alter the properties and permeability of the BBB, thus facilitating the entry of components of the adaptive immune system and molecules usually excluded from the brain parenchyma. These phenomena may consolidate and perpetuate inflammatory reactions in the brain of an affected individual and exacerbate brain damage, thus contributing to brain atrophy. It is still unknown which mechanism ultimately leads to the autoimmune process: viral infection (Xiong et al., 2003), head trauma, or even seizures per se; knowledge of the factors that precipitate the disease can enable prevention of the future development of chronic epilepsy. These recent findings recall attention to the possibility that a viral antigen may act as the initiating event in the complex pathogenetic mechanism leading to brain damage in RE. A cytotoxic T-cell response is in fact compatible with a viral infection, and a viral infection could explain the peculiar hemispheric distribution with centrifugal expansion observed in RE. Previous studies failed to conclusively link a specific virus to RE, but this of course does not rule out the possible role of an unknown virus.

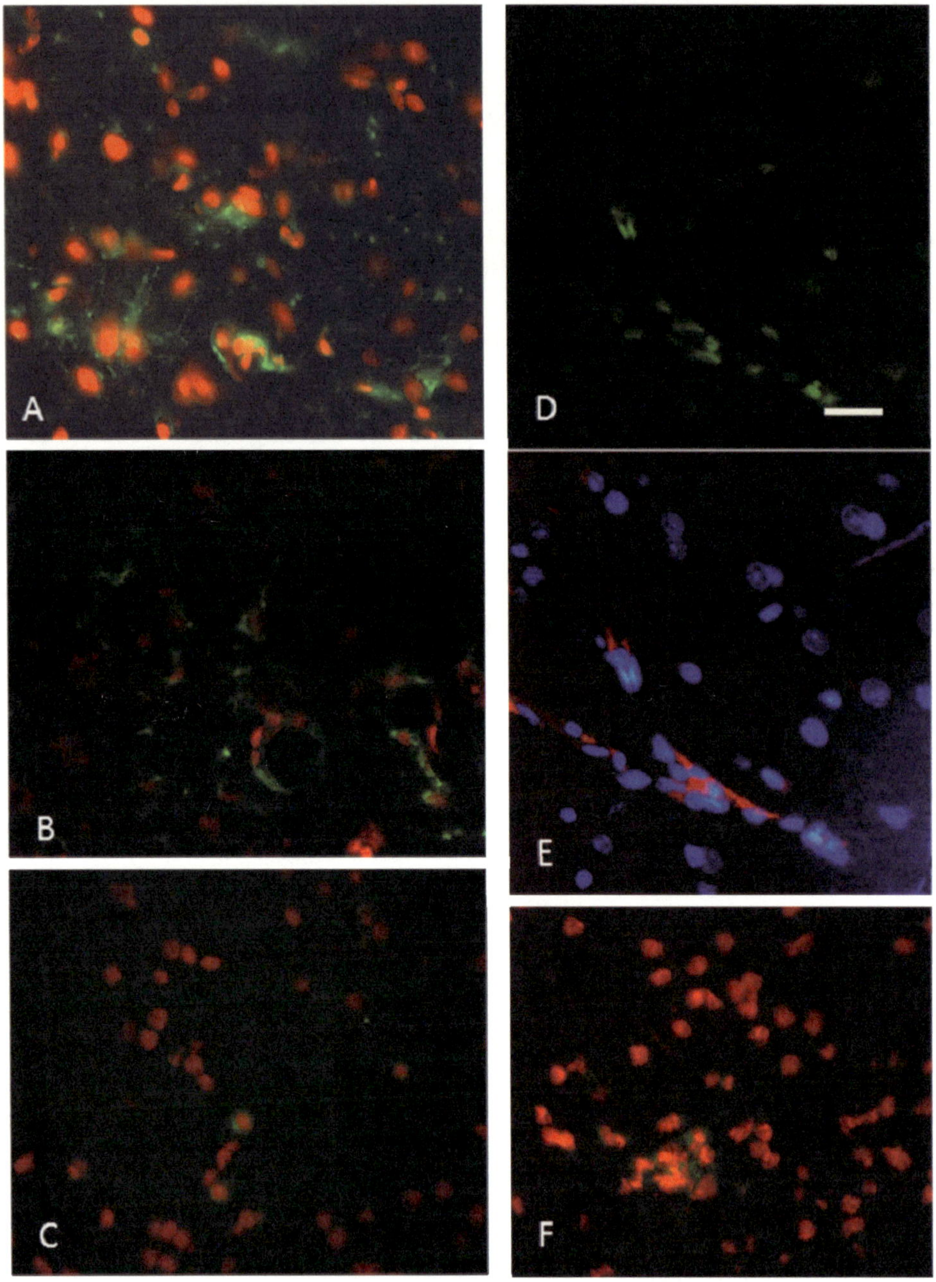

Fig. 3. Photomicrographs of activated microglia (HLA-Dr positive cells, green), A) nodules of microglia in Rasmussen syndrome, B) cortical dysplasia. Cytotoxic T lymphocytes (CD8 +, green) in dysplasia and TLE in (F). Coexpression in capillary of P-glycoprotein (green) and Cox-2 (red) in D and E in Rasmussen syndrome. (scale bar 20 μm D-F)

4.5 West syndrome (WS)

WS is an age-related epileptic encephalopathy with onset in the first year of life, featuring clustered spasms and hypsarrhythmia. It may occur in previously healthy children (cryptogenic WS) but more frequently is a symptom of different congenital or acquired diseases (symptomatic WS). Regardless of the etiology, WS patients benefit most from steroid treatment. Steroid efficacy, together with the possibility of spasm disappearance after viral infections (Hattori, 2001), has long been considered an index for an inflammatory or immune-mediated pathogenesis. A recent report (You et al., 2009). of increased serum levels of IL-2, TNF-*a*, and IFN-*a* in both cryptogenic and symptomatic WS reinforce this hypothesis. These cytokines are produced by monocytes and lymphocytes, and TNF-*a* is also produced by brain glial cells; all three have effects that may contribute to seizures and neuronal cell damage (Brunson et al., 1991). The presence of proinflammatory molecules in both cryptogenic and symptomatic WS patients suggests that cytokine changes are likely to be related to epilepsy rather than to the underlying etiology. However, symptomatic patients displayed a greater elevation of IL-2 levels, which varied depending on the underlying disorder (Prasad et al., 1996). If the extent of the inflammatory reaction depends also on the underlying disease, this could partly explain the different efficacies of steroid treatment in selected etiologic subgroups of symptomatic WS patients. For example, treatment with steroids and adrenocorticotropic hormone ACTH prevents patients with SW from developing Lenox-Gastau (Klein & Livingston, 1950). However, the mechanism underlying the anticonvulsant action of corticosteroids or ACTH remains elusive. Observations from animal models suggest that ACTH acts to repress infantile spasms by suppressing the level of endogenous corticotrophin releasing hormone (CRH) because stress receptors are located in areas of the brain known to be involved in seizure generation (Klein, 1950). It is postulated that the stimulation of synthesis of glucocorticoids that interact with CNS steroid receptors, which then influence voltage-dependent calcium channels, stimulates neurosteroid synthesis in glia and neurons that modulate GABAA receptors, down-regulating CRH, which has pro-convulsant activity in the immature brain, and immunomodulation (Joels, 1991)

4.6 Febrile seizures (FS)

FS are the most common cause of seizures in children, affecting 2 to 5% of children. The threshold to febrile seizures is dependent on body temperature, but the threshold varies with individuals and according to age and maturation (Millichap, 1959). A genetic susceptibility to inflammation may influence the threshold convulsive temperature. Seventeen to 30% of febrile seizure patients have a family history of febrile seizures (Millichap, 1959). A biallelic polymorphism in the promoter region of IL-1 at β the -511 position that can increase IL-1β production occurs more frequently in patients with prolonged febrile convulsions (Virta et al., 2002; Kanemoto et al., 2003). In experimental animals, intraventricular injection of IL-1β reduce the seizure threshold in 14-day old mice subjected to hyperthermia, while IL-1receptor knock-out mice have higher seizure thresholds, supporting the role of proinflammatory cytokines in triggering febrile seizures (Dubé et al., 2005)

Viruses are being increasingly implicated as causative agents of febrile seizures. Neurotropic viruses, such as the herpesviruses and influenza A, are commonly associated with febrile seizures in the United States and Asia (Hall et al., 1994; Chiu et al., 2001). Fever induced by viral infection is regulated by components of the immune response, particularly proinflammatory cytokines. Proinflammatory cytokines are higher in influenza-associated febrile seizures, further suggesting a causative role for cytokines in the pathogenesis of febrile seizures.

5. Anti-inflammatory treatments in epilepsy

Nearly 30% of epilepsy patients are refractory to conventional anti-epileptic drugs, and many alternative treatments have been tried to control epilepsy.(Prasad et al 1996). Immunotherapy, such as corticosteroids and ACTH, has been used to treat epilepsy since ACTH was first reported to have beneficial effects in the treatment of infantile spasms in 1950 (Klein, 1950 & Livingston,1950). For example there is no effective medical treatment for Rasmussen's encephalitis, except perhaps steroids,which can be useful when given early in the course of the disease(Bahi-Buisson et al., 2007), A long term follow-up of 11 Rasmussen's encephalitis patients who received steroids showed that 45% of patients had significant improvement of motor function and reduction of seizure frequency with disappearance of epilepsia partialis continua, while 55% patients had no benefit from steroid therapy and ultimately underwent hemispherotomy. Two initial responders to steroid treatment experienced progressive recurrence of seizures one to four years after the discontinuation of steroids and received a hemispherotomy. ACTH is a well-known effective treatment for infantile spasms that not only results in seizure control, but also improves both behavior and background EEG (Low, 1958). Meta-analysis reveals that ACTH is probably effective for short-term treatment of infantile spasms and leads to resolution of hypsarrhythmia (Mackay et al., 2004). Time to response is usually two weeks. Oral steroids can render 30 to 40% of patients seizure-free (Baram et al., 1996; Hrachovy et al., 1983). Further, early use of steroids is more effective; patients treated within one month of spasm onset had a better outcome than those treated after more than one month (Lombroso et al., 1983). The mechanism behind the anticonvulsant action of corticosteroids or ACTH remains elusive. Possibilities include (1) stimulation of glucocorticoid synthesis that interacts with CNS steroid receptors, which then influences voltage-dependent calcium channels; (2) stimulation of neurosteroid synthesis in glia and neurons that modulate GABAA receptors; (3) down-regulation of corticotrophin releasing hormone (CRH) that has proconvulsant activity in the immature brain; or (4) immunomodulation (Hrachovy et al.,1994; Baram et al., 1998; Reddy et al., 2000; Joëls, 2001).

On the other hand, various classes of specific anti-inflammatory drugs have been studied using models of status epilepticus or in kindling. The outcome measures were affected differently by inhibition of specific inflammatory pathways depending on the experimental model and the treatment schedule. For example non steroidal anti-inflammatory drugs (NSAIDs) NSAIDs act as inhibitors of constitutive COX-1 and inducible COX-2 enzymes. COX-2 selective inhibitors, such as celecoxib, parecoxib and SC58236, have been used to interfere with status epilepticus-induced epileptogenesis that was provoked either by electrical stimulation or systemic injection of pilocarpine in rats. These effects were observed under celecoxib treatment, thus a direct anticonvulsant action of this drug cannot be excluded.

Clinical phase	Drug/treatment	Animal models or Seizure type	Mechanism	References
Experimental (I)	Methanolic extract of *Asparagus pubescens*	PTZ-induced seizures	Inhibits inflammation and seizures	Nwafor et al., 2003
Experimental(I)	Aqueous and ethanolic extract of Solanum nigrum	Picrotoxin, pentylenetetrazole, and electroshocks induced seizures	Immunomodulatory activity	Jain et al, 2011., Ravi et al., 2009
Experimental(I)	Pralnacasan or VX-765	Kainic acid induced seizures	Interleukina converting enzyme/caspase 1 inhibitors and IL-1beta receptor antagonists	Vezzani et al., 2010
Experimental(I)	Naringin	kainic acid-induced status epilepticus in rats	Attenuated the TNF-α and malondialdehyde levels.	Golechha et al, 2011
Experimental(I)	Dexamethasone	Lithium and pilocarpine induced status epilepticus	IL-1 type 1 receptor antagonist and reduction in the number of circulating T-cells (CD3+)	Marchi et al, 2009
Experimental(I)	Naringin, a bioflavanoid	kainic acid (KA)-induced seizures	Antioxidant and anti-inflammatory activity.	Golechha et al., 2011
Experimental(I)	SC-58236, Celecoxib	electrically induced SE, Rat model of pharmacoresistant epilepsy	Selective inhibition of cyclooxygenase-2	Holtman et al., 2010, Schlichtiger et al, 2010
Experimental(I)	Minozac	Electroconvulsive shock	Suppression of proinflammatory cytokine	Somera-Molina et al., 2009; Chrzaszcz et al., 2010
Phase II/III	VX-765	Resistant partial epilepsy	ICE/caspase-1 blockade	Clinical trials gov.
In use	ACTH, prednisolone, and prednisone	Several epileptic syndromes	Antiinflammatory effects	Özkara Ç and Vigevano, 2011
In use	Dexamethasone, methylprednisolone and hydrocortisone	West, Landau-Kleffner or Lennox-Gastaut syndromes and Rasmussen encephalitis	Antiinflammatory effects and improvement of BBB integrity	Marchi et al., 2011
In use	Vigabatrin /and ACTH	Infantile spasms	Interfere with the cellular immune response	Ibrahim et al., 2010

Table 1. Immunotherapy treatments in epilepsy

Daily celecoxib treatment, starting 24 h post-status epilepticus for 42 days, resulted in reduction in the number and frequency of video-monitored spontaneous seizures (Jung, 2006). Other COX-2 inhibitors including nimesulide and rofecoxib, nonselective COX inhibitors such as paracetamol, naproxen, ibuprofen,mefenamic acid and indomethacin, and one selective COX-1 inhibitor SC560, have been tested in the kindling model of epileptogenesis, induced either by repetitive PTZ injections or by electrical stimulation. A significant delay in stage 5 seizure acquisition (i.e. delay in kindling development) was shown in NSAIDs-treated animals, with the exception of ibuprofen, which was found to be ineffective (Tanaka et al., 2009).

Three classical immunosuppressant agents have been used, namely cyclosporine A, FK-506 also known as Tacrolimus, and rapamycin. Their mechanisms of action include inhibition of T lymphocyte activation, although rapamycin alters multiple cellular functions by inhibiting mTOR kinase. Daily systemic injection of cyclosporine A or FK-506 during electrical amygdala kindling prevented the acquisition of stage 5 seizures in rats (Moia et al., 1994). Similar effects of FK-506 were shown in PTZ mkindling in mice(Singh, 2003). However, after drug withdrawal, stimulated animals showed stage 5 seizures, indicating that the treatments failed to inhibit epileptogenesis while providing anticonvulsant effects (Moia et al., 1994). Opposite effects were reported by Suzuki et al. (2001), showing acceleration of PTZ kindling in rats treated with FK-506. The pretreatment with VID-82925" kinase inhibitor molecule in 4-AP induced seizures model which revealed antiepileptogenic effect and it significantly suppressed the manifestation of epileptiform activity and was also effective against ictogenesis during the stable phase of focus (Gajda et al., 2011). Overall, these data indicate that the efficacy of immunosuppressant in kindling epileptogenesis is still controversial and requires further investigation, possibly using similar treatment protocols in the same kindling models. More consistent data are obtained in models of status epilepticus-induced epileptogenesis where T-cells do not appear to play a major role. Future studies are needed to target specific molecules involved in some of the pathways of the inflammatory process and to reduce adverse effects.

6. Concluding remarks

Accumulating evidence suggests that inflammatory and immune reactions may play an important role in promoting increased neuronal excitability, decreasing seizure threshold and is likely to be involved in the molecular, structural and synaptic changes characterizing epileptogenesis. Also, brain inflammation may contribute to the intractability of seizures and comorbidity in chronic epilepsy patients. Histologic analysis of the human brain from individuals with epilepsy of various etiologies strongly suggests the existence of a chronic inflammatory state in the brain almost invariably associated with neuronal loss, reactive gliosis, and activation of microglia. This observation, together with reports that anti-inflammatory drugs have anticonvulsant efficacy in some cases of drug-refractory epilepsies, suggests the possibility that chronic inflammation in the brain may be implicated in the etiopathogenesis of seizures and the associated long-term events. This hypothesis is supported by functional studies in experimental models of seizures, showing that some proinflammatory molecules exacerbate seizures, decrease the threshold for inducing convulsions, or cause seizures, per se.

Anti-inflammatory therapy may be particularly helpful when given during the latency period shortly after the initial neurologic insult, but prior to the onset of epilepsy, before permanent changes can occur in the neuronal aggregates that promote hyperexcitability and seizure spread. It is necessary to confirm with laboratory tests in serum and blood-cerebrospinal fluid to know the immune response of the epilepsy patient to give pharmacological therapy when the immune response is exacerbated. The causative role of inflammation in the pathogenesis of chronic intractable epilepsy needs to be established and requires further investigation from both the clinical and basic sciences. Pharmacological experiments in animal models suggest that antiepileptogenic effects might be achieved by interfering with specific pro-inflammatory pathways post-injury, although further studies are required to characterize the best targets and protocols for successful pharmacological intervention with limited side-effects.

7. Acknowledgment

This work was supported by National Council for Sciences and Technology grants (-52955-M and 98386) and Science and Technology Institute PIFUT -08/027

8. References

Alder MN, Rogozin IB, Iyer LM, Glazko GV, Cooper MD. & Pancer Z. (2005). Diversity and function of adaptive immune receptors in a jawless vertebrate. *Science,* 310,(5756), 1970-3. ISSN 0036-8075.

Aronica E, Boer K, van Vliet EA, Redeker S, Baayen JC, Spliet WG, van Rijen PC, Troost D, da Silva FH, Wadman WJ. & Gorter JA. (2007). Complement activation in experimental and human temporal lobe epilepsy. *Neurobiol Dis,* 26(3),497-511. ISSN 0969-9961.

Avignone E, Ulmann L, Levavasseur F, Rassendren F. & Audinat E. (2008). Status epilepticus induces a particular microglial activation state characterized by enhanced purinergic signaling. *J Neurosci,* 28(37), 9133–44. ISSN 0270-6474.

Bahi-Buisson N, Villanueva V, Bulteau C, Delalande O, Dulac O, Chiron C. & Nabbout R .(2007). Long term response to steroid therapy in Rasmussen encephalitis. *Seizure,* 1, 485-92. ISSN:1059-1311

Baram TZ, Mitchell WG, Tournay A, Snead OC, Hanson RA. & Horton EJ. (1996). High-dose corticotropin (ACTH) versus prednisone for infantile spasms a prospective, randomized, blinded study. *Pediatrics,* 97,375-9. ISSN 0031-4005.

Baram TZ. & Hatalski CG. (1998). Neuropeptide-mediated excitability: a key triggering mechanism for seizure generation in the developing brain. *Trends Neurosci,* 21, 471-6. ISSN 0166-2236.

Bauer J, Bien CG. & Lassmann H. (2002). Rasmussen's encephalitis a role for autoimmune cytotoxic T lymphocytes. *Curr Opin Neurol,* 15(2), 197–200. ISSN, 1350-7540.

Bauer J, Elger CE, Hans VH, Schramm J, Urbach H, Lassmann H. & Bien CG. (2007). Astrocytes are a specific immunological target in Rasmussen's encephalitis. *Ann Neurol,* 62,67–80. ISSN 0364-5134.

Bauer S, Cepok S, Todorova-Rudolph A, Nowak M, Koller M, Lorenz R, Oertel WH, Rosenow F, Hemmer B.& Hamer HM.(2009). Etiology and site of temporal lobe epilepsy influence postictal cytokine release. *Epilepsy Res,* 86, 82-88. ISSN 0920-1211

Beutler B. (2004). Innate immunity: an overview. *Mol Immunol,* 40(12), 845-59. ISSN 0161-5890.

Bezzi P, Carmignoto G, Pasti L, Vesce S, Rossi D, Rizzini BL, Pozzan T. &. Volterra A. (1998). Prostaglandins stimulate calcium-dependent glutamate release in astrocytes. *Nature,* 391,281–285. ISSN 0028-0836.

Bien CG, Bauer J, Deckwerth TL, Wiendl H., Wiestler OD, Schramm J, Elger CE. & Lassmann H. (2002). Destruction of neurons by cytotoxic T cells: a new pathogenic mechanism in Rasmussen's encephalitis. *Ann Neurol,* 51(3), 311–18. ISSN 0364-5134.

Bien CG, Granata T, Antozzi C, Cross JH, Dulac O, Kurthen M, Lassmann H, Mantegazza R. Villemure JG, Spreafico R. & Elger CE. (2005). Pathogenesis, diagnosis and treatment of Rasmussen encephalitis: a European consensus statement. *Brain,* 128(Pt 3), 454–471. ISSN 0006-8950

Bien CG, Urbach H, Schramm J, Soeder BM, Becker AJ, Voltz R, Vincent A. & Elger CE. (2007). Limbic encephalitis as a precipitating even in adult-onset temporal lobe epilepsy. *Neurology,* 69(12), 1236–44. ISSN 0028-3878.

Brunson KL, Khan N, Eghbal-Ahmadi M. & Baram TZ. (2001). Corticotropin (ACTH) acts directly on amygdala neurons to down regulate corticotropin-releasing hormone gene expression. *Ann Neurol,* 49(3), 304–12. ISSN 0364-5134.

Bsibsi M, Ravid R, Gveric D. & van Noort JM. (2002). Broad expression of Toll-like receptors in the human central nervous system. *J Neuropathol Exp Neurol,* 61(11), 1013–21. ISSN 0022-3069.

Cabaniols JP, Fazilleau N, Casrouge A, Kourilsky P, Kanellopoulos JM. (2001). Most alpha/beta T cell receptor diversity is due to terminal deoxynucleotidyl transferase. *J Exp Med,* 194(9), 1385–1390. ISSN 0022-1007

Carson MJ, Doose JM, Melchior B, Schmid CD. & Ploix CC. (2006). CNS immune privilege: hiding in plain sight. *Immunol Rev,* 213, 48–65. ISSN 0105-2896.

Chiu SS, Tse CY, Lau YL. & Peiris M. (2001). Influenza A infection is an important cause of febrile seizures. *Pediatrics,* 108(4), E63. ISSN 0031-4005.

Chrzaszcz M, Venkatesan C, Dragisic T, Watterson DM, & Wainwright MS. (2010).Minozac treatment prevents increased seizure susceptibility in a mouse "two-hit" model of closed skull traumatic brain injury and electroconvulsive shock-induced seizures. *J Neurotrauma,* 27(7), 1283-95.ISSN 0897-7151.

ClinicalTrials.gov. (2010). Study of VX-765 in subjects with treatmentresistant partial epilepsy. Available at http://clinicaltrials.gov/ct2/ show/NCT01048255.

Condie RM, Zak SJ. & Good RA. (1995). Effect of meningococcal endotoxin on the immune response. *Proc Soc Exp Biol Med,* 90(2), 355-60. ISSN 0037-9727.

Crespel A,Coubes P,Rousset MC, Brana C, Rougier A,Rondouin G,Bockaert J,Baldy-Moulinier M. & Lerner-Natoli M. (2002). Inflammatory reactions in human medial temporal lobe epilepsy with hippocampal sclerosis. *Brain Res,* 952(2), 159–69. ISSN 0006-8993.

Davis MM, Bjorkman PJ. (1988). T-cell antigen receptor genes and T-cell recognition. *Nature,* 334(6181), 395–402.ISSN 0028-0836

De Simoni MG, Perego C, Ravizza T, Moneta D, Conti M, Marchesi F, De Luigi A, Garattini S &Vezzani A. (2000). Inflammatory cytokines and related genes are induced in the rat hippocampus by limbic status epilepticus. *Eur J Neurosci,* 12(7), 2623-33. ISNN 0953-816X.

Dinarello CA. (2000). Proinflammatory cytokines. *Chest,* 118(2), 503–8. ISSN 0012-3692.
Dubé C, Vezzani A, Behrens M, Bartfai T. & Baram TZ. (2005). Interleukin-1beta contributes to the generation of experimental febrile seizures. *Ann Neurol,* 57(1), 152-5. ISSN 0364-5134.
Engel J Jr. (2004). Models of focal epilepsy. *Suppl Clin Neurophysiol,* 57, 392-9. ISSN 1567-424X.
Gahring LC, White HS, Skradski SL, Carlson NG. & Rogers SW. (1997). Interleukin-1alpha in the brain is induced by audiogenic seizure. *Neurobiol Dis,* 3(4), 263–9. ISSN 0969-9961.
Gahring L, Carlson NG, Meyer EL. & Rogers SW. (2001). Granzyme B proteolysis of a neuronal glutamate receptor generates an autoantigen and is modulated by glycosylation. *J Immunol,* 166(3), 1433–8. ISSN 0022-1767.
Gajda Z, Török R, Horváth Z, Szántai-Kis C, Orfi L, Kéri G, & Szente M.(2011). Protein kinase inhibitor as a potential candidate for epilepsy treatment. *Epilepsia,* 52(3), 579-588. ISSN0013-9580
Gasque P, Singhrao SK, Neal JW, Götze O. & Morgan BP. (1997). Expression of the receptor for complement C5a (CD88) is up-regulated on reactive astrocytes, microglia, and endothelial cells in the inflamed human central nervous system. *Am J Pathol,* 150(1), 31–41. ISSN 0002-9440.
Gellert, M. (2002). V(D)J recombination: RAG proteins, repair factors, and regulation. *Annu. Rev. Biochem,* 71, 101–132. ISSN 0066-4154.
Golechha M, Chaudhry U, Bhatia J, Saluja D, Arya DS. (2011).Naringin protects against kainic acid-induced status epilepticus in rats: evidence for an antioxidant, anti-inflammatory and neuroprotective intervention. *Biol Pharm Bull,* 34(3), 360-5. ISSN 0918-6158
Gorter JA, van Vliet EA, Aronica E, Breit T, Rauwerda H, Lopes da Silva FH. & Wadman WJ. (2006). Potential New Antiepileptogenic Targets Indicated by Microarray Analysis in a Rat Model for Temporal Lobe Epilepsy. *J Neurosci,* 26(43), 11083–110. ISSN 0270-6474.
Hall CB, Long CE, Schnabel KC, Caserta MT, McIntyre KM, Costanzo MA, Knott A, Dewhurst S, Insel RA. & Epstein LG. (1994). Human herpesvirus-6 infection in children. A prospective study of complications and reactivation. *N Engl J Med,* 331(7), 432-8. ISSN 0028-4793.
Han BW, Herrin BR, Cooper MD. & Wilson IA. (2008). Antigen recognition by variable lymphocyte receptors. *Science,* 321(5897), 1834-7. ISSN 0036-8075.
Hattori H. (2001). Spontaneous remission of spasms in West syndrome--implications of viral infection. *Brain Dev,* 23(7), 705–7. ISSN 0387-7604.
He XP, Patel M, Whitney KD, Janumpalli S, Tenner A. & McNamara JO. (1998). Glutamate receptor GluR3 antibodies and death of cortical cells. *Neuron,* 20(1), 153–63. ISSN 0896-6273.
Holtman L, van Vliet EA, Edelbroek PM, Aronica E, & Gorter JA. (2010).Cox-2 inhibition can lead to adverse effects in a rat model for temporal lobe epilepsy. *Epilepsy Res,* 2010; 91(1), 49-56. ISSN0920-1211
Hosokawa M, Klegeris A, Maguire J. & McGeer PL. (2003). Expression of complement messenger RNAs and proteins by human oligodendroglial cells. *Glia,* 42(4), 417–23. ISSN 089-1491.

Hrachovy RA, Frost JD Jr. & Glaze DG. (1994). High-dose, long-duration versus low-dose, short-duration corticotrophin therapy for infantile spasms. *J Pediatr*, 124(5 Pt 1),803-6. ISSN 0022-3476.

Hrachovy RA, Frost JD Jr., Kellaway P. & Zion TE. (1983). Double-blind study of ACTH vs prednisone therapy in infantile spasms. *J Pediatr*, 103(4), 641-5. ISSN 0022-3476.

Ibrahim S, Gulab S, Ishaque S, & Saleem T.(2010). Clinical profile and treatment of infantile spasms using vigabatrin and ACTH—a developing country perspective. *BMC Pediatr*,.10, 1,5-40.ISSN1471-2431-

Iwasaki A. & Medzhitov R. (2010). Regulation of adaptive immunity by the innate immune system. *Science*, 327(5963), 291-5. ISSN 0036-8075.

Jackson AC, Rossiter JP. & Lafon M. (2006). Expression of Toll-like receptor 3 in the human cerebellar cortex in rabies, herpes simplex encephalitis, and other neurological diseases. *J Neurovirol*, 12(3),229–34. ISSN, 1355-0284.

Jain R, Sharma A, Gupta S, Sarethy IP, & Gabrani R. (2011).Solanum nigrum: current perspectives on therapeutic properties. *Altern Med Rev*, 16(1),78-85. ISSN 10895159

Jankowsky JL. & Patterson PH. (2001). The role of cytokines and growth factors in seizures and their sequelae. *Prog Neurobiol*, 63(2), 125–49. ISSN 0301-0082.

Joëls M. (2001). Corticosteroid actions in the hippocampus. *J Neuroendocrinol*. 13(8),657-69. ISSN 0953-8194.

Jung H, K. Chu, S.T. Lee, J. Kim, D.I. Sinn, J.M. Kim, D.K. Park, J.J. Lee, S.U. Kim, M. Kim, S.K. Lee &. Roh J.(2006), Cyclooxygenase-2 inhibitor, celecoxib, inhibits the altered hippocampal neurogenesis with attenuation of spontaneous recurrent seizures following pilocarpine-induced status epilepticus. *Neurobiol Dis*, 23 237–246. ISSN0969-9961

Kanemoto K, Kawasaki J, Yuasa S, Kumaki T, Tomohiro O. & Kaji R. (2003). Increased frequency of interleukin-1beta-511T allele in patients with temporal lobe epilepsy, hippocampal sclerosis, and prolonged febrile convulsion. *Epilepsia*, 44, 796-9. ISSN0013-9580

Klein R. & Livingston S. (1950).The effect of adrenocorticotropic hormone in epilepsy. *J Pediatr*, 37, 733-42. ISSN0022-3476

Kubera M, Budziszewska B, Basta-Kaiml A, Zajicova A, Holan V. &Lasoń W.(2001).Immunoreactivity in kainate model of epilepsy. *Pol J Pharmacol*. 53(5), 541-5.

Letiembre M, Liu Y, Walter S, Hao W, Pfander T, Wrede A, Schulz-Schaeffer W. & Fassbender K. (2009).Screening of innate immune receptors in neurodegenerative diseases: a similar pattern. *Neurobiol Aging*, 30, 759–68. ISSN. 0197-4580

Lee CH, Hwang IK, Lee IS, Lee IS, Yoo KY, Choi JH, Lee BH. & Won MH. (2008).Differential immunoreactivity of microglial and astrocytic marker protein in the hippocampus of the seizure resistant and sensitive gerbils. *J Vet Med Sci*, 70(12), 1405–11 ISSN0916-7250

Li Z, Woo CJ, Iglesias-Ussel MD, Ronai D,&Scharff MD. (2004). The generation of antibody diversity through somatic hypermutation and class switch recombination. *Genes Dev*. 18(1),1-11. ISSN 0890-9369

Lieber MR. (1991). Site-specific recombination in the immune system. *FASEB J*, 5(14), 2934–2944.ISSN 0892-6638

Litman GW, Rast JP.& Fugmann SD. (2010).The origins of vertebrate adaptive immunity. *Nat Rev Immunol.*, 10(8), 543-53. ISSN 1474-1733

Lombroso CT. (1983). A prospective study of infantile spasms: clinical and therapeutic correlations. *Epilepsia*, 24, 135-58. ISSN0013-9580

Lorigados-Pedre L., Morales-Chacón L, Pavón-Fuentes N. Serrano-Sánchez T, Robinson-Agramonte MA, García-Navarro ME, & Bender-del Busto JE. (2004).Alteraciones inmunológicas en pacientes epilépticos asociadas a la localización del foco epileptogénico. *Rev neurol*, 39(2), 101-4. ISSN0210-0010 .

Low NL.(1958). Infantile spasms with mental retardation. II. Treatment with cortisone and adrenocorticotropin. *Pediatrics*, 22, 1165-9. ISSN0031-4005

Mackay MT, Weiss SK, Adams-Webber T, Ashwal S,Stephens D, Ballaban-Gill K, Baram TZ, Duchowny M, Hirtz D, Pellock JM, Shields WD, Shinnar S. & Wyllie E. (2004). Practice parameter: medical treatment of infantile spasms: report of theAmerican Academy of Neurology and the Child Neurology Society. *Neurology*, 62, 1668-81. ISSN0028-3878

MacLennan IC. (1994). Germinal centers. Ann Rev Immunol, 12, 117–139.ISSN 0732-0582

Maldonado M, BaybisM, NewmanD, Kolson DL, Chen W, McKhann G 2nd, Gutmann DH. & Crino PB.(2003). Expression of ICAM-1 TNF-alpha, NF kappa B, and MAP kinase in tubers of the tuberous sclerosis complex. *Neurobiol Dis*, 14(2), 279–90. ISSN0969-9961.

Marchi N, Granata T, Freri E, Ciusani E, Ragona F, Puvenna V, Teng Q, Alexopolous A, & Janigro D. (2011).Efficacy of anti-inflammatory therapy in a model of acute seizures and in a population of pediatric drug resistant epileptics. PLoS One, 6(3), 18200. ISSN-1932-6203

Mantegazza R, Bernasconi P, Baggi F, Spreafico R, Ragona F, Antozzi C, Bernardi G & Granata T (2002).Antibodies against GluR3 peptides are not specific for Rasmussen's encephalitis but are also present in epilepsy patients with severe, early onset disease and intractable seizures. J *Neuroimmunol*, 131(1-2), 179-85. ISSN 0165-5728.

Meador KJ,Loring DW, Ray PG, Helman SW, Vazquez BR. & Neveu PJ.(2004). Role of cerebral lateralization in control of immune processes in humans. *Ann Neurol*, 55, 840-844.ISSN 0364-5134

Miles JJ, Bulek AM, Cole DK, Gostick E, Schauenburg AJ, Dolton G, Venturi V, Davenport MP, Tan MP, Burrows SR, Wooldridge L, Price DA, Rizkallah P &, Sewell.(2010). Genetic and structural basis for selection of a ubiquitous T cell receptor deployed in Epstein-Barr virus infection. *PLoS Pathog*, 6(11), e1001198. ISSN 1553-7366

Millichap JG. (1959).Studies in febrile seizures. I. Height of body temperature as a measure of the febrile-seizure threshold. *Pediatrics*, 23 (1 Pt 1), 76-85. ISSN0031-4005.

Minami M, Kuraishi Y, Yamaguchi T, Nakai S, Hirai Y. & Satoh M. (1990). Convulsants induce interleukin-1 beta messenger RNA in rat brain. *Biochem Biophys Res Commun*, 171(2), 832–7. ISSN0006-291X

Minami M, Kuraishi Y, Satoh M. (1991). Effects of kainic acid on messenger RNA levels of IL-1 beta, IL-6, TNF alpha and LIF in the rat brain. *Biochem Biophys Res Commun,*. 176(2), 593–8. ISSN0006-291X

Mix E, Goertsches U, Zettl K. (2007). Immunology and neurology. *J Neurol*, 254, (Suppl 2). II/2–7. ISSN0340-5354

Moia, L.J. Matsui, Hde Barros, G.A. Tomizawa, K. Miyamoto K., Kuwata, Y. Tokuda, M.. Itano, T & Hatase O.(1994). Immunosuppressants and calcineurin inhibitors, cyclosporin A and FK506, reversibly inhibit epileptogenesis in amygdaloid kindled rat. *Brain Res*, 648, 337–341. ISSN 0006-8993

Nagawa F, Kishishita N, Shimizu K, Hirose S, Miyoshi M, Nezu J, Nishimura T, Nishizumi H, Takahashi Y, Hashimoto S, Takeuchi M, Miyajima A, Takemori T, Otsuka AJ. & Sakano H. (2007).Antigen-receptor genes of the agnathan lamprey are assembled by a process involving copy choice. *Nat Immunol*, 8(2), 206-13. ISSN 1529-2908

Neumann H, Medana IM, Bauer J. & Lassmann H. (2002).Cytotoxic T lymphocytes in autoimmune and degenerative CNS diseases. *Trends Neurosci*, 25(6), 313–9. ISSN 0166-2236

Nwafor PA, & Okwuasaba FK. (2003).Anti-nociceptive and anti-inflammatory effects of methanolic extract of Asparagus pubescens root in rodents. *J Ethnopharmacol*, 84(2-3),125-9. ISSN 0378-8741

Oby E. & Janigro D. (2006). The Blood–Brain Barrier and Epilepsy. *Epilepsia*, 47(11), 1761–74. ISSN 0013-9580

Okun E, Griffioen KJ, Lathia JD, Tang SC, Mattson MP. & Arumugam TV. (2009). Toll-like receptors in neurodegeneration. *Brain Res Rev*, 59, 278–92. ISSN 0165-0173

Oprica M, Eriksson C. & Schultzberg M. (2003).Inflammatory mechanisms associated with brain damage induced by kainic acid with special reference to the interleukin-1 system. *J Cell Mol Med*, 7(2), 127–40. ISSN 1582-1838.

Özkara Ç, & Vigevano F. (2011).Immuno- and antiinflammatory therapies in epileptic disorders. *Epilepsia*, 2011, 52 Suppl 3, 45-51. ISSN 0013-9580

Owens T, Bechmann I, Engelhardt B. (2008).Perivascular spaces and the two steps to neuroinflammation. *J Neuropathol Exp Neurol*, 67,1113–21. ISSN 0022-3069

Pacifici R, Paris L, Di Carlo S, Bacosi A, Pichini S. & Zuccaro P. (1995). Cytokine production in blood mononuclear cells from epileptic patients. *Epilepsia*, 36(4), 384–7. ISSN 0013-9580

Pardo CA, Vining EP, Guo L, Skolasky RL, Carson BS. & Freeman JM. (2004). The pathology of Rasmussen syndrome stages of cortical involvement and neuropathological studies in 45 hemispherectomies. *Epilepsia*, 45(5), 516–26. ISSN 0013-9580

Peltola J, Hurme M, Miettinen A. & Keränen T. (1998).Elevated levels of interleukin-6 may occur in cerebrospinal fluid from patients with recent epileptic seizures. *Epilepsy Res*, 31(2), 129–33. ISSN 0920-1211

Plata-Salamán CR, Ilyin SE, Turrin NP, Gayle D, Flynn MC, Romanovitch AE, Kelly ME, Bureau Y, Anisman H. & McIntyre DC. (2000). Kindling modulates the IL-1beta system, TNF-alpha, TGF-beta1, and neuropeptide mRNAs in specific brain regions. *Brain Res Mol Brain Res*, 75(2), 248–58. ISSN 0169-328X

Prasad AN, Stafstrom CF. & Holmes GL. (1996).Alternative epilepsy therapies : the ketogenic diet, immunoglobulins,and steroids. *Epilepsia*,37, Suppl 1, S81-95. ISSN 0013-9580

Rast JP, Anderson MK, Strong SJ, Luer C, Litman RT. & Litman GW.(1997).α, β, γ, and δ T cell antigen receptor genes arose early in vertebrate phylogeny. *Immunity*, 6 (1), 1–11. ISSN1074-7613

Ravi V, Saleem TSM, & Patel SS. (2009). Anti-inflammatory effect of methanolic extract of Solanum nigrum Linn berries. *Int J Appl Res Nat Prod*, 2,33-36. ISSN 1940-6223

Ravizza T, Boer K, Redeker S, Spliet WG, van Rijen PC, Troost D, Vezzani A. & Aronica E. (2006).The IL-1β system in epilepsy associated malformations of cortical development. *Neurobiol Dis*, 24, 128–43. ISSN 0969-9961

Ravizza T, Gagliardi B, Noé F, Boer K, Aronica E. & Vezzani A. (2008). Innate and adaptive immunity during epileptogenesis and spontaneous seizures: evidence from experimental models and human temporal lobe epilepsy. *Neurobiol Dis*, 29(1), 142-60. ISSN 0969-9961

Ravizza T, Balosso S. & Vezzani AM. (2011).Inflammation and prevention of epileptogenesis. *Neurosci lett*, 2011, 497, 223–230. ISSN 0304-3940

Reddy DS. & Rogawski MA. (2000).Enhanced anticonvulsant activity of ganaxolone after neurosteroid withdrawal in a rat model of catamenial epilepsy. *J Pharmacol Exp Ther*, 294, 909-15. ISSN 0022-3565

Rivest S, Lacroix S, Vallières L, Nadeau S, Zhang J. & Laflamme N. (2000).How the blood talks to the brain parenchyma and the paraventricular nucleus of the hypothalamus during systemic inflammatory and infectious stimuli. *Proc Soc Exp Biol Med*, 223(1), 22–38. ISSN 0037-9727

Robitaille Y. (1991).Neuropathologic aspects of chronic encephalitis. In: Andermann F Ed., Chronic encephalitis and epilepsy: Rasmussen`s syndrome. ISBN2-7420-0569-2, Boston:, Butterworth-Heinermann. Pp. 79-110.

Schlichtiger J, Pekcec A, Bartmann H, Winter P, Fuest C, Soerensen J, & Potschka H. (2010).Celecoxib treatment restores pharmacosensitivity in a rat model of pharmacoresistant epilepsy. *Br J Pharmacol*, 160(5), 1062-71. ISSN 0007-1188

Sheng JG, Boop FA, Mrak RE. & Griffin WS. (1994). Increased neuronal beta amyloid precursor protein expression in human temporal lobe epilepsy: association with interleukin-1 alpha immunoreactivity. J *Neurochem*, 63(5), 1872–9. ISSN 0022-3042.

Singh A., Kumar G., Naidu P.S. & Kulkarni S.K. (2003) Protective effect of FK506 (tacrolimus) in pentylenetetrazol-induced kindling in mice. *Pharmacol Biochem. Behav*, 75, 853–860. ISSN 0091-3057.

Sinhaa,S, ,Patil S, Jayalekshmyb V. & Satishchandraa P. (2008). Do cytokines have any role in epilepsy?. *Epilepsy Research*, 82, 171—176. ISSN 0920-1211.

Somera-Molina KC, Nair S, Van Eldik LJ, Watterson DM, & Wainwright MS.(2009). Enhanced microglial activation and proinflammatory cytokine upregulation are linked to increased susceptibility to seizures and neurologic injury in a 'two-hit' seizure model. *Brain Res*, 1282162-72. ISSN 0006-8993

Shortman K, Egerton M, Spangrude GJ, Scollay R. (1990). The generation and fate of thymocytes. *Semin Immunol*, 2(1),3–12. ISSN 1044-5323

Rozovsky I, Margan TE, Willoughby DA, Dugich-Djordjevich MM, Pasinetti GM, Johnson SA. & Finch CE.(1994). Selective expression of clusterin (SGP-2) and complement C1qB and C4 during responses to neurotoxins in vivo and in vitro. *Neuroscience*, 62(3), 741–58. ISSN 0306-4522

Stephens D, Ballaban-Gill K, et al.(2004). Practice parameter medical treatment of infantile spasms: report of theAmerican Academy of Neurology and the Child Neurology Society. *Neurology*, 62, 1668-81. ISSN 0028-3878

Suzuki K, Omura S., Ohashi Y., Kawai M., Iwata Y., Tani K., Sekine Y. Takei N. & Mori N (2001).FK506 facilitates chemical kindling induced by pentylenetetrazole in rats. *Epilepsy Res*, 46, 279–282. ISSN 0920-1211

Tanaka S, Nakamura, K. Sumitani F. Takahashi, R. Konishi, Itano T.& Miyamoto O. (2009). Stage and region-specific cyclooxygenase expression and effects of a selective COX-1 inhibitor in the mouse amygdala kindling model, *Neurosci Res,* 65, 79–87. ISSN 0077-7846

Tian L, Rauvala H.& Gahmberg CG. (2009). Neuronal regulation of immune responses in the central nervous system. *Trends Immunol,* 2009, 30, 91–9. ISSN 1471-4906

Tonegawa S. (1983).Somatic generation of antibody diversity. *Nature,* 302(5909), 575–81. ISSN 0028-0836

Tracey KJ.(2009). Reflex control of immunity. *Nat Rev Immunol,* 2009, 9(6), 418-28. ISSN 1474-1733

Turrin NP, Rivest S. Innate immune reaction in response to seizures: implications for the neuropathology associated with epilepsy. *Neurobiol Dis,* 2004, 16(2), 321–34. ISSN 0969-9961

Vezzani A. & Granata T. (2005).Brain inflammation in epilepsy: experimental and clinical evidence. *Epilepsia,* 46(11), 1724-43. ISSN 0013-9580

van Gassen KL, de Wit M, Koerkamp MJ, Rensen MG, van Rijen PC, Holstege FC, Lindhout D &de Graan PN (2008).Possible role of the innate immunity in temporal lobe epilepsy. *Epilepsia,* 49(6), 1055-65. ISSN 0013-9580

van Noort JM. (2007). Toll-like receptors as targets for inflammation,development and repair in the central nervous system. *Curr Opin Investig Drugs,* 8, 60–5. ISSN1472-4472

Vezzani A.(2008). Innate immunity and inflammation in temporal lobe epilepsy:new emphasis on the role of complement activation. *Epilepsy Currents,* 8(3), 75–7. ISSN 1535-7597

Vezzani A, Balosso S, Maroso M, Zardoni D, Noé F,& Ravizza T.(2010).ICE/caspase 1 inhibitors and IL-1beta receptor antagonists as potential therapeutics in epilepsy. *Curr Opin Investig Drugs,* 11(1),43-50. ISSN 1472-4472.

Visser L, Melief MJ, van Riel D, van Meurs M, Sick EA, Inamura S, Bajramovic JJ, Amor S, Hintzen RQ, Boven LA, 't Hart BA, & Laman JD. (2006).Phagocytes containing a disease-promoting Toll-like receptor/Nod ligand are present inthe brain during demyelinating disease in primates. *Am J Pathol,* 169, 1671–85. ISSN 0002-9440

Virta M, Hurme M. & Helminen M. (2002).Increased frequency of interleukin-1beta (-511) allele 2 in febrile seizures. *Pediatr Neurol,*26,192-5. ISSN 0887-8994

Weichhart,T. & Saemann M.D. (2009). The multiple facets of mTOR in immunity. *Trends Immunol,* 30, 218–226. ISSN 1471-4906

Weill JC, Reynaud CA. (1996). Rearrangement/hypermutation/gene conversion: When, where and why. *Immunol Today,* 17(2), 92–97. ISSN 0167-5699.

Xiong ZQ, Qian W, Suzuki K. & McNamara JO. (2003).Formation of complement membrane attack complex in mammalian cerebral cortex evokes seizures and neurodegeneration. *J Neurosci.* 23(9), 955–60 ISSN 0270-6474.

Yin L, Huseby E, Scott-Browne J, Rubtsova K, Pinilla C, Crawford F, Marrack P, Dai S. & Kappler JW. (2011).A single T cell receptor bound to major histocompatibility complex class I and class II glycoproteins reveals switchable TCR conformers. *Immunity,* 35(1), 23-33. ISSN 1074-7613.

You SJ, Kim HD. & Kang HC. (2009).Factors influencing the evolution of West syndrome to Lennox-Gastaut syndrome. *Pediatr Neurol,* 41(2), 111-3. ISSN 0887-8994

8

Plasma Exchange in Severe Attacks Associated with Neuromyelitis Optica Spectrum Disorder

Bonnan Mickael and Cabre Philippe
Service de Neurologie, Centre Hospitalier Universitaire Zobda Quitman, Fort-de-France, French West Indies

1. Introduction

Neuromyelitis optica (NMO) is an inflammatory disorder restricted to the spinal cord and optic nerves. Contrary to multiple sclerosis (MS), relapses of NMO are often strikingly severe and most NMO patients present stepwise neurological impairments. NMO treatments are aimed to prevent the relapses with the administration of various promising immunosuppressive drugs. However, relapse treatment is still a tricky problem. Since the largely used steroid treatment usually fails to control severe attacks, specific add-on treatments have to be considered in order to limit the stepwise increase of residual impairment. Given that a strong humoral response characterizes NMO physiology, one might assume plasma exchange (PLEX) to be particularly well adapted in severe NMO relapses.

This chapter will analyze the relevant data of PLEX in the setting of NMO spectrum disorder. We will first outline the physiological grounds leading to the rationale of the PLEX treatment and the technical aspects of the procedure. Then we will assess the clinical results obtained in each type of attacks. Finally we will try to build an original concept linking the clinical results and the timing of PLEX onset with the dynamic of the inflammation inside the lesions.

2. Physiopathology of NMO

The physiopathology of demyelinating disorders is complex and may grossly be divided in two distinct parts: a cellular response implying lymphocytes, macrophages and granulocytes in NMO; and a humoral response involving many circulating components including antibodies, complement and cytokines which will be extravasated into the inflammatory sites where they will participate to the inflammatory cascade of events leading to the local lesion. We will briefly review the main physiopathological aspects of NMO and focus on the humoral response, which is especially suitable to be eliminated by PLEX upstream to the lesion.

2.1 Physiopathology of NMO lesions

2.1.1 Pathology

A characteristic pathological pattern has been described in NMO (Lucchinetti et al., 2002). Lesions are infiltrated by neutrophils and eosinophils and wall capillaries are hyalinized. A vasculocentric pattern of activated complement and immunoglobulin of IgG and IgM types is observed that mirrors the normal expression of AQP4. AQP4 expression is definitely reduced in normal appearing white matter and lost throughout the lesions. These modifications are the hallmark of NMO and could occur alone or associated with a wide range of lesions from mild demyelination to large necrosis. This pattern of lesion was classified in the pattern II of the Lassmann's classification of the inflammatory lesions (Lucchinetti et al., 2000, 2002).

Contrary to MS, T cells are rare in NMO lesions and probably had no major effect on the formation of the lesions (Saadoun et al., 2011). However T cells are probably involved upstream in physiopathological cascade in the earlier phases of the disease where a complex interplay leads to antigen sensitization and possibly in the initial opening of the blood-brain barrier (BBB) (Pohl et al., 2011).

2.1.2 Specific antibodies and their epitopes

The NMO-IgG antibody is an IgG1 directed against a surface epitope of the protein aquaporin-4 (AQP4) (Lennon et al., 2005). This antibody is detected with tissue-based immunofluorescence assays with a sensitivity and specificity for clinically defined NMO of more than respectively 60% and 90%. NMO-IgM theoretically coexits with NMO-IgG in about 10% of cases but significance is poorly known (Jarius et al., 2010a). Clinically diagnosed NMO patients share common clinical and evolutional characteristics according to the NMO-IgG status. Beyond the surrogate marker value of NMO-IgG, this marker is now used as a major diagnostic criterion (Wingerchuk et al., 2006) and delineates the *NMO spectrum disorders* that gather in a same entity both typical NMO and unusual or truncated clinical forms (Wingerchuk et al., 2007).

Astrocytes closely interact with endothelial cells to maintain the CNS BBB. These cells express AQP4 in the apical domain of the membrane feet expansions situated close to the surrounded blood vessels. They are generally found as single tetramers, closely arranged in orthogonal arrays. This transmembrane protein is critically involved in the homeostasis of the water in the brain and interfaces with blood vessels, especially in the clearance of free water. Loss of perivascular AQP4 in the basal state results in cellular swelling, ostensibly due to a failure to eliminate water generated from cellular metabolism (Amiry-Moghaddam et al., 2003). Thus in NMO, since the interaction of NMO-IgG and AQP4 leads to a functional knock-out phenotype of AQP4, edema develops as a result of functional impairment of AQP4 although BBB is expected to be still intact, which may explain the paradoxical lack of gadolinium enhancement in most NMO lesions. Apart from water homeostasis, the removal of AQP4 from astrocytes membrane is associated with an impaired homeostasis of glutamate via the loss of function of EAAT2, a major glutamate transporter associated with AQP4 in a macromolecular complex (Hinson et al., 2008). The disruption of glutamate homeostasis initiates an excitotoxic mechanism damaging oligodendrocytes and ultimately leading to demyelination (Marignier et al., 2010).

Virtually all the CNS astrocytes express AQP4, however some regions are enriched in AQP4. Those regions are the spinal cord gray matter, the posterior optic nerve, the floor of the fourth ventricle and the circum ventricular organs especially the area postrema, explaining the restriction of the sites of lesion characterizing NMO (Pittock et al., 2006a). Interestingly circumventricular organs are also the only sites of the CNS expressing fenestrated capillaries favoring local passive diffusion of circulating antibodies.

2.1.3 NMO-IgG and complement as key factors

Clinical activity may correlate with the underlying NMO-IgG titres. NMO-IgG detection is a strong predictor of recurrence after an initial spinal or optic attack (Jarius et al., 2008, 2010b; Weinshenker, et al 2006). In few patients, NMO-IgG was high during flares and became negative during the stabilized disease following treatment, and in contrary, an initially seronegative patient became positive during a further attack (Weinstock-Guttman et al., 2008). In the seminal work of Takahashi et al. (2007), NMO-IgG levels were positively correlated with both clinical severity (i.e. blindness) and radiological severity. Moreover a strong positive correlation was obtained between the NMO-IgG titres at the nadir of exacerbations and the spinal cord lesion length on MRI (Takahashi et al., 2007). In contrast, low NMO-IgG titres were observed during remission induced by immunosuppressive maintenance therapy (Jarius et al., 2008).

In vitro, the binding of NMO-IgG to the extracellular domain of AQP4 reversibly down-regulates its plasma expression. In the presence of active complement, this binding leads to strong complement activation and rapid cell destruction. NMO serum IgM is not AQP4-specific and abundant IgM deposits in the NMO lesions may have passively diffused after the BBB disruption by the seminal focal complement activation initiated by NMO-IgG (Hinson et al., 2007).

In an animal model of EAE with passive transfer of NMO-IgG, the transfer exacerbated EAE signs and the typical pathological characteristics were reproduced in treated rats (Kinoshita et al., 2009; Bradl et al., 2009). Direct injection of NMO-IgG in rat brains could reproduce the pathology but only when complement is coinjected (Saadoun et al., 2010)

The NMO-IgG ability to lesion AQP4-transfected cells in the presence of complement was assessed with serum drawn from patients with mild and severe attacks. The percentage of cells lesioned by complement was strongly higher in presence of sera from patients with severe attacks, although lesion induced by sera from patients with mild attacks did not differ from negative controls or MS patients (Hinson et al., 2009). Thus the severity of the disease may be partly determined by intrinsic NMO-IgG characteristics to activate the complement.

2.2 Proof of concept of PLEX in NMO

As we already described, NMO lesions are associated with a strong IgG, IgM and complement deposition, typical of the pattern II in Lassmann's classification. The NMO-IgG is involved in a complement-dependant toxicity against the astrocytes. All of these components -IgG, IgM, and complement- are targeted by plasma exchanges. By means of 5 exchanges, all the exchanged molecules will drop to less than 20% of their initial level. By this way, antibodies and complement, which are the core of the pattern II lesions, are excluded from the circulating pool and cannot migrate anymore to the lesions.

Although PLEX has long been used in various demyelinating disorders (Keegan et al., 2002), there is some clue that the pattern is a key determinant of PLEX efficiency. In a retrospective study, Keegan et al. (2005) reported that all the patients suffering from demyelinating disorders and improved by PLEX had a biopsy proven pattern II lesion. None of the patients with any other kind of lesion improved. However all these patients were MS without NMO-IgG and none were NMO (Keegan et al., 2005; Kale et al., 2009).

All the aforementioned findings stress that circulating NMO-IgG and complements are the two main actors of the NMO pathogeny and why clearing them from blood with PLEX should be appropriate for special benefits.

3. Plasma exchange procédure

3.1 Principles and goals

Basically, the goal of PLEX (or plasmapheresis) is to remove a given volume of patient's plasma containing harmful targeted substances and to reinfuse an artificial plasma substitute in its place -*the plasma exchange* (Brecher, 2002).

3.2 Technique

PLEX are carried on in a nephrology or a resuscitation ward. Two high flow rate accesses are mandatory: an input line from patient to device ('artery') and a return line from device to patient ('vein'). In continuous filtration, two needles are placed in both arms or groins in order to drawn out the blood of the body through an extracorporeal line connected to one needle, then blood is processed and reinfused continuously through the other needle. In case of discontinuous filtration, the separation and remixing are done in small batches through a single venous access in the groin where in and out cycles may alternate. Anticoagulation (citrate or heparin) is added to the blood pre-plasma filter to prevent from clotting. The removed blood is processed (*apheresis procedure*) in a cell separator that continuously separates plasma from cellular components (consisting of red and white blood cells and platelets) either by a centrifugation ring with permanent in and out flow, or by filtration through a porous membrane. Small molecules like cytokines as well as large molecules, such as albumin and immunoglobulin, are easily extruded from the blood compartment with a reported sieving coefficient >0.95 at a blood flow rate of 100 mL/min. The cleared cellular components are then combined with the replacement fluid (donor plasma or artificial albumin mixed with a saline solution) and returned to the patient through the needle in the other arm. A PLEX session is usually performed in 2 to 6 hours, depending on patient's height, weight, viscosity of the blood and technical parameters.

3.3 Kinetics of the target exchanged components.

All the targeted components are distributed in the interstitium (extra-vascular compartment) by variable part. Large molecular weight compounds equilibrate slowly between the vascular space and the interstitium. Calculations of the rate of removal are simplified to first order kinetics. The relation curve of the achieved concentration of a plasma component [C] after a unique exchange of a given plasma volume V is an exponential inverse: $[C] = [C_0].e^{-Y}$. The whole plasma volume can be approximated in an adult with the following formula:

Estimated plasma volume (liters)= 0.07 x weight (kg) x (1-hematocrit).

The larger volume of plasma exchanged during each session clears a larger amount targeted circulating component. An exchange of one body plasma volume leads to the immediate clearance of 50% of the circulating component. A 1.3 body mass volume exchange that removes about 72% of C is generally agreed. Beyond, the volume to process increases massively for too little gain. However, according to the distribution of C in the interstitium, the achievement of the clearance of C will necessitate the use of multiple PLEX sessions separated by the time necessary for the equilibration of C concentration between interstitium and vascular spaces. The number and frequency of sessions should be evaluated according to the biological characteristics of the components to remove (synthesis level, vascular distribution, diffusion ability). An empirically driven number of 4 to 6 sessions is usually scheduled. The durability of the immunomodulatory effect after PLEX is difficult to assess and will depend on the turnover rate of the targeted humoral components. Concomitant intensive immunosuppressive therapy (i.e. steroids, mitoxantrone, mycophenolate mofetil, rituximab) will be required to sustain the obtained depletive effect.

3.4 Risks and side effects

PLEX are contraindicated in case of ongoing infectious disease, precarious hemodynamics and active hemorrhage (heparin). Immediate side effects are related to the extracorporeal line: hemodynamic instability, vaso-vagal syndrome, numbness or tingling, venous puncture hazards with excessive local bleeding, septicemia or allergy. Since blood coagulation factors are all depleted by PLEX, hemostasis is affected in variable ways: first, a hypocoagulation state is immediately achieved by the global depletion of all the coagulation factors for half a day; at day 2, short life pro-coagulant factors are regained but antithrombin-III synthesis is delayed leading to a hypercoagulable state until day 3. Preventive anticoagulation with heparin is always required since the high risk of thrombosis. Persistently low fibrinogen levels have been described with the concomitant use of high dosage steroid infusion. In summary PLEX are generally well tolerated and now commonly and safely used.

4. PLEX in severe attacks

Various regimens of high doses of intravenous methylprednisolone are used in first line of treatment ranging from 3 g infused in 3 days, to 10 g in 5 to 10 days, depending on authors. There is no evidence in favor of one regimen or another and efficacy assessment has never been addressed. Moreover, even if steroids reduce the inflammatory cellular response by triggering apoptosis of lymphocytes, they are clearly not sufficient because poor outcomes are still a common issue even when steroid treatment is given immediately after onset. We wish to develop here the evidence for the effectiveness of PLEX that we have been largely using as an add-on therapy for more than 10 years.

Of note, steroids were always used to treat relapse. When used the same day as PLEX procedure, steroids were infused at the end of each PLEX session. However methylprednisolone pharmacokinetics is characterized by a short half-life and PLEX demonstrated to have no effect on steroids biodisponibility (Assogba et al., 1988; Stigelman et al, 1984).

4.1 Spinal attacks

PLEX proved to be efficient in central demyelinating diseases in a randomized sham-controlled study (Weinshenker et al., 1999, 2001). Keegan et al. (2002) reviewed the clinical data from 59 patients who received PLEX for inflammatory demyelinating diseases, including 10 NMO and 6 acute transverse myelitis (ATM) cases. A moderate or marked improvement was obtained in half of NMO and ATM patient groups. The late final outcome at one year was more or less obtained during the first month after treatment in both groups, without regard to success or failure of treatment (Keegan et al., 2002; Brunot et al., 2011). A small number of case reports and few small studies were reported with variable issues. Judging improvement is even more complex due to the subjective classification of improvement in mild/moderate/marked instead of a quantified clinical exam (Brunot et al., 2011; Keegan et al., 2002; Munemoto et al., 2011; Llufriu et al., 2009). Moreover the natural history of single spinal relapse in NMO has never been addressed, so any improvement bias after PLEX is inappreciable in the absence of a control group. Finally, most authors used PLEX as a rescue treatment given late after the onset. For example PLEX was delayed from onset by a mean of 33±30 days in Brunot et al. (2011) and a median of 30 days [6 to 90 days] in Llufiru et al. (2009).

Although a synergistic effect of steroids and PLEX was long expected due to their complementary action, none of these studies compared PLEX-treated attacks with conventional steroid treatment given alone with add-on PLEX-treated attacks.

We previously refined these results in a study of outcome after severe spinal attacks associated with NMO spectrum disorders (Bonnan et al., 2009a). We included 96 spinal attacks from 43 patients, divided in two groups: 1) a steroid-only group designed from historical patients treated with steroids alone; 2) an active group treated both with PLEX and steroids. Steroid infusion was started immediately after patient admission. PLEX decision was raised at the same time and started as soon as possible during the two days later. As a major difference with other groups, PLEX was never initiated as a delayed rescue treatment after a standard steroid treatment failure. Since PLEX therapy is mainly expected to minimize residual impairment, we used the ΔEDSS (calculated as the difference between residual and basal EDSS) as the main outcome.

If we except 5 PLEX delayed due to difficult medevac reasons, PLEX were initiated by a mean of 5.4 ± 3.1 days after attack onset with a median of 4 sessions.

There was no significant difference between the PLEX-treated and steroid-only groups for basal and acute EDSS (3.9 ± 2.9 vs 4.2 ± 2.9, and 7.9 ± 1.0 vs 8.0 ± 1.4; p=NS), however residual EDSS (5.1 ± 2.4 vs 6.8 ± 1.9, $p<0.01$) and mean ΔEDSS (1.2 ± 1.6 vs 2.6 ± 2.4, $p<0.01$) were significantly lower in the PLEX-treated group than in the steroid-only group.

Basal EDSS dramatically influenced therapy outcome as shown in Table 1. During the first attack, although acute EDSS were similar in both groups (7.6 ± 1.2 vs 7.1 ± 1.5, p=NS), ΔEDSS and residual EDSS were dramatically reduced in the PLEX-treated group (2.1 ± 1.9 vs 5.8 ± 2.0, $p<0.01$) given that acute EDSS was similar in this sub-group. In the two other sub-groups of basal impairment (EDSS 1.0 to 5.5 and EDSS ≥6.0), residual EDSS and ΔEDSS tended to be lower in PLEX-treated attacks but no statistical signification could be obtained due to the small size of these groups.

EDSS	Basal EDSS null St (n=17)	St+PLEX (n=7)	*p*	Basal EDSS 1.0 to 5.5 St (n=26)	St+PLEX (n=13)	*p*	Basal EDSS ≥ 6.0 St (n=24)	St+PLEX (n=9)	*p*
Basal	**0**	**0**	*0.99*	**3.9±0.8**	**3.9±1.6**	*0.59*	**7.4±1.0**	**7.1±0.8**	*0.52*
Acute	**7.1±1.5**	**7.6±1.2**	*0.52*	**7.6±1.3**	**7.6±1.1**	*0.67*	**8.9±0.9**	**8.6±0.6**	*0.24*
Residual	**5.9±1.9)**	**2.1±1.9**	*<.01*	**5.8±1.6**	**5.1±1.1**	*0.21*	**8.5±1.1**	**7.6±1.0**	*0.05*
ΔEDSS	**5.9±1.9**	**2.1±1.9**	*<.01*	**2.0±1.5**	**1.2±1.6**	*0.10*	**1.1±0.8**	**0.5±0.8**	*0.11*

Table 1. Disability measured as EDSS during spinal attacks stratified with basal impairment. St: steroid-only treated group; St+PLEX: steroid and PLEX-treated group. Values are given as mean±SD (from Bonnan et al., 2009a).

The classical Lazarus effect, defined as a very short-term dramatic improvement (Weinshenker et al., 2000), was rather unusual in our group but our study was not designed to analyse short-term improvement. The patients who experienced this effect have all received a very early treatment (less than 2 days). In Magana et al. (2011), patients who exhibited functional improvement did so within a median of 4 days (third PLEX), although a minority (6%) exhibited a delayed response (more than 2 months).

Minor side effects occurred in 24% of PLEX treated attacks and resulted in PLEX interruption once (84-year-old patient with pulmonary embolism).

In summary, PLEX-treated patients achieved a significantly better outcome after a spinal attack, especially if PLEX was given during the first attack. The exact effect of PLEX in previously impaired patients should be validated in a larger multicentric cohort. As PLEX proved to be a promising treatment in spinal attacks, it would now be unethical to design a study with a sham-treated control group.

Predictors of good outcome were studied in a large group of PLEX including 26 NMO patients (Bonnan et al., 2009a). The only good outcome predictor was normal or brisk reflexes in acute phase (Magana et al., 2011). Surprisingly a short PLEX delay was associated with a good outcome in a first study (Keegan et al., 2002) but had no effect in a second study, although one should remind that median PLEX delay (23 days) was delayed in this later compared to our group. The same PLEX response rate was obtained irrespective of NMO-IgG serostatus in our cohort and in the Mayo Clinic cohort (Magana et al., 2011).

As a practical consequence, faced with a patient suffering from a severe relapse, the knowledge of NMO-IgG status should not be required to start PLEX as soon as possible, since PLEX was found efficient in NMO-IgG negative patients.

4.2 Optic attacks

Visual impairment in NMO is very severe. We previously showed that an immediate unilateral blindness occurred in a third of patients after the first optic neuritis (ON), and generally two attacks are sufficient to cause a definitive loss of vision (Merle et al., 2007). Few PLEX were undertaken after ON and a quick dramatic recovery is usual as we also observed (Bonnan et al., 2009b; unpublished results). Depending authors, PLEX were used immediately (Bonnan et al., 2009b) or as a delayed add-on therapy (Schilling et al., 2006;

Watanabe et al., 2007a; Trebst et al., 2009; Yoshida et al., 2010). After pooling severe ON patients (acute visual acuity<1/10°) from available studies (Schilling et al., 2006; Ruprecht et al., 2004; Trebst et al., 2009) with ours (Bonnan et al., 2009b and unpublished results), data were gathered for 39 eyes. PLEX were given in median of 19 days in patients who recovered a visual acuity more than 1/10° (considered here as a treatment success) but 41 days in treatment failure. A clear effect of PLEX delay was observed since success rate was 8/8 (100%) during the first 11 days, than 4/7 (57%) from days 12 to 22, and 7/13 (53%) from days 23 to 73. Moreover, even when patients recovered, averaged residual VA tended to be lower in delayed PLEX patients (Figure 1).

Interestingly, the spontaneous recovery (>1/10°) after severe ON treated by steroids alone was about 40% in our cohort (from Merle et al., 2007), which is very close to the recovery obtained in the two last groups of late PLEX. In conclusion, strong clues support that PLEX change the outcome of severe ON only when they are given early, however broader studies are still lacking to confirm this hypothesis.

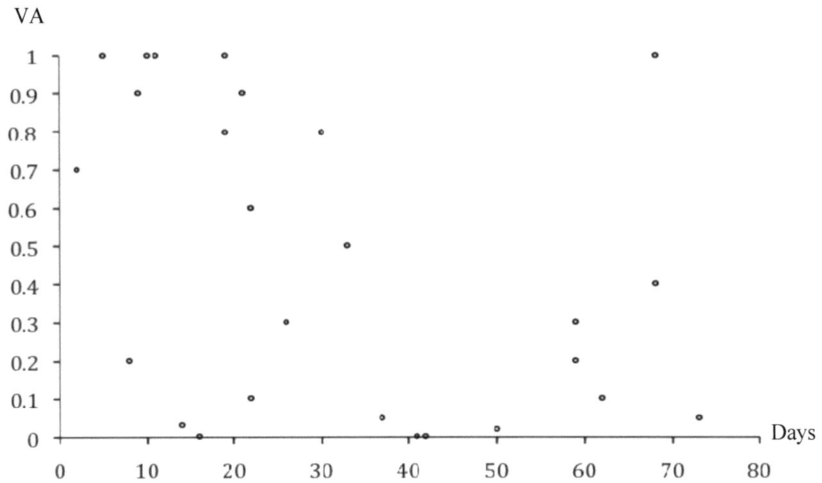

Fig. 1. Metanalysis of residual Visual Acuity as a function of PLEX delay (days) in severe ON attacks (acute VA<1/10°). See text.

4.3 Brain attacks

Apart from optico-spinal attacks, severe brain attacks are described in NMO, especially involving hypothalamus and medulla. Those lesions are usually severe and associated with blindness, central endocrine disorders or quadriplegia with respiratory failure. Brain lesions are common but are mostly asymptomatic (Pittock et al., 2006b). However symptomatic lesions involving supratentorial white matter are exceptional and extensive (Pittock et al., 2006b). Even if a favourable outcome after PLEX has been reported in a few severe cases (Viegas et al., 2009; Watanabe et al., 2009ab), comparative data are still lacking.

Posterior reversible encephalopathy syndrome (PRES) is an encephalopathy with consciousness and visual disturbances with rapidly reversible changes on MRI consistent with vasogenic edema. PRES are triggered by blood pressure instability or fluid stresses due to various causes. It seems to occur more often than coincidental in NMO patients: 5 out of 70 consecutive NMO-IgG patients evaluated at Mayo Clinic (Magana et al., 2009); 2 out of 5 in Hadassah Medical School, Israel (Eichel et al., 2008). Authors proposed that the auto-immune mediated disruption of the AQP4 water channel function may predisposes to PRES at comparable levels of acute illness (Magana et al., 2009). PLEX was involved as a trigger in one case with a good final outcome. In few cases, PLEX were implemented as curative treatment with an overall good outcome (Eichel et al., 2008; Magana et al., 2009).

5. Timing of PLEX: evolving to a key concept

Besides knowing PLEX are effective and safe, the central question remains: is PLEX necessary as-soon-as and as-often-as possible? Prospective, randomised, multi-centre clinical trials would be required to definitively answer the question. For most authors, to date PLEX are considered as an add-on rescue treatment after steroid failure. The European recommendation from EFNS is to start with an early steroid course no matter the severity (Sellner et al., 2010). Early escalation with PLEX is only recommended after a failure of a second course of steroids, that is to say that PLEX initiation may be postponed for more than a week. As we demonstrated before, PLEX efficiency is depends on the timing of initiation, ranging from immediate dramatic improvement (the *Lazarus effect*) to no effect according to whether they are given early or very late. We propose to regress to the dynamic of the inflammatory NMO lesions to explain why PLEX efficiency is strongly dependant of the timing of their onset.

5.1 Evidence for reversible dysfunction preceding irreversible tissue loss.

As we described above, the lesion is the consequence of a cascade of reversible events, susceptible to an external action. One could abruptly divide this cascade in two main points: a direct toxic action upon astrocytes and a bystander effect on oligodendrocytes and axons. Astrocyte dysfunction is initiated by the binding of NMO-IgG to the extracellular domain of AQP4 on the foot of the astrocyte membrane. In vitro, this binding reversibly down-regulates AQP4 plasma expression. The presence of fresh complement leads to a strong complement activation and a rapid cell destruction. IgG titres strongly correlates with the cytotoxic effect (Kalluri et al., 2010). By the other way, the removal of AQP4 from astrocytes membrane, due to internalization or cell death, impairs the clearance of free glutamate due to the dysfunction of the transporter EAAT2. The glutamate progressively accumulates and initiates an excito-toxic mechanism upon oligodendrocytes, ultimately leading to demyelination (Marignier et al., 2010).

The time sequence of these events was studied in lesions induced by direct mouse brain injection with NMO-IgG and complement (Saadoun et al., 2010). Loss of AQP4 and GFAP, and myelin breakdown were evident 7h following the injection. The inflammatory cells infiltration became evident later. Within 12h, axonal injury became prominent. By day 7, axonal loss and dying neurons were evident. Finally, one could suppose that a very early intervention targeting astrocytes dysfunction may prevent the progression to the bystander effect.

5.2 Evidence supporting an early treatment

The influence of treatment delay upon outcome has been addressed in a single study of first ON receiving steroid treatments (Nakamura et al., 2010). The outcomes were both visual acuity and the width of the retinal fibers layer evaluated with optic tomography (OCT). Patients were divided into two groups: one group with a good visual outcome, including a high residual visual acuity and high RFL; and a second group with a poor visual outcome in terms of low acuity and low RFL. Very interestingly, the two groups were similar in all the parameters except one: patients with a good outcome received steroids with a lower mean delay after ON onset, by a mean of 1.8±1.1 days compared to 7.8±3.8 in patients with a poor outcome. This study is the first proof that a delayed infusion of steroids is associated with a poorer outcome. A similar effect of treatment delay, although unknown, should be expected in spinal attacks. Even if no proof is yet available after a PLEX treatment, these clues could be gathered that early PLEX would improve the prognosis (see above).

In spinal attacks treated with PLEX, early initiation of treatment was one out of the predictors of good outcome (Keegan et al., 2002). In a larger study encompassing attacks from various demyelinating disorders, success rates were stratified by delay: improvement occurred in 83% when given before day 15, but fell to 43 after 2 months (Llufriu et al., 2009). Moreover the dramatically very short-term improvement, called Lazarus effect (Weinshenker et al., 2000), is sometimes observed after severe attacks receiving a very early treatment with PLEX and steroids. However, this earliness responsibility on the Lazarus effect remains elusive since no study is available on this rather unusual effect.

5.3 Lesion stages and PLEX action: 'time is cord and eyes'

In the light of the available data, we postulate a link between the staging of NMO lesion and the PLEX effect upon clinical and radiological outcome (Figure 2).

Stage 1 (first hours): acute attack provokes for hours an astrocyte dysfunction (by NMO-IgG binding on AQP4 leading to internalization) mainly expressed by an edema. This purely edematous lesion could be immediately reversible by the clearance of NMO-IgG preventing the loss of astrocytes and the excitotoxic cascade. Clinical and radiological recovery after PLEX is dramatic and explains the Lazarus effect. **Stage 2 (days):** the loss of EAAT2 induces an excitotoxic effect of glutamate on oligodendrocytes leading progressively to demyelination and axonal loss. Astrocytes loss initiates a self-sustained excitotoxic process henceforth independent from NMO-IgG persistence. Even if the extraction of NMO-IgG and complement by PLEX ends the astrocytes aggression. A variable amount of them has been already lost and excitotoxic effects upon oligodendrocytes are evident. Variable amount of tissue is lost as visible on MRI and recovery is incomplete. **Stage 3 (weeks):** atrocytes, oligodendrocytes and axonal loss is prominent, engulfed in large areas of necrosis. PLEX is almost useless. Neural tissue remains cavitated or atrophic on MRI and no recovery will be expected.

We propose to reconsider PLEX as a major part of the treatment of severe NMO attacks and suggest that PLEX could be given systematically in severe relapses of NMO, extended transverse myelitis or bilateral severe ON resistant to steroids. Moreover, when given they should be started as soon as possible with steroids.

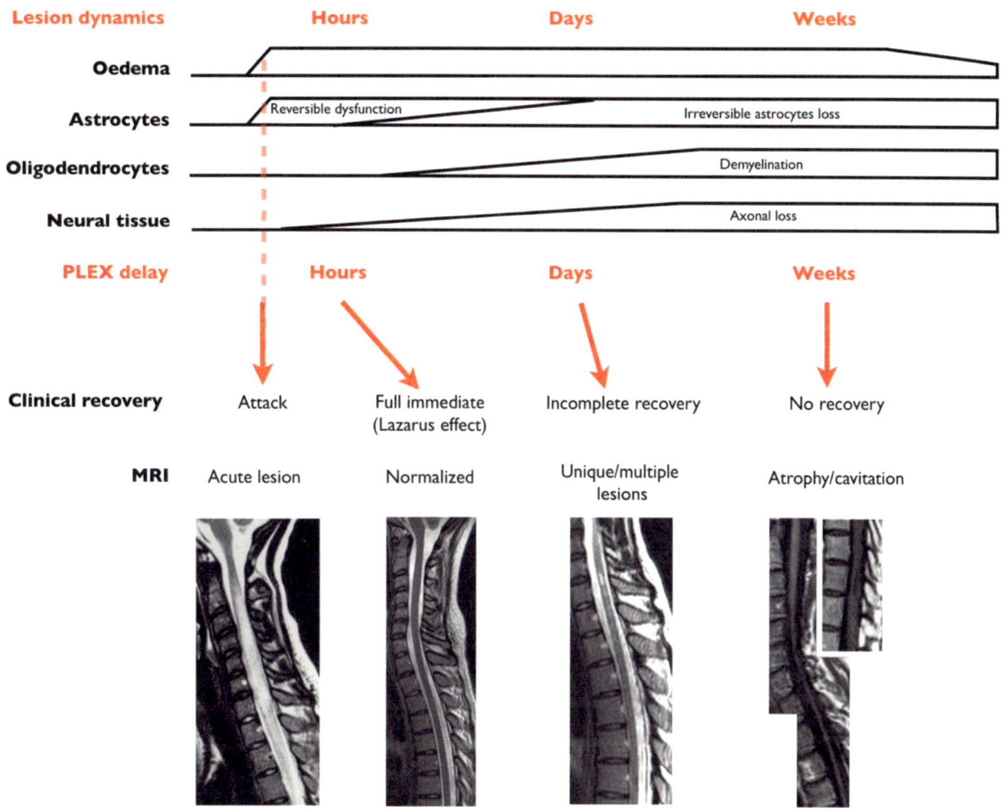

Fig. 2. Putative PLEX effect depending of the three main stages of the lesion.

6. PLEX as preventive treatment

Since NMO-IgG positivity is both predictive of attacks and severity, achieving a low concentration of plasmatic antibodies remains a goal to achieve. Besides immunosuppressive drugs, PLEX have been used to achieve a sustained depletion of NMO-IgG and complement. Favourable cases have been reported but studies are lacking (Miyamoto et al., 2009). Miyamoto et al. (2009) proposed to use PLEX as preventive treatment as an add-on therapy after immunosuppressive drugs failure.

7. Preventive treatments and future avenues

The natural history of NMO leads all the patients to a deep impairment in a stepwise fashion without progressive phase. In our study, 5 years after the onset, 70% of patients suffered from a unilateral loss of vision and almost half of them from a bilateral loss of vision (Merle et al., 2007). After 8 years, half of the patients had suffered from a severe myelitis and become chair-bound (Cabrera-Gomez et al., 2009). The mortality rate was very high before immunosuppressive drugs but dropped since they are largely used (Cabre et al., 2009). The exact role of recurring PLEX along the remaining attacks to tune the outcome to a low impairment has not yet been addressed but remains most probable considering this striking epidemiological change of mortality in French West Indies.

7.1 Immunosuppressive maintenance

Contrary to MS, cumulative evidence accumulates that interferon beta had no effect on activity rate and worsens some patients, especially in lupus-associated NMO (Uzawa et al., 2010). When IFN is compared to immunosuppressive drugs, a dramatic reduction of annualized relapse rate (ARR) is obtained (Papeix et al., 2007). Rituximab and mycophenolate mofetil were well tolerated and dramatically reduced ARR (Jacob et al., 2008; Jacob et al., 2009). A favorable action of mitoxantrone was reported in few cases (Weinstock-Guttman et al., 2006). In a group of 32 patients treated with mitoxantrone in our centre, a dramatic drop in ARR was obtained from a mean rate of 1.8 to 0.3 and sustained over 5 years (Cabre, personal communication). The choice in one these three drugs should mostly be driven by safety concerns since no comparative study or recommendation is readily available. Low dose steroids were reported to be effective in a few patients, however these data needs further studies with more patients. Various others treatments (cyclophosphamide, azathioprine, venous immuno-globulins) have been used in isolated cases where no general conclusion could be drawn upon ARR action. However cyclophosphamide is commonly used to treat lupus in overlapping cases of NMO (Polgar et al., 2011).

7.2 New strategies for the future

Since the lesion severity mostly depends on the initial and definitive depth of the loss of AQP4 and astrocytes, future treatments strategies may be directed upon AQP4 preservation. Small molecules or monoclonal antibodies could be used to prevent NMO-IgG binding to AQP4 and to block the physiopathological cascade upstream (Verkman et al., 2011; Yu et al., 2011). Another strategy may deplete pathogenic antibodies by apheresis using dedicated immunoadsorption systems as previously described in myasthenia gravis (Zisimopoulou et al., 2008) and in various extra neurological disorders. However the value of this technique is less clear in disorders like MS (De Andres et al., 2000; Moldenhauer et al., 2005) where pathology is broader than a specific antibody. No experience is yet available in the NMO setting. Lymphocytapheresis was successfully described in isolated cases of resistant attacks (Aguilera et al., 1984, Nozaki et al., 2006). A complementary approach may target the complement system with newly developed anti-complement recombinant antibodies at various levels, with preliminary promising results (Saadoun et al., 2010). Such future treatments may be aimed at preventing or curing the attacks. During attacks, neuroprotective treatments could be used to prevent the oligodendrocytes loss induced by the excitotoxic action of glutamate.

Animal models gave clues to dynamic mechanisms evolving over time and appear suitable to address the effect of those various early therapeutic interventions directed to halt or prevent ongoing lesions (Saadoun et al., 2010).

8. Conclusion

PLEX, in synergy with steroids, could be a major treatment of relapses, aimed at preventing cumulative disability. PLEX is a safe and efficient add-on therapy in NMO. Since PLEX proved to be effective regardless of NMO-IgG status, NMO-IgG status should not be required to initiate PLEX. These preliminary results suggest that PLEX may modify the short prognostic of NMO relapses. Immunosuppressive drugs are necessary to prevent further relapses but no recommendation is yet available.

Animal models have confirmed that mechanisms leading to lesion evolve over hours and days. Those models should be able to confirm that early therapeutic intervention directed to halt the ongoing lesions should be even more dramatic in an early narrow therapeutic window.

The next steps should be to concentrate upon large multicentric therapeutic trials in order to validate the therapeutic procedure. However we are aware that good trials against placebo could be difficult to accept since this is an extremely devastating disease. The take-away messages are: undertaking PLEX in severe relapses and the importance of starting treatment as soon as possible.

9. References

Aguilera AJ, Carlow TJ, Smith KJ & Simon TL. (1985). Lympho-cytaplasmapheresis in Devic's syndrome. *Transfusion,* Vol. 25, No. 1, pp. 54-6.

Amiry-Moghaddam M, Otsuka T, Hurn PD, Traystman RJ, Haug FM, Froehner SC, & al. (2003). An alpha-syntrophin-dependent pool of AQP4 in astroglial end-feet confers bidirectional water flow between blood and brain. *Proc Natl Acad Sci USA,* Vol.100, pp. 2106-11.

Assogba U, Baumelou A, Pecquinot MA, Raymond F, Durande JP, Lenoir G et al. (1988) Removal of prednisone and prednisolone during plasma exchange. *Ann Med Interne,* Vol. 139, pp. 38-9.

Bonnan M, Valentino R, Olindo S, Mehdaoui H, Smadja D & Cabre P. (2009). Plasma exchange in severe spinal attacks associated with neuromyelitis optica Spectrum disorder. *Mult Scler,* Vol.15, No. 4, pp. 487-92.

Bonnan M, Brasme H, Diaby MM, Vlaicu M, Le Guern V & Zuber M. (2009). Severe bouts of neuromyelitis optica: dramatic improvement after plasma exchanges. *Rev Neurol,* Vol.165, No. 5, pp. 479-81.

Bradl M, Misu T, Takahashi T, Watanabe M, Mader S, Reindl M, & al. (2009). Neuromyelitis optica: pathogenicity of patient immunoglobulin in vivo. *Ann Neurol,* Vol.66, No.5, pp. 630-43.

Brecher ME. Plasma exchange: why we do what we do. (2002). *J Clin Apher,* Vol.17, No.4, pp. 207-11.

Brunot S, Vukusic S, Fromont A, Couvreur G, Mousson C, Giroud M, Confavreux C & Moreau T. (2011). Plasma exchanges in severe and acute inflammatory demyelinating attacks of the central nervous system. *Presse Med,* Vol.40, No.5, pp. e271-8.

Cabre P, Gonzalez-Quevedo A, Lannuzel A, Bonnan M, Merle H, Olindo S, & al. (2009). Descriptive epidemiology of neuromyelitis optica in the Caribbean basin. *Rev Neurol,* Vol.165, pp. 676-83.

Cabrera-Gomez JA, Bonnan M, Gonzalez-Quevedo A, Saiz Hinajeros A, Marignier R, Graus F, & al. (2009). Neuromyelitis optica positive antibodies confer a worse course in relapsing-neuromyelitis optica in Cuba and French West Indies. *Mult Scler*, Vol.15, pp. 828-33.

de Andrès C, Anaya F & Gimenez-Rolden S. (2000). Plasma immunoadsorption treatment of malignant multiple sclerosis with severe and prolonged relapses. *Rev Neurol.* 2000, Vol.30, No.7, pp. 601-5.

Eichel R, Meiner Z, Abramsky O & Gotkine M. (2008). Acute disseminating encephalomyelitis in neuromyelitis optica: closing the floodgates. *Arch Neurol*, Vol.65, No.2, pp. 267-71.

Hinson SR, Pittock SJ, Lucchinetti CF, Roemer SF, Fryer JP, Kryzer TJ & Lennon VA. (2007). Pathogenic potential of IgG binding to water channel extracellular domain in neuromyelitis optica. *Neurology*, Vol.69, No.24, pp. 2221-31.

Hinson SR, Roemer SF, Lucchinetti CF, Fryer JP, Kryzer TJ, Chamberlain JL, Howe CL, Pittock SJ & Lennon VA. (2008). Aquaporin-4-binding autoantibodies in patients with neuromyelitis optica impair glutamate transport by down-regulating EAAT2. *J Exp Med*, Vol.205, No.11, pp. 2473-81.

Hinson SR, McKeon A, Fryer JP, Apiwattanakul M, Lennon VA & Pittock SJ. (2009). Prediction of neuromyelitis optica attack severity by quantitation of complement-mediated injury to aquaporin-4-expressing cells. *Arch Neurol*, Vol.66, pp. 1164-7.

Jacob A, Matiello M, Weinshenker BG, Wingerchuk DM, Lucchinetti C, Shuster E, Carter J, Keegan BM, Kantarci OH & Pittock SJ. (2009). Treatment of neuromyelitis optica with mycophenolate mofetil: retrospective analysis of 24 patients. *Arch Neurol*, Vol.66, No.9, pp. 1128-33.

Jacob A, Weinshenker BG, Violich I, McLinskey N, Krupp L, Fox RJ, Wingerchuk DM, Boggild M, Constantinescu CS, Miller A, De Angelis T, Matiello M & Cree BA. (2008). Treatment of neuromyelitis optica with rituximab: retrospective analysis of 25 patients. *Arch Neurol*, Vol.65, No.11, pp. 1443-8.

Jarius S, Aboul-Enein F, Waters P, Kuenz B, Hauser A, Berger T, Lang W, Reindl M, Vincent A & Kristoferitsch W. (2008). Antibody to aquaporin-4 in the long-term course of neuromyelitis optica. *Brain*, Vol.131, No.11, pp. 3072-80.

Jarius S, Franciotta D, Bergamaschi R, Wildemann B & Wandinger KP. (2010). Immunoglobulin M antibodies to aquaporin-4 in neuromyelitis optica and related disorders. *Clin Chem Lab Med*, Vol.48, No.5, pp. 659-63.

Jarius S, Frederikson J, Waters P, Paul F, Akman-Demir G, Marignier R, Franciotta D, Ruprecht K, Kuenz B, Rommer P, Kristoferitsch W, Wildemann B & Vincent A. (2010). Frequency and prognostic impact of antibodies to aquaporin-4 in patients with optic neuritis. *J Neurol Sci*, Vol.298, No. 1-2, pp. 158-62.

Kale N, Pittock SJ, Lennon VA, Thomsen K, Roemer S, McKeon A & Lucchinetti CF. (2009). Humoral pattern II multiple sclerosis pathology not associated with neuromyelitis Optica IgG. *Arch Neurol*, Vol.66, No.10, pp. 1298-9.

Kalluri SR, Illes Z, Srivastava R, Cree B, Menge T, Bennett JL, Berthele & Hemmer B. (2010). Quantification and functional characterization of antibodies to native aquaporin 4 in neuromyelitis optica. *Arch Neurol*, Vol.67, No.10, pp. 1201-8.

Keegan M, Pineda AA, McClelland RL, Darby CH, Rodriguez M & Weinshenker BG. (2002). Plasma exchange for severe attacks of CNS demyelination: predictors of response. *Neurology*, Vol.58, No.1, pp. 143-6.

Keegan M, Konig F, McClelland R, Bruck W, Morales Y, Bitsch A, Panitch H, Lassmann H, Weinshenker B, Rodriguez M, Parisi J & Lucchinetti CF. (2005). Relation between humoral pathological changes in multiple sclerosis and response to therapeutic plasma exchange. *Lancet*, Vol.366, No.9485, pp. 579-82.

Kinoshita M, Nakatsuji Y, Kimura T, Moriya M, Takata K, Okuno T, Kumanogoh A, Kajiyama K, Yoshikawa H & Sakoda S. (2009). Neuromyelitis optica: Passive transfer to rats by human immunoglobulin. *Biochem Biophys Res Commun*, Vol.386, No.4, pp. 623-7.

Lennon VA, Kryzer TJ, Pittock SJ, Verkman AS & Hinson SR. (2005). IgG marker of optic-spinal multiple sclerosis binds to the aquaporin-4 water channel. *J Exp Med*, Vol.202, No.4, pp. 473-7.

Llufriu S, Castillo J, Blanco Y, Ramio-Torrenta L, Rio J, Valles M, Lozano M & al. (2009). Plasma exchange for acute attacks of CNS demyelination: Predictors of improvement at 6 months. *Neurology*, Vol.73, pp. 949-53.

Lucchinetti CF, Mandler RN, McGavern D, Bruck W, Gleich G, Ransohoff RM, Trebst C, Weinshenker B, Wingerchuk D, Parisi JE & Lassmann H. (2002). A role for humoral mechanisms in the pathogenesis of Devic's neuromyelitis optica. Brain, Vol.125, No.7, pp. 1450-61.

Lucchinetti C, Brück W, Parisi J, Scheithauer B, Rodriguez M & Lassmann H. (2000). Heterogeneity of multiple sclerosis lesions: implications for the pathogenesis of demyelination. *Ann Neurol*, Vol.47, No.6, pp. 707-17.

Magana SM, Matiello M, Pittock SJ, McKeon A, Lennon VA, Rabinstein AA, Shuster E, Kantarci OH, Lucchinetti CF & Weinshenker BG. (2009). Posterior reversible encephalopathy syndrome in neuromyelitis optica spectrum disorders. *Neurology*, Vol.72, No.8, pp. 712-7.

Magana SM, Keegan BM, Weinshenker BG, Erickson BJ, Pittock SJ, Lennon VA & al. (2011). Beneficial plasma exchange response in central nervous system inflammatory demyelination. *Arch Neurol*, Vol.68, pp. 870-8.

Marignier R, Nicolle A, Watrin C, Touret M, Cavagna S, Varrin-Doyer M, Cavillon G, Rogemond V, Confavreux C, Honnorat J & Giraudon P. (2010). Oligodendrocytes are damaged by neuromyelitis optica immunoglobulin G via astrocyte injury. *Brain*, Vol.133, No.9, pp. 2578-91.

Merle H, Olindo S, Bonnan M, Donnio A, Richer R, Smadja D & Cabre P. (2007). Natural history of the visual impairment of relapsing neuromyelitis optica. *Ophthalmology*, Vol.114, No.4, pp. 810-5.

Miyamoto, K. & Kusunoki, S. (2009). Intermittent plasmapheresis prevents recurrence in neuromyelitis optica. *Ther Apher Dial*, Vol.13, pp. 505–8.

Moldenhauer A, Haas J, Wascher C, Derfuss T, Hoffmann KT, Kiesewetter H & Salama A. (2005). Immunoadsorption patients with multiple sclerosis: an open-label pilot study. *Eur J Clin Invest*, Vol.35, No.8, pp. 523-30.

Munemoto M, Otaki Y, Kasama S, Nanami M, Tokuyama M, Yahiro M, Hasuike Y, Kuragano T, Yoshikawa H, Nonoguchi H & Nakanishi T. (2011). Therapeutic efficacy of double filtration plasmapheresis in patients with anti-aquaporin-4 antibody-positive multiple sclerosis. *J Clin Neurosci*, Vol.18, No.4, pp. 478-80.

Nakamura M, Nakazawa T, Doi H, Hariya T, Omodaka K, Misu T, Takahashi T, Fujihara K & Nishida K. (2010). Early high-dose intravenous methylprednisolone is effective in preserving rétinal nerve fiber layer thickness in patients with neuromyelitis optica. *Graefes Arch Clin Exp Ophthalmol*, Vol.248, No.12, pp. 1777-85.

Nozaki I, Hamaguchi T, Komai K & Yamada M. (2006). Fulminant Devic disease successfully treated by lymphocytapheresis. *J Neurol Neurosurg Psychiatry*, Vol.77, No.9, pp. 1094-5.

Papeix C, Vidal JS, de Seze J, Pierrot-Deseilligny C, Tourbah A, Stankoff B, Lebrun C, Moreau T, Vermersch P, Fontaine B, Lyon-Caen O & Gout O. (2007). Immunosuppressive therapy is more effective than interferon in neuromyelitis optica. *Mult Scler*, Vol.13, No.2, pp. 256-9.

Pittock SJ, Weinshenker BG, Lucchinetti CF, Wingerchuk DM, Corboy JR & Lennon VA. (2006). Neuromyelitis optica brain lesions localized at sites of high aquaporin 4 expression. *Arch Neurol*, Vol.63, No.7, pp. 964-8.

Pittock SJ, Lennon VA, Krecke K, Wingerchuk DM, Lucchinetti CF & Weinshenker BG. (2006). Brain abnormalities in neuromyelitis optica. *Arch Neurol*, Vol.63, No.3, pp. 390-6.

Pohl M, Fischer MT, Mader S, Schanda K, Kitic M, Sharma R, Wimmer I, Misu T, Fujihara K, Reindl M, Lassmann H & Bradl M. (2011). Pathogenic T cell responses against aquaporin 4. *Acta Neuropathol*, Vol.122, No.1, pp. 21-34.

Polgar A, Rosa C, Muller V, Matolcsi J, Poor G & Kiss EV. (2011). Devic's syndrome and SLE: challenges in diagnosis and therapeutic possibilities based on two overlapping cases. *Autoimmun Rev*, Vol.10, No.3, pp. 171-4.

Ruprecht K, Klinker E, Dintelmann T, Rieckmann P & Gold R. (2004). Plasma exchange for severe optic neuritis: treatment of 10 patients. *Neurology*, Vol.63, No.6, pp. 1081-3.

Saadoun S., Waters P., Bell BA., Vincent A., Verkman AS. & Papadopoulos MC. (2010). Intra-cerebral injection of neuromyelitis optica immunoglobulin G and human complement produces neuromyelitis optica lesions in mice. *Brain*, Vol.133, pp. 349–61.

Saadoun S, Waters P, Macdonald C, Bridges LR, Bell BA, Vincent A & al. (2011). T cell deficiency does not reduce lesions in mice produced by intracerebral injection of NMO-IgG and complement. *J Neuroimmunol*, Vol.235, pp. 27-32.

Schilling S, Linker RA, Konig FB, Koziolek M, Bahr M, Muller GA & al. (2006). Plasma exchange therapy for steroid-unresponsive multiple sclerosis relapses: clinical experience with 16 patients. *Nervenarzt*, Vol.77, pp. 430-8.

Sellner J, Boggild M, Clanet M, Hintzen RQ, Illes Z, Montalban X, Du Pasquier RA, Polman CH, Sorensen PS & Hemmer B. (2010). EFNS guidelines on diagnosis and management of neuromyelitis optica. *Eur J Neurol*, Vol.17, No.8, pp. 1019-32.

Stigelman WH Jr, Henry DH, Talbert RL, (1984) Townsend RJ. Removal of prednisone and prednisolone by plasma exchange. *Clin Pharm*, Vol.3, pp. 402-7.

Takahashi T, Fujihara K, Nakashima I, Misu T, Miyazawa I, Nakamura M, Watanabe S, Shiga Y, Kanaoka C, Fujimori J, Sato S & Itoyama Y. (2007). Anti-aquaporin-4 antibody is involved in the pathogenesis of NMO: a study on antibody titre. *Brain*, Vol.130, No.5, pp. 1235-43.

Trebst C, Reising A, Kielstein JT, Hafer C & Stangel M. (2009). Plasma exchange therapy in steroid-unresponsive relapses in patients with multiple sclerosis. *Blood Purif*, Vol.28, No.2, pp. 108-15.

Uzawa A, Mori M, Hayakawa S, Masuda S & Kuwabara S. (2010). Different responses to interferon beta-1b treatment in patients with neuromyelitis optica and multiple sclerosis. *Eur J Neurol*, Vol.17, No.5, pp. 672-6.

Verkman AS, Ratelade J, Rossi A, Zhang H & Tradtrantip L. (2011). Aquaporin-4: orthogonal array assembly, CNS functions, and role in neuromyelitis optica. *Acta Pharmacol Sin*, Vol.32, pp. 702-10.

Viegas S, Weir A, Esiri M, Kuker W, Waters P, Leite MI & al. (2009). Symptomatic, radiological and pathological involvement of the hypothalamus in neuromyelitis optica. *J Neurol Neurosurg Psychiatry*, Vol.80, pp. 679-82.

Watanabe S, Nakashima I, Miyazawa I, Misu T, Shiga Y, Nakagawa Y, Fujihara K & Itoyama Y. (2007). Successful treatment of a hypothalamic lesion in neuromyelitis optica by plasma exchange. *J Neurol*, Vol.254, No.5, pp. 670-1.

Watanabe S, Nakashima I, Misu T, Miyazawa I, Shiga Y, Fujihara K & Itoyama Y. (2007). Therapeutic efficacy of plasma exchange in NMO-IgG-positive patients with neuromyelitis optica. *Mult Scler*, Vol.13, No.1, pp. 128-32.

Weinshenker BG, O'Brien PC, Petterson TM, Noseworthy JH, Lucchinetti CF, Dodick DW, Pineda AA, Stevens LN & Rodriguez M. (1999). A randomized trial of plasma exchange in acute central nervous system inflammatory demyelinating disease. *Ann Neurol*, Vol.46, No.6, pp. 878-86.

Weinshenker BG. (2001). Plasma exchange for severe attacks of inflammatory demyelinating diseases of the central nervous system. *J Clin Apher*, Vol.16, No.1, pp. 39-42.

Weinshenker BG, Wingerchuk DM, Vukusic S, Linbo L, Pittock SJ, Lucchinetti CF & Lennon VA. (2006). Neuromyelitis optica IgG predicts relapse after longitudinally extensive transverse myelitis. *Ann Neurol*, Vol.59, No.3, pp. 566-9.

Weinshenker BG. (2000). Plasma exchange for acute attacks of demyelinating disease: detecting a Lazarus effect. *Ther Apher*, Vol.4, No.3, pp. 187-9.

Weinstock-Guttman B, Ramanathan M, Lincoff N, Napoli SQ, Sharma J, Feichter J & Bakshi R. (2006). Study of mitoxantrone for the treatment of recurrent neuromyelitis optica (Devic disease). *Arch Neurol*, Vol.63, No.7, pp. 957-63.

Weinstock-Guttman B, Miller C, Yeh E, Stosic M, Umhauer M, Batra N, Munschauer F, Zivadinov R & Ramanathan M. (2008). Neuromyelitis optica immunoglobulins as a marker of disease activity and response to therapy in patients with neuromyelitis optica. *Mult Scler*, Vol.14, No.8, pp. 1061-7.

Wingerchuk DM, Lennon VA, Lucchinetti CF, Pittock SJ & Weinshenker BG. (2007). The spectrum of neuromyelitis optica. *Lancet Neurol*, Vol.6, No.9, pp. 805-15.

Wingerchuk DM, Lennon VA, Pittock SJ, Lucchinetti CF & Weinshenker BG. (2006). Revised diagnostic criteria for neuromyelitis optica. *Neurology*, Vol;66, No.10, pp. 1485-9.

Yoshida H, Ando A, Sho K, Akioka M, Kawai E, Arai E, Nishimura T, Shinde A, Masaki H, Takahashi K, Takagi M & Tanaka K. (2010). Anti-aquaporin-4 antibody-positive optic neuritis treated with double-filtration plasmapheresis. *J Ocul Pharmacol Ther*, Vol.26, No.4, pp. 381-5.

Yu X, Green M, Gilden D, Lam C, Bautista K & Bennett JL. (2011). Identification of peptide targets in neuromyelitis optica. *J Neuroimmunol*, Vol.236, No.1-2, pp. 65-71.

Zisimopoulou P., Lagoumintzis G., Kostelidou K., Bitzopoulou K., Kordas G., Trakas N. & al. (2008) Towards antigen-specific apheresis of pathogenic autoantibodies as a further step in the treatment of myasthenia gravis by plasmapheresis. *J Neuroimmunol*, Vol. 201-2, pp. 95–103.

9

Regulatory B Cells - Implications in Autoimmune and Allergic Disorders

Susanne Sattler[1*], Luciën E.P.M. van der Vlugt[2], Leonie Hussaarts[2], Hermelijn H. Smits[2] and Fang-Ping Huang[1]
[1]Imperial College London,
[2]Leiden University Medical Center,
[1]UK
[2]The Netherlands

1. Introduction

B lymphocytes represent a major component of the immune system and their best understood effector functions are antibody production, presentation of antigens to T cells and the modulation of immune responses via cytokine production. Although most of these functions serve to amplify immune responses, B cells have also been demonstrated to downregulate inflammatory reactions and induce tolerance. As such, regulatory B (Breg) cells have been implicated in various inflammatory conditions. There is evidence for Breg cell deficiencies in human autoimmune diseases and various adoptive transfer experiments in mouse models of autoimmune and allergic conditions indicate that Breg cells are capable of suppressing disease development. In this review we endeavour to give an overview of the current knowledge about regulatory B cell immunobiology and their implications in autoimmune and allergic disorders.

2. Regulatory B cells

B cells with regulatory capacity have become the focus of intense investigations in recent years. However, the general concept that B cells might have the ability to induce tolerance, was introduced already in the 1970s by Katz et al., who demonstrated that depletion of B cells from splenocytes abolished their ability to inhibit an inflammatory reaction in a delayed type hypersensitivity (DTH) model (Katz, Parker et al. 1974; Mauri and Ehrenstein 2008). More than 20 years later, Janeway and co-workers were the first to demonstrate a role of B cells in protection from autoimmunity, showing that B cell-deficient mice failed to undergo spontaneous remission from experimental autoimmune encephalomyelitis (EAE) (Wolf, Dittel et al. 1996). The term 'regulatory B cells' was introduced shortly afterwards, by Mizoguchi and Bhan, who identified an IL-10 producing B cell subset in gut-associated lymphoid tissues (GALT) with upregulated CD1d expression, which suppressed progression of intestinal inflammation by downregulating inflammatory cascades (Mizoguchi, Mizoguchi et al. 2002). Breg cells are now considered a key regulatory cell type

---

[*] SS and LvdV contributed equally to this work

capable of suppressing effector functions of various target cells including T cells, dendritic cells (DC) and macrophages, and can even convert effector T cells into regulatory T cells (Tian, Zekzer et al. 2001; Matsushita, Horikawa et al. 2010; Ronet, Hauyon-La Torre et al. 2010; Wong, Puaux et al. 2010).

2.1 Breg cell populations in mice and humans

Although the existence of a regulatory subset of B cells is generally accepted, there is still some controversy concerning their origin and relationship to other B cell populations (Vitale, Mion et al. 2010). In mice, B cells are classified according to their developmental origin, into B1 and B2 cells. B1 lymphocytes are considered an innate type of lymphocytes and appear early in life. They produce antibodies with a limited diversity to common pathogens and can respond quickly and independently of T cells. B2 lymphocytes on the other hand are further subdivided into marginal zone (MZ) and follicular B cells in the spleen and circulating B cells in the peripheral blood, each with very specific characteristics and functions (Hardy and Hayakawa 2001). Regulatory B cells or their precursors seem to be able to arise from different subpopulations of both B1 and B2 cells. As shown in Table 1, several Breg cell populations with varying surface phenotypes have been identified in various mouse model systems as well as in different human disease conditions. Some regulatory B cell populations have also been shown to be induced in diverse disease settings and in response to many different exogenous and endogenous stimuli. Toll-like receptor (TLR) signalling via TLR-2, 4 and 9 as well as B cell receptor (BCR) signalling and co-stimulation mediated by CD40, CD80/CD86 or B-cell activating factor (BAFF) has been demonstrated to induce B cells with suppressive activity (Fillatreau, Sweenie et al. 2002; Mauri, Gray et al. 2003; Blair, Chavez-Rueda et al. 2009; Kala, Rhodes et al. 2010; Lampropoulou, Calderon-Gomez et al. 2010; Yang, Sun et al. 2010). One prominent type of 'natural' B cells with regulatory capacity has been isolated from naive mouse spleens and termed B10 cells by reason of their IL-10-dependent suppressive function. Phenotypically these B cells seem to be predominantly $CD1d^{hi}CD5^{+}$, thus they share surface markers with $CD5^{+}$ B1 cells ($CD21^{hi}CD23^{+}IgM^{hi}CD1d^{hi}Cd93^{int}$), MZ B cells ($CD1d^{hi}CD21^{hi}CD23^{lo}IgM^{hi}$) and transitional 2 (T2)-MZ precursor B cells ($CD1d^{hi}CD21^{hi}CD23^{hi}IgM^{hi}$), but do not exclusively belong to one of these B cell subpopulations (Yanaba, Bouaziz et al. 2008). The human equivalent to mouse B10 cells has been identified recently as a small population within peripheral blood $CD24^{hi}CD27^{+}$B cells (Iwata, Matsushita et al. 2011). In analogy to regulatory-type T cells, which can been subdivided into Treg, Tr1 and Th3 according to their expression of FoxP3, IL-10 and transforming growth factor (TGF)-β, respectively, it has been proposed to classify human regulatory B cells into 'Breg', Br1 (B10) and Br3 (Noh and Lee 2011).

Because of the variety of Breg cell populations and inducing factors, several models have been proposed that try to explain their origin and development. The first model put forward by Mizoguchi et al. states that distinct Breg cell populations are generated from already existing B cell subsets depending on distinct activation processes (Mizoguchi and Bhan 2006). According to this hypothesis, innate type regulatory B cells are generated from MZ B cells in the spleen upon stimulation with inflammatory signals such as lipopolysaccharides (LPS) or CpG via toll-like receptors (TLR). On the other hand, acquired type regulatory B cells develop from follicular B cells following activation with CD40 ligand and/or B cell receptor (BCR) ligation with self-antigen. A second model proposed by Lampropoulou et al. states that B cells acquire suppressive function due to a hierarchical process of stepwise B

species	phenotype	initial identification	organ of origin	major effector function	disease condition
mouse	B10	(Yanaba, Bouaziz et al. 2008)	spleen	IL-10	CHS
mouse	T2 MZ	(Carter, Vasconcellos et al. 2011) (Evans, Chavez-Rueda et al. 2007)	spleen	IL-10	arthritis
mouse	MZ	(Gray, Miles et al. 2007)	spleen	IL-10	CIA
mouse	B1	(Nakashima, Hamaguchi et al. 2010)	peri-toneum	IL-10	CHS
mouse	CD1d^{hi}	(Amu, Saunders et al. 2010) (Mizoguchi, Mizoguchi et al. 2002)	spleen	IL-10	AAI, IBD anaphylaxis
mouse	CD23^{+}	(Wilson, Taylor et al. 2010)	mes. LN	?	AAI, EAE
sheep	CD21^{+} B2	(Booth, Griebel et al. 2009)	Peyer's patches	IL-10	healthy
human	immature trans B	(Blair, Norena et al. 2010)	blood	IL-10 CD80/ CD86	SLE
human	'B10 (Br1)'	(Iwata, Matsushita et al. 2011)	blood	IL-10	healthy and autoimmune
human	CD1d^{hi}	(Correale, Farez et al. 2008)		IL-10	
human	'Br3'	(Lotz, Ranheim et al. 1994)	blood	TGF-β	CLL
human	'Breg'	(Noh, Choi et al. 2010)	blood	FoxP3	healthy

Table 1. B cell populations with regulatory phenotypes in different species. B cell populations with regulatory capacity have been identified in various different experimental settings or disease conditions in mice, humans and sheep. CHS: contact hypersensitivity, T2-MZ: transitional 2 marginal zone, CIA: collagen induced arthritis, AAI: allergic airway inflammation, IBD: inflammatory bowel disease, mes.LN: mesenteric lymphnodes, EAE: experimental autoimmune encephalomyelitis, SLE: systemic lupus erythematosus, CLL: chronic lymphocytic leukemia.

cell activation, with TLR ligands initiating the process and BCR and CD40 engagement serving to further reinforce this differentiation. According to this model, all activated B cells have the capacity to become regulatory B cells after activation (Lampropoulou, Calderon-Gomez et al. 2010). A third model, based on shared phenotypic markers between most described IL-10 producing B cell populations, claims that all different B cell populations contain distinct Breg cell precursors, which mature to IL-10 producing cells upon activation (DiLillo, Matsushita et al. 2010). Taken together, currently available information suggests, that in addition to distinct 'natural' Breg cell populations arising from specific Breg cell progenitors, members of many B cells subsets are potentially able to acquire suppressive functions as a negative feedback mechanism in response to activation.

2.2 Immunological effector functions of regulatory B cells

Regulatory B cells employ a variety of mechanisms to modulate immune responses and target many different immune cell types, such as dendritic cells (DC) (Matsushita, Horikawa et al. 2010), macrophages (Wong, Puaux et al. 2010) as well as both T helper 1 (Th1) and Th2 cells (Tian, Zekzer et al. 2001; Ronet, Hauyon-La Torre et al. 2010). Their most prominent effector function is the production of the potent immunosupressive cytokine IL-10, however different subsets also produce TGF-β (Fig. 1) or suppress target cells via cell contact-dependent mechanisms (Fig. 2).

2.2.1 Release of cytokines

As depicted in figure 1, many Breg cell functions have been demonstrated to be mediated by the release of immunosuppressive cytokines. **IL-10** is the hallmark cytokine of regulatory B cells. It has been shown to be essential for the Breg cell suppressive functions in many autoimmune models. Accordingly, the protective function of Breg cells in collagen induced arthritis (CIA), experimental autoimmune encephalomyelitis (EAE), non-obese diabetes (NOD) and inflammatory bowel disease (IBD) is abrogated if B cells are deficient in IL-10 production (Fillatreau, Sweenie et al. 2002; Dalwadi, Wei et al. 2003; Mauri, Gray et al. 2003; Hussain and Delovitch 2007; Booth, Griebel et al. 2009). B cell derived IL-10 efficiently suppresses proliferation and inflammatory cytokine production of T cells (Fillatreau, Sweenie et al. 2002; Mauri, Gray et al. 2003) and can also induce forkhead box P3 (FoxP3) positive regulatory T cells (Gray, Miles et al. 2007; Blair, Chavez-Rueda et al. 2009). Some of these effects might be indirect and due to the effects of IL-10 on innate cell types, as IL-10 is well known to inhibit antigen presentation and pro-inflammatory cytokine production by DC, monocytes and macrophages (Moore, de Waal Malefyt et al. 2001).

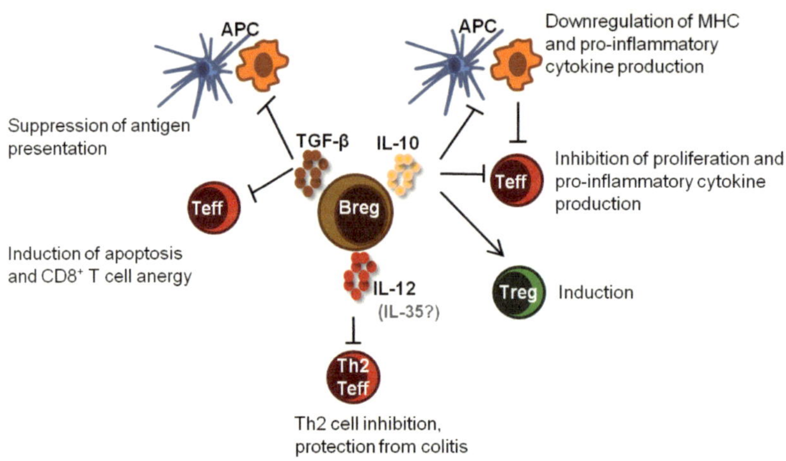

Fig. 1. Suppressive functions of Breg cells mediated by the release of cytokines. Breg cells secrete immunosuppressive cytokines causing downregulation of antigen presenting cell (APC) function, inhibition of T effector cell function and induction of regulatory T cells. Breg: regulatory B cells, Teff/reg: effector/regulatory T cells, APC: antigen presenting cells.

IL-10, **TGF-β** is the second immunosuppressive cytokine found to be secreted by some Breg cell populations to downregulate inflammatory immune responses (Tian, Zekzer et al. 2001; Parekh, Prasad et al. 2003). Similar to IL-10, TGF-β suppresses inflammatory cytokine production by T cells and inhibits the function of antigen presenting cells (APC). In addition, TGF-β induces apoptosis in target effector cells and acts as a negative regulator of mucosal immune responses (Takenoshita, Fukushima et al. 2002).

Interestingly, although not generally considered suppressive, **IL-12** production by B cells has also been demonstrated to have immunomodulatory capacity in a T cell receptor (TCR)α knockout mouse model of Th2-mediated colitis. In this model, IL-10 mediated induction of IL-12 secreting B cells is involved in protection from colitis, as IL-12p35-deficient double knockout mice as well as mice treated with anti-IL-12p40 antibodies developed a more severe colitis compared to control mice (Sugimoto, Ogawa et al. 2007).

2.2.2 Cell contact-dependent suppressive mechanisms

Independent of cytokine secretion, several B cell surface molecules have been implicated in the suppressive functions of regulatory B cells (Fig. 2). **CD1d** is not only a major phenotypic marker highly expressed on many Breg cell populations, it has also been suggested to have an active role in Breg cell-mediated suppression. CD1d is a major histocompatibility complex (MHC) class I-like molecule and is responsible for the presentation of lipid antigens to Natural Killer T (NKT) cells (Chiu, Park et al. 2002; Borg, Wun et al. 2007). Mizoguchi et al. showed that upregulation of CD1d on B cells is associated with B cell-mediated protection against intestinal mucosal inflammation (Mizoguchi, Mizoguchi et al. 2002).

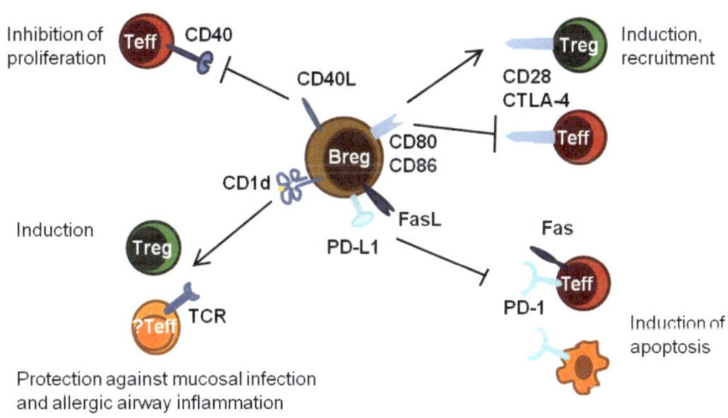

Fig. 2. Suppressive functions of Breg cells mediated by cell contact-dependent mechanisms. Breg cells express several cell surface molecules that cause inhibition of T effector cell function, induction of target cell apoptosis and induction of regulatory T cells. Breg: regulatory B cells, Teff/reg: effector/regulatory T cells, TCR: T cell receptor, PD-1: programmed death-1, PD-L1: programmed death-ligand1, FasL: Fas-Ligand, CTLA-4: cytotoxic T-lymphocyte protein 4, CD40L: CD40-Ligand.

As NKT cells had earlier been shown to be protective in mouse models of diabetes (Lehuen, Lantz et al. 1998) and colitis (Saubermann, Beck et al. 2000), it was feasible to assume that the activation of NKT cells was the underlying mechanism of protection in these models. However, as the TCRα knockout mice used in the studies by Mizoguchi et al., do not have NKT cells, the protective effect in this experimental setting has to be mediated by another CD1d responsive cell type. Amu et al. later confirmed a CD1d^{high} Breg cell-dependent, but

NKT cell-independent mechanism of protection in a model of worm mediated protection from allergic airway inflammation (Amu, Saunders et al. 2010). Another group reported, that CD1d expression on APC and splenic MZ B cells was necessary for efficient generation of regulatory T cells in CD1d-reactive NKT cell-dependent tolerance in immune privileged sites such as the eye (Sonoda and Stein-Streilein 2002).

As described earlier, **CD40-CD40L** interaction seems to play an important role in the differentiation of regulatory B cells. In addition, there are reports indicating that CD40 signalling on target cells might also be involved in the suppressive mechanisms of B cells. Upon activation, B cells express CD40L on their surface (Wykes, Poudrier et al. 1998) and CD40-CD40L interaction has been shown to mediate suppression of colonic inflammation by inhibition of T cells (Bhan, Mizoguchi et al. 2000). Other costimulatory molecules involved in cell contact-dependent suppressive functions of B cells, are the B7 costimulatory receptors **CD80 and CD86.** Interaction of B7 surface receptors with their inhibitory ligands cytotoxic T-lymphocyte protein 4 (CTLA-4) or CD28 on target cells is crucial in regulating T cell activation and peripheral tolerance (Fife and Bluestone 2008). Expression of B7 molecules has been shown to be essential for recovery from EAE due to B cell-mediated generation and recruitment of regulatory T cells (Mann, Maresz et al. 2007) as well as for the suppression of colonic inflammation through inhibition of effector T cell proliferation (Bhan, Mizoguchi et al. 2000).

Moreover, evidence exists that Breg cells upregulate surface molecules like Fas ligand (FasL) and programmed death-ligand 1 (PDL-1), which upon interaction with their receptors can directly induce apoptosis in target cells. Lundy and Fox demonstrated that in a mouse model of rheumatoid arthritis, splenic $CD5^+$ B cells express high levels of FasL and that induced T cell apoptosis indeed was due to FasL-mediated direct killing by B cells (Lundy and Fox 2009). In EAE, Bodhankar et al. showed that the well established protective effect of estrogen is mediated by B cells. The treatment, besides increasing the percentage of IL-10-producing regulatory B cells, also induced upregulation of **PD-L1** expression on B cells (Bodhankar, Wang et al. 2011). Furthermore, in murine experimental stroke, PD-L1 and PD-L2 expressing B cells were found to be protective due to their capacity to inhibit the activation of inflammatory T cells, macrophages and microglial cells through upregulation of PD-1 expression (Ren, Akiyoshi et al. 2011).

3. Regulatory B cells in autoimmune diseases

In homeostasis as well as during acute immune responses a delicate balance between activating and suppressing subsets of immune cells has to be maintained. Disrupting this balance often leads to immunodeficiencies or autoimmune diseases. In particular, the balanced ratio between effector and regulatory T cells has been demonstrated to be of crucial importance in maintaining immune homeostasis, and the role of Treg cells has been well established in autoimmune diseases (O'Connor and Anderton 2008; Yang, Tian et al. 2008; Huang and Sattler 2011). Recently, various studies have also found critical roles and possible clinical relevance of regulatory B cells in both systemic and organ-specific autoimmune diseases (Lemoine, Morva et al. 2009).

3.1 Regulatory B cells in systemic autoimmune diseases

Systemic autoimmune diseases are defined by their multi-organ involvement. Antibodies reactive to a wide variety of ubiquitous autoantigens including DNA, cell surface molecules as well as intracellular matrix proteins can cause tissue damage in various target organs. Although the underlying cause leading to systemic autoimmunity remains unclear, several genetic and environmental factors and immunological mechanisms have been implicated.

3.1.1 Systemic lupus erythematosus

Systemic lupus erythematosus (SLE) is a systemic autoimmune condition often considered the prototype of autoimmune diseases. It is mainly characterised by the presence of auto-antibodies to a variety of self antigens, particularly against nuclear components (Mills 1994). Because of the high production of pathogenic auto-antibodies, B cells are considered a major contributor to SLE pathogenesis and several therapies targeting B cells in SLE patients have been introduced (Sabahi and Anolik 2006). In addition however, there is evidence for the existence of a subset of B cells with regulatory capacity in lupus (Amano, Amano et al. 2003). Furthermore, human SLE patients have been shown to have an increased percentage of B10 and B10pro cells in peripheral blood (Iwata, Matsushita et al. 2011). However, regulatory B cells isolated from the peripheral blood of SLE patients might be functionally impaired, as they appeared to be unresponsive to CD40 stimulation, produced less IL-10 and lacked the capacity to suppress T cells (Blair, Norena et al. 2010).

Interesting insights into a possible dual role of B cells in lupus were obtained from CD19 deficient lupus-prone mice (NZB/W mice). Although, auto-antibody accumulation was significantly delayed in these mice, nephritis appeared earlier and survival was reduced compared to wild type NZB/W mice. Adoptive transfer of wild type $CD1d^{hi}CD5^{+}$ splenic B cells containing IL-10 producing regulatory B cells into CD19 deficient recipients significantly prolonged survival (Watanabe, Ishiura et al. 2010). Adoptive transfer of *in vitro* anti-CD40 stimulated T2 B cells into lupus-prone mice also improved renal disease and survival by an IL-10-dependent mechanism. This effect was explained by the suppression of Th1 responses and the induction of IL-10 producing and regulatory T cells. Direct *in vivo* administration of anti-CD40 also reversed established lupus disease (Blair, Chavez-Rueda et al. 2009). A possible role for innate immune signalling in the pathogenesis of SLE has been suggested previously (Lenert, Goeken et al. 2003) and TLR-9 signalling in marginal zone B cells has been demonstrated to induce higher IL-10 production in lupus-prone mice compared to controls. These high levels of B cell derived IL-10 inhibits the production of IL-12 by macrophages and DC and consequently can modulate T cell mediated inflammatory responses (Lenert, Brummel et al. 2005).

3.1.2 Rheumatoid arthritis

Rheumatoid arthritis (RA) is a common T cell-dependent chronic inflammatory disease characterised by synovial proliferation and excessive pro-inflammatory cytokine production, resulting in cartilage and bone destruction (Firestein 2003). Data available on Breg cells in human rheumatoid arthritis are limited, however similar to lupus patients, an increased percentage of B10 and B10pro cells in the peripheral blood of rheumatoid arthritis patients has been observed, indicating that regulatory B cells might play a role in this autoimmune condition too (Iwata, Matsushita et al. 2011). To date, the majority of the experimental data available on arthritis, has been obtained from the murine model of collagen-induced arthritis (CIA), which mimics the immunopathogenesis of human rheumatoid arthritis (Trentham, Townes et al. 1977). Using this model, adoptive transfer of

IL-10 producing B cells has been demonstrated by different groups to prevent the development of arthritis as well as to ameliorate already established disease (Mauri, Gray et al. 2003; Evans, Chavez-Rueda et al. 2007; Gray, Miles et al. 2007).

Mauri and co-workers were the first to show that adoptive transfer of *in vitro* anti-CD40 activated splenic B cells prevented the development of arthritis. The B cells used in these experiments were shown to produce increased amounts of IL-10 and inhibited Th1 differentiation (Mauri, Gray et al. 2003). Work by Evans et al. demonstrated that the number of endogenous IL-10 producing MZ and their precursors T2 MZP B cells were increased during the remission phase of arthritis and that adoptive transfer of T2 MZP to CIA mice prevented disease progression and alleviated established disease. Again, the underlying mechanism seemed to be the reduction of a Th1 type immune response in the presence of immunosuppressive cytokines, rather than cell contact-dependent mechanisms (Evans, Chavez-Rueda et al. 2007). Gray et al. induced IL-10 producing regulatory B cells in the spleen of CIA mice by administration of apoptotic thymocytes. Regulatory B cells induced in this manner *in vivo* as well as upon passive transfer after *in vitro* induction, were effective in protecting mice from autoimmune joint inflammation (Gray, Miles et al. 2007).

3.2 Regulatory B cells in organ-specific autoimmune diseases

In contrast to systemic autoimmune diseases, organ-specific autoimmune conditions are characterised by cell- and auto-antibody-mediated immune responses directed specifically against antigens which are only localised in a particular organ such as the pancreatic islets in type I diabetes or the central nervous system in multiple sclerosis.

3.2.1 Inflammatory bowel disease

Inflammatory Bowel Disease (IBD) refers to a group of conditions characterised by inflammation in the intestinal tract, with Crohn's disease (CD) and ulcerative colitis (UC) accounting for the majority of cases. While in CD chronic inflammation is mainly mediated by the Th1 pathway, UC is also associated with the presence of auto-antibodies, leading to the initial assumption that B cells might play a role in disease initiation (Mizoguchi, Mizoguchi et al. 1996; Bhan, Mizoguchi et al. 1999).

Studies in various mouse models of IBD demonstrating the protective roles of B cells, were among the earliest publications to document the existence and relevance of regulatory B cells. Mizoguchi et al. used a mouse model deficient in TCRα that spontaneously develops UC-like chronic colitis and demonstrated that B cells were not required to initiate disease at all, but could actually suppress colitis (Mizoguchi, Mizoguchi et al. 1997). These B cells were later shown to appear during chronic intestinal inflammation, exhibit upregulated CD1d expression and release IL-10 (Mizoguchi, Mizoguchi et al. 2002). Furthermore, adoptive transfer experiments confirmed a protective role of B cells via mechanisms like IL-10 production and induction of regulatory T cells (Bhan, Mizoguchi et al. 2000; Mizoguchi, Mizoguchi et al. 2002; Wei, Velazquez et al. 2005). Several additional studies performed by different groups using various mouse models have confirmed that B cells can regulate UC-like intestinal inflammation (Gerth, Lin et al. 2004; Hokama, Mizoguchi et al. 2004; Su, Guo et al. 2004; Sugimoto, Ogawa et al. 2007) as well as Crohn's disease-like conditions (Dalwadi, Wei et al. 2003; Wei, Velazquez et al. 2005; Ostanin, Pavlick et al. 2006).

Interestingly, B cells producing IL-12 in an IL-10-dependent manner, have also been demonstrated to be protective in a mouse model of UC-like Th2-mediated colitis (Sugimoto, Ogawa et al. 2007). In Crohn's disease-like Th1-mediated colitis, IL-12 was initially considered to be pathogenic, however a recent report suggests that IL-23 sharing the common subunit p40 (p19/p40) rather than IL-12 (p35/p40) is pro-inflammatory and the one to mediate disease (Cua, Sherlock et al. 2003; Yen, Cheung et al. 2006). Importantly, both IL-12 subunits p35 and p40 have been demonstrated to be crucial in B cell mediated attenuation of colitis (Sugimoto, Ogawa et al. 2007). However, it needs to be noted that a possible contribution of another potent suppressive cytokine sharing the p35 subunit, namely IL-35, has not been taken into account (Collison, Workman et al. 2007; Niedbala, Wei et al. 2007).

3.2.2 Multiple sclerosis

Multiple sclerosis (MS) is considered a T cell-mediated autoimmune condition that results in inflammatory lesions, demyelination and axonal damage in the central nervous system (CNS). A mouse model mimicking human MS, experimental autoimmune encephalomyelitis (EAE) has been used widely to investigate the underlying immunological mechanisms and the components of the immune system involved in disease pathogenesis (Baxter 2007). Similar to other autoimmune diseases, clonal expansion of B cells and the production of auto-antibodies, indicate that B cells contribute to the pathogenesis of MS (Colombo, Dono et al. 2000; Fraussen, Vrolix et al. 2009). However, the effects of anti-CD20-mediated B cell depletion in the EAE model depend crucially on timing, as treatment shortly after disease onset reduced disease severity, while depletion prior to disease induction or at the peak of disease did not change the disease course or even led to disease exacerbation (Matsushita, Yanaba et al. 2008). Exacerbation of disease indicates a protective role of B cells and Wolf et al. were one of the first groups to show that there might indeed be an additional protective function of B cells in EAE. They demonstrated that although the incidence and severity of disease was comparable between mice genetically deficient in mature B cells and wild type control mice, B cell deficient mice failed to undergo spontaneous recovery and developed chronic disease instead (Wolf, Dittel et al. 1996).

Several recent studies confirm these findings showing in addition that IL-10 producing B cells are responsible for this protective effect (Fillatreau, Sweenie et al. 2002; Matsushita, Fujimoto et al. 2006; Lampropoulou, Hoehlig et al. 2008). Furthermore, adoptive transfer experiments revealed a possible therapeutic potential of isolated regulatory B cells in EAE (Mann, Maresz et al. 2007; Matsushita, Yanaba et al. 2008; Rafei, Hsieh et al. 2009; Kala, Rhodes et al. 2010). Considering the extensive use of MS treatments that are dependent on B cell depletion, it seems crucial to define this dual role of B cells in the progression of disease. Lee-Chang et al. demonstrated that homeostasis of the B cell subsets is altered during the preclinical and acute phases of EAE, where the percentage of B cells with regulatory phenotype are significantly reduced (Lee-Chang, Lefranc et al. 2011), indicating again that timing is an important consideration when targeting B cells during therapy. It was also shown that B cell depletion reduced the frequency of regulatory T cells, and increased the pro-inflammatory polarising capacity of the remaining myeloid APC (Weber, Prod'homme et al. 2010).

Interestingly, in human MS patients, peripheral blood B cells produced less IL-10 in response to TLR-9 as well as CD40 and BCR stimulation compared to healthy controls (Duddy, Niino et al. 2007; Hirotani, Niino et al. 2010). This might indicate that Breg cells in human MS patients are functionally impaired, or simply exhausted due to chronic pro-inflammatory stimulation, and thereby are implicated in disease development.

3.2.3 Type 1 diabetes

Type 1 diabetes (T1D) and the spontaneous disease that develops in the corresponding mouse model (non-obese diabetic (NOD) mouse), is characterised by autoimmune destruction of the insulin-producing pancreatic β cells. Attack on β cells is primarily mediated by T cells (Anderson and Bluestone 2005), however B cells and humoral immunity also play a role, especially in disease initiation (Silveira and Grey 2006; Xiu, Wong et al. 2008). Despite the pathogenic role of B cells in disease initiation, B cells activated *in vitro* can maintain tolerance and transfer protection from disease in NOD mice (Tian, Zekzer et al. 2001; Hussain and Delovitch 2007). Transfusion of BCR-stimulated B cells reduced the incidence and delayed the onset of disease, when given repeatedly starting at a young age before disease onset. Disease protection was dependent on IL-10 and correlated with the polarisation of T cells towards a Th2 phenotype (Hussain and Delovitch 2007). In a different experimental setting, transfer of *in vitro* LPS-stimulated B cells protected NOD mice from spontaneous diabetes. As these B cells were shown to express FasL and secrete TGF-β, this effect was attributed to the triggering of apoptosis in Th1 cells and/or the inhibition of APC activity (Tian, Zekzer et al. 2001).

4. Regulatory B cells in allergic diseases

The vast majority of studies on regulatory B cells has been focused on autoimmunity models. However, recent studies indicate that Breg cells may also be instrumental in reducing T-helper 2 (Th2) skewed immune diseases, such as allergies. Allergies are dysregulated immune responses towards normally harmless allergens that result in an expansion of polarised Th2 cells, elevated immunoglobulin E (IgE) production and eosinophilia (Kay 2000). Common allergic diseases include allergic asthma, rhinitis, atopic dermatitis, and food allergies. Allergic asthma is characterised by reversible airway obstruction and airway remodelling upon exposure to inhaled aeroallergens such as house dust mite (HDM), grass pollen, or pet dander. In allergic rhinitis (hay fever), allergen exposure leads to irritation and inflammation of the nasal airways, whereas atopic dermatitis is an inflammatory, chronically relapsing, non-contagious and pruritic skin disorder. In food allergies, exposure to food products such as peanuts, fruits or milk may lead to allergic symptoms including gastrointestinal and respiratory distress, or life-threatening anaphylactic responses (Kay 2000).

Traditionally, B cells have been known for their capacity to produce antibodies, thereby contributing to humoral immunity and clearance of pathogens. During allergic disorders, B cells are driven to preferentially class-switch to IgE isotypes in the presence of local IL-4 and this forms a central element in the acute inflammatory responses to allergens. Allergen-specific IgE binds to Fc-receptors (FcR) on mast cells and basophils and subsequent exposure to the same allergen leads to degranulation and inflammation. So far, reports evaluating B cell function other than Ig(E) production in allergies are limited. Nevertheless, a few reports suggest that in allergic inflammation, like in autoimmunity, B cells can have a regulatory role (Hussaarts, van der Vlugt et al. 2011). For example, B cells isolated from OVA tolerant mice were able to dampen acute allergic airway inflammation via the TGF-β induced conversion of $CD4^+CD25^-$T cells into functionally suppressive $CD4^+CD25^+FoxP3^+$ T regulatory cells (Singh, Carson et al. 2008). In addition, B cells were also shown to control experimental cockroach allergen-induced inflammation by the induction of FasL-mediated apoptosis of $CD4^+$ T cells. In mice lacking B1a B cells, it was demonstrated that in particular the $CD5^+$ B1a B cell population was important for protective $CD4^+$ T cell apoptosis (Lundy, Berlin et al. 2005). Furthermore, two reports have studied the presence of human IL-10 or TGF-β producing B cells in non-IgE mediated food allergy. In response to the milk antigen, casein, the frequency of IL-10 or TGF-β producing $CD5^+$ peripheral blood B cells increased in healthy donors whereas the frequency declined in allergic donors (Noh, Choi et al. 2010; Lee, Noh et al. 2011). In addition, our group observed less IL-10 producing B cells in response to LPS in house dust mite allergic asthma patients compared to healthy controls (Mlejnek and van der Vlugt 2012). These findings support the notion that Breg cells may form an important regulatory arm of the immune system and seem to be dysfunctional in allergic disorders.

5. Implications of pathogen-induced Breg cells in autoimmunity and allergy

The onset of hyperinflammatory disorders such as allergies and autoimmunities seems to be partly genetic, as the risk for developing disease increases when a parent or a sibling is affected (Mariani 2004; von Mutius 2009). However, the steep increase in the incidence of hyperinflammatory disorders over the last few decades in the Western world has suggested that environmental factors may also have a major impact. Fast changes in lifestyle, housing, improved hygiene and vaccinations in industrialised countries have resulted in reduced microbial exposure during early childhood (Wills-Karp, Santeliz et al. 2001; Yazdanbakhsh, Kremsner et al. 2002), which may allow for uncontrolled inflammatory responses against either innocuous or self-antigens later in life. In support of this 'hygiene' hypothesis, several epidemiological studies have pointed towards a reversed relationship between hyperinflammatory disorders and microbial exposure, such as bacterial, viral and helminth infections.

5.1 Hyperinflammatory disorders and the 'hygiene hypothesis'

Parasites are regarded to be master manipulators of the host immune system. A negative correlation between the rates of parasitic infections in developing countries and the prevalence of allergic symptoms and atopic sensitisation in children has been highlighted in a number of studies in different geographical areas (Flohr, Quinnell et al. 2009). Strikingly, long-term anti-helminth treatment resulted in increased atopic reactivity to house dust mite, supporting a direct link between helminth exposure and protection against allergic diseases (Lynch, Hagel et al. 1993; van den Biggelaar, Rodrigues et al. 2004). In addition, helminth infected MS patients showed better clinical disease outcome compared to control MS patients (Correale, Farez et al. 2008). A relationship between helminth infections and protection against hyperinflammatory disorders has also been established in various mouse models for food allergy (Nagler-Anderson 2006), asthma (Smits, Hammad et al. 2007; Amu, Saunders et al. 2010), T1D (Zaccone, Fehervari et al. 2003; Liu, Sundar et al. 2009), CIA

(Osada, Shimizu et al. 2009) and EAE (La Flamme, Ruddenklau et al. 2003; Wilson, Taylor et al. 2010). Furthermore, different cross-sectional studies show that children living in farming environments are protected from childhood asthma and atopy and this correlation has been attributed to contact with livestock (Ege, Frei et al. 2007) and hay and the consumption of raw cow's milk (Douwes, Cheng et al. 2008; Loss, Apprich et al. 2011). In farming environments, both outdoor and indoor microbial exposure are higher and more diverse compared to nonfarming environments (von Mutius, Braun-Fahrlander et al. 2000; Ege, Mayer et al. 2011). More detailed analysis of the dust composition showed that a lower risk of asthma was associated with Gram-negative bacteria and fungi of the *Eurotium* and *Penicillium* species (Ege, Frei et al. 2007; Ege, Mayer et al. 2011). Inhalation is a main route of exposure to pathogens, but ingestion of orofecal microbes (Matricardi, Rosmini et al. 1997) or colonization of certain probiotic bacteria stimulating the gut associated lymphoid tissue (GALT) may also help to avoid allergic responses or certain autoimmune conditions. A direct association between the composition of the gastrointestinal microbiome and the risk of developing allergies has been described in several studies, suggesting that *Lactobacilli* and *Bifidobacterium bifidum* have a protective effect (Bjorksten, Sepp et al. 2001; Johansson, Sjogren et al. 2011). Also in line with this data, changes in faecal microbiota were detected in autoimmune patients suffering from Crohn's disease and ulcerative colitis (Manichanh, Rigottier-Gois et al. 2006; Frank, St Amand et al. 2007).

Altogether these findings indicate that microbial exposure during early life seems to be important to prevent hyperinflammatory conditions. Various studies have indicated that the development of the regulatory arm of the immune system is instrumental for this protection, and so far have highlighted a role for Treg cells (Wohlfert and Belkaid 2008). However, there is a growing amount of evidence showing a protective role for Breg cells induced by infectious agents.

5.2 Pathogen-induced Breg cells are protective in autoimmune and allergic conditions

One of the first observations that helminths, such as *Schisostoma mansoni*, could induce suppressive B cells was made in µMT mice, which lack mature B cells. These mice show increased *S.mansoni*-induced tissue pathology compared to infected wild-type mice (Jankovic, Cheever et al. 1998). Subsequent studies with *S. mansoni* demonstrated that B cells isolated from helminth-infected mice could play a protective role in allergy, as transfer of B cells protected recipient mice against systemic fatal anaphylaxis or OVA-induced airway inflammation via the production of IL-10 (Mangan, Fallon et al. 2004; Mangan, van Rooijen et al. 2006; Amu, Saunders et al. 2010). Interestingly, these regulatory mechanisms were only active during the chronic phase of infection (Smits, Hammad et al. 2007). Similar results were obtained in *Heligosomoides polygyrus*-infected mice, where $CD19^{+}CD5^{-}CD23^{hi}$ B cells isolated from mesenteric lymph nodes of chronically infected mice were able to suppress Derp1-induced airway inflammation, although independently of IL-10 (Wilson, Taylor et al. 2010). Interestingly, *S. mansoni*-induced Breg cells also incurred protection against allergic airway inflammation via the induction of regulatory T cells (Amu, Saunders et al. 2010). However, Breg-induced immune regulation was only partially dependent on Treg cell induction as we could demonstrate in conditional FoxP3 knockout mice (van der Vlugt and Labuda 2012). In addition, B cell induced FasL-mediated apoptosis of $CD4^{+}$ T cells appeared to be another mechanism used by Breg cells to control inflammation during schistosome infections (Lundy and Boros 2002). Helminth-induced Breg cells also ameliorated symptoms of several autoimmune diseases. Adoptive transfer of B cells isolated from *H. polygyrus* infected mice, dramatically reduced EAE severity in uninfected recipients (Wilson, Taylor et al. 2010) and B cells from helminth infected MS patients suppressed T cell activation *in vitro* (Correale, Farez et al. 2008). The production of B cell IL-10 and the induction of Treg cells were important in the reduction of inflammation. Treg cell induction was further shown to be dependent on expression of B7 costimulatory molecules, as B7 deficient B cells failed to efficiently recruit Treg cells into the CNS and mediate recovery from EAE clinical disease (Mann, Maresz et al. 2007). In addition to helminthic infection, bacterial exposure may also enhance the activity of Breg cells. For example, TLR signaling on B cells is required for the recovery from EAE. Interestingly, although both TLR-4 (LPS) and TLR-9 (CpG) signaling induced IL-10 expression in B cells, only LPS stimulation via TLR-2/4 was capable of inducing recovery from EAE (Lampropoulou, Hoehlig et al. 2008). Furthermore, tissue damage as a result of invading pathogens may induce apoptosis and can influence the development of Breg cells. Injection of apoptotic cells into mice has been shown to induce Breg cells and reduce inflammatory processes in a collagen-induced arthritis model (Gray, Miles et al. 2007). Overall, there is a strong case for the capacity of various pathogens to induce functional Breg cells that are protective against inflammation-driven pathology.

6. Possible therapeutic applications targeting Breg cells in autoimmune and allergic disorders

Several studies have highlighted the relevance of Breg cells in downmodulating inflammation in autoimmune and allergic disorders. In addition to the direct effects via cytokine production, Breg cells also function indirectly via the induction or recruitment of regulatory T cells and therefore may have promising therapeutic potential. However, the mechanism underlying the formation of regulatory B cells and their implications in existing therapies must be fully understood, before these pathways can be exploited for therapeutic purposes.

6.1 Pathogen-driven pathways for the induction and expansion of Breg cells

As demonstrated in figure 3, Breg cells can be induced by bacterial or parasitic infections. Therefore, the identification of the secreted or excreted pathogenic compound(s) driving Breg cell induction provides useful information for the development of therapeutic interventions. Indeed, the fact that live schistosome worms could induce IL-10 producing Breg cells from splenic B cells in an *in vitro* culture system, suggests that helminth antigens have a direct effect on B cells (Amu, Saunders et al. 2010). Helminth-related TLR ligands may be a likely candidate responsible for helminth-induced Breg cell formation, given the implication of certain TLR ligands in the induction of Breg cells in autoimmune models (as discussed above). Notably, lacto-N-fucopentaose-III (LNFPIII), a sugar found on soluble egg antigens (SEA) interacts with TLR-4 and stimulates splenic B cells to produce IL-10 (Velupillai and Harn 1994). Likewise, microfilarial extracts from *Leishmania major*, and *Brugia malayi*, which both bind to TLR-4, can induce IL-10 production by B cells (Palanivel, Posey et al. 1996). Furthermore, lyso-phosphatidylserine, a lipid derived from *S. mansoni* worms ligated TLR-2 on human monocyte-derived DC and promoted Treg cell activity (van der Kleij, Latz et al. 2002). Although it is unclear whether this TLR-2 ligating molecule has an effect on the formation of Breg cells, SEA stimulation of human B cells did result in TLR-2 mediated elevated IL-10 production (Correale and Farez 2009).

Bacterial infections such as *Helicobacter felis* induced IL-10 producing B cells via TLR-2 signalling and were also able to suppress *Helicobacter*-induced pathology via the induction of IL-10 producing T cells (Sayi, Kohler et al. 2011). Other bacterial structures, such as CpG oligonucleotides (ODN) binding to TLR-9, are also well known to be strong inducers of B cell IL-10 production (Barr, Brown et al. 2007; Bouaziz, Calbo et al. 2010). Interestingly, administration of CpG ODN to mice potently inhibited acute and established asthma, allergic rhinitis and conjunctivitis (Fonseca and Kline 2009). Additionally, human clinical trials with CpG ODN conjugated with ragweed antigen revealed that ragweed allergy subjects developed a shift in immune response from Th2 towards a dominant Th1 profile (Simons, Shikishima et al. 2004) and a decrease in clinical allergy symptoms two years after treatment (Tulic, Fiset et al. 2004). Although the role of IL-10 producing B cells was not studied in those clinical trials, a recent study in mice clearly showed that immunosuppressive IL-10 producing follicular B cells appeared after CpG treatment. These Breg cells were responsible for the reduction in late phase experimental allergic conjunctivitis (Miyazaki, Kuo et al. 2009), suggesting that the administration of CpG can also form an important therapeutic approach to induce Breg cell activity.

6.2 Induction and expansion of Breg cells by chemical drugs used in medical treatment

Clonal expansion of B cells and the production of auto-antibodies indicate that B cells contribute to the pathogenesis of several autoimmune diseases. Accordingly, B cell depletion therapy using Rituximab (anti-CD20) has shown promising effects in clinical trials (Bar-Or, Calabresi et al. 2008; Hauser, Waubant et al. 2008). However, possible implications for regulatory B cells in the treatment of human autoimmune diseases have been indicated by recent studies investigating the immunological mechanisms of drugs already used for medical treatment of human patients (Fig. 3). A very recent report shows that an antibody acting as an IL-6R antagonist (Tocilizumab), which has recently been introduced as therapy for rheumatoid arthritis, causes regulatory $CD25^+$ B cells to increase their TGF-β expression and alter their activation status, indicating that the beneficial effects of Tocilizumab are due to an induction or expansion of regulatory B cells (Snir, Kessel et al. 2011).

Beneficial effects of several drugs used in the treatment of multiple sclerosis also seem to be mediated by regulatory B cells. Glatiramer acetate (GA) is a drug safely used in MS patients, and it has been demonstrated that the beneficial effects of GA were abrogated in B cell-deficient mice. Furthermore, adoptive transfer of B cells from GA-treated mice inhibited the proliferation of autoreactive T cells as well as the development of Th1 and Th17 cells, but promoted IL-10 production in recipient mice (Kala, Rhodes et al. 2010; Begum-Haque, Christy et al. 2011). Estrogen, a hormone drug with well established therapeutic effects on MS, was shown to depend on B cells as well. In EAE, estrogen-mediated protection from disease was associated with a general increase in the percentage of IL-10-producing regulatory B cells as well as an upregulation of PD-L1 expression on B cells, possibly leading

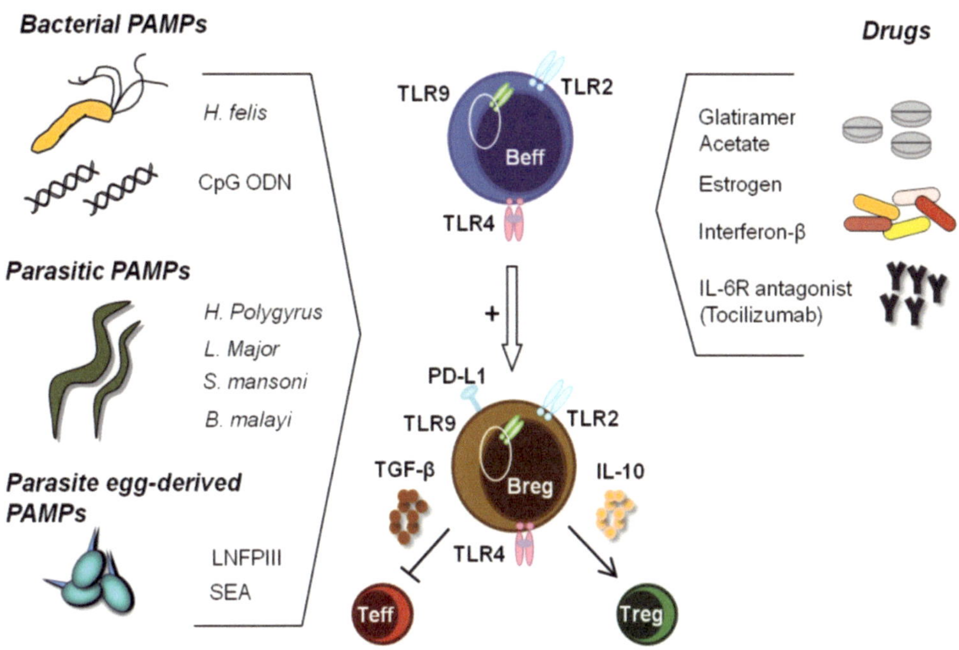

Fig. 3. Pathways for the induction and expansion of Breg cells. Different secreted or excreted (non)pathogenic compounds of bacteria, parasites or their eggs can drive Breg cell induction. These compounds have been shown to bind to TLR and thereby induce Breg cell development. Additionally, Breg cell promoting activities were found in several registered drug-based treatments for autoimmune diseases. As a consequence, Breg cells start to produce anti-inflammatory cytokines IL-10 and TGF-β, inhibit Teff cell proliferation and induce Treg cells. PAMPs: pathogen associated molecular patterns, TLR: Toll-like receptor, Breg: regulatory B cells, Teff/reg: effector/regulatory T cells, LNFPIII: lacto-N-fucopentaose-III, SEA: soluble egg antigens.

to direct target cell apoptosis (Bodhankar, Wang et al. 2011). As previous studies on B cells from human MS patients have demonstrated a defective IL-10 producing capacity (Duddy, Niino et al. 2007; Hirotani, Niino et al. 2010), upregulation of IL-10 production by B cells might be of importance in disease resolution in MS patients undergoing treatment. Indeed, a study on human patients treated with IFN-β demonstrated that their B cells showed a lower proliferative response *in vitro* than B cells from untreated patients. *In vitro* IFN-β treatment of B cells shifted their cytokine profile and induced IL-10 secretion (Ramgolam, Sha et al. 2011).

7. Concluding remarks

The underlying mechanisms leading to inflammatory conditions such as autoimmune diseases and allergies are diverse and far from being fully understood. However, it has become obvious that a balance between effector and regulatory functions of different subsets of immune cells is crucially important in the maintenance of a healthy steady-state situation.

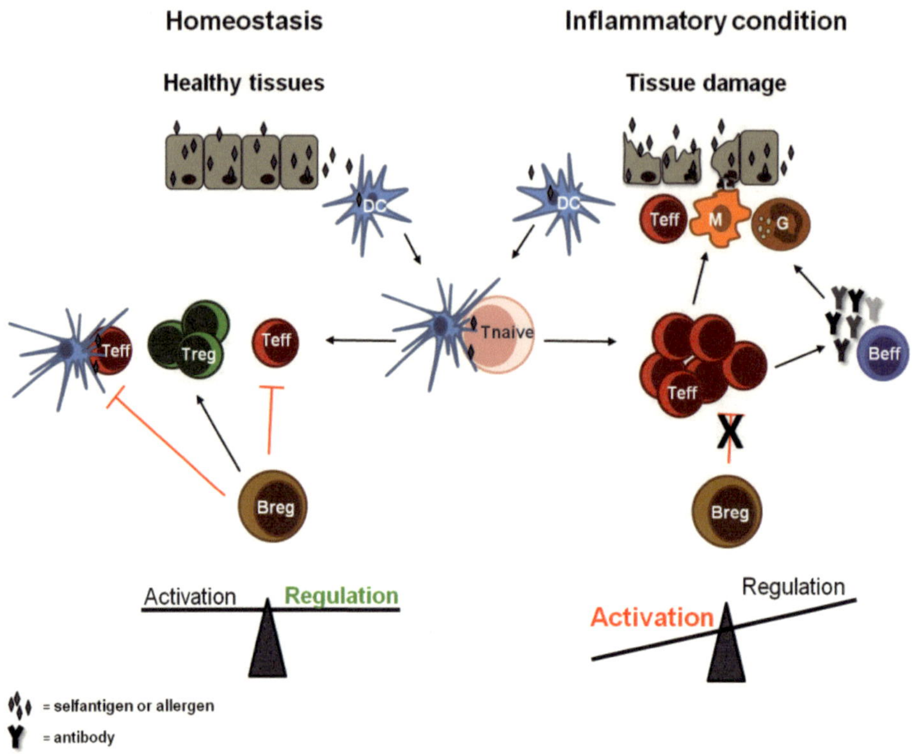

Fig. 4. Regulatory B cells in homeostasis and disease. Under normal conditions regulatory B cells control T effector cell activation and proliferation in response to harmless self antigens and allergens, and induce and activate regulatory T cells. If Breg cell mediated control fails, effector T cells can proliferate and activate antibody producing B cells as well as innate immune cell types causing tissue damage. Beff/reg: effector/regulatory B cells, Teff/reg: effector/regulatory T cells, Tnaive: naive T cells, DC: dendritic cells, M: macrophages, G: granulocytes.

Regulatory B cells are an exciting new player on the regulatory side of this constant struggle for balance. As depicted in figure 4, in the healthy immune system Breg cells help to control effector cell activation, by releasing immunosuppressive cytokines and inducing target cell apoptosis. The broad target cell range of their cytokines allows them to inhibit pro-inflammatory functions of both innate immune cells, such as DC and macrophages as well as cells of the adaptive immune system, such as effector T cells of both the Th1 and Th2 lineage. On the other hand they also amplify the regulatory arm of immune responses by inducing regulatory T cells. Impaired regulatory capacity of Breg cells might play a role in the development of inflammatory diseases. Uncontrolled effector T and B cell activation can ultimately lead to inflammation and tissue damage in various target organs. Correspondingly, several treatments demonstrated to be beneficial in autoimmune and allergic diseases seem to affect the immune system at the level of B cells by amplifying their regulatory capacity. Currently much effort is put into therapies aiming to induce regulatory T cells. However, targeting regulatory B cells instead holds the added benefit of indirectly affecting all target cell types of Breg cells, including regulatory T cells, making it a more efficient approach. Therefore, further research is needed to increase our understanding of Breg cell biology in health and disease, as targeting Breg cells for therapeutic applications holds great promise for the future treatment of autoimmune and allergic inflammatory conditions.

8. References

Amano, H., E. Amano, et al. (2003). "The Yaa mutation promoting murine lupus causes defective development of marginal zone B cells." *J Immunol* 170(5): 2293-2301.

Amu, S., S. P. Saunders, et al. (2010). "Regulatory B cells prevent and reverse allergic airway inflammation via FoxP3-positive T regulatory cells in a murine model." *J Allergy Clin Immunol* 125(5): 1114-1124 e1118.

Anderson, M. S. and J. A. Bluestone (2005). "The NOD mouse: a model of immune dysregulation." *Annu Rev Immunol* 23: 447-485.

Bar-Or, A., P. A. Calabresi, et al. (2008). "Rituximab in relapsing-remitting multiple sclerosis: a 72-week, open-label, phase I trial." *Ann Neurol* 63(3): 395-400.

Barr, T. A., S. Brown, et al. (2007). "TLR-mediated stimulation of APC: Distinct cytokine responses of B cells and dendritic cells." *Eur J Immunol* 37(11): 3040-3053.

Baxter, A. G. (2007). "The origin and application of experimental autoimmune encephalomyelitis." *Nat Rev Immunol* 7(11): 904-912.

Begum-Haque, S., M. Christy, et al. (2011). "Augmentation of regulatory B cell activity in experimental allergic encephalomyelitis by glatiramer acetate." *J Neuroimmunol* 232(1-2): 136-144.

Bhan, A. K., E. Mizoguchi, et al. (2000). "Regulatory role of mature B cells in a murine model of inflammatory bowel disease." *International Immunology* 12(5): 597-605.

Bhan, A. K., E. Mizoguchi, et al. (1999). "Colitis in transgenic and knockout animals as models of human inflammatory bowel disease." *Immunol Rev* 169: 195-207.

Bjorksten, B., E. Sepp, et al. (2001). "Allergy development and the intestinal microflora during the first year of life." *J Allergy Clin Immunol* 108(4): 516-520.

Blair, P. A., K. A. Chavez-Rueda, et al. (2009). "Selective targeting of B cells with agonistic anti-CD40 is an efficacious strategy for the generation of induced regulatory T2-like B cells and for the suppression of lupus in MRL/lpr mice." *J Immunol* 182(6): 3492-3502.

Blair, P. A., L. Y. Norena, et al. (2010). "CD19(+)CD24(hi)CD38(hi) B cells exhibit regulatory capacity in healthy individuals but are functionally impaired in systemic Lupus Erythematosus patients." *Immunity* 32(1): 129-140.

Bodhankar, S., C. Wang, et al. (2011). "Estrogen-induced protection against experimental autoimmune encephalomyelitis is abrogated in the absence of B cells." *Eur J Immunol* 41(4): 1165-1175.

Booth, J. S., P. J. Griebel, et al. (2009). "A novel regulatory B-cell population in sheep Peyer's patches spontaneously secretes IL-10 and downregulates TLR9-induced IFNalpha responses." *Mucosal Immunol* 2(3): 265-275.

Borg, N. A., K. S. Wun, et al. (2007). "CD1d-lipid-antigen recognition by the semi-invariant NKT T-cell receptor." *Nature* 448(7149): 44-49.

Bouaziz, J. D., S. Calbo, et al. (2010). "IL-10 produced by activated human B cells regulates CD4(+) T-cell activation in vitro." *Eur J Immunol* 40(10): 2686-2691.

Carter, N. A., R. Vasconcellos, et al. (2011). "Mice lacking endogenous IL-10-producing regulatory B cells develop exacerbated disease and present with an increased frequency of Th1/Th17 but a decrease in regulatory T cells." *J Immunol* 186(10): 5569-5579.

Chiu, Y. H., S. H. Park, et al. (2002). "Multiple defects in antigen presentation and T cell development by mice expressing cytoplasmic tail-truncated CD1d." *Nat Immunol* 3(1): 55-60.

Collison, L. W., C. J. Workman, et al. (2007). "The inhibitory cytokine IL-35 contributes to regulatory T-cell function." *Nature* 450(7169): 566-569.

Colombo, M., M. Dono, et al. (2000). "Accumulation of clonally related B lymphocytes in the cerebrospinal fluid of multiple sclerosis patients." *J Immunol* 164(5): 2782-2789.

Correale, J. and M. Farez (2009). "Helminth antigens modulate immune responses in cells from multiple sclerosis patients through TLR2-dependent mechanisms." *J Immunol* 183(9): 5999-6012.

Correale, J., M. Farez, et al. (2008). "Helminth infections associated with multiple sclerosis induce regulatory B cells." *Ann Neurol* 64(2): 187-199.

Cua, D. J., J. Sherlock, et al. (2003). "Interleukin-23 rather than interleukin-12 is the critical cytokine for autoimmune inflammation of the brain." *Nature* 421(6924): 744-748.

Dalwadi, H., B. Wei, et al. (2003). "B cell developmental requirement for the G alpha i2 gene." *J Immunol* 170(4): 1707-1715.

DiLillo, D. J., T. Matsushita, et al. (2010). "B10 cells and regulatory B cells balance immune responses during inflammation, autoimmunity, and cancer." *Ann N Y Acad Sci* 1183: 38-57.

Douwes, J., S. Cheng, et al. (2008). "Farm exposure in utero may protect against asthma, hay fever and eczema." *Eur Respir J* 32(3): 603-611.

Duddy, M., M. Niino, et al. (2007). "Distinct effector cytokine profiles of memory and naive human B cell subsets and implication in multiple sclerosis." *J Immunol* 178(10): 6092-6099.

Ege, M. J., R. Frei, et al. (2007). "Not all farming environments protect against the development of asthma and wheeze in children." *J Allergy Clin Immunol* 119(5): 1140-1147.

Ege, M. J., M. Mayer, et al. (2011). "Exposure to environmental microorganisms and childhood asthma." *N Engl J Med* 364(8): 701-709.

Evans, J. G., K. A. Chavez-Rueda, et al. (2007). "Novel suppressive function of transitional 2 B cells in experimental arthritis." *J Immunol* 178(12): 7868-7878.

Fife, B. T. and J. A. Bluestone (2008). "Control of peripheral T-cell tolerance and autoimmunity via the CTLA-4 and PD-1 pathways." *Immunol Rev* 224: 166-182.

Fillatreau, S., C. H. Sweenie, et al. (2002). "B cells regulate autoimmunity by provision of IL-10." *Nat Immunol* 3(10): 944-950.

Firestein, G. S. (2003). "Evolving concepts of rheumatoid arthritis." *Nature* 423(6937): 356-361.

Flohr, C., R. J. Quinnell, et al. (2009). "Do helminth parasites protect against atopy and allergic disease?" *Clin Exp Allergy* 39(1): 20-32.

Fonseca, D. E. and J. N. Kline (2009). "Use of CpG oligonucleotides in treatment of asthma and allergic disease." *Adv Drug Deliv Rev* 61(3): 256-262.

Frank, D. N., A. L. St Amand, et al. (2007). "Molecular-phylogenetic characterization of microbial community imbalances in human inflammatory bowel diseases." *Proc Natl Acad Sci U S A* 104(34): 13780-13785.

Fraussen, J., K. Vrolix, et al. (2009). "B cell characterization and reactivity analysis in multiple sclerosis." *Autoimmun Rev* 8(8): 654-658.

Gerth, A. J., L. Lin, et al. (2004). "An innate cell-mediated, murine ulcerative colitis-like syndrome in the absence of nuclear factor of activated T cells." *Gastroenterology* 126(4): 1115-1121.

Gray, M., K. Miles, et al. (2007). "Apoptotic cells protect mice from autoimmune inflammation by the induction of regulatory B cells." *Proc Natl Acad Sci U S A* 104(35): 14080-14085.

Hardy, R. R. and K. Hayakawa (2001). "B cell development pathways." *Annu Rev Immunol* 19: 595-621.

Hauser, S. L., E. Waubant, et al. (2008). "B-cell depletion with rituximab in relapsing-remitting multiple sclerosis." *N Engl J Med* 358(7): 676-688.

Hirotani, M., M. Niino, et al. (2010). "Decreased IL-10 production mediated by Toll-like receptor 9 in B cells in multiple sclerosis." *J Neuroimmunol* 221(1-2): 95-100.

Hokama, A., E. Mizoguchi, et al. (2004). "Induced reactivity of intestinal CD4(+) T cells with an epithelial cell lectin, galectin-4, contributes to exacerbation of intestinal inflammation." *Immunity* 20(6): 681-693.

Huang, F.-P. and S. Sattler (2011). "Regulatory T Cell Deficiency in Systemic Autoimmune Disorders - Causal Relationship and Underlying Immunological Mechanisms." *Autoimmune Disorders - Pathogenetic Aspects, Mavragani Clio (Ed.), ISBN 978-953-307-643-0, InTech.*

Hussaarts, L., L. E. van der Vlugt, et al. (2011). "Regulatory B-cell induction by helminths: Implications for allergic disease." *J Allergy Clin Immunol* 128(4): 733-739.

Hussain, S. and T. L. Delovitch (2007). "Intravenous transfusion of BCR-activated B cells protects NOD mice from type 1 diabetes in an IL-10-dependent manner." *J Immunol* 179(11): 7225-7232.

Iwata, Y., T. Matsushita, et al. (2011). "Characterization of a rare IL-10-competent B-cell subset in humans that parallels mouse regulatory B10 cells." *Blood* 117(2): 530-541.

Jankovic, D., A. W. Cheever, et al. (1998). "CD4+ T cell-mediated granulomatous pathology in schistosomiasis is downregulated by a B cell-dependent mechanism requiring Fc receptor signaling." *J Exp Med* 187(4): 619-629.

Johansson, M. A., Y. M. Sjogren, et al. (2011). "Early colonization with a group of Lactobacilli decreases the risk for allergy at five years of age despite allergic heredity." *PLoS One* 6(8): e23031.

Kala, M., S. N. Rhodes, et al. (2010). "B cells from glatiramer acetate-treated mice suppress experimental autoimmune encephalomyelitis." *Exp Neurol* 221(1): 136-145.

Katz, S. I., D. Parker, et al. (1974). "B-cell suppression of delayed hypersensitivity reactions." *Nature* 251(5475): 550-551.

Kay, A. B. (2000). "Overview of 'allergy and allergic diseases: with a view to the future'." *Br Med Bull* 56(4): 843-864.

La Flamme, A. C., K. Ruddenklau, et al. (2003). "Schistosomiasis decreases central nervous system inflammation and alters the progression of experimental autoimmune encephalomyelitis." *Infect Immun* 71(9): 4996-5004.

Lampropoulou, V., E. Calderon-Gomez, et al. (2010). "Suppressive functions of activated B cells in autoimmune diseases reveal the dual roles of Toll-like receptors in immunity." *Immunol Rev* 233(1): 146-161.

Lampropoulou, V., K. Hoehlig, et al. (2008). "TLR-activated B cells suppress T cell-mediated autoimmunity." *J Immunol* 180(7): 4763-4773.

Lee-Chang, C., D. Lefranc, et al. (2011). "Susceptibility to experimental autoimmune encephalomyelitis is associated with altered B-cell subsets distribution and decreased serum BAFF levels." *Immunol Lett* 135(1-2): 108-117.

Lee, J. H., J. Noh, et al. (2011). "Allergen-specific transforming growth factor-beta-producing CD19+CD5+ regulatory B-cell (Br3) responses in human late eczematous allergic reactions to cow's milk." *J Interferon Cytokine Res* 31(5): 441-449.

Lehuen, A., O. Lantz, et al. (1998). "Overexpression of natural killer T cells protects Valpha14- Jalpha281 transgenic nonobese diabetic mice against diabetes." *J Exp Med* 188(10): 1831-1839.

Lemoine, S., A. Morva, et al. (2009). "Regulatory B cells in autoimmune diseases: how do they work?" *Ann N Y Acad Sci* 1173: 260-267.

Lenert, P., R. Brummel, et al. (2005). "TLR-9 activation of marginal zone B cells in lupus mice regulates immunity through increased IL-10 production." *J Clin Immunol* 25(1): 29-40.

Lenert, P., A. Goeken, et al. (2003). "Innate immune responses in lupus-prone Palmerston North mice: differential responses to LPS and bacterial DNA/CpG oligonucleotides." *J Clin Immunol* 23(3): 202-213.

Liu, Q., K. Sundar, et al. (2009). "Helminth infection can reduce insulitis and type 1 diabetes through CD25- and IL-10-independent mechanisms." *Infect Immun* 77(12): 5347-5358.

Loss, G., S. Apprich, et al. (2011). "The protective effect of farm milk consumption on childhood asthma and atopy: The GABRIELA study." *J Allergy Clin Immunol* 128(4): 766-773 e764.

Lotz, M., E. Ranheim, et al. (1994). "Transforming growth factor beta as endogenous growth inhibitor of chronic lymphocytic leukemia B cells." *J Exp Med* 179(3): 999-1004.

Lundy, S. K., A. A. Berlin, et al. (2005). "Deficiency of regulatory B cells increases allergic airway inflammation." *Inflamm Res* 54(12): 514-521.

Lundy, S. K. and D. L. Boros (2002). "Fas ligand-expressing B-1a lymphocytes mediate CD4(+)-T-cell apoptosis during schistosomal infection: induction by interleukin 4 (IL-4) and IL-10." *Infect Immun* 70(2): 812-819.

Lundy, S. K. and D. A. Fox (2009). "Reduced Fas ligand-expressing splenic CD5+ B lymphocytes in severe collagen-induced arthritis." *Arthritis Res Ther* 11(4): R128.

Lynch, N. R., I. Hagel, et al. (1993). "Effect of anthelmintic treatment on the allergic reactivity of children in a tropical slum." *J Allergy Clin Immunol* 92(3): 404-411.

Mangan, N. E., R. E. Fallon, et al. (2004). "Helminth infection protects mice from anaphylaxis via IL-10-producing B cells." *J Immunol* 173(10): 6346-6356.

Mangan, N. E., N. van Rooijen, et al. (2006). "Helminth-modified pulmonary immune response protects mice from allergen-induced airway hyperresponsiveness." *J Immunol* 176(1): 138-147.

Manichanh, C., L. Rigottier-Gois, et al. (2006). "Reduced diversity of faecal microbiota in Crohn's disease revealed by a metagenomic approach." *Gut* 55(2): 205-211.

Mann, M. K., K. Maresz, et al. (2007). "B cell regulation of CD4+CD25+ T regulatory cells and IL-10 via B7 is essential for recovery from experimental autoimmune encephalomyelitis." *J Immunol* 178(6): 3447-3456.

Mariani, S. M. (2004). "Genes and autoimmune diseases - a complex inheritance." *MedGenMed* 6(4): 18.

Matricardi, P. M., F. Rosmini, et al. (1997). "Cross sectional retrospective study of prevalence of atopy among Italian military students with antibodies against hepatitis A virus." *BMJ* 314(7086): 999-1003.

Matsushita, T., M. Fujimoto, et al. (2006). "Inhibitory role of CD19 in the progression of experimental autoimmune encephalomyelitis by regulating cytokine response." *Am J Pathol* 168(3): 812-821.

Matsushita, T., M. Horikawa, et al. (2010). "Regulatory B cells (B10 cells) and regulatory T cells have independent roles in controlling experimental autoimmune encephalomyelitis initiation and late-phase immunopathogenesis." *J Immunol* 185(4): 2240-2252.

Matsushita, T., K. Yanaba, et al. (2008). "Regulatory B cells inhibit EAE initiation in mice while other B cells promote disease progression." *J Clin Invest* 118(10): 3420-3430.

Mauri, C. and M. R. Ehrenstein (2008). "The 'short' history of regulatory B cells." *Trends Immunol* 29(1): 34-40.

Mauri, C., D. Gray, et al. (2003). "Prevention of arthritis by interleukin 10-producing B cells." *J Exp Med* 197(4): 489-501.

Mills, J. A. (1994). "Systemic lupus erythematosus." *N Engl J Med* 330(26): 1871-1879.

Miyazaki, D., C. H. Kuo, et al. (2009). "Regulatory function of CpG-activated B cells in late-phase experimental allergic conjunctivitis." *Invest Ophthalmol Vis Sci* 50(4): 1626-1635.

Mizoguchi, A. and A. K. Bhan (2006). "A case for regulatory B cells." *J Immunol* 176(2): 705-710.

Mizoguchi, A., E. Mizoguchi, et al. (1996). "Cytokine imbalance and autoantibody production in T cell receptor-alpha mutant mice with inflammatory bowel disease." *J Exp Med* 183(3): 847-856.

Mizoguchi, A., E. Mizoguchi, et al. (1997). "Suppressive role of B cells in chronic colitis of T cell receptor alpha mutant mice." *J Exp Med* 186(10): 1749-1756.

Mizoguchi, A., E. Mizoguchi, et al. (2002). "Chronic intestinal inflammatory condition generates IL-10-producing regulatory B cell subset characterized by CD1d upregulation." *Immunity* 16(2): 219-230.

Mlejnek, E. and L.E.P.M. van der Vlugt (2012). "Impaired IL-10 expression by CD24hiCD27+ regulatory B cells in response to LPS in allergic asthmatic patients." *submitted*.

Moore, K. W., R. de Waal Malefyt, et al. (2001). "Interleukin-10 and the interleukin-10 receptor." *Annu Rev Immunol* 19: 683-765.

Nagler-Anderson, C. (2006). "Helminth-induced immunoregulation of an allergic response to food." *Chem Immunol Allergy* 90: 1-13.

Nakashima, H., Y. Hamaguchi, et al. (2010). "CD22 expression mediates the regulatory functions of peritoneal B-1a cells during the remission phase of contact hypersensitivity reactions." *J Immunol* 184(9): 4637-4645.

Niedbala, W., X. Q. Wei, et al. (2007). "IL-35 is a novel cytokine with therapeutic effects against collagen-induced arthritis through the expansion of regulatory T cells and suppression of Th17 cells." *Eur J Immunol* 37(11): 3021-3029.

Noh, G. and J. H. Lee (2011). "Regulatory B cells and allergic diseases." *Allergy Asthma Immunol Res* 3(3): 168-177.

Noh, J., W. S. Choi, et al. (2010). "Presence of Foxp3-expressing CD19(+)CD5(+) B Cells in Human Peripheral Blood Mononuclear Cells: Human CD19(+)CD5(+)Foxp3(+) Regulatory B Cell (Breg)." *Immune Netw* 10(6): 247-249.

O'Connor, R. A. and S. M. Anderton (2008). "Multi-faceted control of autoaggression: Foxp3+ regulatory T cells in murine models of organ-specific autoimmune disease." *Cell Immunol* 251(1): 8-18.

Osada, Y., S. Shimizu, et al. (2009). "Schistosoma mansoni infection reduces severity of collagen-induced arthritis via down-regulation of pro-inflammatory mediators." *Int J Parasitol* 39(4): 457-464.

Ostanin, D. V., K. P. Pavlick, et al. (2006). "T cell-induced inflammation of the small and large intestine in immunodeficient mice." *Am J Physiol Gastrointest Liver Physiol* 290(1): G109-119.

Palanivel, V., C. Posey, et al. (1996). "B-cell outgrowth and ligand-specific production of IL-10 correlate with Th2 dominance in certain parasitic diseases." *Exp Parasitol* 84(2): 168-177.

Parekh, V. V., D. V. Prasad, et al. (2003). "B cells activated by lipopolysaccharide, but not by anti-Ig and anti-CD40 antibody, induce anergy in CD8+ T cells: role of TGF-beta 1." *J Immunol* 170(12): 5897-5911.

Rafei, M., J. Hsieh, et al. (2009). "A granulocyte-macrophage colony-stimulating factor and interleukin-15 fusokine induces a regulatory B cell population with immune suppressive properties." *Nat Med* 15(9): 1038-1045.

Ramgolam, V. S., Y. Sha, et al. (2011). "B cells as a therapeutic target for IFN-beta in relapsing-remitting multiple sclerosis." *J Immunol* 186(7): 4518-4526.

Ren, X., K. Akiyoshi, et al. (2011). "Programmed Death-1 Pathway Limits Central Nervous System Inflammation and Neurologic Deficits in Murine Experimental Stroke." *Stroke.*

Ronet, C., Y. Hauyon-La Torre, et al. (2010). "Regulatory B cells shape the development of Th2 immune responses in BALB/c mice infected with Leishmania major through IL-10 production." *J Immunol* 184(2): 886-894.

Sabahi, R. and J. H. Anolik (2006). "B-cell-targeted therapy for systemic lupus erythematosus." *Drugs* 66(15): 1933-1948.

Saubermann, L. J., P. Beck, et al. (2000). "Activation of natural killer T cells by alpha-galactosylceramide in the presence of CD1d provides protection against colitis in mice." *Gastroenterology* 119(1): 119-128.

Sayi, A., E. Kohler, et al. (2011). "TLR-2-activated B cells suppress Helicobacter-induced preneoplastic gastric immunopathology by inducing T regulatory-1 cells." *J Immunol* 186(2): 878-890.

Silveira, P. A. and S. T. Grey (2006). "B cells in the spotlight: innocent bystanders or major players in the pathogenesis of type 1 diabetes." *Trends Endocrinol Metab* 17(4): 128-135.

Simons, F. E., Y. Shikishima, et al. (2004). "Selective immune redirection in humans with ragweed allergy by injecting Amb a 1 linked to immunostimulatory DNA." *J Allergy Clin Immunol* 113(6): 1144-1151.

Singh, A., W. F. t. Carson, et al. (2008). "Regulatory role of B cells in a murine model of allergic airway disease." *J Immunol* 180(11): 7318-7326.

Smits, H. H., H. Hammad, et al. (2007). "Protective effect of Schistosoma mansoni infection on allergic airway inflammation depends on the intensity and chronicity of infection." *J Allergy Clin Immunol* 120(4): 932-940.

Snir, A., A. Kessel, et al. (2011). "Anti-IL-6 receptor antibody (tocilizumab): a B cell targeting therapy." *Clin Exp Rheumatol*.

Sonoda, K. H. and J. Stein-Streilein (2002). "CD1d on antigen-transporting APC and splenic marginal zone B cells promotes NKT cell-dependent tolerance." *Eur J Immunol* 32(3): 848-857.

Su, T. T., B. Guo, et al. (2004). "Signaling in transitional type 2 B cells is critical for peripheral B-cell development." *Immunol Rev* 197: 161-178.

Sugimoto, K., A. Ogawa, et al. (2007). "Inducible IL-12-producing B cells regulate Th2-mediated intestinal inflammation." *Gastroenterology* 133(1): 124-136.

Takenoshita, S., T. Fukushima, et al. (2002). "The role of TGF-beta in digestive organ disease." *J Gastroenterol* 37(12): 991-999.

Tian, J., D. Zekzer, et al. (2001). "Lipopolysaccharide-activated B cells down-regulate Th1 immunity and prevent autoimmune diabetes in nonobese diabetic mice." *J Immunol* 167(2): 1081-1089.

Trentham, D. E., A. S. Townes, et al. (1977). "Autoimmunity to type II collagen an experimental model of arthritis." *J Exp Med* 146(3): 857-868.

Tulic, M. K., P. O. Fiset, et al. (2004). "Role of toll-like receptor 4 in protection by bacterial lipopolysaccharide in the nasal mucosa of atopic children but not adults." *Lancet* 363(9422): 1689-1697.

van den Biggelaar, A. H., L. C. Rodrigues, et al. (2004). "Long-term treatment of intestinal helminths increases mite skin-test reactivity in Gabonese schoolchildren." *J Infect Dis* 189(5): 892-900.

van der Kleij, D., E. Latz, et al. (2002). "A novel host-parasite lipid cross-talk. Schistosomal lyso-phosphatidylserine activates toll-like receptor 2 and affects immune polarization." *J Biol Chem* 277(50): 48122-48129.

van der Vlugt, L. E. P. M. and L. A. Labuda (2012). "Schistosomes induce regulatory features in human and mouse CD1dhi B cells: inhibition of allergic inflammation by IL-10 and regulatory T cells." PloS One. *Accepted.*

Velupillai, P. and D. A. Harn (1994). "Oligosaccharide-specific induction of interleukin 10 production by B220+ cells from schistosome-infected mice: a mechanism for regulation of CD4+ T-cell subsets." *Proc Natl Acad Sci U S A* 91(1): 18-22.

Vitale, G., F. Mion, et al. (2010). "Regulatory B cells: evidence, developmental origin and population diversity." *Mol Immunol* 48(1-3): 1-8.

von Mutius, E. (2009). "Gene-environment interactions in asthma." *J Allergy Clin Immunol* 123(1): 3-11; quiz 12-13.

von Mutius, E., C. Braun-Fahrlander, et al. (2000). "Exposure to endotoxin or other bacterial components might protect against the development of atopy." *Clin Exp Allergy* 30(9): 1230-1234.

Watanabe, R., N. Ishiura, et al. (2010). "Regulatory B cells (B10 cells) have a suppressive role in murine lupus: CD19 and B10 cell deficiency exacerbates systemic autoimmunity." *J Immunol* 184(9): 4801-4809.

Weber, M. S., T. Prod'homme, et al. (2010). "B-cell activation influences T-cell polarization and outcome of anti-CD20 B-cell depletion in central nervous system autoimmunity." *Ann Neurol* 68(3): 369-383.

Wei, B., P. Velazquez, et al. (2005). "Mesenteric B cells centrally inhibit CD4+ T cell colitis through interaction with regulatory T cell subsets." *Proc Natl Acad Sci U S A* 102(6): 2010-2015.

Wills-Karp, M., J. Santeliz, et al. (2001). "The germless theory of allergic disease: revisiting the hygiene hypothesis." *Nat Rev Immunol* 1(1): 69-75.

Wilson, M. S., M. D. Taylor, et al. (2010). "Helminth-induced CD19+CD23hi B cells modulate experimental allergic and autoimmune inflammation." *Eur J Immunol* 40(6): 1682-1696.

Wohlfert, E. and Y. Belkaid (2008). "Role of endogenous and induced regulatory T cells during infections." *J Clin Immunol* 28(6): 707-715.

Wolf, S. D., B. N. Dittel, et al. (1996). "Experimental autoimmune encephalomyelitis induction in genetically B cell-deficient mice." *J Exp Med* 184(6): 2271-2278.

Wong, S. C., A. L. Puaux, et al. (2010). "Macrophage polarization to a unique phenotype driven by B cells." *Eur J Immunol* 40(8): 2296-2307.

Wykes, M., J. Poudrier, et al. (1998). "Regulation of cytoplasmic, surface and soluble forms of CD40 ligand in mouse B cells." *Eur J Immunol* 28(2): 548-559.

Xiu, Y., C. P. Wong, et al. (2008). "B lymphocyte depletion by CD20 monoclonal antibody prevents diabetes in nonobese diabetic mice despite isotype-specific differences in Fc gamma R effector functions." *J Immunol* 180(5): 2863-2875.

Yanaba, K., J. D. Bouaziz, et al. (2008). "A regulatory B cell subset with a unique CD1dhiCD5+ phenotype controls T cell-dependent inflammatory responses." *Immunity* 28(5): 639-650.

Yang, C. H., L. Tian, et al. (2008). "Immunological mechanisms and clinical implications of regulatory T cell deficiency in a systemic autoimmune disorder: roles of IL-2 versus IL-15." *Eur J Immunol* 38(6): 1664-1676.

Yang, M., L. Sun, et al. (2010). "Novel function of B cell-activating factor in the induction of IL-10-producing regulatory B cells." *J Immunol* 184(7): 3321-3325.

Yazdanbakhsh, M., P. G. Kremsner, et al. (2002). "Allergy, parasites, and the hygiene hypothesis." *Science* 296(5567): 490-494.

Yen, D., J. Cheung, et al. (2006). "IL-23 is essential for T cell-mediated colitis and promotes inflammation via IL-17 and IL-6." *J Clin Invest* 116(5): 1310-1316.

Zaccone, P., Z. Fehervari, et al. (2003). "Schistosoma mansoni antigens modulate the activity of the innate immune response and prevent onset of type 1 diabetes." *Eur J Immunol* 33(5): 1439-1449.

10

The CNS Innate Immune System and the Emerging Roles of the Neuroimmune Regulators (NIRegs) in Response to Infection, Neoplasia and Neurodegeneration

J. W. Neal[2], M. Denizot[1], J. J. Hoarau[1] and P. Gasque[1]
[1]*GRI, Immunopathology and Infectious Disease Research Grouping (IRG, GRI), University of La Reunion,*
[2]*Neuropathology Laboratory, Dept. of Histopathology, Cardiff University Medical School,*
[1]*Reunion Island*
[2]*UK*

1. Introduction

The mammalian CNS relies upon the ancient, innate immune system, to provide defence against attack by pathogens (virus, bacteria, fungi and parasites) and the clearance of both neurotoxic proteins and apoptotic cells. The main function(s) of the CNS innate immune system can be summarised as the detection of "non self"(pathogens) and " altered self " (neurotoxic proteins and apoptotic cells), with their subsequent clearance, designed to facilitate tissue repair and rapid return to normal function. The failure to express an effective protective response to detect and remove a pathogen (non -self) prolongs the innate immune response and this is associated with autoimmunity, chronic inflammatory diseases (Multiple sclerosis) and neuro degeneration (Alzheimer's and Prion disease) (Hauwel et al., 2005 Griffiths et al., 2009). The failure to detect and clear apoptotic cells results in their accumulation and subsequent release of neurotoxic proteins and enzymes, contributing to excessive tissue damage (Griffiths et al., 2009).

2. The blood brain barrier and immuno privilege

Insects, have a brain lymph barrier, whereas, the vertebrate blood brain barrier (BBB) evolved 50-100 million years before the appearance of the adaptive immune system (Abbot 1995; Lowenstein 2002). For this reason, the CNS immune response against pathogens relies upon the ancient and highly conserved innate immune system that first appeared in limited form in the Agnatha, 500 million years ago and almost 100 million years before the emergence of the systemic adaptive immune system in bony fish. (Lowenstein 2002). The vertebrate type BBB, was therefore present, long before the adaptive immune system and this barrier provide some immunoregulatory control of the CNS response to pathogens (Abbot 1995; Lowenstein 2002).

Other protective physical barriers, are the choroid plexus between the systemic circulation and ventricular CSF (cerebro spinal fluid) and the specialized, ciliated ependymal (glia) layer, that lines ventricles containing the CSF(Martino et al., 2001). Both these epithelial layers express highly conserved receptors that are able to detect pathogens in the CSF and regulate intra CSF inflammation (McMenamin., 1999; Laflamme and Rivest 2001; Canova et al., 2006; Rivest 2009).

The presence of a BBB composed of endothelial cells linked by tight junctions and surrounded by astrocyte foot processes (Pachter et al., 2003) contributed to the development of homeostatic systems to preserve CNS electrolyte and hydrostatic pressure gradients (Abott 1995). To some extent, this also prevented infiltration into the brain by systemic cells (lymphocytes, myeloid related cells) of the more recent adaptive immune system and provided some evidence of immuno regulatory function. Once the vertebrate BBB had developed, the brain relied upon the resident glia and neurons (also perivascular cells and choroid plexus) to deliver the CNS immune response against pathogen invasion (Lowenstein 2002).

To reflect this function, the resident glial cells have been termed" amateur "innate immune cells, in contrast with the" professional" innate immune system cells such as macrophages, dendritic cells and natural killer cells (Hauwel et al., 2005).

3. The CNS innate immune response involves detection of " non self" and clearance of dangerous pathogens, neurotoxic proteins and apoptotic cells

The cells responsible for delivering the CNS innate immune response are microglia, astrocytes, endothelial cells, ependymal cells and to a lesser extent neurons (Rivest 2009). Of great importance, is the capacity of these cells to discriminate between" non –self"defined by pathogens and "altered self " (apoptotic cells and dangerous proteins)from "self " (host cells) (Takeuchi et al., 2010; Elward and Gasque 2003). This discrimination relies upon the expression by microglia and the other glia of ancient, highly conserved, pattern recognition receptors PRR (TLR, RLR, NRL) that are localized upon the cell membrane, within endosomes and also released in soluble form (Jane way 1992; Kawai and Akira 2010).

PRR, are able to detect unique, pathogen associated molecular patterns or PAMPs as represented by bacterial cell wall constituents, such as lipopolysaccharide (LPS). (Medzithov and Janeway 200). This property of the PRR is important for the danger theory as proposed by Matzinger; that while the immune system distinguishes between "self "and "non –self", it also must discriminate dangerous from non -dangerous signals (Matzinger 1994). Endogenous molecules such as S-100 proteins (Foell et al., 2007) and high mobility box group I (HMBG1) (Bianchi 2007; Castiglioni et al., 2011) are released during non -apoptotic cell injury and initiate host tissue inflammation: they are regarded as either "alarmins" or "danger signals "and are identified by the PRR of the innate immune system, because they express, damage associated molecular patterns or DAMPs (Klune et al., 2008; Biannchi 2007).

Apoptotic cells express a range of "altered self "molecules on their surface, so called apoptotic cell associated molecular patterns or ACAMPs (Elward and Gasque 2003; Gregory and Devitt 2004; Griffiths et al., 2009). The detection of " altered self" by PRR as defined by DAMPS and ACAMPs, results in the activation of signalling pathways composed of intra cellular adaptor proteins regulating the expression of pro inflammatory cytokines such as the interferons (INFα/β), interleukins (IL) and tumour necrosis factor (TNFα) (Griffiths et al 2009).

Scavenger receptors (SR), Mannose macrophage receptor (MMR), CD14, CD36, CD91(α2 macroglobulin or LRP low density lipoprotein receptor) and phosphatidylserine recepotor (PRS) are present on the host cell membrane or intracellular endosomes. These receptors are multifunctional because they detect PAMPS, ACAMPs and DAMPs to initiate engulfment and phagocytosis of pathogens or apoptotic cells (Stahl and Ezekowitz., 1998. Fadok et al., 2000 and b, Hanayama et al., 2002; Gregory and Devitt 2004; Mukhopadhyay et al., 2004.)

The resident cells of the CNS express two of the three complement pathways(CP) the classical and alternative, but not the lectin activated pathway (Gasque P et al., 2000; Morgan and Gasque 1996). The first complement component, C1q, functions as a PRR, a property shared with a wide range of other C lectins including, mannan binding protein (MBL) and the pentraxins; all these molecules are able to function as both opsonins and PRR capable of detecting PAMPS and ACAMPs. (Tenner AJ 1999; Lu et al., 2002; Thielens et al 2002; Ogden et al., 2005).

After binding to either an apoptotic cell (by detecting ACAMPS) or bacteria (through PAMPS), the opsonins provide a signal on a phagocytic cell that enhances phagcoytosis, either through activation of the complement C pathway or facilitating binding to a PRR such as the β2 integrin, CR3/CR4, receptors (Ehlers et al., 2000; Gasque et al 2000; Gasque 2004). Phagocytosis of opsonized pathogens, neurotoxic proteins and apoptotic cells by microglia and macrophages will promote a reduction in local inflammation (non -phlogistic response) stimulating the recruitment of stem cells from a distance niche and assisting tissue repair (Griffiths et al., 2009).

4. Regulatory pathways prevent an uncontrolled innate immune response; the Neuro immuno-regulatory molecules (NIRegs)

The uncontrolled activation of the innate immune response results in the production of neurotoxic factors and unregulated inflammatory cytokine release. These two factors contribute to any indiscriminate bystander damage and the amplification of underlying disease state. For this reason, the innate immune response must be regulated in order to prevent bystander neuron loss and an uncontrolled inflammatory response. There is now evidence of a group of neuro immuno regulatory (NIRegs) molecules, that by analogy are similar to T reg lymphocytes (Griffiths al., 2007; Hoarau et al., 2011). These T cells are responsible for regulating /controlling the innate immune response and for shaping the resident cells towards a protective phenotype. Several NIRegs, CD47 and CD 200, are capable of acting as "don't eat me "signals allowing host cells to evade detection and phagocytosis by microglia and macrophages (Elward and Gasque 2003; Barclay et al., 2002; Brown and Frazier., 2001; Hoek et al., 2000). The Siglecs, a family of lectins, also detect cells expressing "don't eat me" signals in the form of sialic acid containing molecules (Crocker and Varki 2005). Pathogens do not generally express sialic acid residues and the absence of sialic acids provides a " non -self " signal, sometimes referred to as an "eat me signal "and this is detected by lectins, including Siglecs, and complement proteins.

The CP is also strictly regulated by a series of complement regulatory proteins CRP (FH, CD55, CD46) preventing inappropriate activation and host destruction (Elward et al., 2005; Griffiths et al., 2009; Zipfel et al., 2009). Furthermore, components of the CP including C3a, are also capable of recruiting stem cells into areas of tissue damage and increasing growth factor expression, both facilitating tissue repair (Griffiths et al., 2010).

5. Toll like receptors (TLRs) are PRR with multiple roles in infection including pathogen detection and inflammatory response

The TLR are an ancient, highly conserved family of PRR, which belong to the type-1 trans membrane receptors. They are characterized by a cytosolic C-terminal signalling domain – Toll/interleukin -1receptor (TIR) required for intracellular signal transduction and terminal LRR(leucine rich repeats) domain that mediates the recognition of PAMPs (Kawai and Akira 2010). This family of PRR are vital for the detection of PAMPs, including cell wall lipoproteins and nucleic acids, derived from bacteria, viruses, parasites and fungi (Iwaski and Medhitov 2010).

TLR 4, or heterodimers TLR2-TLR1, TLR2-TLR6 and TLR5 (but notTLR3) binds to a ligand such as a PAMP or DAMP, the complex is internailized within the endosome and this triggers intracellular transduction pathways by recruiting the TIR interaction domain that forms multimers with, a number of adaptor proteins such as myeloid differentiation primary response protein, My D88, My D88 adaptor like (Mal, also TIR domain containing adaptor protein, TIRAP), TIR domain containing adaptor inducing IFN–γ(TRIF) and TRIF – related adaptor molecule TRAM. Activation of TLR by PAMPS recruits one of the above adaptor molecules and activates the My D 88 dependent pathway with NF- kB activation. An alternative signalling pathway following TLR binding to a ligand involves the activation of the TRIF -dependent pathway, with the induction of the type I interferon (anti -virus) response, with the expression of IFNβ and inflammatory cytokines (Netea et al., 2004 Creagh and O Neill 2006).

Mice deficient in the individual TRL negative regulatory proteins, such as zinc finger proteins, autophagy related molecules and ubiquitin are unable to regulate the inflammatory response subsequent to TLR ligand binding. This uncontrolled inflammatory response results in multi organ inflammation such as, chronic inflammatory bowel disease and auto immune arthritis. Conversly, MyD 88 deficiency reduces inflammation (Kwai and Akira 2010 for detailed discussion).

A detailed review of the intra cellular signalling pathways linked to TLR activation by viral nucleic acids, bacterial lipo proteins and other ligands, with subsequent inflammatory cytokine synthesis is outside the scope of this review, but see Takeuchi and Akira 2007; Iwaski and Medhitov 2010; Kawai and Akira 2010)

5.1 TLR act in combination with other PRRs and not always alone

Interestingly, TLR2, forms hetero dimers with TLR-1 and this combination is able to detect Gram negative bacteria, whereas the heterodimer TLR-2-TLR-6 combination recognizes Gram positive organisms. Further cooperation between TLR -4 and the SR co -receptors, CD14 and CD36, together with the C lectin receptor, dendritic cell –specific intercellular molecule -3 grabbing non –integrin (DC -SIGN), detects glucuronoxylmannans found on the cell wall of fungi (Kumar et al 2010).

5.2 TLR distribution in the CNS

Ten functional TLRs have been identified in humans, of these, nine are conserved in both humans and mice. In the human and mouse CNS, TLR 3, , TLR 7 and TLR 8 are located on the cell surface of neurons (Bisibi et al., 2002; Prehaud et al., 2005; Jackson et al., 2006), microglia (Alexopoulou et al., 2001; Olson et al., 2004; Jack 2005), astrocytes (Bsibi et al., 2001; Bisibi et al 2006 Farina et al., 2005; Rivieccio et al., 2006; Carpentier et al., 2007) ependyma and oligodendrocytes (Bsibi 2002). TLR 7 and 8 on microglia (Olson et al., 2004), astrocytes (Buchiet al., 2008) neurons (Ma et al., 2006), TLR 9 on microglia (Mc Kimme et al., 2006). Cells of the meninges, choroid plexus and circum ventricular organs are all exposed to the systemic circulation and express TLR 2 and TLR 4 (Lafalamme and Rivest 2001; Bowman et al., 2003; Laflamme et al., 2003;) see table1

TLR, 3 TLR7, TLR8 and TLR 9 are distributed within intracellular organelles, endoplasmic reticulum, lysosomes and endolysosomes so they are strategically placed to detect intra cytoplasmic viral nucleic acids, both RNA and DNA (Griffin 2003; Kumar et al., 2011). Conversly, TLR2, TLR5 and TLR 6, are present on the cell surface and detect various bacterial components (Kumar et al., 2011; Iwasaki and Medzhitov 2010)

TLRs11-13 have been described in neurons, astrocytes, ependymal and endothelial cells(Mishra er al., 2008). see table 1

5.3 TLRs; Innate immune response to bacterial infection

TLRs are expressed by glial and choroid plexus cells following bacterial infection (Bowman et al., 2003 Carpentier et al., 2008). TLR- 4 forms a complex with MD2 on the host cell surface and they provide the main Lipopolysaccharide (LPS), binding site. Further interaction between LPS binding protein with CD14, a glycophosphatidylinositol protein (GPI) with leucine repeat protein, delivers LPS to the TLR4-MD2 complex, this is internalized into endosomes and through the My88 protein intracellular signalling pathway eventually results in cytokine expression. TLR4 also detects virus envelope proteins and *Streptococcus pneumoniae* pneumolysin (Kwai and Akira 2010. Akira and Uematas., 2006).

TLR2, is able to detect a wide range of bacterial wall PAMPS, including peptidoglycan, Mycobacteria (lipoarabinomannan mycobcateria), fungal (zymosan), haemagluttin on influenza virus, together with mucin molecules from *Trypanosoma cruzei.* The glucans are a main constituent of the fungal cell wall and in association with dectins -1(a C type - lectin)are detected by the TLR2 receptor and internalized to produce a protective inflammatory response (Netea et al., 2004). TLR2 is not able to detect viral nucleic acids.

TLR5 and TLR9 detect a different range of bacterial constituents; TLR5 recognizes the flagellin protein expressed by flagellated bacteria, whereas TLR9, detects bacterial and viral DNA, especially CpG DNA motifs, that are rarely found in mammalian cells (Kawai and Akira 2010). (see table 1). TRL 11, recognizes bacteria found in the genitourinary tract as well as a profilin, a molecule expressed by *Toxoplasmosis gondii* (Yarovinsky et al., 2005), and also neurocysticercosis (Mishra er al 2008).

5.4 TLR; virus detection and the anti virus response

TLR3 detects double stranded (ds) RNA formed during replication of RNAand DNA viruses (Alexopoulou et al., 2001; Wang T et al., 2004; Daffis et al., 2008) the viral nucleic acid binds to N and C terminal sites on the TLR3 ectodomain activating the TRIF and NF- kB dependent pathways to produce an interferon type 1 anti- virus (IFN type -1) response (Paul et al., 2007)

Conversly, TLR7 and TLR 9 detect single stranded viral (ss)RNA and DNA respectively, and signal through the adaptor protein (MyD88) to initiate intracellular signalling by activating transcription factors NF-kB and the interferon regulatory factors (IRFs).

IRFs are translocated to the host cell nucleus where they regulate inflammatory cytokine synthesis and stimulate IFN type I interferon synthesis(IFNα/β expression) resulting in a protective response in adjacent cells, uninfected with a virus (Katze et al., 2002; Paul et al 2007). IFNα/βbinds to the IFN surface receptor (IFNAR) on an uninfected host cell leading to the activation of Janus kinases (JAK) with phosphorylation of transcription factors Signal Transducer and Activation of Signal (STAT1 and STAT2). These two proteins enter the host nucleus to drive the expression of IFN stimulated genes (ISGs)to intiate the anti virus host response.

Many of the emerging RNA viruses responsible for encephalitis express viral proteins that inhibit the host's innate anti -virus response by inhibiting specific steps in the pathway for IFN α/β synthesis, namely the ISGs and several anti -virus proteins blocking the hosts anti virus response (Type 1 interferon) (Griffin 2003; Paul et al., 2007) Examples of viruses and their individual proteins that block the host's IFN expression include, West Nile Fever (Envelope protein E), Influenza (Non Structual protein -1), Ebola (VP 24, VP35) Rabies (Rabies virus phosphoprotein), Enterovirus (structural protein 3C).

5.5 TLR detection of DAMPs in the absence of infection promotes inflammation

Necrotic cells release a range of endogenous proteins such as, heat shock proteins (HSP), S - 100, High mobility group box 1 Interleukin (HMGB1), ATP and mitochondrial proteins that are all regarded as DAMPS, because they can initiate an inflammatory response. (Roth et al., 2003; Lotze et al 2005; Krysko et al., 2010).

Several PRR including TLR-3, TLR-7 and TLR-9 function as sensors of tissue necrosis (Cavassani et al., 2008; Marshak- Rothstein and Rifkin 2007). Chromatin –DNA and ribonucleoprotein complexes all of which contain "self"nucleotides that activate the intracellular PRRs, TLR 7and TLR 9, resulting in an autoimmune disease(Tian et al 2010). Self nucleic acids are usually unable to activate the innate immune system, but after degradation by serum nucleases they are detected by TLRs in endolysosomes resulting in a further inflammatory response (Cavassani et al., 2008) In Systemic lupus erythematosus SLE, (a chronic inflammatory multi-organ disease charachterized by antibody production against self antigens such as DNA). On this basis SLE is regarded as a typical autoimmune disease because serum auto antibodies bind to " self" nucleic acids and are internalized by FcγR IIIa receptors on DC. These complexes are detected by TLR7 and 9, leading to interferon type I response and persistent autoimmune inflammation (Marshak- Rothstein and Rifkin 2007).

HMBG1 is an important DAMP, because it can bind to self DNA and pathogens. The receptor for activated glycation endproducts (RAGE) is also a PRR, and binds with HMBG1 to form a complex. This is delivered to endosomes containing TLR9, activating both DC and

B lymphocytes, with an up regulation of inflammatory cytokines (Tian et al., 2007). The regulation of HMGBI is clearly an important factor contributing to reducing DAMP initiated inflammation. One regulator of this interaction is Thrombomodulin (CD141); it is expressed by microglia and has been shown to bind to HMBG before it can form a complex with RAGE, to prevent this complex being detected by TLR and promoting an inflammatory response. (Abeyama et al 2005).

Heat shock proteins (HSP) and S-100, are important DAMPs and also interact with TLR 2-4 /CD91 and the RAGE receptor. This complex also signals through the NF-kB pathway to activate proinflammatory cytokine expression (Foell et al., 2007; Yu et al., 2006). The regulation of DAMP initiated inflammation is not well understood; however two macrophage (and possibly microglial) related lectins, MINCL and Clec9A, both bind to ribonucleoproteins, SAP 130, released by necrotic cells preventing DAMPS binding to TLR, with a down regulation of cytokine expression (Sancho et al 2009).

6. Non-TLR PRRs in pathogen detection

6.1 RIG like receptor; RIG -1 and MDA5 receptors detect intracellular viral nucleic acids and initiate interferon synthesis

Retinoic acid inducible agent -1 and melanoma differentiation associated gene 5 (MDA5) are both RIG-1 -like receptors (RLRs) , are helicases and signal through the adaptor molecule IPS-1 (Yoneyama et al., 2004; Kato et al 2006; Kwaki and Akiar 2010). They are expressed by microglia and astrocytes, and are located in the cytosol (Miranada et al., 2009). RLRs detect mainly virus RNA, both short and long ds and ss RNA (. Fur et al., 2008; Yoshida et al., 2007) RIG-1 detects short double stranded RNA; negative sense single strand, Influenza A and Ebola viruses and positive sense single strand RNA, Japanese encephalitis and Hepatitis C (Yoneyama et al., 2004; Fuijita et al 2007., Mohamadzadeh et al., 2007) whereas, MDA-5 detects cytoplasmic positive sense RNA, for example Poliovirus. (Griffin 2003; Kato et al 2008)

6.2 RiG-1 and MDA-5 anti virus response

RIG-1 and MDA-5 contain caspase recruitment domains (CARDS) essential for down stream signalling and an intermediate DEeD/H-box RNA Helicase domain, essential for ligand binding and recognition. (Parisien et al., 2003) The interaction between the RIG-1 and MDA-5 with nucleic acid from a pathogen activates the CARD containing adaptor (IPS-1) known as Cardif, MAVS and VISA, resulting in the up regulation of interleukins and a range of anti -virus proteins (Kumar et al 2010: Kato 2006) promoting the IFN type I response, capable of inhibiting viral replication(Paul et al 2007). See table 1.

6.3 ND LR receptors; roles in the innate response against infection

The NDLR (nucleotide -binding domain leucine rich repeat) are a group of highly conserved proteins found in diverse species, including sea urchins and humans. They (twenty two have been identified in humans and thirty four in mice) are a family of intracellular cytoplasmic PRR that represent sensors for detecting Gram negative and Gram positive bacteria, mycobacteria and DAMPs (Karaparakis et al 2007: ; Ting et al., 2010; Kumar et al., 2011).

These receptors are characterized by an N -terminal effector domain caspase recruitment domain (CARD), a centrally located nucleoside binding domain NACHT (or NOD) domain for nucleotide binding and a C terminal of leucine rich (LRR) mediating PAMP ligand recognition, e. g peptioglycan and flagellin in the bacterial cell wall (Sterka and Marriott 2006: Kaparakis et al., 2007 Proell et al 2008).

The actual process wherby an NLR detects either a PAMP or DAMP, is not understood. However, the C terminal LRR region recognizes PAMPS, but the crucial step in NLR activation is the oligomerization of NACHT domain and this permits binding to a series of intracellular adaptor proteins and eventually the intiation of IFN synthesis as the inflammatory response. (Proel2008)Further information about potential homo and heterotypical interactions between NLR s is needed to determine whether or not different combinations of NLRS demonstrate functional differences. Mutations in the genes encoding individual NLR have been linked to several chronic inflammatory disorders (such as Crohn's disease and asthma) underlying the potential importance of NLR in human disease (Tinget al 2010).

The expression of the NLR in the CNS is not clearly defined, although NOD 2 is expressed by monocytes, microglia and astrocytes (Chauhan et al; 2009)

NOD1 and 2 are cytosol proteins, they are able to detect major components of bacteria cell walls, g –D glutamyl –meso –diaminopimelic acid (iE- DAP) present in numerous organisms including Listeria Bacillus subtilis, Shigella Flexneri, Campylobacter jejuni and, Helicobacter pylori; NOD-2 detects murmayl dipepetide from Salmonella Typhimurium, Mycobacteria tuberculosis, Listeria monocytogenes, Saphylococcus aureus and Neiseeria menigitidis (Sterka et al., 2006) Kumar et al 2011). Uncontrolled NOD-2 activation can, however, result in demyelinization, representing the detrimental effects of unregulated activation of the innate immune system against pathogen invasion. (Proell et al., 2008).

NLR3, is a key component of NLR- 3 inflammosome (NLR 3, ASC and procaspase -1) because it is able to detect a wide range of PAMPs including viruses (adeno and influenzaviruses), bacteria (Staphylococcus aureus) and fungi (Candida albicans) (Osawa et al., 2010) and various DAMPs (HSP and BCL-2)(Schroder 2010). Of interest, is the association between a mutation in the nucleotide –binding oligomerization domain gene 2(NOD2) and Crohn's disease, an inflammatory bowel disease (Rehaume et al; ., 2010; Ting et al., 2010).

The explanation for the role of NOD2 in some forms of bowel inflammation (Crohn's disease) provides several insights into the more general immuno regulatory roles for NOD - 2. Firstly, as an activator of the transcription factor NF-kB, to increase cytokine synthesis, or as a negative regulator of the host TLR response to pathogens, thirdly, a capacity to increase host defence by up regulating the expression of small molecular weight (18-45 amino acids) molecules called the α defensins in Paneth cells. The defensins assist with the intracellular lysis of phagocytosed bacteria, therfore regulating the severity of inflammation in the intestine wall (Rehaume et al., 2010).

The precise mechanism by which intra cellular sensing of PAMPs, such as bacterial peptidoglycan derived molecules, meso –diaminopimelic acid and muramyl dipeptide is carried out is as yet, not known (Ting et al 2010). Once a PAMP or DAMP is detected by the NLR this activates the inflammasome pathway (a complex composed of NLR, the adaptor

ASC (apoptotic speck-containing protein) with a CARD and procaspase -1 increasing the expression of proinflammatory cytokines IL-β and IL-18. (Royet et al., 2007; Hoarau et al., 2011).

The involvement of NLR in virus infection requires the mitochondrial located anti virus signalling protein, MAVS (also Cardif, IPS-1, VISA), that is responsible for type I interferon response. An NLR protein family member, NLRX1, regulates the interferon type 1 response by inhibiting the interaction between RIG-1 and MAVS, whereas NOD 2, also inhibits RNA virus production through its interaction with the anti- viral protein, 2-5 oligodenylate synthase type 2 (OAS2) (Ting et al 2010). see table 1.

7. Scavenger Receptors (SR) detect pathogens, apoptotic cells and endogenous proteins; vital components of the innate immune response

7.1 CD14, CD36 and SCARB

CD14 is expressed by microglia and is both a membrane anchored glycophosphatidylinositol protein (GPI) and soluble PRR. It has a co-operative interaction with TLR- 4 to facilitate bacterial LPS detection and it interacts with apoptotic lymphocytes, via the intercellular adhesion molecule(ICAM-3) to facilitate their phagocytosis (Gregory 2000). Clearance of apoptotic cells by CD14, depends upon detection of ACAMPS and this is also an anti -inflammatory response, reducing tissue damage, because the soluble form CD14 switches off activated T cells (Pender 2001).

7.2 Scavenger receptors class A (SRAI, SRABI/II) and class B, CD36

The best characterised SR is CD36, a multifunctional receptor, expressed by microglia and astrocytes (Husemann etal., 2002). It is able to bind to phosphatidyl (PS) and oxidized low density lipoprotein, both present on apoptotic cells (as ACAMPs) as well as neurotoxic proteins such as Aβ4 (Ren et al., 1995; Coraci et al., 2002). Macrophage, CD36, co-operates with the vitronectin receptor $\alpha v\beta_3$ (CD51/CD61) to increase phagocytosis, because this complex recognizes the protein thrombospondin (TSP) located on the surface of apoptotic cells. (Lamy et al 2007: Fadok et al., 1998).

A further receptor, Scavenger receptor B, SCARB (Lysosomal integral membrane protein II or CD36b like-2) is expressed by many different tissues and has also been identified as a receptor for the enterovirus EV71and coxsackie virus A16, although only EV71 is responsible for encephalitis. SCARB is expressed in most tissues, so it not possible to explain the neurotophic effect of EV71 as the result of this virus binding this new receptor. (Yamayoshi et al, 2009).

7.3 CD91; a multi functional PRR

The α2 macroglobulin LRP receptor-related or the lipoprotein low density lipoprotein receptor (CD91) is expressed by microglia and neurons (Marzolo et al., 2000), and functions as an entry receptor for both bacteria and viruses. HIV-1 utilizes CD91 as a docking receptor to enter the CNS via endocytosis; the toxin of the bacterium Pseudomonas is taken up by CD91 (Herz et al., 2001). Despite this evidence, the contribution made by this SR in defending against neuro infection is not yet clarified; CD91 is also able to bind toAβ4 amyloid and apoptotic cells (Marzolo et al., 2000). As the result of apoptosis, calreticulin, a soluble protein located on the endoplasmic reticulum migrates to the cell surface and becomes a potentially important ligand for phagocyte receptors, including mannan binding lectin (MBL), the first complement proteinC1q and the CD91 complex. (Ogden et al., 2001; Gardai et al., 2005)

7.4 TREM -2; a new scavenger receptor

Triggering receptor expressed by myeloid cells (TREM-2) and is an SR expressed on monocyte derived dendritic cells, osteoclasts and microglia (Takahashiet al., 2007). The TREM-2 receptor is expressed by microglia in conjunction with the receptor DAP-12 that shares many features with Draper, an ancient phagocytic receptor found in *Drosphila*. The microglial, DAP-12 receptor and Draper, both contain ITAM (immuno receptor tyrosine based activation motifs) and stimulation of this signalling pathway increases microglial phagocytosis and pro inflammatory cytokine expression. (Linnaetz et al., 2010). In vitro, microglia expressing TREM -2 demonstrated increased phagocytosis of membrane fragments from apoptotic neurons. This effect was also reproduced in experimental autoimmune encephalomyelitis(EAE)following the intravenous administration of TREM-2 in bone marrow precursor cells and was accompanied by a down regulation of tumour necrosis factor (TNFα). A loss of function mutation in both TREM-2 and Draper proteins are associated with a chronic neurodegenerative disease, Nasu-Hakola, characterized by the failure to clear neurotoxic proteins, representing a contributory factor in this form of early onset dementia (Colonna M et al., 2003). The TREM -2 mediated apoptotic response was inhibited by inflammatory signals activating the ITIM (immuno receptor tyrosine based inhibitory motifs) leading to the recruitment src homology 2 (SH) domains of syk protein kinases, preventing phagocytosis and down regulating both the microglial inflammatory and anti -pathogen responses.

7.5 Lectins as PRR in the innate immune response to infection and injury

The lectins are a range of carbohydrate binding proteins and glycoproteins, either homo or hetero oligomers of non -covalently bound, polypeptide units and carbohydrate recognition domains (CRD) that bind to a sugar molecule in a Ca 2+ dependent manner (Cambi et al., 2005). One important role for the lectins is to establish tolerance between bacteria living inside the host through molecular mimicry. Bacteria display surface lectin molecules similar to those present on host cells so bacterial lectins are detected as " self " by the host immune system, allowing them to remain in the gut with mutual benefit to both host and bacteria.

The innate immune response also includes the C- type lectins (acting as PRRs) to detect PAMPS (Endo et al., 2006; Geijten beek et al., 2009). The most important families of lectins are the Pentraxins (extracellular), the Macrophage mannose receptor (MMR) located on the endoplasmic reticulum)(Stahl and Ezowitz 1998), the non classical C-type lectins, dectins 1and 2, expressed by microglia (Brown G et al., 2006) Siglecs (cell membrane)(Crocker and Varki, 2001) and the newly identified C –type lectin member 4E (Clec4) (Sancho et al., 2009). The galectins, expressed by cerebral blood vessels, are an increasingly important family of lectins, functioning as a PRR to detect both intracranial l PAMPs and DAMPs (Sato et al., 2009; Vasa, 2009).

7.6 MMR and DC-SIGN are PRR for "non self", complex carbohydrates

Glia, express trans membrane C- type lectins (Burundi et al., 1999) namely MMR (microglia, astrocytes and peri vascular cells) (Linehan et al., 1999) and DC- SIGN receptor that recognizes "self "intercellular adhesion glycoproteins ICAM. (van Kooyk et al., 2003). The DC-SIGN receptor is expressed by peri vascular cells and a population of dendritic cells, both associated with cerebral blood vessels (Mukhtar et al., 2002; Schwartz et al., 2002; Greter., 2005). MMR and DC- SIGN function as PRRs binding to and internalising viruses by endocytosis, promoting their degradation and antigen presentation to T cells in association with MHC (Stahl et al 1998; van Kooyk et al., 2003).

Both, MMR and DC-SIGN, also recognize "non self" molecules containing a high mannose content (functioning as PAMPs), as found on enveloped viruses. Both MMR and DC-SIGN receptors provide a pathway for a virus to enter the CNS (le Cabec et al., 2005) and this is the case for Dengue (Miller et al 2008), HIV, Ebola and Marburg (both ss RNA Filo viruses), West Nile Fever virus (WNFV), Influenza A, all target MMR (Upham et al 2010.). Whereas, WNV and Ebola virus target the DC- SIGN receptor (Alvarez et al., 2002; Schwartz et al., 2002; Mohameazah et al., 2007)

7.7 Pentraxins

The pentraxins are highly conserved proteins with a cyclic multimeric structure and include the acute phase reactant C protein (CRP) and serum amyloid protein (SAP). Microglia and neurons express CRP and SAP, both of which are capable of opsonising apoptotic cells with subsequent binding to the collectin, C1q, the first C pathway protein to stimulate phagocytosis. (Elward and Gasque 2003; Nauta et al 2003). CRP recognizes apoptotic cells through binding to phosphorylcholine found in oxidized lipids which are regarded as ACAMPs (Chang et al., 2002). Pentraxins, as opsonins, also initiate phagocytosis of apoptotic cells as they are capable of binding directly to microglial Ig (FcγR) receptors and C1q (Chang et al 2002: Nauta et al., 2003) Despite this evidence, the contribution of the pentraxins to the removal of apoptotic cells from the CNS in neurodegenerative and inflammatory disease is yet to be defined.

7.8 Galectins are lectins and PRR with multiple roles

Most galectins are non - glycosylated, soluble proteins, distributed in most mammalian tissues, including the innate and adaptive immune systems (Sato et al., 2010: Vasta 2010). Glactins(previously known as S- type lectins) are expressed by cerebral vessel wall endothelium (Joubert et al., 1998). They are also examples of PRR capable of binding to viruses, bacteria (*Streptococcus pneumonia, Neisseria meningitides, Haemophilus influenza* and fungi *Candida albicans,* the protozoan *Trypanosoma cruzi* and parasite *Toxoplasmosis gondii.* Glactins are able to prevent Nipah virus entry in to endothelial cells by preventing virus fusion with ephrin B2 and B3 receptors on endothelial cell surface (Lo et al., 2010; Garner et al., 2010) However, this protective function of glactein is exploited by the HIV -1 virus, because it binds to glactin -1 and enters host cells. Organs that represent reservoirs for HIV-1 infection express abundant glactin –1 on their cell surface, confirming glactins are " non self" detecting PRR. (Sato 2009).

7.9 Defense collagens or collectins (MBL and SPA)

These are soluble molecules expressed by the liver, lungs and astrocytes (Kuraya et al., 2003; Wagner et al 2003)and include mannose binding lectin (MBL) and Lung surfactant protein A (SPA). Both these collectins are capable of recognizing carbohydrate patterns containing large numbers of mannose and fucose molecules characterized as PAMPs, and found in the cell wall of bacteria and viruses (non self), but not expressed by mammalian cells (Tenner AJ 1999; Elward Gasque 2003). The globular carboxyl C terminal of the defence collagen acts as PRR recognizes PAMPs and potentially ACAMPs, whereas the N -terminal domain links defence collagen to a receptor on phagocytic cells e. g microglia. MBL binds to Ebola and Marburg envelope gylco proteins, preventing these viruses gaining "subversive "entry to the host cell through the DC -SIGN receptor (Ji et al 2005). SPA and MBL are capable of binding to apoptotic cells and neutrophils, functioning as a bridging molecules, between the apoptotic cell and the phagocyte receptor CD91 (Vandivier et al., 2002).

7.10 Siglecs detect sialic residues as markers of "self"

Siglecs (sialic acid -binding immunoglobulin like lectins) are a subgroup of the Ig super family, type 1 membrane proteins with an amino terminal V -set immunoglobulin domain; they represent a family of receptors that detect sialylated glycoproteins and glycolipids (Crocker and Varki 2001 Crocker etal., 2007). Two group of Siglecs can be identified; Siglecs common to mammals Siglec -1(sialoahesin, CD169) (Delputte et al., 2011), Siglec 2 (CD22), myelin associated siglec 4 and those Siglecs related to the CD33 family including siglec -10, 11 and 16 (Lock et al., 2009 Mott et al., 2004). Most siglecs, are present on haemopoietic tissue however, sialoadhesin is expressed only on macrophages as a specific adhesion molecule, whereas siglec -11 is expressed by microglia (Angata et al., 2002). The CD33 family of siglecs are expressed on most mammalian cells, with each siglec having a unique specificity for a sialylated ligands (sialic acid), so there is room for overlapping functions within the family of Siglec receptors (Cao and Crocker 2010). Their main function is the detection of "self " indicated by sialic acid residues and the suppression of inappropriate microglial directed host cell phagocytosis.

7.11 Complement system provides first line defence against pathogens PAMPS, DAMPs and ACAMPs

The C system is an extremely ancient component of the innate immune system. It is thought to have evolved 300 million years ago, as part of the coagulation protein pathway. The complement system comprises of three pathways, the classical, alternative and lectin activated pathways. (Sjoberg et al., 2008; Gasque 2004; Gasque et al., 2000)

The first component of the classical C pathway, C1q, has a multimeric structure, that represents a PRR and is expressed by astrocytes and neurons (Gasque et al., 2000). C1q is able to detect a variety of pathogens, apoptotic cells and neurotoxic misfolded proteins (mutant Prions, fibrillary amyloid), antigen -antibody complexes and DNA (Nauata et al 2002; Korb et al., 1997). The identity of the C1q receptor is not well defined, but candidates include, CD93, expressed by microglia or C1qRp (Dean et al 2000 Webster et al., 2002. ; Elward and Gasque 2003).

The activation of the classical C pathway generates two anaphylotoxins (C3a, C5a) responsible for recruiting inflammatory cells into areas of tissue injury, as welll as opsonins (iC3b and C3) and the cytolytic membrane activation complex (MAC). With regards to pathogens such as bacteria and fungi, the opsonins (C3b and iC3b) coat the pathogen making it a more attractive target for microglia expressing the β2 integrin (CR3 /CR4)receptors (Akiyma and Mc Geer 1990: Ehlers 2000; Reichart et al., 2003). Apoptotic cells contain activated DNA and this enables C1q to directly bind to apoptotic cells, activating the classical C pathway with the generation of opsonins C3b and iC3b, again providing targets for phagocytosis by CR3 and CR4 to reduce host cell damage (Mevorach et al., 1998; Korb et al., 1997). There is also evidence that the Ficolins (lectins) bind to ACAMPs expressed by apoptotic cells, activate complement and generate the opsonin C3, facilitating phagocytosis (Matsushita., 2010)

8. Neurodegeneration; The detection and clearance of Pathogen protein associated molecular patterns (PPAMPS) and innate immune system activation

Neurodegeneration produces neuronal loss and is characterized by intra and extra neuronal accumulation of dangerous(neurotoxic) intrinsic proteins (fibrillary amyloid, mutant prions, α–synuclein, mutant tau) classified as PPAMPs(pathogen protein associated molecular patterns) regarded as a sub type of DAMPS. PPAMPs are detected by a range of PRRs with resulting proinflammatory cytokine expression (Wyss-Coray and Mucke 2002). During chronic CNS inflammation, the accumulation of endogenous protein aggregates is perceived by the innate immune system as "stranger" or "danger" signals (DAMPs). In AD, it has been suggested that a variety of glial related PRR (CD14, TLR, CD36, CD91) with opsonins(C 1q, iC3b, C3) derived from C activation contribute to the removal of Aβ4amyloid fibrils (Coraci et al., 2002: Elkhoury et al., 2003; Fassbender et al., 2004; Alarcon et al 2005: Tahara et al., 2006; Landreth et al., 2009)The SR, CD36, facilitates the assembly of a heteromeric complex composed of CD36, TLR4 and TLR6 following binding to Aβ 4 (Stewart et al., 2010).

Aβ fibrils can activate microglia and astrocytes through TLR4 (together with CD14 and MD2 in microglia), leading to the activation of downstream inflammatory response genes (Reed - Geaghan et al., 2009; Walter et al., 2007; Chen et al., 2006: Lehnardt et al., 2003, Bamberger et al., 2003). This explanation is consistent with mice carrying a nonfunctional TLR4 crossed with a mouse model of AD (APP/PS1 double transgenic mice) having a lower level of inflammatory cytokines than wild type animals (Walter et al., 2007; Jin et al., 2008). A TLR4 polymorphism was shown to be associated with protection against late-onset AD in an Italian population, suggesting that theTLR4–mediated innate immune inflammation could influence AD pathology (Minorettiet al., 2006). TLR2 also may be a sensor for fibrillar Aβ (Chen K et al., 2006; Jana et al 2008). Blocking TLR2 signaling with antibody or by knockdown of the receptor gene *in vitro* suggested that TLR2 stimulation by Aβ promotes neurotoxic inflammation. However, mice lacking TLR2 crossed with APP/PS1 transgenic AD mice were reported to show a delay in Aβ deposition and improved behavior on memory tests (Richard et al., 2008) These apparently contradictory functions of TLR could be due to differences in the cell types as well as signaling pathways that are engaged by the amyloid peptides and/or fibrils. (Tahara et al., 2006)

NOD-like receptors (NLRs) are also involved in Aβ-induced inflammatory response. In AD, Aβ oligomers and fibrils induce lysosomal damage and trigger NALP3, a member of the NLR family that is expressed in microglia (Halle et al., 2008) NALPs activate downstream signaling proteins, such as ASC and this will lead to caspase 1 activation and increased processing of proinflammatory mediators like IL-1β and IL-18.

Fibrillary amyloid and aggregated forms of mutant prion protein are opsonized by complement components (C1q, C3) to promote clearance by macrophages and microglia CR3/CR4(Tenner 2001: Kovacs et al., 2004). In AD as the result of C1q binding to fibrillary Aβ4, the C pathway is activated increasing C3 and C5 as part of the protective response promoting clearance of the amyloid plaque (Mc Geer et al., 1989; Jian et al., 1994; Eikelenboom et al., 2002); inhibition of the complement cascade increased amyloid plaque burden (Wyss Coray and Mucke., 2002). However, in the context of acute inflammation, microglia and astrocytes express complement and it is plausible C activation on myelin/ neuronal debris contributes to secondary brain injury. The formation of the MAC and non-specific binding to host cells would cause bystander damage.

In Huntington's disease the expression of C1q, C3, iC3b and C4 is increased on microglia and astrocytes, C activation is also present in experimental models of ischaemia (van Beek et al., 2000; van Beek et al., 2001: Singhrao et al., 1999). Interestingly, administration of a C1q inhibitor C1-INH, resulted in neuron protection after experimental ischaemia, but its protective effect was interpreted as independent of C1q activation of the complement pathway (De Simoni et al., 2004).

A further sensing system for Aβ, is provided by RAGE (receptor for advanced glycation endproducts) a PRR and trans membrane receptor of the immunoglobulin super family RAGE is expressed on the surface of microglia, astrocytes, vascular endothelial cells, and particularly on neurons (Fang F et al 2010). Several reports suggest that Aβ peptide as well as Aβ oligomers bind to RAGE and contributing to the activation of microglia and the production of proinflammatory mediator (Yan et al., 2006). RAGE is also suggested to play an important role in the clearance of Aβ4 and to be involved in cellular processing and signaling (Origlia et al, 2008; Takuma et al 2009). The role of the SRs, CD36, CD14 and particularly CD91, in AD is ambiguous; studies indicate that CD91 has the capacity to influence both the production and the clearance of Aβ. CD91 is a receptor for APP, apoE, and α2M, which all have been genetically linked to AD (. Bu, 2006). Clearance of Aβ complexed to these ligands could contribute to a reduction in amyloid plaque burden (Herz et al., 2001).

8.1 Phagocytosis of apoptotic cells (altered self) reduces local inflammation (the non phlogistic response)

Apoptotic cells result from the consquences of infection, ischaemic infarction and neurodegeneration; they express a range of apoptotic cell associated molecular patterns or ACAMPs on their surface. In general phagocytosis of apoptotic cells reduces local tissue inflammation, as the so called "non pholgistic response", providing some degree of local immunoregulation. (Chan et al., 2001: Chang et al., 2001; Magus et al., 2002; Griffith set al., 2009. The result of clearing apoptotic cells reduces local inflammation (non phlogistic response) and this is in contrast to the increase inflammatory response, following attempted clearance of pathogens (phlogistic response). The clearance of apoptotic cells by CD14 is anti-inflammatory (non phlogistic) as it binds to and switches off T cells (Gold1991), releases the anti-inflammatory cytokines TGFβ and prostaglandin E2, together with growth factors such as Vascular endothelial growth factor (VEGF), all reducing local inflammation and promoting tissue repair (Griffiths., 2009 et al, Golpon HA et al., 2004, Huynh et al., 2002, Voll R et al., 1997)

ACAMPs include nucleic acids and sugars, the best characterized ACAMPs are, phosphatidyl serine (PS) and calreticulin (Fadok et al., 2000: Hoffman et al 2001; Gardai et al., 2005; Gardai et al., 2006).

Glia and macrophages express PRRs that recognize ACAMPS, including the PS receptor (PSR), CD14 (in conjunction with ICAM), LRP, CD36, the soluble bridging molecules milk - fat gobulin (MFG -EGF 8), growth arrest –specific gene 6, and TREM-2 (Prieto et al., 1999, Gregory 2000; Hanayama et al., 2002; Leonardi –Essman et al., 2005 Gardaiet al., 2006). Thrombospondin, a protein expressed by glia, acts as a bridging molecule between an as yet undefined ligand on the apoptotic cell and CD36, to promote phagocytic clearance (Lamy et al., 2007). PS on apoptotic cells and IgM both bind to C1q to activate C pathway and opsonin (C3b iC3b) synthesis, to provide targets for CR3 and CR4 (Kim et al., 2002).

Animals deficient in C1q accumulate apoptotic cells, resulting in glomerulonephritis and an (SLE)- like disease, because the accumulated DNA and RNA both function as DAMPs and trigger autoimmune inflammation (Botto et al 1998). Activated microglial and Kolmer cells in the choroid plexus (Singhrao et al., 1999) express C3R /CR4 and both detect C1q, C3b, C3b as well as MBL, underlining the importance of glia for removing apoptotic cells opsonised with C from the CSF (Mevorach et al., 1998; Reichart et al., 2003). The lectins, Ficolins and MBL, are capable of interacting with ACAMPs such as calcireticulin, to initiate clearance of apoptotic cells (Ogden et al., 2001).

Phagocytes involved in apoptotic cell clearance also express, the T cell immunoglobulin domain mucin domain protein 4 receptor (TIM4) and the TAM receptors (Tyro2, Axland Mer) which bind to Gas 6 both are expressed by neurons (Lemke and Rothlin 2008). These receptors regulate the effects of TLR mediated response by inducing the expression of Suppressor of Cytokine Signalling proteins (SOCS 1 and 3), a family of intracellular inducible proteins, that inhibit cytokine synthesis. (Baker et al., 2009).

8.2 Neuroimmunoregulatory molecules (NIRegs) regulate the innate immune response and prevents inappropriate activation

One basic property of the NIRegs is their expression by host cells, but neither by pathogens nor by apoptotic cells. NIRegs interact with either macrophages or microglia to provide immuno regulation, promoting a reduction in the severity of inflammation and facilitating tissue repair (Hoarau et al., 2011).

Examples of NIRegs, include CD200 and CD47; these two molecules both represent "don't eat me" signals cells, to prevent un warranted phagocytosis, whereas the Siglecs detect sialic acid (a "don't eat me" signal) on host cells resulting in immuno regulation and inhibition of microglial activation. CRProteins modulate complement activation whereas, the the CD24/siglec 10 pathway inhibits DAMPs initiated inflammatory response (Chen et al., 2009). see table 2, for a summary of the current NIreg s.

8.3 Complement regulatory proteins (CRP) as NIRegs

To avoid self-destruction, host cells employ a range of regulatory molecules, including the CRP, which inhibit assembly of either the C3-cleaving enzymes or the formation of the membrane attack complex (MAC) on host cell surface. As pathogens lack these inhibitors, activation of the complement cascade can proceed and results in lysis or phagocytosis of microbial intruders. (Zipfle and Skerka 2009). However, animals deficient in CRP are also likely to experience severe inflammation, because unregulated activation of the C system will generate C3a and C5a, both anaphylatoxins(chemotaxis of macrophages and neutrophils) with uncontrolled activation of MAC.

Similarly, as "self" cells progress to "altered self" (apoptotic cells), there is a down-regulation of complement inhibitors (including CRP) at the cell surface including a low sialic acid content and the loss of the CRP, FH(Crocker and Verki 2001). The loss of CRP based membrane inhibitors, such as CD46, can lead to moderate and limited opsinonisation of apoptotic cells with the complement proteins (C3b, iC3b) with the promotion of phagocytosis by CR3/CR4. (Elward et al., 2005)

The soluble C1 inhibitor (C1-INH), C4b-binding protein (C4bp), factor H (fH), factor I (fI), S protein (Sp) and clusterin are all CRP, expressed by glia and neurons (Gasque 2004). C4bp is an important NIReg, because it is able to inhibit the DAMP effect of DNA released from necrotic cells and has been detected upon amyloid plaques in AD, potentially limiting C activation (Torouw et al., 2007; Torouw et al., 2005).

The other CRP are expressed on the cell membrane and include two trans membrane proteins CR1, membrane cofactor protein (MCP, CD46) and two GPI-anchored proteins, Decay Accelerating Factor (DAF, CD55) and CD59 (see comprehensive review Zipel and Skerka., 2009). Moreover, since CD55 is a ligand for CD97 on macrophages it is tantalizing to speculate that CD55-CD97 interactions could play an important role regulating phagocytosis (Hamann et al., 1996).

FH, CD55 and CD59, fulfill the criteria for an NIReg given that they are broadly expressed and extremely important in the control of complement activation on self-cells. Neurons also express NIRegs in the form of the CRP, Factor H. This CRP is able to reduce axonal degeneration (self injury) in a MOG induced EAE model, as the result of inhibiting C pathway activation. (Griffiths et al., 2009)

8.4 Siglecs are an emerging NIReg

The Siglecs, are expressed by monocytes, microglia and macrophages; they have a potentially important immuno regulatory function in the CNS (Linnartz et al., 2010) The absence of sialic acid expression on micro-organsims or apoptotic cells is detected by siglecs as a signal of "missing self "and this promotes phagocytosis (Crocker and Virki 2001). To emphasize the importance of sialic acid residues as a signal of "self", over twenty, pathogens have evolved the capacity to synthesize or capture sialic acids, providing molecular mimics of host ("self ") and thus avoiding detection by their host (Jones et al., 2003). This possibility is supported by evidence showing Group B Streptocci with siaylated surface molecules bind to neutrophils expressing siglec 9, with reduction in their killing response aiding the survival of bacteria (CaoCrocker 2010).

The CD33 related sub-family of Siglecs (includes human Siglec 10, Siglec 11, Siglec 16) and the CD22 related Siglecs, both signal through cytosolic ITIM (immuno receptor tyrosine based inhibitory motifs) that provide inhibitory regulation of receptor pathways (Crocker and Varki 2003; Lemke and Rothlin 2008). This association strengths the potential NIReg regulatory role for both CD33 and CD22 siglecs on the basis of their capacity to detect sialylated glycans (α-2, 6 α–2, 3 and α–2, 8 linked sialic acids) representing markers of" self "on host cells.

The interaction between CD22 and B cells results in a phosphorylation of ITIMS with the recruitment of the Src homology 2 domain -containing protein tyrosine phophatases(SHP-1 and SHP-2 proteins) with a down regulation of inflammatory signalling. (Crocker 2007).

Cortical neurons express high levels of CD 22 and on ligation with microglial CD45 it reduced LPS induced microglial expression of TNF–α acting as a negative regulator of microglial cytokine release (Mott et al., 2004). Siglec 11, expressing microglia have a reduced neurotoxic capacity and fail to phagocytose apoptotic material in micro glial- neuron co culture experiments. (Wang et al., 2010: Toguchi et al 2009).

CD33 related Siglecs inhibit cell proliferation, negatively regulate TLR, increase apoptosis and reduce IFN production, again through ITIM signalling pathways (Cao and Crocker 2010). The absence of sialic acid in the cell wall of a pathogen will prevent the interaction with CD22, CD33, resulting in the failure to promote an ITIM related inhibitory response with an increased host " protective " inflammatory response (Crocker 2010). The presence of sialic acid residues defines host cell as "self" and initiates an inhibitory signal to down regulate any inflammatory response and prevent inappropriate phagocytosis of host cells. A further immunoregulatory role for Siglecs is their inhibitory response to TLR signalling activated by DAMPs.

8.5 CD24/siglec 10; an NIReg pathway that regulates DAMPS and reduces tissue injury

The successful resolution of pathogen invasion of the CNS requires the detection of PAMPs and also DAMPs released by tissue injury. HMBG, S100 and HSP are all examples of a DAMPand released from cells after injury. The innate immune system can be activated by DAMPs as a consequence of being detected by a RAGE and TLRs and triggering the TLR - MyD88 -NFkB pathway (Liu et al., 2009). Of interest, is the relatively low level inflammatory response elicted by DAMPs, raising the possibility that DAMPS are capable of regulating the inflammatory response.

One pathway, capable of imunoregulating DAMPS involves, CD24, a heat stable antigen and GPI anchored protein, that binds to HMBG, reducing the pro inflammatory properties of this DAMP. Two lines of evidence support the regulatory role of CD24; individuals with polymorphisms of CD24 appear to at risk of developing so called autoimune disease involving inflammation and when T cells are introduced into CD24 deficient mice, they undergo rapid proliferation. Furthermore CD24, is expressed in the developing CNS and by stem cells; although not fully characterized, it is known to regulate cell proliferation and neuritic outgrowth (Kleene et al., 2001: Shewan et al., 1996).

CD24 detect s DAMPs, but not PAMPS and the CD24- DAMP complex binds to the Siglec 10, which has an ITIM motif and recruits SHP-1 SHP-2 and SHIP complexes. The presence of

Siglec 10- SHIP-1 compex inhibits the DAMP-TLR /NLR based activation of the NF-kB pathway, reducing DAMP activated inflammatory cytokine expression. PAMP activation of the TLR -MyD88 -Nf-kB pathway remains intact and inflammatory cytokines are synthesised. This proposed pathway, based upon CD24 binding to DAMPS, but not PAMPS, allows the host to regulate endogenous protein activation of inflammation following infection and neuro degeneration, adding a further protective pathway to reduce the severity of tissue injury.

Mice deficient in the human homologue of siglec 10 have an increased proinflammatory response to pathogens (Chen et al., 2009). Further evidence, that the CD24/siglec 10 interaction presents an NIReg pathway is the inhibition of the inflammatory response initiated by the DAMPS, HSP 70 and HSP90 (Liu et al., 2009). The CD24 /Siglec 10 pathway represent an NIReg pathway capable of regulating endogenous DAMPs released during injury, neurodegeneration and infection. (Liu et al 2009; Hoarau et al., 20011)

8.6 CD200-200R an NIReg pathway for evasion of phagocytosis

CD200, is a well defined member of the NIRegs family it is expressed by reactive astrocytes; its counter receptor, C200R is expressed by microglia and perivascular macrophages (Barclay et al., 2002; Broderick et al., 2002 Lyons et al., 2007). The interaction between CD200 and CD200R results in down regulation of microglial phagcocytosis, preventing "self" attack (Barclay et al., 2002: Hoek et al., 2000). CD200 is a 41-47kD surface molecule and a member of the immunoglobulin Ig supergene family, characterized by two IgSF domains (Barclay et al., 2002; Wright et al., 2001). It is a highly conserved and found in invertebrates and vertebrates; like many of the glycoproteins containing this molecular arrangement they are involved with regulation of the immune system.

In the brain CD200, is expressed by microglia, cerebellar and retinal neurons, together with vascular endothelium. (Broderick et al., 2002). The counter receptor to CD200, CD200R, also contains two IgSF domains and is expressed by myeloid cells and brain microglia (Koning et al., 2009; Koning et al., 2007). In CD200 deficient mice, the number of activated microglia and macrophages were more numerous after an experimental lesion, as compared to wild type animals, providing evidence that the CD200/CD200R interaction is related to regulation of microglial activation and regulation of local inflammation (Hoek et al., 2000). This interpretation is supported by experiments in CD200 -/-mice inoculated with myelin oligodendrocyte glycoprotein MOG peptide to induce EAE. In these experiments the severity of the EAE was increased owing to the loss of CD200 regulation of microglial activity (Hoeket al., 2000). The contribution made by the CD200 (astrocytes)-CD200R (microglia) interaction on microglia in MS and AD remains to be established, although evidence for a dysregulation of CD200-CD200R pathway as a contributory factor to increase the severity of inflammation in MS has been proposed (Koning et al., 2009).

8.7 CD47-C172 an NIReg pathway as a marker of " self" or "don't eat me".

CD47, is expressed by astrocytes, neurons, macrophages and endothelium. The interaction between CD47 with the counter receptor CD172a, down regulates microglial activity, complement activation and cytokine expression, overall reducing the severity of the inflammatory response (deVries et al., 2002 Reinholdet al., 1995)

CD47 has five trans membrane regions with alternatively spliced isoforms of CD47 having a tissue specific expression, form 2 is present in bone marrow, whereas form 4 is highly expressed in brain (Reinhold et al., 1995). CD47, has two counter receptors; CD172a is expressed by myeloid cells, microglia and neurons a plasma membrane protein with three Ig domains in its extracellular component (Brown et al., 2001) and thrombospondin TSP (Lamy et al., 2007).

The interaction between CD47 with CD172a, recruits tyrosine phosphotases SHP-1 and SHP-2, with down regulation of macrophage phagocytosis, complement activation and cytokine synthesis including (Vernon -Wilson et al 2001: Brown et al., 2001: Oldenborg et al., 2001: Seiffertet al., 2001. The protective activity of CD47 could also be extended to its beneficial role in supporting neural development and promoting clearance of amyloid fibrils, albeit by mechanisms that remain ill-characterized (Bamberger et al., 2003).

The interaction between CD47 and CD172a has been shown to reduce neutrophil migration across endothelium and blocking CD47 induced expression of inflammatory cytokines by dendritic cells. CD47 is capable of inducing apoptosis in both T cells and cells deficient in CD47 i. e. loss of "self" identity, these cells are subsequently cleared rapidly from the systemic circulation by the spleen. (Oldenborg et al., 2001). The interaction between CD47 and thrombospondin promotes apoptosis of activated T cells, therefore, reducing inflammation by terminating T cell activation (Lamy et al., 2007: Sarati et al., 2008).

Hence, CD47, represents an important "don't eat me signal", preventing inappropriate phagocytosis of host cells (Elward and Gasque 2003). Apoptotic cells rapidly loose CD47, reducing its ability to bind and phosphorylate CD172a to recruit inhibitory signals and increasing their clearance through phagocytosis. The presence of CD47 on neurons and T cells is capable of promoting apoptosis through the CD95/Fas and caspase independent pathways (Manna et al., 2005). In MS, CD47, but not CD172a expression, is reduced at the edge of a chronic plaque, contributing to the loss of immuno regulation of microglia in this chronic inflammatory disease(Koning et al 2009).

The finding that viable cells are readily ingested if 'don't eat me signals' are disrupted raises the intriguing possibility that recognition and removal by phagocytosis is a default process that is actively prevented by inhibitory ligands on viable cells. Whether or not the CD47-CD172a pathway is capable of regulating microglial activity in disease remains to be determined. (Hoarau et al., 2011)

9. Emerging NIRegs; semaphorins and suppressor of cytokine signalling proteins (SOCS)

9.1 Semaphorins and microglia represent a potential pathway to regulate the host inflammatory response

The semaphorins are a diverse group of highly conserved trans membrane and extra cellular proteins with an extra cellular, 500 amino acid cysteine rich, semaphorine domains. Semaphorins bind to a diverse range of receptors; in the brain, plexins and neuropilins whereas in the immune system, the C -type lectin, CD72 is expressed mainly by T cells, but also on DC and macrophages. The functional importance of the semaphorins was initially directed towards control of axon growth, but it is now apparent these molecules are important immuno regulators in the CNS (Takegahara et al., 2005).

The interaction between Sema 4D (originally CD100), a trans membrane semaphorine, and the immune system CD72 results in an increased expression of cytokines by B cells, because Sema 4D turns off the inhibitory ITIM associated pathway (Suzuki et al., 2008). In the CNS microglia are activated by Sema 4D binding to plexin B1, rather than the CD72 molecule that is also expressed by microglia (Okuno et al; 2009)

Interestingly, plexin B1 and Sema 4D deficient mice are resistant to EAE induced by MOG derived peptide, because of the failure to generate MOG –specific T cells, emphasising the importance of functional Sema 4D for T cell activation and differentiation within the CNS (Takegahara et al., 2005). Antibodies raised against Sema 4D reduced inflammation during EAE, this was explained as the result of blocking T cells expressing Sema 4D interacting with microglial plexin to promote expression of pro inflammatory cytokines (Okuno et al., 2009).

In contrast to the other NIReg pathways, Sema 4D, increases the host inflammatory response by upregulating the level of cytokine expression and microglial activation. The regulation provided by Sema4D ensures the host inflammatory response is approporiate to counter the effects of pathogens and neurtoxic proteins. Conversly inhibition of the SEMA 4D-plexin pathway represents a potential new target to suppress and regulate neuro inflammation.

9.2 Suppressor of cytokine signalling proteins (SOCS)

SOCS, are a family of eight intracellular, cytokine inducible proteins, expressed by CNS cells (microglia, astrocytes and neurons) that inhibit IFN signalling in CNS cells (Baker etal., 2010). Through activation of STAT transcription factors the C terminal of the SOCS binds to and inhibits phosphorylated tyrosine residues on Janus kinases (JAK), in addition the of the N terminus contains a kinase inhibitory region, and this also inhibits INF synthesis and blocks the NF-kB pathway. In the brain, SOCS1 and 3 are induced by a variety of inflammatory cytokines including INF$\gamma$and LPS. Overall, SOCS 1and 3 are examples of NIRegs because they block the JAK/STAT pathway regulating glial and neuron inflammatory cytokine synthesis.

SOCS1 and SOCS3 have potentially important clinical applications. Administration of SOCS-1 to experimental animals prevents EAE by inhibiting JAK-2 mediated phosphorylation reducing the expression of inflammatory cytokines IL-2, IL -5 and TNFα raising the possibility that SOCS-1 is a potential therapeutic agent to treat inflammatory mediated demyelination (Baker et al 2010)Furthermore, the level of SOCS 3 exppressed by T cells in relapsed MS was less than in remission and this correlated with STAT levels, such that reduced SOCS allowed STAT to rise increasing inflammatory cytokine levels and increasing the likelihood of relapse. (Baker et al 2009 for review of clinical studies involving SOCS)

9.3 Loss of immuno surveillance, NIRegs and CNS neoplasia

Glioblastoma (GBM), is the most common primary brain tumour in adults, it is highly aggressive and infiltrates throughout the brain. These tumours have developed the capacity to escape immune surveillance by suppressing the host anti -glioma response. Failure to promote an anti glioma response is associated with an accumulation of immunosuppressive, CD4-Fox P3+ regulatory T cells, both within and surrounding the tumour (Sonabend et al.,

2008). Glioma stem cells and macrophages are also capable of inducing immuno supression in host microglia, because they express the anti -inflammatory cytokines TGF-1β MIC-1macrophage inhibitory factor and also inhibit microglial phagocytosis (Wu et al., 2010; Hussain et al., 2006). A pivotal role in this apparent loss of anti- glioma response is the inhibition of the JAK/STAT signalling pathway in glioma cells with resulting cell proliferation, inhibition of both host cell inflammatory response and tumour immuno surveillance (Brantley et al., 2008). The inhibition of STAT signalling pathway in GBM is thought to result from an over expression of the NIReg, SOCS -1that inhibits STAT and function as an immuno-modulatory molecule by blocking IFNβ and CD40, with the down regulation of both MHC I and II expression in GBM. However, the function role of the other SOCS proteins (SCOCS- 3) in GBM remains to be clarified; in vitro SOCS -3 increases the IL-10 mediated anti-inflammatory response and radio resistance, but therapeutic inhibition of STATalso promotes microglial recognition of glioma cells (Baker et al., 2009).

Glioma cells express a limited range of TLR and application of various ligands including LPS and Poly I; C did not have any therapeutic effect, probably due to the failure to stimulate intra tumour Antigen Presenting Cells. (Grauner et al., 2008. However, the injection of the TLR9 ligand, CpG, an oligonucleotide, resulted in effective anti glioma response with inhibition of local Tregs, together with an T effector cell mediated anti - glioma respons. TLR9 is not present in host cells surrounding the glioma, providing an explanation for the apparent failure of host cell to produce an effective T cell response (Grauner et al., 2008). The intra tumour injection of ligands such as CpG to selectively stimulate host expression of TLR is of potential therapeutic importance.

One further protective strategy employed by gliomas to evade imuno surveillance is the expression of C regulator proteins. Activation of C pathway is potentially able to lyse tumour cells, but several glioma cells lines have been shown to express complement regulators CD59, CD55, CD46 and FH on their cell surface, preventing C attack and generation of lytic MAC(Maenpaa A et al., 1996, Junnikkala S et al., 2000). One possible therapeutic route is infact, the use of surface CD46, this Creg is very similar to the adenovirus receptors (adenovirus serotype 3) and provides a target to deliver an adenovirus containing anti- glioma therapy. (Ulasov et al 2006)

Outside the CNS, squamous cell carcinoma of the skin, leukaemias and myeloma cells up regulate surface expression of the NIReg, CD200, and this inhibits local immune detection promoting metastatic potential. After spreading to local lymph nodes, metastatic tumour cells that are CD200+ interact with local CD200R+ myeloid drived cells such as macrophages and potentially microglia, enhancing their survival, conversely loss of CD200 reduces metastatic tumour survival. The expression of CD200 is a property of the primary tumour and this expression did not vary according the type of tissue infiltrated by metastatic tumour (Stumpova et al., 2010).

10. Conclusion

The host inflammatory reaction is required to counter the detrimental effects of pathogen invasion (encephalitis and meningitis) and the accumulation of amyloid, mutant prions (neurodegenerative disease). One consequence of the host's protective inflammatory reaction is an inevitable amount of associated tissue injury. The detrimental effects of tissue injury have to be to be balanced against the, consequences of not removing a pathogen (or clearing neurotoxic proteins), usually this leads to peristent inflammation preventing any tissue repair. This balance between protective and destructive consquences is the so called "double edged sword"effect, that accompanies brain inflammation (Wyss- Coray and Mucke 2002). The role of the NIRegs is to modulate the level of the protective inflammatory response, in order to provide the "appropriate amount " of inflammation to allow the efficent clearance of pathogens and neurotoxic proteins from the brain.

The immune response against "non self" (pathogens, neurotoxic protiens) must be critically regulated in order to provide conditions of tissue repair without excessive destruction of "self "or host cells. Self (host) must be distinguish from " non –self "as defined by, pathogens PAMPs, apoptotic cells ACAMPs and "danger proteins" (HMGB1, HSP and S100) classified as (DAMPs). Non self (PAMPS, DAMPS), is detected by a range of intracellular and trans membrane PRR (TLR, RIG, NDLR,) whereas the scavenger receptors CD14, CD36, C lectins and TREM-2 provide a clerance pathway for apoptotic cells and neurotoxic proteins. Activation of the complement pathway by pathogens and neurotoxic proteins (Fibrillary Amyloid and mutant prion protein) results in MAC formation and anaphylotoxins C3a and C5a, all promoting inflammation and tissue destruction. The C pathway also assists the SR clear apoptotic cells through opsonins C3 and C4 localization on the surface of apoptotic cells.

To prevent excessive host tissue destruction, (NIRegs) must control the proinflammatory response and efficiently clear apoptotic cells (non-phlogistic response), before they are able to release neurotoxic enzymes to increase host tissue destruction. NIRegs, provide cell surface signals (CD200, CD47, sialic acid, CD46,) to identify "self " and through interaction with counter receptors (CD200R, CD172a, FH, Siglecs, CD24 –Siglec,) utilizing ITAM /ITIM pathways, inhibit microglial activation and phagocytosis of host cells. The C pathway is regulated by a series of CRP also regarded as NIRegs, because they reduce C activation and excessive host tissue destruction. The inhibiton of CRPs on tumour cells could provide a mechanism to increase host anti -tumour cell lysis as well as providing receptors for the delivery of viruses carrying anti glioma reagents. One emerging pathway controls, microglial activation as the result of T cells expressing Sema 4D; inhibiton of this pathway resulted in a down regulation of the severity of inflammation in MOG induced EAE. Similarly, the contribution made by the SOCS family of intracellular proteins to regulating the innate immune response in a diverse range of neuroinflammatory conditions requires clarification.

The therapeutic benefit of NIRegs is apparent, but to date, there is only limited evidence for their influence in clinical examples of neuro-degneration and neuro-inflammation. CD200-CD200R, CD47 and SOCS have been detected in MS tissue providing evidence for dys regulation of the host inflammatory response. There is some experimental evidence to show PAMPS and DAMPs can be distinguished by the host and DAMP initiated inflammation is regulated by the emerging NIReg, CD24/Siglec, pathway. The cellular localization and functional importance for each of the NIRegs is summarised in table 2.

It is highly likely the NIRegs provide a range of potentially important therapeutic reagents that selectively regulate the host immune response and promote tissue repair in a variety of brain infections (viral and bacterial), neurodegerative diseases and neoplasia. The opportunity presented by the NIRegs as the means to selectively regulate the CNS immune response to a wide range of pathogens and neurotoxic proteins should be exploited as a matter of some importance.

Pattern Recognition Receptor PRR	Ligand detected	PRR and CNS cell expression	Function	Host Innate immune response
TLR2	Bacterial cell wall peptidoglycan Zymosan (Fungi) Haemagluttin (Measles virus)	Microglia Astrocytes Choroid plexus	Form hetero dimres with TLR-1 to detect Gram neg ative bacteria Co operates with Dectin -1to detect fungi	Microglia increased pro inflammatory cytokines Phagocytosis
TLR3	ds RNA	Neurons microglia astrocytes oligodendroglia	West Nile Virus Detect necrosis and danger signals (HMGB, HSP)	Microglial IFNβ TNFα IL-6 Systemic cytokines and BBB receptor
TLR4	Bacteria Lipopolysacahride LPS	Microglia, astrocytes ependyma Choroid plexus	Cooperates with CD36, CD14 and DC-SIGN to detect fungi and *Streptococcus pneumonia*	Microglia and astrocyte inflammatory cytokines phagocytosis of apoptotic cells
TLR 5	Flagellin, bacterial protein	Macrophage		
TLR7	ssRNA	Microglia, astrocytes ependyma, neurons	Influenza A Detect necrosis and "danger signal "HMGB, HSP	Astrocytes increased TNFα IFNβ MCP-1
TLR8	ssRNA	Neurons	RNA viruses	Astrocytes increased TNF α, IFNβ, MCP-1
TLR9	CpG DNA	Microglia, astrocytes	Detect necrosis and "danger signals" HMBG-1	Microglia express TNFα, IL-12, NO HMBG-1 /RAGE detected by TLR-9
TLR11	Profilin, bacterial protein	Genitourinary Neurons	Detects Toxoplasmosis Neurocysticerosis	Inflammatory cytokines
RIG-1	Short dsRNA	Microglia, astrocytes	Japanese encephalitis virus Influenza A, Ebola virus	Astrocytes express IFNβ, IL-6, IL-8 RANTES
MDA-5	Long dsRNA	Microglia astrocytes	?Nipah virus, polio virus,	Microglia express IFNβ
NOD like	Bacterial cell wall		*Listeria bacillius Shigella*	

Receptors NOD-1 and NOD-2		?Microglia, astrocytes	*Flexneri* *Helicobacter pylori* *Mycobacterium tuberculosis*	
NLR -3 (NLP-3)	Bacterial cell wall peptidglycan peptidoglycan and virus proteins	? in CNS	Bacteria Viruses Crohn's disease	Inflammasome(NLR ASC, procaspase -1) is engaged to produce inflammatory cytokines

Table 1. Shows the individual ligands detected by TLR and Non- TLR (R LR MDA and NLR), Pattern Recognition Receptors PRR in the CNS. The cellular distribution of each of these receptors in the CNS is provided together with their contribution to host CNS innate immune system in response to pathogens(PAMPS and danger signals (DAMPS).

Neuroimmuoregulatory (NIReg)	**NIReg- receptor/ligand**	**Cell -cell interaction**	**Mechanism of immune regulation**	**Human disease**
CD200 Astrocyte	CD200R microglia	Astrocyte - microglia	Reduce phagocytosis	Alzheimer's (AD) Multiple sclerosis (MS)
CD47 Astrocyte Endothelium neuron	CD172a myeloid cells microglia	Astrocyte - microglia	Reduce phagocytosis and cytokine expression	Multiple sclerosis
Complement regulators FH, CD46, CD55, CD59 C4bp CD46 (MCP) CD55(DAF)	Sialic acid Complement proteins	Astrocytes Microglia Neurons	Reduce C activation	Neurodegenerative disease AD Huntington's disease Inhibits complement regulation of glioma lysis
Siglecs CD33 family Siglec 10 Siglec 11	Sialic acid Detect absence of sialic acids " non self"	NK cells Microglia	Reduces inflammation ITIM pathway	Bacterial infection; bacteria mimic sialic acids to become " self "
CD24 -Siglec 10 pathway	DAMPs HMGB-1	microglia stem cells	Binds with SHP - 1, this complex inhibits DAMPS activation of NF-kB	Reduces DAMP associated inflammation Polymorphisms in CD24 associated with autoimmune disease
Suppressor of cytokine synthesis SOCS1 SOCS3	Inhibits IFN and IL cytokine stimulation of cytokine expression	Microglia astrocytes neurons	Blocks JAK/STAT cytokine pathway	Glioblastoma SOCS increased SOCS reduced in relapsed MS

Thrombomodulin CD141	HMBG1/ DAMPS	Microglia	Blocks HMBG binding to RAGE and TLR activation	
Semaphorin SEMA4	CD72 on T cells Plexin B1 on microglia	T cell with microglia	Blocks ITIM increases cytokine expression	Sema4D deficiency reduced EAE severity

Table 2. The potential of NIRegs and their cellular localization, ligands and mechanism whereby they produce immuno regulation. In the final column there is information relating to their contribution to infection, neurodegeneration and neuro inflammation as well as neoplasia, in the human CNS.

11. References

Abbot, NJ. Morphology of non mammalian glial cells; functional implications. Chapter 4. in Neuroglia ed Kettleman H, Ransom BR. Oxford University Press 1995

Abeyama, K, D. M Stren, Y Ito, K Kawahara, Y. Yoshimoto, M. Tanka, T. Uchmura, N. Ida, Y. Yamakazi, S. Ymada, Y. Yamamoto, H. Yamamoto, S, Iino, N Taniguchi I. Maruyama. 2005. The terminal domain of thrombomodulin sequesters high mobility group B-1 protein, a novel anit inflammatory mechanism. J Clin. Invest. 115: 1267-1274.

Akira, S, S. Uematsu, O. Takeuchi. 2006. Pathogen recognition and innate immunity. Cell 124: 783-801.

Akiyma, H, Mc Geer. 1990. Brain microglia constitutively express beta -2 integrins. J Neuroimmunology. ; 39: 81-93.

Alexopoulou, L., A. C. Holt, R. Medzhitov, and R. A. Flavell. 2001. Recognition of double-stranded RNA and activation of NF-kappaB by Toll- like receptor 3. Nature 413: 732-738. 39.

Alarcon R, C. Fuenzalida, M. Santibanez, and R von Bernardi. 2005. Expression of scavenger receptors in glial cells. Comparing the adhesion of astrocytes and microglia from neonatal rats to surface bound beta amyloid. J Biol Chem. ; 280: 30406- 30415.

Alvarez, C., , F. Lasala, J. Carrillo, O. Munz, A. L. Corbi and R. Delgado. 2002. C Type le ctins DC In-SIGN and L-SIGN mediate cellular entry y Ebola virus in *cis* and *trans*. J Virol 76 (13); 6841-6844.

Angata, T., S. C. Kerr, D. R. Greaves, N. M. Varki, P. R. Crocker, and A. Varki. 2002. Cloning and characterization of human Siglec-11. A recently evolved signaling that can interact with SHP-1 and SHP-2 and is expressed by tissue macrophages, including brain microglia. J Biol Chem 277: 24466-24474.

Babcock, A. A., M. Wirenfeldt, T. Holm, H. H. Nielsen, L. Dissing-Olesen, H. Toft-Hansen, J. M. Millward, R. Landmann, S. Rivest, B. Finsen, and T. Owens. 2006. Toll-like receptor 2 signaling in response to brain injury: an innate bridge to neuroinflammation. J Neurosci 26: 12826-12837

Baker, B. J. L. Nowoslawski -Akhtar and E. N. Benveniste. 2009. SOCS1 and SOCS3 in the control of CNS immunity. TIMS 30 (8): 392-400

Bamberger, M. E., M. E. Harris, D. R. McDonald, J. Husemann, and G. E. Landreth. 2003. A cell surface receptor complex for fibrillar beta-amyloid mediates microglial activation. J Neurosci 23: 2665-2674.

Barclay, A. N., G. J. Wright, G. Brooke, and M. H. Brown. 2002. CD200 and membrane protein E interactions in the control of myeloid cells. Trends in Immunology 23: 285-290.

Bianchi, M. E, 2007. DAMPSs, PAMPS and alarmins: all we need to know about danger. Journ Leukocyte Biology 81: 1-5.

Botto, M, E. M. Dell, 'Angnola EM, Golay J, et al. 1998. Homozygous C1q deficiency causes glomerulonephritis associated with multiple apoptotic bodies. Nat Genetics. 19: 1956-59

Bowman, C. C., A. Rasley, S. L. Tranguch, and I. Marriott. 2003. Cultured astrocytes express toll-like receptors for bacterial products. Glia 43: 281-291.

Bsibsi, M., R. Ravid, D. Gveric, and J. M. van Noort. 2002. Broad expression of Toll-like receptors in the human central nervous system. Journal of Neuropathology and Experimental Neurology 61: 1013-1021.

Broderick, C., R. M. Hoek, J. V. Forrester, J. Liversidge, J. Sedgwick, A. D. Dick. 2002. Constitutive retinal expression of CD200 regulates resident microglial and activation state of inflammatory cells during experimental autoimmune uveoretinitis Am J Path 1612: 1669-1677.

Brown, E. J., and W. A. Frazier. 2001. Integrin-associated protein (CD47) and its ligands. 11: 130-135.

Brown, G. 2006 Dectin -1 a signaling non TLR pattern recognition receptor. Nature Rev Immunol 6: 33-43.

Bsibsi, M., C. Persoon-Deen, R. W. Verwer, S. Meeuwsen, R. Ravid, and J. M. Van Noort. 2006. Toll-like receptor 3 on adult human astrocytes triggers production of neuron protective mediators. Glia 53: 688-695.

Brantley, E. C, and E. N. Benveniste, 2008. Signal transducer and activator of transcription - 3: a molecular hub for signaling pathways in gliomas. Mol Cancer Res: 6(5): 675-684

Bu, G., J. Cam, and C. Zerbinatti. 2006. LRP in amyloid-beta production and metabolism. Ann N Y Acad. Sci. 1086: 35-53.

Burudi, E. M, P. D Stahl and A. Regnier-Vigouroux. 1999. Identification and functional characterization of the mannose receptor in astrocytes. *Glia* 25: 44-55.

Butchi, N. B., S. Pourciau, M. Du, T. W. Morgan, and K. E. Peterson. 2008. Analysis of the neuroinflammatory response to TLR7 stimulation in the brain: comparison of multiple TLR7 and/or TLR8 agonists. J Immunol 180: 7604-7612.

Cambi, A., M. Koopman, C. G Figdor. 2005. C type lectins detect pathogens. Cell Microbiol 7(4): 481-488.

Cameron, J. S., L. Alexopoulou, J. A. Sloane, A. B. DiBernardo, Y. Ma, B. Kosaras, R. Flavell, S. M. Strittmatter, J. Volpe, R. Sidman, and T. Vartanian. 2007. Toll-like receptor 3 is a potent negative regulator of axonal growth in mammals. J Neurosci 27: 13033-13041.

Canova, C., J. W. Neal, and P. Gasque. 2006. Expression of innate immune complement regulators on brain epithelial cells during human bacterial meningitis. J Neuroinflammation 3: 22.

Cao, H, and P. R. Crocker. 2010. Evolution of CD33 -related siglecs: regulating host immune functions and escaping pathogen exploitation. Immunology 132: 18-26.

Carpentier, P. A., W. S. Begolka, J. K. Olson, A. Elhofy, W. J. Karpus, and S. D. Miller. 2005. Differential activation of astrocytes by innate and adaptive immune stimuli. Glia 49: 360-374.

Carpentier, P. A., D. S. Duncan, and S. D. Miller. 2008. Glial toll-like receptor signaling in central nervous system infection and autoimmunity.

Carpentier, P. A., B. R. Williams, and S. D. Miller. 2007. Distinct roles of protein kinase R and toll-like receptor 3 in the activation of astrocytes by viral stimuli. Glia 55: 239-252.

Castiglioni, A, V Canti, P. Rovere-Queriniand, A. A, Manfredi. 2011. High mobility box 1(HGBM1) as a master regulator of innate immunity. Cell Tis Res 343: 189-199.

Cavassani, K. A., M. Ishii, H. Wen, M. A. Schaller, P. M. Lincoln, N. W. Lukacs, C. M. Hogaboam, and S. L. Kunkel. 2008. TLR3 is an endogenous sensor of tissue necrosis during acute inflammatory events. J Exp Med 205: 2609-2621.

Chan A, T. Magus, and R Gold R. 2001. Phagocytosis of apoptotic inflammatory cells by microglia and modulation by different cytokines; mechanism for removal of apoptotic cells in the inflamed nervous system. Glia; 33: 87-95.

Chang G, N. M. Barbaro, R. O Pieper. 2002. Phosphatidylserine- dependent phagocytosis of cells by normal human microglia, astrocytes and glioma cells. Neuro oncol 2002; 3: 174-183.

Chauhan, V. S., D. G. Sterka, Jr., S. R. Furr, A. B. Young, and I. Marriott. 2009. NOD2 plays an important role in the inflammatory responses of microglia and astrocytes to bacterial CNS pathogens. Glia 57: 414-423.

Chen, GY, J Tang P, L Zheng, Y Liu. 2009. CD24 and siglec 10 selectively repress tissue damage- induced immune responses. Science 323: 1722-1725.

Chen, K., P. Iribarren, J. Hu, J. Chen, W. Gong, E. H. Cho, S. Lockett, N. M. Dunlop, and J. M. Wang. 2006. Activation of Toll-like receptor 2 on microglia promotes cell uptake of Alzheimer disease-associated amyloid beta peptide. J Biol Chem 281: 3651-3659.

Colonna, M, . 2003. TREMs in the immune system and beyond. Nat Rev Immunol 6: 445-453.

Coraci, I. S, H. J., Berman, J. W, Hulette, C. Dufour, J. H. Campanella, G. K, Luster, AD, Silverstein, J. B. El Khoury. 2002. CD36, a Class B Scavenger Receptor, is expressed on Microglia in Alzheimer's disease brains and can mediate production of reactive oxygen species in response to beta-amyloid fibrils. Am J Pathol 160: 101-112.

Creagh, E. M, L. A. J O'NEIL. 2006. TLRs, NLRs and RLRs; a trinity of pathogen sensors that cooperate in innate immunity. Trends in Immunology 277: 352-357.

Crocker, P. R., A. Varki. 2001. Siglecs, sialic acids and innate immunity Trends in Immunology 22 6: 337-342.

Crocker, P. R, J. C. Paulson and A. Varki. 2007. Siglecsand their roles in the immune system. Nature reviews in Immunol; 7 255-266

Daffis, S., M. A. Samuel, M. S. Suthar, M. Gale, Jr., and M. S. Diamond. 2008. Toll-like receptor 3 has a protective role against West Nile virus infection. J Virol 82: 10349-10358.

Dean, Y D, McGreal EP, Akatsu H, et al. Molecular and cellular properties of the rat AA4 antigen, a C type lectin -like receptor with structural homolgy to thrombomodulin. J Biol Chem 2000; 275: 34382 -34392

Delputte, P. L, H. Van Gorp, H. W. Favoreel, I. Hoebeke, I. Delrule, H. Dewerchin, , F Verdnock, B. Verhasselt, E. Cox, H. J. Nauwynck. 2011 Porcine Siaoladhesin (CD 169/Siglec -1) is an endocytic receptor that allows targeted delivery of toxins and antigens to macrophages PLos ONE 6: e1682

De Simoni, M. G., E. Rossi, C. Storini, S. Pizzimenti, C. Echart, and L. Bergamaschini. 2004. The powerful neuron protective action of C1-inhibitor on brain ischemia-reperfusion injury does not require C1q. Am J Pathol 164: 1857-1863.

de Vries, H. E., J. J. Hendriks, H. Honing, C. R. De Lavalette, S. M. van der Pol, E. Hooijberg, C. D. Dijkstra, and T. K. van den Berg. 2002. Signal-regulatory protein alpha-CD47 interactions are required for the transmigration of monocytes across cerebral endothelium. J Immunol 168: 5832-5839.

Ehlers, M. R. 2000. CR3: a general purpose adhesion-recognition receptor essential for innate immunity. Microbes Infect 2: 289-294.

Eikelenboom, P., C. Bate, W. A. Van Gool, J. J. Hoozemans, J. M. Rozemuller, R. Veerhuis, and A. Williams. 2002. Neuroinflammation in Alzheimer's disease and prion disease. Glia 40: 232-239.

El Khoury, J. B., K. J. Moore, T. K. Means, J. Leung, K. Terada, M. Toft, M. W. Freeman, and A. D. Luster. 2003. CD36 mediates the innate host response to beta-amyloid. J Exp Med 197: 1657-1666.

Elward, K., and P. Gasque. 2003. "Eat me" and "don't eat me" signals govern the innate immune response and tissue repair in the CNS: emphasis on the critical role of the complement system. Mol Immunol 40: 85-94.

Elward, K., M. Griffiths, M. Mizuno, C. L. Harris, J. W. Neal, B. P. Morgan, and P. Gasque. 2005. CD46 plays a key role in tailoring innate immune recognition of apoptotic and necrotic cells. J Biol Chem 280: 36342-36354.

Endo, Y, M., Takahashi, T. Fujita. 2006. Lectin complement system and pattern recognition. Immunobiology 211(4): 283-293.

Fadok, V. A, B. D. L. Rose, D. M, Pearson, A. B Ezekewitz, P. M. Henson. 2000. A receptor for phosphatidylserine specific clearance of apoptotic cells. Nature 405: 85-90.

Fadok, V. A, W. M. Bratton, P. M. Henson PM. 1998. CD36 is required for phagocytosis of apoptotic cells by human macrophages that use either a phosphatidylserine receptor or the vitronectin receptor (alpha v beta 3). J Immunol 161: 6350-6357.

Fang F, L. F. Lue, S. Yan, H. Xu, J. S. Luddy, D. Chen, D. GWalkr D. M. Stern, S. Yan, A. N. Schmidt, J. X. Chen and S. S. Yan. 2010. RAGE- dependent signaling in microglia contributes to neuroinflammation, A beta accumulation, and impaired learning memory in a mouse model of Alzheimer's disease Faseb 4: 1043-105

Farina, C., M. Krumbholz, T. Giese, G. Hartmann, F. Aloisi, and E. Meinl. 2005. Preferential expression and function of Toll-like receptor 3 in human astrocytes. J Neuroimmunol 159: 12-19.

Fassbender, K., S. Walter, S. Kuhl, R. Landmann, K. Ishii, T. Bertsch, A. K. Stalder, F. Muehlhauser, Y. Liu, A. J. Ulmer, S. Rivest, A. Lentschat, E. Gulbins, M. Jucker, M. Staufenbiel, K. Brechtel, J. Walter, G. Multhaup, B. Penke, Y. Adachi, T. Hartmann, and K. Beyreuther. 2004. The LPS receptor (CD14) links innate immunity with Alzheimer's disease. Faseb J 18: 203-205.

Foell, D., H. Wittkowski, T. Vogl, and J. Roth. 2007. S100 proteins expressed in phagocytes: a novel group of damage-associated molecular pattern molecules. J Leukoc Biol 81: 28-37.

Fujita, T., K. Onoguchi, K. Onomoto, R. Hirai, and M. Yoneyama. 2007. Triggering antiviral response by RIG-I-related RNA helicases. Biochimie 89: 754-760.

Furr, S. R, V. S. Chauhan, D. Sterka Jr, V. Grdzelishvilli and I Marriot. 2008. Characterization of retinoic acid-inducible gene-I expression in primary murine glia following exposure to vesicular stomatitis virus. J Neurovirol; : 1-11.

Gardai, S, D. L. Bratton, C. AOgden, P. M. Henson. 2006. Recognition ligands on apoptotic cells; a perspective. J Leukco Biol 2006; 79: 896-903

Gardai, S. J., K. A. McPhillips, S. C. Frasch, W. J. Janssen, A. Starefeldt, J. E. Murphy-Ullrich, D. L. Bratton, P. A. Oldenborg, M. Michalak, and P. M. Henson. 2005. Cell-surface calreticulin initiates clearance of viable or apoptotic cells through trans-activation of LRP on the phagocyte. Cell 123: 321-334.

Garner, O. B, HC Aguilar JA, Fulcher, EL, Levroney R, Harrison, L. L. Wright, V Robinson, Aspericueta, M Panico, SM Hasalam, HR Morris A Dell, B. Lee and L. G. Baum 2010. Endothelial galectin -1 binds to specific glycans on nipah virus fusion protein and inhibits maturation mobility and functions to block syncytia formation. PloS Pathog; 15; 6 e10000993

Gasque, P. 2004. Complement: a unique innate immune sensor for danger signals. Mol Immunol 41: 1089-1098.

Gasque, P., Y. D. Dean, E. P. McGreal, J. VanBeek, and B. P. Morgan. 2000. Complement components of the innate immune system in health and disease in the CNS. Immunopharmacology 49: 171-186. 56.

Geijtenbeek, T. B., and S. I. Gringhuis. 2009. Signalling through C-type lectin receptors: shaping immune responses. Nat Rev Immunol 9: 465-47

Golpon, H,A.,V.A.Fadok.,LTaraseviciene. -Stewart 2004 Life after corpse engulfment, phagocytosis of apoptotic cells leads to VEGF secretionand cell growth Faseb 18; 1716-1718

Gregory, C. D. 2000. CD14 dependent clearance of apoptotic cells: relevance to the immune system. Current Opinions in Immunology 12: 27-34.

Gregory, C. D., and A. Devitt. 2004. The macrophage and the apoptotic cell: an innate immune interaction viewed simplistically? Immunology 113: 1-14.

Greter, M, Heppner FL, Lemos MP, Odermatt BM, Goebels N, Laufer T, et al. 2005 Dendritic cells permit immune invasion of the CNS in an animal model of multiple sclerosis. Nature Medicine; 11: 328-334

Griffin, D. E. 2003. Immune responses to RNA-virus infections ofthe CNS. Nat Rev Immunol 3: 493-502.

Griffiths, M. R, , J. W. Neal, P. Gasque. 2007. Innate immunity and protective neuroninflammation new emphasis on the role of neuroimmune regulatory proteins. Int Rev Neurobiol 82: 29-55

Griffiths, M. R., P. Gasque, and J. W. Neal. 2009. The multiple roles of the innate immune system in the regulation of apoptosis and inflammation in the brain. J Neuropathol Exp Neurol 68: 217-226.

Griffiths, M. R, J. W. Neal, M. Fontaine, T. Das, P. Gasque. 2009. Complement factor H, a marker of self protects against experimental autoimmune encephalomyelitis. J Immunol. 182: 4368-4377.

Grauer, OM, JW Molling, E. Bennink, L. W. J Toonen, R. M. P Sutmuller, S. Nierkens and G. J, Adema, 2008. TLR Ligands in the local treatment of established murine gliomas. JI 181: 6720-6729.

Halle, A., V. Hornung, G. C. Petzold, C. R. Stewart, B. G. Monks, T. Reinheckel, K. A. Fitzgerald, E. Latz, K. J. Moore, and D. T. Golenbock. 2008. The NALP3 inflammasome is involved in the innate immune response to amyloid-beta. Nat Immunol 9: 857-865.

Hanayama, R., M. Tanaka, K. Miwa, A. Shinohara, A. Iwamatsu, and S. Nagata. 2002. Identification of a factor that links apoptotic cells to phagocytes. Nature 417: 182-187.

Hamann, J., B. Vogel, G. M. van Schijndel, and R. A. van Lier. 1996. The seven-span transmembrane receptor CD97 has a cellular ligand (CD55, DAF). J Exp Med 184: 1185-1189.

Hauwel, M., E. Furon, C. Canova, M. R. Griffiths, J. W. Neal, and P. Gasque. 2005. Innate (inherent) control of brain infection, brain inflammation and brain repair: the role of microglia, astrocytes, "protective" glial stem cells and stromal ependymal cells. Brain Res Brain Res Rev 48: 220-233.

Helmy, K. Y., K. J. Katschke, Jr., N. N. Gorgani, N. M. Kljavin, J. M. Elliott, L. Diehl, S. J. Scales, N. Ghilardi, and M. van Lookeren Campagne. 2006. CRIg: a macrophage complement receptor required for phagocytosis of circulating pathogens. Cell 124: 915-927

Herz, J., and D. K. Strickland. 2001. LRP: a multifunctional scavenger and signaling receptor. J Clin Invest 108: 779-784.

Hoek RM, R. S., Murphy CA, Wright GJ, Goddard R, Zurawski SM, Blom B, Homola ME, Streit WJ, Brown MH, Barclay AN, Sedgwick JD. 2000. Down-regulation of the Macrophage Lineage Through Interaction with OX2 (CD200). Science 290: 1768.

Hoffman PR de Cathelineau AN Ogden CA et al, et al 2001. Phosphatidyl serine(PS) inducesPS receptor mediated macropinocytosis and promoted clearance of apoptotic cells. J Cell Biol; 155: 649-660

Hoarau, J. J, . Krejbich-Troto, M. C. Jaffar –Bandjee, T. Das, V. Thon-Hon, S. Kumar J. W. Neal, P. Gasque. 2011 The natural healing properties of innate immune receptors and neuroimmune regulatory proteins (NIRegs) in the CNS. CNS Drug Targets 10(1): 25-43

Husemann, J., J. D. Loike, R. Anankov, M. Febbraio, and S. C. Silverstein. 2002. Scavenger receptors in neurobiology and neuropathology: their role on microglia and other cells of the nervous system. Glia 40: 195-205.

Hussain, S. F, D. Yeng, D. Suki, K. Aldape, A. B Heimberger. 2006. The role of human glioma infiltrating microglia/macrophages in mediating antitumour -immune resonse. Neuro Oncol 8 (3) 261-279

Iwasski A, Medzhitov 2010 Regulation of adaptive immunity by the innate system Science 327: 291-295.

Jack, C. S., N. Arbour, J. Manusow, V. Montgrain, M. Blain, E. McCrea, A. ShapiJack and J. P. Antel. 2005. TLR signaling tailors innate immune responses in human microglia and astrocytes. J Immunol 175: 4320-4330.

Jackson, A. C., J. P. Rossiter, and M. Lafon. 2006. Expression of Toll-like receptor 3 in the human cerebellar cortex in rabies, herpes simplex encephalitis, and other neurological diseases. J Neurovirol 12: 229-234.

Jana, M., C. A. Palencia, and K. Pahan. 2008. Fibrillar amyloid-beta peptides activate microglia via TLR2: implications for Alzheimer's disease. J Immunol 181: 7254-7262.

Janeway, Jr, CA 1992 The immune system evolved to discriminate infectious nonself from non infectious self. Immunol Today; 13: 11-16.

Ji- X, Gg. Olinger, S. Aris, Y. Chen, H. Gewurz, and G. T. Spear. 2005 Mannose binding lectin binds to Ebola and Marburg envelope glycoproteins resulting in blocking of virus interaction with DC-SIGN and complement -mediated virus neutralization. J Gen Virol; 86: 2535-2542.

Jin, J. J., H. D. Kim, J. A. Maxwell, L. Li, and K. Fukuchi. 2008. Toll-like receptor 4-dependent upregulation of cytokines in a transgenic mouse model of Alzheimer's disease. J Neuroinflammation 5: 23.

Jones, C., M. Virji, and P. R. Crocker. 2003. Recognition of sialylated meningococcal lipopolysaccharide by siglecs expressed on myeloid cells leads to enhanced bacterial uptake. Mol Microbiol 49: 1213-1225.

Joubert ,RS Kuchler,J. Zanetta P. Bladier ,D V Avellana-Adalid V M Caron M, Doinel C , CVincedon -galactoside binding lectin in. 1989. Immunohistochemical localization of a rat central nervous system 1. Light -and electron microscopical studies on developing cerebral cortex and corpus callosum. Dev Neuroci 1989 11: 397-413.

Karaparakis, M, D. J, Philpott, and R. L. Ferrero. 2007 Mammalian NLR proteins; discriminating foe from friend. Immuno Cell Biol 85(6): 495-502.

Kato, H, O. Takeguchi and S. Sato et al Differential roles of MDA5 and RIG-1 helicases in the recognition of RNA viruses. Nature: 441: 101-105.

Katze, M. G., Y. He, and M. Gale, Jr. 2002. Viruses and interferon: a fight for supremacy. Nat Rev Immunol 2: 675-687.

Kawai, T, S. Akira. 2010. The role of pattern - recognition receptors in innate immunity Update on Toll-like receptors. Nat Immunol 11: 373-384.

Kim, S. J, D. Gershov, X. Ma, N. Brot, and K. B. Elkon. 2002. I PLA -2 activation during apoptosis promotes the exposure of membrane lysophosphatidylcholine leading to binding by natural immunoglobulin M antibodies and complement activation. J Exp Med; 196: 655-665.

Kleene, R, H. Yang, M. Kutscheand, M. Schachner. 2001The neural recognition molecule is a sialic binding lectin for CD24, which induces promotion and inhibition of neurite outgrowth. J Biol Chem 276: 21656-21663.

Klune, J. R, R. Dhupar, J. Cardinal, T. R Billiar and A. Tsung. 2008. HMGB-1: Endogenous Danger signalling. Mol Med 14: 476-484

Koning N, D. F. Swab, R. M Hoek, I. Huitinga. 2009. Distribution of the immune inhibitory molecules CD200 and CD200Rin the normal central nervous system and multiple scelrosis lesions suggests neuron-glia and glia glia interactions. J Neuropath Exp Neurol 68(2): 159-167

Koning, N., L. Bo, R. Hoek, . 2007. Down regulation of macrophage inhibitory molecules in Multiple sclerosis lesions. Ann Neurol; 62: 504 -514

van Kooyk, Y. and, T. B. H Geijenbeek. 2003. DC-SIGN: escape mechanism for pathogens. Nature Rev Immunol 3: 697-709

Korb, L. C., and J. M. Ahearn. 1997. C1q binds directly and specifically to surface blebs of apoptotic human keratinocytes: complement deficiency and systemic lupus erythematosus revisited. J Immunol 158: 4525-4528.

Kovacs, G. G., P. Gasque, T. Strobel, E. Lindeck-Pozza, M. Strohschneider, J. W. Ironside, H. Budka, and M. Guentchev. 2004. Complement activation in human prion disease. Neurobiol Dis 15: 21-28.

Krysko, D. V, P Agostinis, O. Krysko, A. D. Garg C. Bachert, B. N Lanbrecht and P. Vanenabeele. 2011. Emerging role of damage-associated molecular patterns derived from mitochondria in inflammation. Trends in Immunol 32: 157-164.

Kumar, H, Kawai T and S Akira 2011 Pathogen Recognition by The Innate Immune system. International reviews of Immunology 30: 16-42

Kuraya, M., M. Matsushita, Y Endo, etal. 2003Expression of H-ficoline / Hahkata antigen mannose, binding lectin associated serine protease (MASP-1) and MASP3 by human glioma cell line T98G. Int Immunol; 15: 109-117

Laflamme, N., and S. Rivest. 2001. Toll-like receptor 4: the missing link of the cerebral innate immune response triggered by circulating gram-negative bacterial cell wall components. Faseb J 15: 155-163.

Laflamme, N., G. Soucy, and S. Rivest. 2001. Circulating cell wall components derived from gram-negative, not gram-positive, bacteria cause a profound induction of the gene-encoding Toll-like receptor 2 in the CNS. J Neurochem 79: 648-657.

Laflamme, N., H. Echchannaoui, R. Landmann, and S. Rivest. 2003. Cooperation between toll-like receptor 2 and 4 in the brain of mice challenged with cell wall components derived from gram-negative and gram-positive bacteria. Eur J Immunol 33: 1127-1138.

le Cabec, . V, L. J. Emorine, I. Toesca, C. Cougoule, I. Maridonneau-Parini. 2005. The human macrophage mannose receptor is not a professional phagocytic receptor. 77: 934-943

Leonardi-Essmann, F., M. Emig, Y. Kitamura, R. Spanagel, and P. J. Gebicke-Haerter. 2005. Fractalkine-up regulated milk-fat globule EGF factor-8 protein in cultured rat microglia. J Neuroimmunol 160: 92-101

Lamy L, Foussat A, Brown EJ, et al. Interactions between CD47 and thrombospondin reduce inflammation. J Immunol 2007; 178: 5930 -5939

Landreth, G. E., and E. G. Reed-Geaghan. 2009. Toll-like receptors in Alzheimer's disease. Curr Top Microbiol Immunol 336: 137-153

Lehnardt, S., L. Massillon, P. Follett, F. E. Jensen, R. Ratan, P. A. Rosenberg, J. J. Volpe, and T. Vartanian. 2003. Activation of innate immunity in the CNS triggers neurodegeneration through a Toll-like receptor 4-dependent pathway. Proc Natl Acad Sci U S A 100: 8514-8519.

Lemke, G, . C. V Rothlin. Immunobiology of the TAM receptor. 2008. Nat Rev Immunol 8(5)327-336.

Linehan, SA, L. Martinez –Pomares, P. G Stahl, and S. Gordon. 1999. Mannose receptor and its putative ligand in normal murine lymphoid and non lymphoid organs; In situ expression of mannose receptor by selected macrophages, endothelial cells perivascular microglia and mesangial cells, but not dendritic cells. J Exp Med 1999; 189: 1961-1972.

Linnartz, B., Y Wang, and H Neumann. 2010. Microglial Immuno receptor Tyrosine –Based activation and Inhibition motif signalling in Neuro inflammtion. International Journal of Alzheimer's disease 10. 4061/2010/587463.

Liu, Y, GY, Chen and P Zheng. 2009. CD24-siglec G/10 discriminates danger from pathogen associated molecular patterns. Trends in Immunol 12: 557-561.

Lo MK, MillerD, Aljofan M, Mungall BA, Rollin PE, Bellini WJ PE Rota 2010 Characterization of the antiviral and inflammatory responses against Nipah virus in endothelial cells and neurons. Virology; 404(1): 78-88

Lock, K., J. Zhang, J. Lu, S. H. Lee, and P. R. Crocker. 2004. Expression of CD33-related siglecs on human mononuclear phagocytes, monocyte-derived dendritic cells and plasmacytoid dendritic cells. Immunobiology 209: 199-207.

Lotze, M. T., and K. J. Tracey. 2005. High-mobility group box 1 protein (HMGB1): nuclear weapon in the immune arsenal. Nat Rev Immunol 5: 331-342.

Lowenstein, PR 2002 Immunology of viral-vector-mediated gene transfer into the brain: an evolutionary developmental perspective. Trends in Immunology 23: 23-3012.

Lyons A, EJ Downer SCrotty, YM Nolan: KHMills MA Lynch 2007 CD200 ligand receptor interaction modulates microglial activation in vivo and in vitro: a role for IL-4. J Neurosci 27: 830-8313

Lu, J., C. Teh, U. Kishore, and K. B. Reid. 2002. Collectins and ficolins: sugar pattern recognition molecules of the mammalian innate immune system. Biochim Biophys Acta 1572: 387-400.

Ma, Y., J. Li, I. Chiu, Y. Wang, J. A. Sloane, J. Lu, B. Kosaras, R. L. Sidman, J. J. Volpe, and T. Vartanian. 2006. Toll-like receptor 8 functions as a negative regulator of neurite outgrowth and inducer of neuronal apoptosis. J Cell Biol 175: 209-215.

Magnus. T. C, O. Grauer, K. V. Toyka, RGold. 2001. Microglial phagocytosis of apoptotic inflammatory T cells leads to down regulation of microglial immune activation. J Immunol; 167; 5004-10.

Martino, G., R. Furlan, G. Comi, and L. Adorini. 2001. The ependymal route to the CNS: an emerging gene-therapy approach for MS. Trends Immunol 22: 483-490.

McGeer, P. L., H. Akiyama, S. Itagaki, and E. G. McGeer. 1989. Activation of the classical complement pathway in brain tissue of Alzheimer patients. Neurosci Lett 107: 341-346.

McKimmie, C. S., D. Roy, T. Forster, and J. K. Fazakerley. 2006. Innate immune response gene expression profiles of N9 microglia are pathogen-type specific. J Neuroimmunol 175: 128-141.

McMenamin, PG Distribution and Phenotype of dendritic cells and resident tissue macrophages in the dura mater. J Comp Neurol 1999; 405: 553-562.

Manna P, J. Dimitry P. E. Oldenborg, W. A. Frazier. 2005. CD 47 augments Fas /CD95 mediated Apoptosis. J Biol Chem; 280: 29637-29644.

Marshak –Rothstein, A and I. R. Rifkin. 2007. Immunologically active autoantigens: the roll of toll like recepotrs in the development of chronic inflammatory disease Ann Rev Immunol 25; 419-441

Marzolo MP, R. von Berhardi, N. C. Inestrosa. 2001. Mannose receptor is present in a functional state in rat microglial cells. J Neuroscience Res 2001; 58: 387-395.

Matushita, M 2009 Ficolins: complement –activating lectins involved in Innate Immunity J Innate Immunity; 2: 24-32

Matzinger, P. 2007. Friendly and dangerous signals: is the tissue in control? Nat Immunol 8: 11-13.

Medzhitov R, and CA Janeway. 2000. Innate immune recognition mechanisms and pathways. Immuno Rev; 173: 89-9.

Mevorach, D, J. O Mascraenhas, D. Gershov and K. B, Elkon. 1998. Complement dependant clearance of apoptotic cells by human macrophages. J Exp Med; 188: 2313-2320.

Miller, J. L., B. J deWet, L. Martinez-Pomares, C. M. Radcliffe, R. W. Dwek, and S Gordon. 2008. The mannose receptor mediates dengue virus infection of macropahges. PlosPathog 4: e17.

Minoretti, P., C. Gazzaruso, C. D. Vito, E. Emanuele, M. Bianchi, E. Coen, M. Reino, and D. Geroldi. 2006. Effect of the functional toll-like receptor 4 Asp299Gly polymorphism on susceptibility to late-onset Alzheimer's disease. Neurosci Lett 391: 147-149.

Miranda, J., K. Yaddanapudi, M. Hornig, and W. I. Lipkin. 2009. Astrocytes recognize intracellular polyinosinic-polycytidylic acid via MDA-5. Faseb J 23: 1064-1071.

Mishra, B. B., U. M. Gundra, J. M. Teale. 2008. Expression and distribution of Toll –like receptors 11-13 in the brain during murine neurocysticercosis. J Neuroinflammation 12: 5 53

Mohamadzadeh, M., L Chen, Schmaljohn AL. 2007. How Ebola and Marburg viruses battle the immune system. Nature Reviews in Immunology; 7: 556-567.

Morgan, B. P., and P. Gasque. 1996. Expression of complement in the brain: role in health and disease. Immunol Today 17: 461-466.

Mott, R. T., G. Ait-Ghezala, T. Town, T. Mori, M. Vendrame, J. Zeng, J. Ehrhart J Mullan and J. Tan 2004 Neuronal expression of CD22: novel mechanism for inhibiting microglial proinflammatory cytokine production. Glia 4: 369-379.

Mukhopadhyay, S., and S. Gordon. 2004. The role of scavenger receptors in pathogen recognition and innate immunity. Immunobiology 209: 39-49.

Mukhtar M., S. Harley, P. Chen M, BouHamdan, C. Patel, E. Acheampong, R. J. Pomerantz. 2002. Primary isolated human brain microvascular endothelial cells express diverse HIV/SIV associated chemokine co receptors and DC-SGN and L-SIGN. Virology: 297(1): 78-88.

Nauta, A. J, M. Daha, R. van Kooten, A. Roos. 2003. Recognition and clearance of apoptotic cells; a role for complement and pentraxins. Trends in Immunol; 24: 148-15425.

Netea, M. G, C. van der Graaf, J. W. M. Van der Meer, B. J. Kulberg. 2004. Toll like receptors and the host defence against microbial pathogens; bringing specificity to the innate -immune system. J Leuk Biol 75: 749-755

Ogden, CA, A. de Cathelineau P. R. D, Hoffman, B. Bratton, B. Ghebrehiwet, V. A. Fadok, P. M. Henson. 2001. C1q and mannose binding lectin engagement of cell surface calreticulin and CD91 initiates micropinocytosis and uptake of apoptotic cells. J Exp Med; 194: 78-795.

Okuno, T., Y. Nakatsuji, M. Moriya, H. Takamatsu, S Nijima, N Takegahara, T. Toyofuku, Ynakagawa, S. Kang, R. H. Friedel, S Sakoda, H Kikutani, and A. Kumangooh. 2010. Roles of Sema 4-D Plexin -B1 interactions in the central nervous system for pathogenesis of Experimental Autoimmune Encephalomyelitis. J Immunol 3: 1499-1506.

Oldenborg, P. A., H. D. Gresham, and F. P. Lindberg. 2001. CD47-signal regulatory protein alpha (SIRPalpha) regulates Fcgamma and complement receptor-mediated phagocytosis. J Exp Med 193: 855-862.

Olson, J. K., and S. D. Miller. 2004. Microglia initiate central nervous system innate and adaptive immune responses through multiple TLRs. J Immunol 173: 3916-3924.

Origlia, N., M. Righi, S. Capsoni, A. Cattaneo, F. Fang, D. M. Stern, J. X. Chen, A. M. Schmidt, O. Arancio, S. D. Yan, and L. Domenici. 2008. Receptor for advanced glycation end product-dependent activation of p38 mitogen-activated protein kinase contributes to amyloid-beta-mediated cortical synaptic dysfunction. J Neurosci 28: 3521-3530.

Osawa, R., K. L. Williams, and N. Singh. 2011. The inflammasome regulatory pathway and infections: Role in patho physiology and clinical implications. J Infection 62; 119-129

Pachter, J. S, H. de Vries and Z. Fabry. 2003. The Blood brain barrier and its Role in the central nervous system. J Neuropath Exp Neurol 62: 593-604

Parisien JP, Bamming D, Komuo A. 2009et al A shared interface mediates paramyxovirus interference with antiviral RNA helicases MDA5 and LGP2. *J Virol* 2009; (14): 7252-7260

Paul, S., C. Ricour, C. Sommereyns, F. Sorgeloos, and T. Michiels. 2007. Type I interferon response in the central nervous system. Biochimie 89: 770-778.

Pender, MP, and Rist MJ Apoptosis of inflammatory cells in immune control of the nervous system; role of glia. Glia 2001; 36: 137- 144.

Prehaud, C., F. Megret, M. Lafage, and M. Lafon. 2005. Virus infection switches TLR-3-positive human neurons to become strong producers of beta interferon. J Virol 79: 12893-12904.

Prieto, A. L., J. L. Weber, S. Tracy, M. J. Heeb, and C. Lai. 1999. Gas6, a ligand for the receptor protein-tyrosine kinase Tyro-3, is widely expressed in the central nervous system. Brain Res 816: 646-661.

Proell, M, SJ Riedl, JH Fritz, AM Rojas, and R Schwarzenbacher. 2008. The Nod -Like Receptor (NLR) family: a tale of similarities and differences. PLos ONE 3 e2119.

Reed-Geaghan, E. G., J. C. Savage, A. G. Hise, and G. E. Landreth. 2009. CD14 and toll-like receptors 2 and 4 are required for fibrillar A{beta}-stimulated microglial activation. J Neurosci 29: 11982-11992.

Reichert, F., and S. Rotshenker. 2003 Complement -receptor 3and scavenger -receptor-AI/ myelin phagocytosis in microglia and macrophages Neurobiology of disease; 12; 65-72

Rehaume, L. M, T. Jouault, M. Chamaillard. 2010. Lessons from the inflammasome: a molecular sentry linking *Candida* and Crohn's disease. Trends in Immunology; 2 171-176.

Reinhold, M. I., F. P. Lindberg, D. Plas, S. Reynolds, M. G. Peters, and E. J. Brown. 1995. In vivo expression of alternatively spliced forms of integrin-associated protein (CD47). J Cell Sci 108 (Pt 11): 3419-3425.

Ren tein R L, J Allen, et al. CD36 gene transfer confers capacity for phagocytosis of cells undergoing apoptosis. J Exp Med 1995; 181: 1857 1872

Richard, K. L., M. Filali, P. Prefontaine, and S. Rivest. 2008. Toll-like receptor 2 acts as a natural innate immune receptor to clear amyloid beta 1-42 and delay the cognitive decline in a mouse model of Alzheimer's disease. J Neurosci 28: 5784-5793.

Rivest. S, Regulation of innate of immune responses in the brain 2009. Nature Rev in Immunol 9: 429-439

Rivieccio, M. A., H. S. Suh, Y. Zhao, M. L. Zhao, K. C. Chin, S. C. Lee, and C. F. Brosnan. 2006. TLR3 ligation activates an antiviral response in human fetal astrocytes: a role for viperin/cig5. J Immunol 177: 4735-4741.

Roth, J., T. Vogl, C. Sorg, and C. Sunderkotter. 2003. Phagocyte-specific S100 proteins: a novel group of proinflammatory molecules. Trends Immunol 24: 155-158.

Royet, J., and R. Dziarski. 2007. Peptidoglycan recognition proteins: pleiotropic sensors and effectors of antimicrobial defenses. Nat Rev Microbiol 5: 264-277.

Sancho, D, O. PJoffre, N. C Rogers, D. Martinez, P. Hernanz-Falcon, I. Rosewell E. Reis and C Sousa. 2009. Identification of a dendritic cell receptor that couples sensing of necrosis to immunity. Nature. 458: 899-903.

Sarati M, G. Fontin, M. Raymond and S. Susin. 2008. CD47 in the immune response: role of thrombospondin and SIRP alpha reveres signaling. Curr Drug Targets ; 9: 842-850.

Sato S., C. St -Pierre, P. Bhaumik, and J. Nieminen. 2009. Galectins in innate immunity: dual functionof host soluble beta galactoside-binding lectins as damage associated molecular patterns(DAMPs) and as receptors for pathogen associated molecular patterns (PAMPs). Imunol Review 230: 172-187.

Schwartz, A. J, X. Alvarez, A. A Lackner. 2002. Distribution and immunophenotype of DC-SIGN -expressing cells in SIV infected and uninfected macaques. AIDS research and Human retroviruses. 2002; 18 (14): 1021-1029

Seiffert, M., P. Brossart, C. Cant, M. Cella, M. Colonna, W. Brugger, L. Kanz, A. Ullrich, and H. J. Buhring. 2001. Signal-regulatory protein alpha (SIRP alpha) but not SIRPbeta is involved in T-cell activation, binds to CD47 with high affinity, and is expressed on immature CD34(+)CD38(-) hematopoietic cells. Blood 97: 2741-2749.

Shewan D V Calaora PNielsen, Cohen, G Rougon, and H Moreau. 1996. mCD24, a glycoprotein transiently expressed by neurons is an inhibitor of neurite growth J Neurosci 16(8): 2624-2634

Singhrao, S. K, J. W Neal., Gasque P, and Newman G. R. 1999. Increased Complement Biosynthesis By Microglia and Complement Activation on Neurons in Huntington's disease. Experimental Neurology 159: 362-376

Singhrao, S. K, J. W. Neal, N. K. Rushmere, B. P Morgan, P. Gasque et al. 1999 Differential expression of individual complement regulators in the brain and choroid plexus. Lab Invests 10: 1247-1259

Sjoberg, A. P, L. A Trouw, A. M Bloom. 2009. Complement activation and inhibition: a delicate balance. Trends in Immunology 30 (92): 83-90.

Schroder, , K., and J. Tschopp. 2010. The inflammasomes. Cell 140: 821-832.

Stahl, P. D, and R. E. Ezekowitz. 1998 The mannose receptor is a pattern recognition receptor involved in host defence. Curr Opin Immunol 10: 50-55.

Stewart, C. R., L. M Stuart, K. Wilkinson, J. M. van Gils, J. Deng, A. Halle, K. J. Rayner, L. Boyer, R. Zhong, W. A. Frazier, A, Lacy -Hulbert, J, El Khoury, D. T. Golenbock, KJ More. 2010. CD36 ligands promote sterile inflammation through assembly of a Toll -like receptor 4and 6 heterodimer. Nat Immunol 12: 155-161.

Sonabend, A. M., C. E Rollc, and M. S Lesniak. 2008. The role of regulatory T cells in malignant gliomas. Anticancer Res 28(2B) 1143-1150.

Sterka, D., Jr., and I. Marriott. 2006. Characterization of nucleotide-binding oligomerization domain (NOD) protein expression in primary murine microglia. J Neuroimmunol 179: 65-75.

Sterka, D., Jr., D. M. Rati, and I. Marriott. 2006. Functional expression of NOD2, a novel pattern recognition receptor for bacterial motifs, in primary murine astrocytes. Glia 53: 322-330.

Stumpova, M., D Ratner, E. B Desciak, Y. D Eliezri and DM Owens. 2010. The immunosuppressive surface ligand CD200 augments the metastatic capcity of Squamous cell carcinomas. Cancer Res. 70: 2962-2972.

Suzuki, K., A. Kumanogoh, H. Kikutani. 2008. Semaphorins and their receptors on immune cell interaction. Nature Immunology: 9 17-27.

Tahara, K., H. D. Kim, J. J. Jin, J. A. Maxwell, L. Li, and K. Fukuchi. 2006. Role of toll-like receptor signaling in A beta uptake and clearance. Brain 129: 3006-3019.

Takahashi, K, C, . D. P. Rochford and H, Neumann. Clearance of apoptotic neurons without inflammation by microglial triggering receptor expressed on myeloid cells -2. J Exp Med 2005; 201: 647-657.

Takegahara, N, A. Kumanogoh, H Kikutani. 2005 Semaphorins: a new class of immunoregulatory molecules Proc. Trans. R Soc B 360: 1673-168

Takeuchi, O., and S. Akira. Pattern recognition receptors and inflammation. Cell 140: 805-820.

Tenner, A. J. 1999. Membrane Receptors for soluble defense collagens. Current Opinion in Immunology 11: 34-41.

Tenner, A. J. 2001. Complement in Alzheimer's disease: opportunities for modulating protective and pathogenic events. Neurobiol Aging 22: 849-861.

Thielens, N. M, P. Tacnet -Delormeand, G. J. Arlaud. 2002. Interaction of C1q and mannan – binding lectin with viruses. Immunology 205: 563-574

Tian, J, A. M. Avalos, S. Y. Mao, B. Chen, , K Senthil, H. Wu, P Parroche, S Drabic, D Golenbock, C. Sirois, J. Hua, L. L. An, L Audoly GLeRosa ABierhaus, P. Naworth, A. Marshak -Rothstein, M. K. Crow, K Fitzgerald E. Latz, P. A Kiener, and A J Coyle. 2007. Toll like receptor 9 –dependent activation by DNA- containing immune coplexes is mediated by HMGB1 and RAGE. Nature Immunol 8: 487-49. .

Ting, J. P. Y, J. A, Duncan, Y. Lei. 2010 How the Non inflammasome NLRS function in the innate immune system. Science 327: 286-290.

Toguchi, M., D. Gonnzalez, S. Furukawa, S. Inagaki. 2009. Involvement of Sema-4D in the control of microglial activation. Neurochem Int 55: 573-580.

Trouw L, A. Bengtssona, K. A, Gelderman, B Dahlback, G. Sturfelt, A. M. Blom 2007. C4b - binding protein and factor H compensate for the loss of membrane bound complement inhibitors to protect apoptotic cells against excessive complement attack. J Biol Chem; 282: 28540-28548

Trouw L, Nielsen HM, Minthon LE Londos, G Landburg Rverhuis, S Janciauskiene, AM Blom, 2008C4b- binding protein in Alzheimer's disease: binding to Abeta 1-42 and to dead cells. Mol Immunol 2008; 45: 3649-3660

Upham JP, Pickett D, Anders T, Reading C. Macrophage receptors for Influenza A virus: role for the macrophage galactose-type lectin and mannose receptor in viral entry. *J Virol* 2010; 84(3): 3730-3737

Van Beek, J., O. Nicole, C. Ali, A. Ischenko, E. T. MacKenzie, A. Buisson, and M. Fontaine. 2001. Complement anaphylatoxin C3a is selectively protective against NMDA-induced neuronal cell death. Neuroreport 12: 289-293.

Van Beek, J., M. Bernaudin, E. Petit, P. Gasque, A. Nouvelot, E. T. MacKenzie, and M. Fontaine. 2000. Expression of receptors for complement anaphylatoxins C3a and C5a following permanent focal cerebral ischemia in the mouse. Exp Neurol 161: 373-382.

van Kooyk, and T. B. H. Geijenbeek. DC-SIGN escape mechanism for pathogens Nat Review Immunol 2003; 3: 697-709.

Vandivier, RW, Ogden CA, Fadok VA, P. R. Hofmann, Brown, M. Botto, M. J. Walport J. H. Fisher, . PM. Henson, K. E. Greene. 2002. Role of surfactant proteins A, D and

C1qin the clearance of apoptotic cells in vivo and in vitro: calcireticulin and CD91 as a common collectin receptor complex. J Immunol; 169: 3978-3986

Vasta, G. Roles of galectins in infection. Nature Reviews in Microbiology; 7: 424-438.

Vernon-Wilson, E. F., W. J. Kee, A. C. Willis, A. N. Barclay, D. L. Simmons and M. H. Brown. 2000. CD47 is a ligand for rat macrophage membrane signal regulatory protein SIRP (OX41) and human SIRPalpha 1. Eur J Immunol 30: 2130-2137.

Voll R, Herrmann, Roth EA. 1997 Immunosuppresive effects of apoptotic cells Nature; 390: 350-351

Wagner, S., Lynch, NJ, Walter W, etal. 2003 Differential expression of the murine mannose-binding lectins A and C in lymphoid and nonlymphoid organs and tissues. J Immunol; 170: 1462-1465.

Walter, S., M. Letiembre, Y. Liu, H. Heine, B. Penke, W. Hao, B. Bode, N. Manietta, J. Walter, W. Schulz-Schuffer, and K. Fassbender. 2007. Role of the toll-like receptor 4 in neuroinflammation in Alzheimer's disease. Cell Physiol Biochem 20: 947-956.

Wang, J., I. and L. Campbell. 2002. Cytokine signaling in the brain: putting a SOCS in it? *J Neurosci Res* 67: 423-427.

Wang, T., T. Town, L. Alexopoulou, J. F. Anderson, E. Fikrig, and R. A. Flavell. 2004. Toll-like receptor 3 mediates West Nile virus entry into the brain causing lethal encephalitis. Nat Med 10: 1366-1373.

Wang. Y, H. Neumann. 2010. Alleviation of neurotoxicity by microglial human Siglec- 11. J Neurosci 30 (9) 3482 -4388.

Webster, S, D, , M. D Galavan, E. Ferran, W. Garzon –Rodriguez, C. G. Glabe, A. J. Tenner Antibody –mediated phagocytosis of the amyloid beta peptide in microglia is differentially modulated by microglia. J Immunol; 12: 7496-74503.

Wu, A, J. Wei, L. Y. Wong, Y. Wang, W. Priebe, W. Qiao, R. Sawaya and A. B Heimbergerg. 2010 Glioma cancer stem cells induce immunosuppressive macrophages /microglia. Neuro Oncol. 12: 113-1125

Wright, G. J., M. Jones, M. J. Puklavec, M. H. Brown, and A. N. Barclay. 2001. The unusual distribution of the neuronal/lymphoid cell surface CD200 (OX2) glycoprotein is conserved in humans. 102: 173-179.

Wyss-Coray, T., and L. Mucke. 2002. Inflammation in neurodegenerative disease. A double-edged sword. Neuron 35: 419-432.

Yagami, T., K. Ueda, K. Asakura, N. Okamura, T. Sakaeda, G. Sakaguchi, N. Itoh, Y. Hashimoto, T. Nakano, and M. Fujimoto. 2003. Effect of Gas6 on secretory phospholipase A(2)-IIA-induced apoptosis in cortical neurons. Brain Res 985: 142-149.

Yamayoshi, S, Y. Yamashita, J. Li, N. Hanagata, TMinowa, T, Takemura, 2009. Scavenger receptor B2 is a cellular receptor for enterovirus 71. Nat Med; 15: 798-801

Yan, S. D, A. Bierhaus, P. P. Naworth, D. M. Stern. 2009. RAGE and Alzheimer's disease: a progression factor for amyloid induced cellular perturbation ?J. Alzheimers Dis 16: 833-843

Yoneyama, M., M. Kikuchi, T. Natsukawa, N. Shinobu, T. Imaizumi, M.

Miyagishi, K. Taira, S. Akira, and T. Fujita. 2004. The RNA helicase RIG-I has an essential function in double-stranded RNA-induced innate antiviral responses. Nat Immunol 5: 730-737.

Yarovinsky, F., D. Zhang, J. F. Andersen, G. L. Bannenberg, C. N. Sheran, M. S. Hayden, S Hieiny, F. S Sutterwala, R. A. Flavell, S. Ghosh, A. Sher. 2005 TRL-11 activation of dendritic cells by a protozoan profilin-like protein. Science 308: 1626-1629.

Yoshida, H., T. Imaizumi, S. J. Lee, K. Tanji, H. Sakaki, T. Matsumiya, A. Ishikawa, K. Taima, E. Yuzawa, F. Mori, K. Wakabayashi, H. Kimura, and K, Satoh. 2007. Retinoicacid-inducible gene-I mediates RANTES/CCL5 expression in U373MG human astrocytoma cells stimulated with double-stranded RN A. Neurosci Res 58: 199-206.

Yu, MH, Wang, A Ding, DT Golenbock, E Latz, CJ Cura, MJ Fenton, K Tracey and H Yang. 2006. HMGB1 signals through toll like receptor (TLR) 4 and TLR 2. Shock 2: 174-179.

Zipfel, P. F., and C. Skerka. 2009. Complement regulators and inhibitory proteins. Nat Rev Immunol 9: 729-740.

11

Regulation of Oligodendrocyte Differentiation: Relevance for Remyelination

Olaf Maier
Institute of Cell Biology and Immunology, University of Stuttgart
Germany

1. Introduction

A major distinguishing feature of the vertebrate nervous system is the formation of myelin sheaths. The myelin sheath has two main functions. First, it electrically insulates the axon thereby enabling saltatory conduction and highly increasing conduction velocity. This also strongly reduces energy consumption since restoration of ion gradients occurs only at the nodes of Ranvier (i.e. at less than 1 % of the axonal surface). Second, the myelin sheath is important for trophic support and protection of the axon (Nave, 2010).

Oligodendrocytes (OLG) are the myelinating cells of the central nervous system (CNS). In contrast to Schwann cells, the myelinating cells of the peripheral nervous system (PNS), OLG form multiple extensions. Each of these extensions forms a myelin sheath after contacting an axon. Due to the synthesis and maintenance of multiple myelin sheaths OLG are highly metabolic active and thus produce large amounts of reactive oxygen species. Moreover, they contain a large amount of iron, which can cause free radical formation. Accordingly, OLG are highly vulnerable to lipid peroxidation and DNA damage due to oxidative stress. It is therefore not surprising that OLG cell death as well as myelin degradation (demyelination) are features of many acute and chronic diseases of the CNS, e.g. trauma, ischemia, spinal cord injury, Alzheimer's Disease and even schizophrenia (McTigue & Tripathi, 2008; Bradl & Lassmann, 2010). Ultimately demyelination results in axonal degeneration and decline of neuronal functions.

Demyelination or dysmyelination (impaired myelin synthesis) are the defining feature of CNS white matter diseases (leukodystrophies). Primary and secondary leukodystrophies can be distinguished. Whereas in primary leukodystrophies, myelin and OLG are directly affected, in secondary leukodystrophies the function of other cells, e.g. astrocytes, is perturbed resulting indirectly in OLG cell death and demyelination. Examples for primary leukodystrophies are Pelizaeus-Merzbacher disease (PMD) and spastic paraplegia type 2 (SPG2), which are characterized by dysmyelination in the CNS (Inoue, 2005), as well as globoid cell leukodystrophy (Krabbe's disease) and metachromatic leukodystrophy. These diseases are caused by impaired degradation of the major myelin lipids galactosylceramide (GalCer) and sulfatide, respectively, and are characterized by progressive demyelination and mental retardation (Wenger et al., 2000; Gieselmann, 2003). The best example for an inherited secondary leukodystrophy is Alexander disease, which is caused by mutation of the astrocytic intermediate filament protein GFAP (Johnson, 2004).

The most common demyelinating diseases are multiple sclerosis (MS) and neuromyelitis optica (NMO), which are both characterized by an autoimmune attack of the immune system on the CNS. Whereas it is generally accepted that, in MS, OLG are the primary target of the immune attack, it has been recently discovered that aquaporin 4, localized in astrocytes, is the primary target in NMO (Roemer et al., 2007; Parratt & Prineas, 2010). The resulting dysfunction and death of astrocytes then causes demyelination and OLG death.

After demyelination the function of the affected area is restored by remyelination, the intrinsic repair mechanism after demyelination. Remyelination of demyelinated axons in the CNS occurs when OLG progenitor cells (OPC) proliferate, migrate to the site of damage, locally differentiate into mature OLG and finally produce new myelin sheaths that are wrapped around the naked axon (C. Zhao et al., 2005). Therefore remyelination largely resembles the developmental myelination process and accordingly knowledge of all steps relevant for developmental OLG differentiation and myelination is essential for potential therapies based on tissue regeneration (Franklin & ffrench-Constant, 2008).

Here I will review main aspects of myelin formation in the CNS starting with the synthesis and transport of myelin components and the morphological differentiation of OLG, which culminates in the formation of multiple myelin sheaths. I will then discuss intrinsic and extrinsic factors that regulate OLG differentiation. Finally, I will address specific aspects of remyelination and will draw attention to differences between developmental myelination and remyelination, e.g. due to changes in the CNS microenvironment.

2. Differentiation of oligodendrocytes

Most aspects of OLG biology have been studied in rodents and in rodent-derived cells. These studies have revealed that the differentiation of OLG is a highly regulated process, in which several stages can be distinguished. During embryonal development neural stem cells in the ventral ventricular zone of the CNS (and later also in more dorsal areas) develop into OPC. These cells are characterized by the expression of the ganglioside A2B5, the chondroitin sulfate proteoglycan NG2 and the platelet-derived growth factor receptor α (PDGFRα; Nishiyama et al., 1999). OPC proliferate and migrate throughout the CNS to their final destination. Around birth the OPC start to differentiate and extend multiple processes. Those branches that do not find an axon retract and OPC that cannot make axonal contact undergo apoptotic cell death. When a process makes contact with an axon, the cell synthesizes myelin components and vast amounts of membrane, which is wrapped several times around the axon. After extrusion of the cytoplasm the formation of the compact myelin sheath is completed (Baumann & Pham-Dinh, 2001; Bradl & Lassmann, 2009). These stages are characterized by the sequential expression of cellular marker molecules. Concomitantly, OPC-specific marker molecules are lost (see Fig. 1).

2.1 Myelin structure and composition

The myelin sheath is not homogeneous. The compact myelin, which is important for the electrical insulation of the axon, can be distinguished from several regions of non-compact myelin (Sherman & Brophy, 2005). These include the adaxonal and abaxonal plasma membranes, which face the axon and the extracellular matrix (ECM), respectively, the radial component, important for energy and metabolite transport within the myelin sheath, and the paranodal loops. These are the main contact sites between myelin and axon and are especially relevant for the functionality as well as structural integrity of the nodes of Ranvier (Tait et al. 2000).

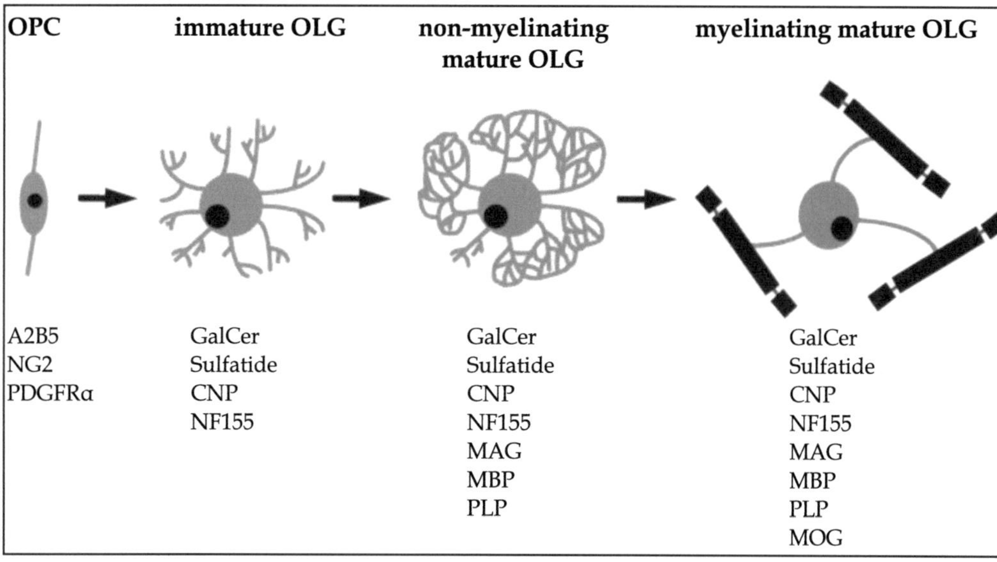

Fig. 1. Schematic representation of OLG developmental stages. Indicated are stages of OLG differentiation ultimately resulting in myelin sheath formation (black) as well as proteins and lipids specific for these developmental stages (adapted from Maier et al., 2005).

To fulfil its function of electrical insulation, the myelin sheath is highly enriched in lipids, which comprise approx. 70 % of its dry weight. The most abundant myelin lipids are cholesterol and the glycosphingolipids GalCer and its sulfated form sulfatide. Cholesterol is essential for myelin formation (Saher et al. 2005) while GalCer and sulfatide are important for the correct formation of the paranodal loops (Dupree et al., 1998; Marcus et al. 2006). The major myelin proteins are proteolipid protein (PLP), its derivative DM20 and myelin basic protein (MBP), which comprise together approx. 80 % of the total myelin proteins (Brunner et al. 1989: Griffiths et al., 1998). PLP/DM20 and MBP are localized in the compact internodal myelin and are required for the compaction of the myelin sheath. Important non-compact myelin proteins are, e.g., 2′3′-cyclic nucleotide 3′-phosphodiesterase (CNP), localized throughout the non-compact myelin, myelin-associated glycoprotein (MAG) in the adaxonal membrane, myelin/oligodendrocyte glycoprotein (MOG) in the abaxonal membrane and the 155 kDa isoform of neurofascin (NF155) in the paranodal loops (Brunner et al., 1989; Schachner & Bartsch, 2000; Tait et al., 2000). For a comprehensive description of myelin composition see, e.g., Baumann & Pham-Dinh, 2001; Aggarwal et al., 2011.

2.2 Synthesis and transport of myelin components

Each OLG myelinates all contacted axons simultaneously and completes the initial wrapping of axons within 12 to 18 hours (Watkins et al., 2008). To achieve this task OLG have to synthesize tremendous amounts of myelin in a very short time (Pfeiffer et al., 1993).

Accordingly, synthesis and transport of myelin components must be highly coordinated in time and space. Moreover, since the composition of the myelin membrane and the membrane of the OLG soma differ significantly, myelin components must be sorted prior to their transport to the myelin sheath. Three main steps required for this polarized transport can be distinguished: i) the sorting of proteins and lipids destined for the different plasma membrane domains, ii) the directed transport towards the different plasma membrane domains along the cytoskeleton and finally iii) the specific targeting to and incorporation into the correct membrane domain. Since these aspects are relevant for the understanding of OLG differentiation, here I will discuss briefly some features of the synthesis and transport of myelin proteins and consequences of incorrect protein synthesis and/or transport, focussing on the major proteins PLP and MBP. Due to space limitations I will not address the directed transport and targeting to the myelin sheath (see, e.g., Krämer et al., 2001, Anitei & Pfeiffer, 2006; Maier et al., 2008)

The exact routes by which transmembrane proteins are transported to the myelin sheath are not well understood and distinct transport pathways towards the myelin sheath have been discussed (Krämer et al., 2001; Anitei & Pfeiffer, 2006; Maier et al., 2008). In general, transmembrane proteins, such as PLP, are synthesized at the endoplasmic reticulum and transported via the Golgi apparatus to the plasma membrane. For PLP there is good evidence that the newly synthesized protein is first transported to the plasma membrane of the cell soma. From there it is internalized and stored in late endosomes before it is finally transported by a transcytotic pathway to the myelin sheath (Trajkovic et al., 2006; Feldmann et al., 2011). Surprisingly, although PLP deletion results in neuronal degeneration, it has only minor effects on myelin formation (Garbern et al. 2002). In contrast, overexpression of PLP causes its accumulation in late endosomes and/or lysosomes together with cholesterol and results in missorting of several membrane markers indicating that major trafficking pathways are affected thereby ultimately interfering with myelination and OLG viability (Simons et al., 2002). Indeed, most cases of PMD are caused by PLP gene duplication resulting in a massive overexpression of PLP demonstrating the relevance of these findings for human disease. In addition, missense mutations in PLP can result in PMD or SPG2 due to the accumulation of PLP in the ER resulting in an unfolded protein response and finally in OLG cell death (Krämer-Albers et al., 2006).

MBP is a multi-functional protein and several isoforms of MBP have been described (Boggs, 2006). In contrast to PLP, MBP is a cytoplasmic protein and is therefore synthesized at free ribosomes in the cytoplasm. Myelin-specific MBP isoforms mediate myelin compaction by interconnecting the cytoplasmic leaflets of the myelin membrane. Accordingly, MBP must have strong adhesive properties. To preclude these adhesive properties taking effect in the cell soma, the MBP messenger RNA (mRNA) is transported into the OLG processes where the protein is synthesized and directly associates with the myelin membrane. To prevent premature MBP protein synthesis the MBP mRNA is incorporated into granules which are transported along microtubules into the OLG branches (Barbarese et al., 1995). This incorporation is mediated by the mRNA binding factor hnRNP A2, which is highly expressed during OLG differentiation (Maggipinto et al., 2004). The importance of correct MBP expression for myelination is demonstrated by the finding that MBP absence causes dysmyelination. This is exemplified by the severe reduction of compact myelin in the so called shiverer mouse due to partial MBP deletion (Roach at al., 1985).

2.3 Morphological differentiation: role of the cytoskeleton

An intact cytoskeleton is essential for all aspects of OLG biology. Both actin filaments and microtubules are essential for the coordinated transport of myelin components to the myelin sheath and the actin cytoskeleton is important for OPC migration. Of particular interest is the role of the cytoskeleton during the morphological differentiation of the OLG.

Each of the multiple branches of the OLG forms a myelin sheath upon axonal contact. One OLG can thus myelinate up to 40 different axons (Pfeiffer et al., 1993). Outgrowth of cellular processes is therefore a fundamental property of OLG and both microtubules and actin filaments are essential to coordinate the morphological changes accompanied with OLG differentiation (Richter-Landsberg, 2008; Bauer et al., 2009). In general, microtubules are especially important for process outgrowth and stabilization whereas actin filaments are more important for the formation of the lamellipodium that initiates the formation of the myelin sheath.

Both depolymerization and stabilization of microtubules perturb the formation of myelin-like membrane sheets *in vitro* indicating that microtubule turnover is required for correct myelination (Benjamins & Nedelkoska, 1994). Nevertheless, a stable microtubular cytoskeleton is required to promote outgrowth and maintenance of cellular processes during OLG differentiation. Indeed, acetylated tubulin, indicative for stable microtubules is present in OLG branches. Moreover, microtubules can be stabilized by associated proteins such as MAP2c and tau (Richter-Landsberg & Gorath, 1999). Tau, in particular, has been implicated in stabilization of microtubules in OLG branches. Whereas OPC express tau isoforms with three microtubule binding domains, differentiating OLG predominantly express tau isoforms containing four microtubule binding domains, which may promote microtubule stability. Moreover, phosphorylation of tau is decreased during OLG differentiation, thereby promoting interaction of tau with microtubules and microtubule stabilization (Richter-Landsberg, 2008). In addition to stabilizing proteins, microtubules are modulated by proteins that promote their disassembly. One prominent protein that mediates microtubule disassembly is stathmin. Accordingly, stathmin expression is downregulated during OLG differentiation (Liu et al., 2003).

Similar to microtubules actin filaments are important for outgrowth and stabilization of OLG extensions. The actin cytoskeleton has been especially implicated in the formation of the lamellipodium, which initiates the enwrapment of the axon. Important regulators of actin cytoskeleton dynamics are proteins of the Rho family of GTPases (Ridley, 2006). Indeed, several members of this family, namely RhoA, Rac and Cdc42 have been implicated in OLG process outgrowth and myelination (Liang et al., 2004, Thurnherr et al., 2007, Rajasekharan et al., 2009). Activation of both Rac and Cdc42 promotes myelination, whereas activation of RhoA inhibits OLG differentiation. An important downstream effector of Rho GTPases that has been implicated in OLG process outgrowth and myelination is the neuronal Wiskott Aldrich Syndrome Protein (nWASP) (Bacon et al. 2007). Activation of nWASP, e.g. by Cdc42, can activate the Arp2/3 complex, which acts as a nucleating factor for actin filament polymerization thereby promoting the formation of the actin network required for lamellipodium formation (Ridley, 2006).

Not surprisingly, several myelin components are interacting with the cytoskeleton thereby facilitating the coordination of the myelination process. Of particular relevance are the cytoplasmic myelin proteins CNP and MBP (Dyer & Benjamins, 1989). CNP can interact with both actin filaments and microtubules and acts as a microtubule assembly protein (De Angelis et al., 1996; Lee et al., 2005). Consequently, CNP is essential for OLG arborization and membrane expansion during myelination. Although cytoplasmic, CNP is anchored to the plasma membrane by isoprenylation and inhibition of CNP isoprenylation perturbs arborization and OLG differentiation (Lee et al., 2005; Smolders et al., 2010). Similar to CNP, MBP can interact with both actin filaments and microtubules and is important for cytoskeleton integrity in OLG. Dephosphorylated MBP, which is predominantly localized in myelin, stabilizes microtubules and enhances microtubule polymerization (Galiano et al., 2006). Moreover, dephosphorylated MBP can act as membrane anchoring protein for actin filaments (Boggs, 2006).

3. Regulation of oligodendrocyte differentiation

OLG differentiation is a highly regulated multistep process. Here I will discuss intrinsic and extrinsic factors that regulate OLG differentiation and myelination. Although the understanding of the interplay between the intrinsic and extrinsic factors that orchestrate OLG myelination is far from complete, I will also address how these factors can initiate and modulate signaling pathways implicated in OLG differentiation.

3.1 Intrinsic factors

In culture, OPC synthesize myelin components and form myelin-like membrane sheets in absence of CNS-derived factors suggesting that differentiation into mature OLG is an intrinsic property of these cells. Differentiation is predominantly regulated on the level of gene transcription and protein translation and much progress has been made in the characterization of these intrinsic factors for OLG differentiation. However, it is still far from understood how the function of these intrinsic factors is coordinated to mediate OLG differentiation.

On the level of gene transcription promoting and repressing transcription factors of OLG differentiation have been identified. Transcription factors that promote differentiation of OPC into mature OLG are, e.g., Olig1, Olig2 and Nkx2.2 and Sox10 (Liu & Casaccia, 2010; Miron et al., 2011). Especially relevant for the initiation of OLG differentiation is the concomitant expression of Olig2 and Nkx2.2 (Zhou et al., 2001). Most transcription factors that promote differentiation are, however, expressed in all stages of OLG development indicating that their presence is not sufficient to induce OLG differentiation. Indeed, several transcription factors that are expressed in OPC, such as Hes5, Id2, Id4, Sox5 and Sox6, strongly inhibit OLG differentiation (Liu & Casaccia, 2010; Miron et al., 2011). Blocking the expression of these inhibitory factors is essential to promote OLG differentiation and there is increasing evidence that this is achieved by epigenetic mechanisms.

In principle, epigenetic inhibition of gene expression can be achieved by two major mechanisms: i) repression of transcription by DNA or histone modification and ii) inhibition of protein translation by microRNAs (miRNAs). Both mechanisms are operational during OLG differentiation. The predominant modification of histones relevant for OLG differentiation is deacetylation, which inhibits gene transcription. Indeed, activity of histone deacetylases is essential for OPC generation and their development into mature OLG. Histone deacetylases can, e.g., bind to the promoter region of OLG differentiation repressors such as Hes5 and Id4 thereby preventing their expression and thus promoting OLG differentiation (Liu & Cassacia, 2010; Copray et al., 2011). In addition, expression of other proteins can be regulated by histone deacetylation. Thus, the expression of stathmin is repressed by this mechanism during OLG differentiation (Liu et al., 2003) thereby promoting microtubule polymerization and stabilization of the outgrowing OLG branches.

MiRNAs are small non-coding RNAs of approximately 23 nucleotides that are processed from larger precursor RNAs by the RNaseIII enzymes Dicer and Drosha. By binding to the 3′ untranslated region of mRNAs one miRNA can inhibit the translation of multiple mRNAs (Bartel, 2004). Expression of Dicer increases during OLG differentiation and conditional knockout of Dicer in OLG results in dys- or demyelination depending on the stage of Dicer repression (Dugas et al., 2010; X. Zhao et al., 2010). In these studies miR219 and miR338 have been identified as important regulators of OLG differentiation. Both miR219 and miR338 can directly suppress the inhibiting transcription factors Sox6 and Hes5 thereby promoting OLG differentiation (Dugas et al., 2010; X. Zhao et al., 2010). An additional target of miR219 is the PDGFRα, (Dugas et al., 2010), which, although important for OPC proliferation and migration, inhibits OLG differentiation (see next section).

3.2 Extrinsic factors

Although *in vitro* OLG can form myelin-like membranes in the absence of axons, there is ample evidence that *in vivo* myelination is coordinated by the presence of axons. However, in contrast to the PNS, where axonal expression of neuregulin-1 type III determines the myelination by Schwann cells (Taveggia et al., 2005), no master regulator for myelination in the CNS has been identified. It is more likely that several factors act together to initiate and promote myelination in the CNS. In general, signals modulating OLG differentiation can be divided into two classes: long-range signals such as growth factors and short-range signals such as ECM and cell adhesion molecules (see Table 1 for important factors regulating OLG behavior). Since the differentiation into a myelinating phenotype is an intrinsic property of OLG while myelination of the axon has to be tightly controlled, it is perhaps not surprising that many axonal factors inhibit OLG differentiation. Here I will address some of the exogenous factors that modulate myelination and subsequently discuss how these signals may be integrated to result in the induction and modulation of myelin formation.

3.2.1 Modulation of oligodendrocyte differentiation by neurons

During embryonic development neurons prevent premature differentiation of OPC. For this purpose they express inhibitory proteins at the axonal surface, e.g. the polysialylated form of the neural cell adhesion molecule (PSA-NCAM), which is a general inhibitor of cell adhesion (Charles et al., 2000). In addition, neurons express molecules that can directly inhibit OLG differentiation. Examples are Jagged and the Leucine-rich repeats and Ig domain-containing, neurite outgrowth inhibitor (Nogo) receptor-interacting protein-1 (LINGO-1). Jagged is the axonal ligand of the Notch receptor in the OLG membrane and activation of the Notch signaling pathway interferes with OLG development (S. Wang et al., 1998). LINGO-1 is part of the Nogo-66 receptor complex in the axonal membrane and interaction of this receptor complex with OLG proteins such as Nogo-A and MAG can inhibit axonal growth. Conversely, inactivation of LINGO-1 promotes myelination suggesting that LINGO-1 is a key inhibitor of OLG differentiation (Mi et al., 2005). Since LINGO-1 is also expressed by OLG, homophilic LINGO-1 interactions may also interfere with OLG development.

An important factor for the induction of OLG differentiation is the electrical activity of neurons (Demerens et al., 1996) most likely by the release of adenosine which may activate purinergic receptors at the OLG surface (Stevens et al., 2002). Very recently it has been shown that also the neurotransmitter glutamate, released at the synapse upon action potentials, can promote OLG differentiation (Wake et al., 2011).

It is likely that *in vivo* the direct contact of an OLG extension with the axon is important to initiate OLG myelination. The best candidate for an axonal molecule required to induce myelination is the ECM molecule laminin-2, since laminin-2 deficiency causes myelination defects in mice and humans (Chun et al., 2003; Colognato et al., 2005). In addition, neuregulin-1 promotes OLG differentiation (Z. Wang et al., 2007). Other molecules that may be involved in the interaction between OLG and axon and thus promote OLG maturation are gangliosides, which can bind to MAG at the OLG cell surface (Yang et al., 1996).

3.2.2 Modulation of oligodendrocyte differentiation by astrocytes

The intimate relationship of OLG with astrocytes is demonstrated by the formation of gap junctions between these cell types (Orthmann-Murphy et al., 2008). In addition to the direct exchange of molecules via these cell-cell interaction sites, astrocytes modulate OLG function by the release of growth factors and by the deposition of ECM molecules.

Astrocytes are the primary source of growth factors in the CNS (Moore et al., 2011). Among these are, e.g., PDGF-AA and fibroblast growth factor-2 (FGF-2), which mediate proliferation and migration of OPC (Milner et al., 1997; Baron et al., 2000). PDGF-AA is also important for OLG survival in presence of laminin-2 (Baron et al., 2003). However, both PDGF-AA and FGF-2 inhibit OLG differentiation at least *in vitro* (Noble et al., 1988; Bansal & Pfeiffer, 1994). Moreover, astrocytes inhibit OLG maturation during CNS development by secretion of bone morphogenetic proteins (BMP), which are strong suppressors of OLG differentiation (See et al., 2004). Besides these inhibitory factors, however, several factors secreted by astrocytes promote OLG differentiation and myelination. Prominent examples are insulin-like growth factor-1 (IGF-1), leukemia inhibitory factor (LIF) and ciliary neurotrophic factor (CNTF) (McMorris et al., 1986; Stankoff et al., 2002). Interestingly, electrical activity of axons causes the release of LIF from astrocytes (Ishibashi et al., 2005), providing a link between neuronal and astrocytic modulation of myelination. Moreover, astrocytes affect OLG function by synthesizing ECM-molecules, such as fibronectin and tenascin C (Price & Hines, 1985; Götz et al., 1997). Fibronectin promotes proliferation and migration of OPC (Milner et al., 1996; Baron et al., 2002), which is important during embryonal development. However, fibronectin impairs morphological differentiation of OLG *in vitro* (Buttery & ffrench-Constant, 1999; Maier et al., 2005). Similarly, tenascin C inhibits process outgrowth and myelin membrane formation of OLG (Czopka et al., 2009).

Factor	Predominant source	Effect on OLG
Soluble Factors		
Adenosine	neurons	promotes differentiation
Glutamate	neurons	promotes differentiation
PDGF-AA	astrocytes	promotes migration and proliferation; inhibits differentiation
FGF-2	astrocytes	promotes migration and proliferation; inhibits differentiation
IGF-1	astrocytes	promotes differentiation
CNTF	astrocytes	promotes differentiation
LIF	astrocytes	promotes differentiation
BMP	astrocytes	inhibits differentiation
Membrane proteins		
LINGO-1	neurons	inhibits differentiation
Jagged	neurons	inhibits differentiation
PSA-NCAM	neurons	inhibits interaction with axon
Neuregulin-1	neurons	promotes myelination
ECM molecules		
Laminin-2	neurons	promotes differentiation
Fibronectin	astrocytes	promotes migration and proliferation; inhibits differentiation
Tenascin C	astrocytes	inhibits migration and differentiation
Other factors		
Electrical activity	neurons	promotes differentiation

Table 1. Neuronal and astrocytic factors that regulate OLG behaviour and differentiation

3.2.3 Modulation of oligodendrocyte signaling pathways by extrinsic factors

It is obviously essential that the signals supplied by these extrinsic factors are integrated at the OLG cell surface, followed by signal transduction into the cell and modulation of signaling pathways resulting in OLG differentiation. Here I will focus on two main aspects that are important to coordinate signaling pathways in the developing OLG. First, the interaction of ECM molecules, in particular laminin-2 and fibronectin, with receptors on the OLG cell surface and the modulation of these interactions by growth factors. Second, the multiple roles of the Src-family non-receptor tyrosine kinase Fyn in OLG maturation.

ECM molecules such as laminin-2 and fibronectin interact predominantly with integrin receptors in the plasma membrane. Integrins are heterodimeric proteins consisting of one α- and one β-subunit. OLG express a limited number of integrins, namely αvβ1-, αvβ3-and αvβ5-integrins, which bind to ECM-molecules containing an RGD-motif such as fibronectin and vitronectin, and α6β1-integrin, which can bind to laminin-2. Proliferation and migration of OPC, stimulated by PDGF, are mediated by activation of αvβ1 and αvβ3-integrins, implicating RGD-containing ECM-molecules in these processes (Milner et al., 1996; Baron et al., 2002). The importance of α6β1 integrin for myelination was indicated by applying antagonists of the β1-subunit, which inhibit myelination *in vitro* and *in vivo* (Buttery and ffrench-Constant, 1999; Relvas et al., 2001). However, the OLG-specific knockout of the β1-subunit does not cause demyelination (Benninger et al., 2006) indicating that another laminin-2 receptor is present in the OLG membrane. Indeed, dystroglycan has been identified as a receptor for laminin-2, which is required for myelination (Colognato et al., 2007). The β1-subunit in OLG is, however, important for cell survival *in vivo* (Benninger et al., 2006). Interestingly, in presence of laminin-2 the PDGFRα dissociates from αv-containing integrins and instead interacts with α6β1-integrin causing a change in signaling from cell proliferation to cell survival (Baron et al., 2003). Similarly, laminin-2 causes the interaction of the neuregulin receptor erbB2 with α6β1-integrin. This causes a switch in neuregulin signaling from cell proliferation towards cell survival and differentiation (Colognato et al., 2004). These examples show how integrins coordinate short range (ECM-mediated) and long range (growth factors, cytokines) signals, which are both required to regulate cell behaviour.

Although it is still far from understood how the signals received at the plasma membrane are further processed to promote OLG differentiation, several signaling pathways have been identified. For example, binding of laminin-2 to α6β1-integrin promotes OLG differentiation and myelination by the activation of integrin-linked kinase (Chun et al., 2003). Moreover, activated α6β1 integrin binds to the Src family kinase Fyn and this interaction is important for the modulation of the PDGF and neuregulin signaling pathways described above and thus for OLG survival and differentiation (Colognato et al., 2004). Indeed, Fyn has been identified as a key regulator of OLG differentiation. The relevance of Fyn for myelination is exemplified by the finding that the OLG-specific knockout of Fyn results in hypomyelination *in vivo* (Biffiger et al., 2000). Fyn has been implicated in various aspects of OLG biology ranging from migration to myelination. Importantly, Fyn kinase activity is activated by interaction with cell adhesion molecules such as NCAM120 and contactin in the OLG membrane which may interact with axonal proteins thereby initiating myelination (Krämer et al, 1999). Moreover, Fyn can act as a bridge between integrins or other membrane receptors and the cytoskeleton and, depending on the developmental stage of the OLG and the corresponding expression of potential interaction partners, Fyn may bind to different proteins thereby explaining its diverse roles in OLG differentiation. In OPC, binding of PDGF to its receptor PDGFRα results in recruitment of Fyn and modulation of the actin cytoskeleton thereby increasing OPC migration (Miyamoto et al., 2008). Later in OLG development, integrin signaling via Fyn promotes morphological differentiation by activating Rac and Cdc42 and inactivating RhoA, again implicating modulation of the actin cytoskeleton in this process (Liang et al., 2004). Interestingly, LINGO-1 suppresses OLG differentiation and myelination by inactivation of Fyn kinase thereby activating RhoA signaling pathways (Mi et al., 2005). Besides modulating the actin cytoskeleton, Fyn can also affect the microtubular network via binding to tau thereby stabilizing microtubules and thus promoting process outgrowth and OLG differentiation (Klein et al., 2002).

4. Remyelination

Remyelination as the natural regenerative mechanism after a demyelinating insult is the basis of the functional recovery of the affected neurons (Bruce et al., 2010). Since mature OLG are incapable to myelinate nude axons (Crang et al., 1998; Watkins et al., 2008), remyelination requires the de novo differentiation of OPC. Importantly, OPC, characterized by the expression of NG2 and PDGFRα, are present throughout the adult CNS (Polito and Reynolds, 2006) and remyelination is usually very effective after transient demyelination. However, the new myelin sheaths are frequently shorter and thinner than the original sheaths thus giving rise to so-called shadow plaques (Franklin and ffrench-Constant, 2008). Moreover, in chronic diseases, such as MS, remyelination is often incomplete and ultimately fails in most patients resulting in increased neurodegeneration and progressive disease. A main goal for the treatment of chronic demyelinating diseases is therefore to increase the remyelination of the affected axons and thus at least partially restore axonal function.

Two main strategies are followed to improve remyelination: promotion of the endogenous remyelinating capacity and transplantation of exogenous stem cells or progenitor cells. Cell transplantation studies are predominantly performed in animals suffering from dysmyelination, such as the shiverer mouse, or by chemically induced demyelination to ensure that the observed myelination is due to the transplanted cells. In such studies it has been shown that several cell types are able to (re)myelinate CNS axons, such as neural stem cells, Schwann cell precursor cells, olfactory ensheathing cells and OPC (J. Yang et al., 2009). Of these, fetal OPC, possibly derived from induced stem cells, are probably suited best for CNS remyelination (Franklin, 2002; Tepavcevic & Blakemore, 2005). One problem in studying the potential of exogenous OPC to differentiate and (re)myelinate axons after transplantation is that endogenous OPC inhibit the migration and survival of transplanted OPC (O'Leary and Blakemore, 1997). Accordingly, endogenous OPCs have to be eliminated, e.g. by X-ray treatment (Hinks et al., 2001), which may cause conditions that differ from those in most demyelinating diseases. Several other obstacles in cell transplantation are: i) finding a cell source that is abundant enough to repopulate the CNS without causing ethical problems, ii) the delivery of the cells to the CNS and iii) their migration through the CNS to the demyelinated areas.

Irrespective of these considerations, the most useful strategy depends predominantly on the disease one wants to treat. Thus in primary inherited leukodystrophies, such as PMD, the most useful therapy would be the transplantation of allogeneic OPC. In contrast, in MS endogenous OPC are present in and around chronic demyelinated lesions indicating that the environment that these OPC encounter is not permissive for differentiation (Wolswijk, 1998). It is therefore unlikely that transplanted cells will be able to sufficiently migrate and differentiate under these conditions. Irrespective of the cellular source it is therefore essential to modulate the environment resulting in conditions that are permissive for remyelination.

4.1 Inhibitors of remyelination in the diseased CNS

Although remyelination does occur in MS and can be very efficient in a subset of MS patients even after a long disease course (Patrikios et al., 2006; Patani et al., 2007), remyelination eventually fails in most patients. Two obvious potential reasons for remyelination failure are axonal loss or depletion of the endogenous OPC pool. Although such a scenario cannot be excluded in some cases, it is unlikely to be the predominant reason for remyelination failure since in most lesions axons are still preserved and OPC are present in or around the lesion site, often in close proximity of a demyelinated axon. This strongly suggests that inhibitory factors are present in the lesion area that impair OLG differentiation and remyelination. Indeed, in MS a block of OLG differentiation in chronic lesions has been observed (Kuhlmann et al., 2008). This impaired remyelination is characterized by the accumulation of OPC that remain in an undifferentiated stage resulting in a failure to generate myelinating OLG (Goldschmidt et al., 2009). In general, disease-dependent and disease-independent factors can be distinguished that may affect remyelination and in this section I will summarize several of these factors.

The demyelinated axons themselves may repress the interaction with OLG branches and thus their remyelination by the expression of inhibitory cell adhesion molecules. Nude axons in chronic MS-lesions re-express PSA-NCAM, which inhibits OLG differentiation during development (Charles et al., 2000, 2002). Similarly, there is good evidence that expression of LINGO-1 in the lesion area inhibits efficient remyelination (Mi et al., 2007). Moreover, OPC functions may be changed in demyelinating diseases. It has, e.g., been shown that stathmin levels are increased in MS patients, which may contribute to reduced OLG differentiation and remyelination failure in MS lesions (Liu et al., 2005).

Several changes in the environment surrounding the recruited OPC may contribute to the inhibition of cell differentiation. Most relevant in the context of demyelinating diseases is that myelin components strongly inhibit OLG differentiation and (re-)myelination, which is at least partially due to inactivation of Fyn kinase activity (Kotter et al., 2006; Baer et al, 2009). Accordingly, it is essential that the myelin debris that is present in the lesion due to the demyelination process is efficiently removed to allow OPC differentiation and thus remyelination to proceed. Clearance of myelin debris is mediated predominantly by activated microglia, the resident immune cells of the CNS, and macrophages that have entered the CNS parenchyma from the periphery (Neumann et al., 2009). However, it should be kept in mind that microglia can act as antigen presenting cells after ingestion of myelin debris and thus may activate myelin-specific T-cells that have entered the CNS. Moreover, reactive microglia can produce proinflammatory cytokines and reactive oxygen species. Therefore activated microglia may actually enhance the demyelination process (Lassmann & van Horssen, 2011).

In addition to activation of microglia, demyelination results in the activation of astrocytes. Depending on the signals that these astrocytes receive, their activation can be beneficial or detrimental for the remyelination process (Williams et al., 2007). Activated astrocytes secrete growth factors and ECM molecules, e.g. PDGF-AA, FGF-2 and fibonectin, which promote proliferation of OPC and their recruitment to the lesion area. Other factors secreted by astrocytes can promote differentiation of these OPC to mature OLG (see section 3.2.2). However, some of these astrocyte-derived factors can have opposing effects. The chemokine CXCL1, e.g., can stimulate OPC proliferation but also acts as a stop signal for OPC migration (Tsai et al., 2002; Filipovic & Zecevic, 2008). Since in MS, astrocytes surrounding chronic lesions can secrete CXCL1 they may therefore repress the recruitment of OPC to the lesion site (Omari et al., 2006). Moreover, the persistent presence of fibronectin and other ECM molecules, e.g. chondroitin sulfates and hyaluronic acid, can impair OLG differentiation and may, together with astrocyte proliferation, result in the formation of a glial scar thus impairing the remyelination process (Kotter et al., 2011; Miron et al., 2011). This is particularly the case in chronic demyelination when repair mechanisms have failed. In this respect, it has been speculated that the formation of a glial scar is the consequence rather than the cause of remyelination failure (Franklin & Kotter, 2008).

The major disease-independent factor that impedes remyelination is age. In general, regenerative mechanisms are less efficient in old animals compared to young animals and this has also been observed for remyelination. This age-related effect is predominantly due to impaired recruitment of the OPC to the lesion area and a delay in their subsequent differentiation to myelinating OLG (Sim et al., 2002). There may be several reasons for this effect. First, OPC themselves may be less efficient in migration and differentiation. Indeed, the response to growth factors differs in adult OPC compared neonatal OPC possibly delaying the recruitment of OPC into lesion areas (Lin et al., 2009; Cui et al., 2010). Furthermore, histone deacetylates are less active in OPC of adult animals. This can impair the repression of inhibitory transcription factors, which is required for OLG differentiation (Shen et al., 2008) and thus result in a delay of OLG differentiation. It should, however, be mentioned that adult OPC are highly efficient in myelination of nude axons when transplanted into the CNS of shiverer mice indicating that the intrinsic myelinating capacity of adult OPC is not reduced compared to neonatal OPC provided they are in an environment that is permissive for myelination (Windrem et al., 2004). It is therefore more likely that age-related changes in the CNS environment result in a delay of OLG differentiation. One likely cause for impaired OLG differentiation in demyelinating diseases is that adult microglia and macrophages are less efficiently recruited to the lesion area resulting in a delayed clearing of myelin debris (Neumann et al., 2009). Accordingly, the prolonged presence of myelin in the lesion prevents OLG differentiation and may even close the therapeutic window in which remyelination can proceed (Kotter et al., 2011).

4.2 Initiation and promotion of remyelination

Although present throughout the CNS, adult OPC do not differentiate spontaneously into myelinating OLG implying that they are in a quiescent stage. Accordingly, OPC have to be activated by extrinsic factors, which are most likely derived from activated microglia and astrocytes, as these cells are highly sensitive to injury-induced environmental changes. Similar to developmental myelination, several stages of OPC activation can be distinguished during remyelination, starting with OPC proliferation and migration to the lesion site followed by cell differentiation (Franklin & ffrench-Constant, 2008).

Major progress in the elucidation of the requirements for remyelination has been done in MS and animal models of MS. In MS, the immune system attacks the OLG resulting in demyelination and neurodegeneration and virtually all components of the innate and adaptive immune system have been implicated in the demyelination and/or neurodegeneration in MS lesions (Gandhi et al., 2009; Kasper & Shoemaker, 2010). Interestingly and perhaps paradoxically, there is increasing evidence that inflammation is also important for remyelination. First, remyelination is abundant in immunologically active MS lesions whereas it is rarely observed in chronic, immunologically less active lesions (Goldschmidt et al., 2009). Second, genome studies of remyelination have revealed that pro-inflammatory cytokines are important for OLG regeneration. Indeed, the pro-inflammatory cytokine tumor necrosis factor (TNF) is important for remyelination after cuprizone-induced demyelination (Arnett et al., 2001, 2003). Third, as mentioned above, activated microglia and macrophages are required to clear the myelin debris from the lesion area, which is a prerequisite for remyelination. Interestingly, clearing of myelin debris by microglia can be enhanced by infiltrating myelin-specific T cells (Nielsen et al., 2009). Fourth, T cells and microglia can promote OLG proliferation and differentiation by producing neurotrophic factors such as brain derived neurotrophic factor (BDNF; Hohlfeld et al. 2006; Neumann et al., 2009). Indeed, T cells are required for efficient remyelination (Bieber et al., 2003).

Although inflammation can promote remyelination and the immune response might therefore be beneficial for neuroregeneration in MS, MS is predominantly an inflammatory disease (Lassmann & van Horssen, 2011). Maintaining an acute inflammatory milieu in order to improve remyelination may therefore be harmful to the patient. Nevertheless, immunomodulation may be a promising immediate approach to promote remyelination. Indeed, glatiramer acetate and FTY720 (fingolimod), two compounds that are approved for MS therapy, may promote remyelination. Glatiramer acetate, a polypeptide resembling MBP, alters the T cell response in MS from a pro-inflammatory Th1 to an anti-inflammatory Th2 phenotype. Interestingly, these glatiramer acetate-specific Th2 cells produce IGF-1 and BDNF and promote oligodendrogenesis and myelin repair in chemically induced demyelination (Skihar et al., 2009). The sphingosine-1-phosphate analogue FTY720 is used predominantly to inhibit the egress of T cells from secondary lymphoid organs. In addition, FTY720 can promote OLG differentiation (Miron et al., 2010) and as FTY720 can enter the CNS parenchyma it may thus directly promote remyelination.

Another direct approach to promote remyelination might be the injection of adult stem cells. Indeed, intracerebal or intraventricular injection of stem cells results in effective myelination in various models of demyelination. However, due to the multiple focal lesions in MS a systemic application is probably required. It is therefore promising that intravenous administration of adult neural and bone-marrow derived stem cells can enhance remyelination and ameliorate symptoms in experimental autoimmune encephalomyelitis (EAE), the animal model of MS (Pluchino et al., 2003; J. Yang et al., 2009). However, there is some evidence that this effect is predominantly due to the immunomodulatory function of stem cells (Pluchino et al., 2005) and it is still a matter of debate whether stem cells can indeed translocate into the CNS parenchyma and directly myelinate demyelinated axons (Franklin and ffrench-Constant, 2008; Franklin & Kotter, 2008).

Since OPC are present in chronic MS lesions but fail to differentiate the most relevant approach to improve remyelination will be to change the environment within the lesion from inhibitory to permissive for myelination. This would largely increase the therapeutic window in which remyelination can occur and thus would be expected to protect axons from further degeneration. Also in this field some promising results have been obtained. Of particular interest is the observation that the inhibitory effect of myelin components on OLG differentiation due to inactivation of Fyn can be antagonized by pharmacological inhibition of the RhoA signaling pathway (Baer et al., 2009). Moreover, suppression of the OLG differentiation inhibitor LINGO-1 by a specific antagonist stimulates OLG differentiation and promotes remyelination and axonal integrity in EAE (Mi et al., 2007, 2009).

5. Conclusion

OLG differentiation and myelination are extremely complex and highly regulated processes and disturbance of myelination is associated with various CNS diseases. Understanding of OLG differentiation is essential to establish neuroprotective therapies that are based on remyelination. Of particular relevance to develop such therapies is a profound knowledge of the intrinsic and extrinsic factors that coordinate myelination. The role of astrocytes and microglia are of special interest in view of their ambiguous role in neurodegenerative diseases. Here the challenge will be to minimize their role in neurodegeneration and maximize their role in neuroprotection and regeneration. A promising approach may therefore be to modulate astrocytes in such a way that the release of pro-myelinating factors is increased whereas the release of molecules detrimental for myelination is reduced. Concerning microglia it will be important to promote their capacity to efficiently clear the myelin debris in the lesions while at the same time minimizing their harmful effects since the presence of myelin debris is arguable the most important inhibitory factor for remyelination.

Much progress has been made to improve remyelination in model systems. Nevertheless currently no therapy directly aimed at improving remyelination exists and it is therefore now the question how this knowledge can be translated into therapeutic approaches. The most effective approach to achieve remyelination therapy will certainly depend on the diseases to treat. The first diseases, in which it is realistic to directly improve remyelination with cell-based therapies, will most likely be leukodystrophies, such as PMD. For chronic MS it is less likely that cell transplantation is a realistic treatment option. Here the promotion of the endogenous remyelination capacity is more promising, which will largely depend on the generation of a permissive environment for OLG differentiation. The progress that has been made in the last decade makes one cautiously optimistic that therapies based on remyelination are becoming a feasible scenario for the treatment of MS-patients.

6. References

Aggarwal, S.; Yurlova, L. & Simons, M. 2011. Central nervous system myelin: structure, synthesis and assembly. *Trends in Cell Biology*, Vol.21, No.10 (October 2011), pp. 585-593. ISSN: 0962-8924.

Anitei, M. & Pfeiffer, S.E. (2006). Myelin biogenesis: sorting out protein trafficking. *Current Biology*, Vol.16, No.11 (June 2006), pp. R418-R421. ISSN: 0960-9822.

Arnett, H.A.; Mason, J.; Marino, M.; Suzuki, K.; Matsushima, G.K. & Ting, J.P. (2001). TNFα promotes proliferation of oligodendrocyte progenitors and remyelination. *Nature Neuroscience*, Vol.4, No.11 (November 2001), pp. 1116-1122. ISSN: 1097-6256.

Arnett, H.; Wang, Y.; Matsushima, G.K.; Suzuki, K. & Ting, J.P. (2003). Functional genomic analysis of remyelination reveals importance of inflammation in oligodendrocyte regeneration. *Journal of Neuroscience*, Vol.23, No.30 (October 2003), pp. 9824-9832. ISSN: 0270-6474.

Bacon, C.; Lakics, V.; Machesky, L. & Rumsby, M. (2007). N-WASP regulates extension of filopodia and processes by oligodendrocyte progenitors, oligodendrocytes, and Schwann cells - implications for axon ensheathment at myelination. *Glia*, Vol.55, No.8 (June 2007), pp. 844-858. ISSN: 0894-1491.

Baer, A.S.; Syed, Y.A.; Kang, S.U.; Mitteregger, D.; Vig, R.; ffrench-Constant, C.; Franklin, R.J.; Altmann, F.; Lubec, G. & Kotter, M.R. (2009). Myelin-mediated inhibition of oligodendrocyte precursor differentiation can be overcome by pharmacological modulation of Fyn-RhoA and protein kinase C signalling. *Brain*, Vol.132, No.2 (February 2009), pp. 465-481. ISSN: 0006-8950.

Bansal, R. & Pfeiffer, S. (1994). Inhibition of protein and lipid sulfation in oligodendrocytes blocks biological responses to FGF-2 and retards cytoarchitectural maturation, but not developmental lineage progression. *Developmental Biology*, Vol. 162, No. 2 (April 1994), pp. 511-524. ISSN: 0012-1606.

Barbarese, E.; Koppel, D.E.; Deutscher, M.P.; Smith, C.L.; Ainger, K.; Morgan, F. & Carson, J.H. (1995). Protein translation components are colocalized in granules in oligodendrocytes. *Journal of Cell Science*, Vol.108, No.8 (August 1995), pp. 2781-2790. ISSN: 0021-9533.

Baron, W.; Metz, B.; Bansal, R.; Hoekstra, D. & de Vries, H. (2000). PDGF and FGF-2 signaling in oligodendrocyte progenitor cells: regulation of proliferation and differentiation by multiple intracellular signaling pathways. *Molecular and Cellular Neuroscience*, Vol.15, No.3 (March 2000), pp. 314-329. ISSN: 1044-7431.

Baron, W.; Shattil, S.J. & ffrench-Constant, C. (2002). The oligodendrocyte precursor mitogen PDGF stimulates proliferation by activation of αvß3 integrins. *The EMBO Journal*, Vol.21, No.8 (April 2002), pp. 1957-1966. ISSN: 0261-4189.

Baron, W.; Decker, L.; Colognato, H. & ffrench-Constant, C. (2003). Regulation of integrin growth factor interactions in oligodendrocytes by lipid raft microdomains. *Current Biology*, Vol.13, No.2 (January 2003), pp. 151-155. ISSN: 0960-9822.

Bartel, D.P. (2004). MicroRNAs: Genomics, biogenesis, mechanism, and function. *Cell*, Vol.116, No.2 (January 2009), pp. 281-297. ISSN: 0092-8674.

Bauer, N.G.; Richter-Landsberg, C. & ffrench-Constant, C. (2009). Role of oligodendroglial cytoskeleton in differentiation and myelination. *Glia*, Vol.57, No.16 (December 2009), pp. 1691-1705. ISSN: 0894-1491.

Baumann, N. & Pham-Dinh, D. (2001). Biology of oligodendrocyte and myelin in the mammalian central nervous system. *Physiological Reviews*, Vol.81, No.2 (April 2001), pp. 871-927, ISSN: 0031-9333.

Benjamins, J.A. & Nedelkoska, L. (1994). Maintenance of membrane sheets by cultured oligodendrocytes requires continuous microtubule turnover and Golgi transport. *Neurochemical Research*, Vol. 19, No.5 (May 1994), pp. 631-639. ISSN: 0364-3190.

Benninger, C.; Colognato, H.; Thurnherr, T.; Franklin,R.J.; Leone, D.P.; Atanasoski, S.; Nave, K.A.; ffrench-Constant, C.; Suter, U. & Relvas, J.B. (2006). β1-integrin signalling mediates premyelinating oligodendrocyte survival but is not required for myelination and remyelination. *Journal of Neuroscience*, Vol.26, No.29 (July 2006), pp. 7665-7673. ISSN: 0270-6474.

Bieber, A.J.; Kerr, S. & Rodriguez, M. (2003). Efficient central nervous system remyelination requires T cells. *Annals of Neurology*, Vo.53, No.3 (May 2003), pp. 680-684. ISSN: 0364-5134.

Biffiger, K.; Bartsch, S.; Montag, D.; Aguzzi, A.; Schachner M. & Bartsch, U. (2000). Severe hypomyelination of the murine CNS in the absence of myelin-associated glycoprotein and Fyn tyrosine kinase. *Journal of Neurosience*, Vol. 20, No.19 (October 2000), pp. 7430-7437. ISSN: 0270-6474.

Boggs, J.M. (2006). Myelin basic protein: a multifunctional protein. *Cellular and Molecular Life Sciences*, Vol.63, No.17 (September 2006), pp. 1945-1961. ISSN: 1420-682X.

Bradl, M. & Lassmann, H. (2010). Oligodendrocytes: biology and pathology. *Acta Neuropathologica*, Vol.119, No.1 (January 2010), pp. 37-53. ISSN: 0001-6322.

Bruce, C.C.; Zhao, C. & Franklin, R.J. (2010). Remyelination - An effective means of neuroprotection. *Hormones and Behavior*, Vol.57, No.1 (January 2010), pp. 56-62. ISSN: 0018-506X.

Brunner, C.; Lassmann, H.; Waehneldt, T.V.; Matthieu, J.M. & Linington, C. (1989). Differential ultrastructural localization of myelin basic protein, myelin/oligodendroglial protein, and 2′,3′-cyclic nucleotide 3′-phosphodiesterase in the CNS of adult rats. *Journal of Neurochemistry*, Vol.52, No.1 (January 1989), pp. 296-304. ISSN: 0022-3042.

Buttery, P.C. & ffrench-Constant, C. (1999). Laminin-2/integrin interactions enhance myelin membrane formation by oligodendrocytes. *Molecular and Cellular Neuroscience*, Vol.14, No.3 (September 1999), pp. 199-212. ISSN: 1044-7431.

Charles, P.; Hernandez, M.P.; Stankoff, B.; Aigrot, M.S.; Colin, C.; Rougon, G.; Zalc, B. & Lubetzki, C. (2000). Negative regulation of central nervous system myelination by polysialylated-neural cell adhesion molecule. *Proceedings of the National Academy of Sciences of the USA*, Vol.97, No.13 (June 2000), pp. 7585-7590. ISSN: 0027-8424.

Charles, P.; Reynolds, R.; Seilhean, D.; Rougon, G.; Aigrot, M.S.; Niezgoda, A.; Zalc, B. & Lubetzki, C. (2002). Re-expression of PSA-NCAM by demyelinated axons: an inhibitor of remyelination in multiple sclerosis? *Brain*, Vol.125, No. 9 (September 2002), pp. 1972-1979. ISSN: 0006-8950.

Chun, S.J.; Rasband, M.N.; Sidman, R.L.; Habib, A.A. & Vartainen, T. (2003). Integrin-linked kinase is required for laminin-2 induced oligodendrocyte cell spreading and CNS myelination. *Journal of Cell Biology*, Vol.163, No.2 (October 2003), pp. 397-408. ISSN: 0021-9525.

Colognato, H.; Baron, W.; Avellana-Adalid, V.; Relvas, J.B.; Baron-Van Evercooren, A.; Georges-Labouesse, E. & ffrench-Constant, C. (2002). CNS integrins switch growth factor signalling to promote target-dependent survival. *Nature Cell Biology*, Vol. 4, No.11 (November 2002), pp. 833-841. ISSN: 1465-7392.

Colognato, H.; Ramachandrappa, S.; Olsen, I.M. & ffrench-Constant, C. (2004). Integrins direct Src family kinases to regulate distinct phases of oligodendrocyte development. *Journal of Cell Biology*, Vol.167, No.2 (October 2004), pp. 365-375. ISSN: 0021-9525.

Colognato, H.; ffrench-Constant, C. & Feltri, M. (2005). Human diseases reveal novel roles for neural laminins. *Trends in Neurosciences*, Vol.28, No.9 (September 2005), pp. 480-486. ISSN: 0166-2236.

Colognato, H.; Galvin, J.; Wang, Z.; Relucio, J.; Nguyen, T.; Harrison, D.; Yurchenco, P.D. & ffrench-Constant, C. (2007). Identification of dystroglycan as a second laminin receptor in oligodendrocytes, with a role in myelination. *Development*, Vol.134, No.9 (May 2007), pp. 1723-1736. ISSN: 1011-6370.

Copray, S.; Huynh, J.L.; Sher, F.; Casaccia-Bonnefil, P. & Boddeke, E. (2009). Epigenetic mechanisms facilitating oligodendroyte development, maturation, and aging. *Glia*, Vol. 57, No.15 (November 2009), pp.1579-1587. ISSN: 0894-1491.

Crang, A.J.; Gilson, J. & Blakemore, W.F. (1998). The demonstration by transplantation of the very restricted remyelinating potential of post-mitotic oligodendrocytes. *Journal of Neurocytology*, Vol.27 (August 1998), No.7, pp. 541-553. ISSN: 0300-4864.

Cui, Q.L.; Fragoso, G.; Miron, V.E.; Darlington, P.J.; Mushynski, W.E.; Antel, J. & Almazan, G. (2010). Response of human oligodendrocyte progenitors to growth factors and axon signals. *Journal of Neuropathology and Experimental Neurology*, Vol. 69, No.9 (September 2010), pp. 930-944. ISSN: 0022-3069.

Czopka, T.; von Holst, A.; Schmidt, G.; ffrench-Constant, C. & Faissner, A. (2009). Tenascin C and tenascin R similarly prevent the formation of myelin membranes in a RhoA-dependent manner, but antagonistically regulate the expression of myelin basic protein via a separate pathway. *Glia*, Vol.57, No.16, (December 2009), pp. 1790-1801. ISSN: 0894-1491.

De Angelis, D.A. & Braun, P.E. (1996) 2',3'-Cyclic nucleotide 3'-phosphodiesterase binds to actin-based cytoskeletal elements in an isoprenylation-independent manner. *Journal of Neurochemistry*, Vol.67, No.3 (September 1996), pp. 943-951. ISSN: 0022-3042.

Demerens, C.; Stankoff, B.; Logak, M.; Anglade, P.; Allinquant, B.; Couraud, F.; Zalc, B. & Lubetzki, C. (1996). Induction of myelination in the central nervous system by electrical activity. *Proceeding of the National Academy of Sciences of the USA*, Vol.93, No.18 (September 1996), pp. 9887-9892. ISSN: 0027-8424.

Dugas, J.C.; Cuellar, T.L.; Scholze, A.; Ason, B.; Ibrahim, A.; Emery, B.; Zamanian, J.L.; Foo, L.C.; McManus, M.T. & Barres, B.A. (2010). Dicer1 and miR-219 are required for normal oligodendrocyte differentiation and myelination. *Neuron*, Vol.65, No.5 (March 2010), pp. 597-611. ISSN: 0896-6273.

Dupree, J.L.; Coetzee, T.; Blight, A.; Suzuki, K. & Popko, B. (1998). Myelin galactolipids are essential for proper node of Ranvier formation in the CNS. *Journal of Neuroscience*, Vol.18, No.5 (March 1998), pp. 1642-1649. ISSN: 0270-6474.

Dyer, C.A. & Benjamins, J.A. (1989). Organization of oligodendroglial membrane sheets. I: Association of myelin basic protein and 2',3'-cyclic nucleotide 3'-phosphohydrolase with cytoskeleton. *Journal of Neuroscience Research*, Vol. 24, No.2 (October 1989), pp. 201-211. ISSN: 0360-4012.

Feldmann, A.; Amphornrat, J.; Schönherr, M.; Winterstein, C.; Möbius, W.; Ruhwedel, T.; Danglot, L.; Nave, K.A.; Galli, T.; Bruns, D.; Trotter, J. & Krämer-Albers, E.M. (2011). Transport of the major myelin proteolipid protein is directed by VAMP3 and VAMP7. *Journal of Neuroscience*, Vol.31, No.15 (April 2011), pp. 5659-5672. ISSN: 0270-6474.

Filipovic, R. & Zecevic, N. (2008). The effect of CXCL1 on fetal oligodendrocyte progenitor cells. *Glia*, Vol.56, No.1 (January 2008), pp. 1-15. ISSN: 0894-1491.

Franklin, R.J. (2002). Remyelination of the demyelinated CNS: the case for and against transplantation of central, peripheral and olfactory glia. *Brain Research Bulletin*, Vol.57, No.6 (April 2002), pp. 827-832. ISSN: 0361-9230.

Franklin, R.J.M. & ffrench-Constant, C. (2008). Remyelination in the CNS: from biology to therapy. *Nature Reviews. Neuroscience*, Vol.9, No. 11 (November 2008), pp. 839-855. ISSN: 1471-0048.

Franklin, R.J. & Kotter, M.R. (2008). The biology of CNS remyelination: the key to therapeutic advances. *Journal of Neurology*, Vol.255, Suppl. 1 (March 2008), pp. 19-25. ISSN: 0340-5354.

Galiano, M.R.; Andrieux, A.; Deloulme, J.C.; Bosc, C.; Schweitzer, A.; Job, D. & Hallak, M.E. (2006). Myelin basic protein functions as a microtubule stabilizing protein in differentiated oligodendrocytes. *Journal of Neuroscience Research*, Vol. 84, No.3 (August 2006), pp. 534-541. ISSN: 0360-4012.

Gandhi, R.; Laroni, A. & Weiner, H.L. (2010). Role of the innate immune system in the pathogenesis of multiple sclerosis. *Journal of Neuroimmunology*, Vol.221, No.1-2 (April 2010), pp. 7-14. ISSN: 0165-5728.

Garbern, J.Y.; Yool, D.A.; Moore, G.J.; Wilds, I.B.; Faulk, M.W.; Klugmann, M.; Nave, K.A.; Sistermans, E.A.; van der Knaap, M.S.; Bird, T.D.; Shy, M.E.; Kamholz, J.A. & Griffiths I.R. (2002). Patients lacking the major CNS myelin protein, proteolipid protein 1, develop length-dependent axonal degeneration in the absence of demyelination and inflammation. *Brain*, Vol.125, No.3 (March 2002), pp. 551-561. ISSN: 0006-8950.

Gieselmann, V. (2003). Metachromatic leukodystrophy: recent research developments. *Journal of Child Neurology*, Vol.18, No.9 (September 2003), 591-594. ISSN: 0883-0738.

Goldschmidt, T.; Antel, J.; König, F.B.; Brück, W. & Kuhlmann T. (2009). Remyelination capacity of the MS brain decreases with disease chronicity. *Neurology*, Vol. 72, No.22 (June 2009), pp. 1914-1921. ISSN: 0028-3878.

Götz, M.; Bolz, J.; Joester, A. & Faissner, A. (1997). Tenascin-C synthesis and influence on axonal growth during rat cortical development. *European Journal of Neuroscience*, Vol. 9, No.3 (March 1997), pp. 496–506. ISSN: 0953-816X.

Giffiths, I.; Klugmann, M.; Andersen, T.; Thomson, C.; Vouykouklis. D. & Nave, K.A. (1998). Current concepts of PLP and its role in the nervous system. *Microscopy Research and Technique*, Vol.41, No.5 (June 1998), pp. 345-358. ISSN: 1059-910X.

Hinks, G.L.; Chari, D.M.; O'Leary, M.T.; Zhao, C.; Keirstead, H.S.; Blakemore, W.F. & Franklin, R.J. (2001). Depletion of endogenous oligodendrocyte progenitors rather than increased availability of survival factors is a likely explanation for enhanced survival of transplanted oligodendrocyte progenitors in X-irradiated compared to normal CNS. *Neuropathology and Applied Neurobiology*, Vol.27, No.1 (February 2001), pp. 59–67. ISSN: 0305-1846.

Hohlfeld, R.; Kerschensteiner, M.; Stadelmann, C.; Lassmann, H. & Wekerle, H. (2006). The neuroprotective effect of inflammation: implications for the therapy of multiple sclerosis. *Neurological Sciences*, Vol.27, Suppl.1 (March 2006), pp. 1-7. ISSN: 1590-1874.

Inoue, K. (2005). PLP1-related inherited dysmyelinating disorders: Pelizaeus-Merzbacher disease and spastic paraplegia type 2. *Neurogenetics*, Vol.6, No.1 (February 2005), pp. 1-6. ISSN: 1364-6745.

Ishibashi, T.; Dakin, K.A.; Stevens, B.; Lee, P.R.; Kozlov, S.V.; Stewart, C.L. & Fields, R.D. (2006). Astrocytes promote myelination in response to electrical impulses. *Neuron*, Vol.49, No.6 (March 2006), pp. 823-832. ISSN: 0896-6273.

Johnson, A.B. (2004). Alexander disease: a leukodystrophy caused by a mutation in GFAP. *Neurochemical Research*, Vol.29, No.5 (May 2004), pp. 961-964. ISSN: 1573-6903.

Kasper, L.H. & Shoemaker, J. (2010). Multiple sclerosis immunology. The healthy immune system vs. the MS immune system. *Neurology*, Vol.74, Suppl. 1 (January 2010), pp. 2-8. ISSN: 0028-3878.

Klein, C.; Krämer, E.M.; Cardine, A.M.; Schraven, B.; Brandt, R. & Trotter, J. (2002). Process outgrowth of oligodendrocytes is promoted by interaction of Fyn kinase with the cytoskeletal protein Tau. *Journal of Neuroscience*, Vol. 22, No.3 (February 2002), pp. 698-707. ISSN: 0270-6474.

Kotter, M.R.; Li, W.W.; Zhao, C. & Franklin, R.J.M. (2006). Myelin impairs CNS remyelination by inhibiting oligodendrocyte precursor cell differentiation. *Journal of Neuroscience*, Vol.26, No.1 (January 2006), pp. 328-332. ISSN: 0270-6474.

Kotter, M.R.; Stadelmann, C. & Hartung, H.P. (2011). Enhancing remyelination in disease – can we wrap it up? *Brain*, Vol.134, No.7 (July 2011), pp. 1882-1900. ISSN: 0006-8950.

Krämer, E.M.; Klein, C.; Koch, T.; Boytinck, M. & Trotter, J. (1999). Compartmentation of Fyn kinase with glycosylphosphatidylinositol-anchored molecules in oligodendrocytes facilitates kinase activation during myelination. *Journal of Biological Chemistry*, Vol.274, No.41 (October 1999), pp. 29042-29049. ISSN: 0021-9258.

Krämer, E.M.; Schardt, A. & Nave, K.A. (2001). Membrane traffic in myelinating oligodendrocytes. *Microscopy Research and Technique*, Vol.52, No.6 (March 2001), pp. 656-671, ISSN: 1059-910X.

Krämer-Albers, E.M.; Gehrig-Burger, T.; Thiele, C.; Trotter, J. & Nave, K.A. (2006). Perturbed interactions of mutant proteolipid protein/DM20 with cholesterol and lipid rafts in oligodendroglia: implications for dysmyelination in spastic paraplegia. *Journal of Neuroscience*, Vol.26, No.45 (November 2006), pp. 11743-11752. ISSN: 0270-6474.

Kuhlmann, T.; Miron, V.; Cui, Q.; Wegner, C.; Antel, J. & Brück, W. (2008). Differentiation block of oligodendroglial progenitor cells as a cause for remyelination failure in chronic multiple sclerosis. *Brain*, Vol.131, No.7 (July 2008) pp. 1749-1758. ISSN: 0006-8950.

Lassmann, H. & van Horssen, J. (2011) The molecular basis of neurodegeneration in multiple sclerosis. *FEBS Letters*, Vol.585, No.23 (December 2011), pp. 3715-3723. ISSN: 0014-5793.

Lee, J.; Gravel, M.; Zhang, R.; Thibault, P. & Braun, P.E. (2005). Process outgrowth in oligodendrocytes is mediated by CNP, a novel microtubule assembly protein. *Journal of Cell Biology*, Vol.170, No.4 (August 2005), pp. 661-673. ISSN: 0021-9525.

Liang, X.; Draghi, N.A. & Resh, M.D. (2004). Signaling from integrins to Fyn to Rho family GTPases regulates morphologic differentiation of oligodendrocytes. *Journal of Neuroscience*, Vol.24, No.32 (August 2004), pp. 7140-7149. ISSN: 0270-6474.

Lin, G.; Mela, A; Guilfoyle, E.M. & Goldman, J.E. (2009). Neonatal and adult O4(+) oligodendrocyte lineage cells display different growth factor responses and different gene expression patterns. *Journal of Neuroscience Research*, Vol.87, No.15 (November 2009), pp. 3390-3402. ISSN: 0360-4012.

Liu, J.; Muggironi, M.; Marin-Husstege, M. & Cassaccia-Bonnefil, P. (2003). Oligodendrocyte process outgrowth in vitro is modulated by epigenetic regulation of cytoskeletal severing proteins. *Glia*, Vol.44, No.3 (December 2003), pp. 264-274. ISSN: 0894-1491.

Liu, J.; Stadelmann, C.; Moscarello, M.; Bruck, W.; Sobel, A.; Mastronardi, F.G. & Cassaccia-Bonnefil. P. (2005). Expression of stathmin, a developmentally controlled cytoskeleton-regulating molecule, in demyelinating disorders. *Journal of Neuroscience*, Vol.25, No.3 (January 2005), pp. 737-747. ISSN: 0270-6474.

Liu, J. & Casaccia, P. (2010). Epigenetic regulation of oligodendrocyte identity. *Trends in Neurosciences*, Vol.33, No.4 (April 2010), pp. 193-201. ISSN: 0166-2236.

Maggipinto, M.; Rabiner C.; Kidd, G.J.; Hawkins, A.J.; Smith, R. & Barbarese, E. (2004). Increased expression of the MBP mRNA binding protein hnRNP A2 during oligodendrocyte differentiation. *Journal of Neuroscience Research*, Vol.75, No.5 (March 2004), pp. 614-623. ISSN: 0360-4012.

Maier, O.; van der Heide, T.; van Dam, A.M.; Baron, W.; de Vries, H. & Hoekstra, D. (2005). Alteration of the extracellular matrix interferes with raft-association of neurofascin in oligodendrocytes. Potential significance for multiple sclerosis? *Molecular and Cellular Neuroscience*, Vol.28, No.2 (February 2005), pp. 390-401. ISSN: 1044-7431.

Maier, O.; Hoekstra, D. & Baron, W. (2008). Polarity development in oligodendrocytes: sorting and trafficking of myelin components. *Journal of Molecular Neuroscience*, Vol.35. No.1 (May 2008), pp. 35-53. ISSN: 0895-8696.

Marcus, J.; Honigbaum, S.; Shroff, S.; Honke, K.; Rosenbluth, J. & Dupree, J.L. (2006). Sulfatide is essential for the maintenance of CNS myelin and axon structure. *Glia*, Vol.53, No.4 (March 2006), pp. 372-381. ISSN 0894-1491.

McMorris, F.A.; Smith, T.M.; DeSalvo, S. & Furlanetto, R.W. (1986). Insulin-like growth factor I/somatomedin C: a potent inducer of oligodendrocyte development. *Proceedings of the National Academy of Sciences of the USA*, Vol.83, No.3 (February 1996), pp. 822-826. ISSN: 0027-8424.

McTigue, D.M. & Tripathi, R.B. (2008). The life, death, and replacement of oligodendrocytes in the adult CNS. *Journal of Neurochemistry* Vol.107, No.1 (October 2008), pp. 1-19. ISSN: 0022-3042.

Mi, S.; Miller, R.H.; Lee, X.; Scott, M.L.; Shulag-Morskaya, S.; Shao, Z.; Chang, J.; Thill, G.; Levesque, M.; Zhang, M.; Hession, C.; Sah, D.; Trapp, B.; He, Z.; Jung, V.; McCoy, J.M. & Pepinsky, R.B. (2005). LINGO-1 negatively regulates myelination by oligodendrocytes. *Nature Neuroscience*, Vol.8, No.6 (June 2005), pp. 745-751. ISSN: 1097-6256.

Mi, S.; Hu, B.; Hahm, K.; Luo, Y.; Kam Hui, E.S.; Yuan, Q.; Wong, W.M.; Wang, L.; Su, H.; Chu, T.H.; Guo, J.; Zhang, W.; So, K.F.; Pepinsky, B.; Shao, Z.; Graff, C.; Garber, E.; Jung, V.; Wu, E.X. & Wu, W. (2007). LINGO-1 antagonist promotes spinal cord remyelination and axonal integrity in MOG-induced experimental autoimmune encephalomyelitis. *Nature Medicine*, Vol.13, No.10 (October 2007), pp. 1228-1233. ISSN: 1078-8956.

Mi, S.; Miller, R.H.; Tang, W.; Lee, X.; Hu, B.; Wu, W.; Zhang, Y.; Shields, C.B.; Zhang, Y.; Miklasz, S.; Shea, D.; Mason, J.; Franklin, R.J.; Ji, B.; Shao, Z.; Chédotal, A.; Bernard, F.; Roulois, A.; Xu, J.; Jung, V. & Pepinsky, B. (2009). Promotion of central nervous system remyelination by induced differentiation of oligodendrocyte precursor cells. *Annals of Neurology*, Vol. 65, No. 3 (March 2009), pp. 304-315. ISSN: 0364-5134.

Milner, R.; Edwards, G.; Streuli, C. & ffrench-Constant, C. (1996). A role in migration for the αvβ1 integrin expressed on oligodendrocyte precursors. *Journal of Neuroscience*, Vol.16, No.22 (November 1996), pp. 7240-7252. ISSN: 0270-6474.

Milner, R.; Anderson, H.J.; Rippon, R.F.; McKaym J.S.; Franklin R.J.; Marchionni, M.A.; Reynolds, R. & ffrench-Constant, C. (1997). Contrasting effects of mitogenic growth factors on oligodendrocyte precursor cell migration. *Glia*, Vol.19, No.1 (January 1997), pp. 85-90. ISSN: 0894-1491.

Miron, V.E.; Ludwin, S.K.; Darlington, P.J.; Jarjour, A.A.; Soliven, B.; Kennedy, T.E. & Antel, J.P. (2010). Fingolimod (FTY720) enhances remyelination following demyelination of organotypic cerebellar slices. *American Journal of Pathology*, Vol.176, No.6, (June 2010), pp. 2682-2694. ISSN: 0002-9440.

Miron, V.E.; Kuhlmann, T. & Antel, J.P. (2011). Cells of the oligodendroglial lineage, myelination, and remyelination. *Biochimica et Biophysica Acta. Molecular Basis of Disease*, Vol.1812, No.2 (February 2011), pp. 184-193. ISSN: 0925-4439.

Miyamoto, Y; Yamauchi, J. & Tanoue, A. (2008). Cdk5 phosphorylation of WAVE2 regulates oligodendrocyte progenitor cell migration through nonreceptor tyrosine kinase Fyn. *Journal of Neuroscience*, Vol. 28, No.33 (August 2008), pp. 8326-8337. ISSN: 0270-6474.

Moore, C.S.; Abdullah, S.L.; Brown, E.; Arulpragasam, A. & Crocker, S.J. (2011). How factors secreted from astrocytes impact myelin repair. *Journal of Neuroscience Research*, Vol. 89, No.1 (January 2011), pp. 13-21. ISSN: 0360-4012.

Nave, K.H. (2010). Myelination and support of axonal integrity by glia. *Nature*, Vol.468, No. 7321 (November 2010), pp. 244-252. ISSN: 0028-0836.

Neumann, H.; Kotter, M.R. & Franklin, R.J.M. (2009). Debris clearance by microglia: an essential link between degeneration and regeneration. *Brain*, Vol.1323, No.2 (February 2009), pp. 288-295. ISSN: 0006-8950.

Nielsen, H.H.; Ladeby, R.; Fenger, C.; Toft-Hansen, H.; Babcock, A.A.; Owens, T. & Finsen, B. (2009) Enhanced microglial clearance of myelin debris in T cell-infiltrated central nervous system. *Journal of Neuropathology and Experimental Neurology*, Vol.68, No.8 (August 2009), pp. 845-856. ISSN: 0022-3069.

Nishiyama, A.; Lin, X.H.; Giese, N.; Heldin, C.H. & Stallcup, W.B. (1996). Colocalization of NG2 proteoglycan and PDGF α-receptor on O-2A progenitor cells in the developing rat brain. *Journal of Neuroscience Research*, Vol.43, No. 3 (February 1996), pp. 299-314. ISSN: 0360-4012.

Noble, M.; Murray, K.; Stroobant, P.; Waterfield, M.D. & Riddle, P. (1988). Platelet-derived growth factor promotes division and motility and inhibits premature differentiation of the oligodendrocyte/type-2 astrocyte progenitor cell. *Nature*, Vol.333, No.6173 (June 1988), pp. 560-562. ISSN: 0028-0836.

O'Leary, M.T. & Blakemore, W.F. (1997). Oligodendrocyte precursors survive poorly and do not migrate following transplantation into the normal adult central nervous system. *Journal of Neuroscience Research*, Vol.48, No.2 (April 1997), pp. 159-167. ISSN: 0360-4012.

Omari, K.M.; John, G.; Lango, R.; Raine, C.S. (2006). Role for CXCR2 and CXCL1 on glia in multiple sclerosis. *Glia*, Vol.53, No. 1 (January 2006), pp. 24-31. ISSN: 0894-1491.

Orthmann-Murphy, J.L.; Abrams, C.K. & Scherer, S.S. (2008). Gap junctions couple astrocytes and oligodendrocytes. *Journal of Molecular Neuroscience*, Vol.35, No.1 (May 2008), pp. 101-116. ISSN: 0895-8696.

Parratt, J.D. & Prineas, J.W. (2010) Neuromyelitis optica: a demyelinating disease characterized by acute destruction and regeneration of perivascular astrocytes. *Multiple Sclerosis Journal*, Vol.16., No.10 (October 2010), pp. 1156-1172. ISSN: 1352-4585.

Patani, R.; Balaratnam, M.; Vora, A. & Reynolds, R. (2007). Remyelination can be extensive in multiple sclerosis despite a long disease course. *Neuropathology and Applied Neurobiology*, Vol.33, No.3 (June 2007), pp. 277-287. ISSN: 0305-1846.

Patrikios, P.; Stadelmann, C.; Kutzelnigg, A.; Rauschka, H.; Schmidbauer, M.; Laursen, H.; Sorensen, P.S.; Brück, W.; Lucchinetti, C. & Lassmann, H. (2006). Remyelination is extensive in a subset of multiple sclerosis patients. *Brain*, Vol.129, No.12 (December 2006), pp. 3165-3172. ISSN: 0006-8950.

Pfeiffer, S.E.; Warrington, A.E. & Bansal, R. (1993). The oligodendrocyte and its many cellular processes. *Trends in Cell Biology*, Vol.3, No.6 (June 1993), pp. 191-197. ISSN: 0962-8924.

Pluchino, S.; Quattrini, A.; Brambilla, E.; Gritti, A.; Salani, G.; Dina, G.; Galli, R.; Del Carro, U.; Amadio, S.; Bergami, A.; Furlan, R.; Comi, G.; Vescovi, A.L. & Martino, G. (2003). Injection of adult neurospheres induces recovery in a chronic model of multiple sclerosis. *Nature*, Vol.422, No.6933 (April 2003), pp. 688-694. ISSN: 0028-0836.

Pluchino, S.; Zanotti, L.; Rossi, B.; Brambilla, E.; Ottoboni, L.; Salani, G.; Martinello, M.; Cattalini, A.; Bergami, A.; Furlan, R.; Comi, G.; Constantin, G. & Martino, G. (2005). Neurosphere-derived multipotent precursors promote neuroprotection by an immunomodulatory mechanism. *Nature*, Vol.436, No.7048 (July 2005), pp. 266-271. ISSN: 0028-0836.

Polito, A. & Reynolds, R. (2006). NG2-expressing cells as oligodendrocyte progenitors in the normal and demyelinated adult central nervous system. *Journal of Anatomy*, Vol. 207, No.6 (December 2006), pp. 707-716. ISSN: 1469-7580.

Price, J. & Hines, R.O. (1985). Astrocytes in culture synthesize and secrete a variant form of fibronectin. *Journal of Neuroscience*, Vol.5, No.8 (August 1985), pp. 2205-2211. ISSN: 0270-6474.

Rajasekharan, S.; Baker, K.A.; Horn, K.E.; Jarjour, A.A; Antel, J.P. & Kennedy TE. (2009). Netrin 1 and Dcc regulate oligodendrocyte process branching and membrane extension via Fyn and RhoA. *Development*, Vol.136, No.3 (February 2009), pp. 415-426. ISSN: 1011-6370.

Relvas, J.B.; Setzu, A.; Baron, W.; Buttery, P.C.; LaFlamme, S.E.; Franklin, R.J. & ffrench-Constant, C. (2001). Expression of dominant-negative and chimeric subunits reveals an essential role for β1 integrin during myelination. *Current Biology*, Vol.11, No.13 (July 2001), pp. 1039-1043. ISSN: 0960-9822.

Richter-Landsberg, C. & Gorath, M. (1999). Developmental regulation of alternatively spliced isoforms of mRNA encoding MAP2 and tau in rat brain oligodendrocytes during culture maturation. *Journal of Neuroscience Research*, Vol.56, No. 3 (May 1999), pp. 259-270. ISSN: 0360-4012.

Richter-Landsberg, C. (2008). The cytoskeleton in oligodendrocytes. Microtubule dynamics in health and disease. *Journal of Molecular Neuroscience*, Vol. 35, No. 1 (May 2008), pp. 55-63. ISSN: 0895-8696.

Ridley, A.J. (2006). Rho GTPases and actin dynamics in membrane protrusions and vesicle trafficking. *Trends in Cell Biology*, Vol.16, No.10 (October 2006), pp. 522-529. ISSN: 0962-8924.

Roach, A.; Takahashi, N.; Pravtcheva, D.; Ruddle, F. & Hood, L.E. (1985). Chromosomal mapping of mouse myelin basic protein gene and structure and transcription of the partially deleted gene in shiverer mutant mice. *Cell*, Vol. 42, No.1 (August 1985), pp. 149-155. ISSN: 0092-8674.

Roemer, S.F.; Parisi, J.E.; Lennon, V.A.; Benarroch, E.E.; Lassmann, H.; Bruck, W.; Mandler, R.N.; Weinshenker, B.G.; Pittock, S.J.; Wingerchuk, D.M. & Lucchinetti, C.F. (2007). Pattern-specific loss of aquaporin-4 immunoreactivity distinguishes neuromyelitis optica from multiple sclerosis. *Brain*, Vol.130, No. 5 (May 2007), pp. 1194-1205. ISSN: 0006-8950.

Saher, G.; Brügger, B.; Lappe-Siefke, C.; Möbius, W.; Tozawa, R.; Wehr, M.C.; Wieland, F.; Ishibashi, S. & Nave, K.A. (2005). High cholesterol level is essential for myelin membrane growth. *Nature Neuroscience,* Vol.8, No.4 (April 2005), pp. 468-475. ISSN: 1097-6256.

Schachner, M. & Bartsch, U. (2000). Multiple functions of the myelin-associated glycoprotein MAG (siglec-4) in formation and maintenance of myelin. *Glia*, Vol.29, No.2 (January 2000), pp. 154-165. ISSN: 0894-1491.

See, J.; Zhang, X.; Eraydin, N.; Mun, S.B.; Mamontov, P.; Golden, J.A. & Grinspan, J.B. (2004). Oligodendrocyte maturation is inhibited by bone morphogenetic protein. *Molecular and Cellular Neuroscience,* Vol.26, No.4 (August 2004), pp. 481-492. ISSN: 1044-7431.

Shen, S.; Sandoval, J.; Swiss, V.A.; Li, J.; Dupree, J.; Franklin, R.J. & Casaccia-Bonnefil, P. (2008). Age-dependent epigenetic control of differentiation inhibitors is critical for remyelination efficiency. *Nature Neuroscience,* Vol.11, No.9 (September 2008), pp. 1024-1034. ISSN: 1097-6256.

Sherman, D.L. & Brophy, P.J. (2005). Mechanisms of axon ensheathment and myelin growth. *Nature Reviews Neuroscience,* Vol.6, No.9 (September 2005), pp. 683-690. ISSN: 1471-0048.

Sim, F.J.; Zhao, C.; Penderis, J. & Franklin, R.J. (2002). The age-related decrease in CNS remyelination efficiency is attributable to an impairment of both oligodendrocyte progenitor recruitment and differentiation. *Journal of Neuroscience,* Vol.22, No.7 (April 2002), pp. 2451-2459. ISSN: 0270-6474.

Simons, M.; Krämer, E.M.; Macchi, P.; Rathke-Hartlieb, S.; Trotter, J.; Nave, K.A. & Schulz, J.B. (2002). Overexpression of the myelin proteolipid protein leads to accumulation of cholesterol and proteolipid protein in endosomes/lysosomes: implications for Pelizaeus-Merzbacher disease. *Journal of Cell Biology,* Vol.157, No.2 (April 2002), pp. 327-336. ISSN: 0021-9525.

Skihar, V.; Silva, C.; Chojnacki, A.; Döring, A.; Stallcup, W.B.; Weiss, S. & Yong, V.W. (2009). Promoting oligodendrogenesis and myelin repair using the multiple sclerosis medication glatiramer acetate. *Proceedings of the National Academy of Sciences of the USA,* Vol.106, No.42 (October 2009), pp. 17992-17997. ISSN: 0027-8424.

Smolders, I.; Smets, I.; Maier, O.; vandeVen, M.; Steels, P. & Ameloot, M. (2010). Simvastatin interferes with process outgrowth and branching of oligodendrocytes. *Journal of Neuroscience Research,* Vol. 88, No.15 (November 2010), pp. 3361-3375. ISSN: 0360-4012.

Stankoff, B.; Aigrot, M.S.; Noel, F.; Wattilliaux, A.; Zalc, B. & Lubetzki, C. (2002). Ciliary neurotrophic factor (CNTF) enhances myelin formation: a novel role for CNTF and CNTF-related molecules. *Journal of Neuroscience,* Vol.22, No.21 (November 2002), pp. 9221-9227. ISSN: 0270-6474.

Stevens, B.; Porta, S.; Haak, L.L.; Gallo, V. & Fields, R.D. (2002) Adenosine: a neuron-glial transmitter promoting myelination in the CNS in response to action potentials. *Neuron,* Vol.36, No.5 (December 2002), pp. 855-868. ISSN: 0896-6273.

Tait, S.; Gunn-Moore, F.; Collinson, J.M.; Huang, J.; Lubetzki, C.; Pedraza, L.; Sherman, D.L.; Colman, D.R. & Brophy, P.J. (2000). An oligodendrocyte cell adhesion molecule at the site of assembly of the paranodal axo-glial junction. *Journal of Cell Biology*, Vol.150, No.3 (August 2000), pp. 657-666. ISSN: 0021-9525.

Taveggia, C.; Zanazzi, G.; Petrylak, A.; Yano, H.; Rosenbluth, J.; Einheber, S.; Xu, X.; Esper, R.M.; Loeb, J.A.; Shrager, P.; Chao, M.V.; Falls, D.L.; Role, L. & Salzer, J.L. (2005). Neuregulin-1 type III determines the ensheathment fate of axons. *Neuron*, Vol.47, No.5 (September 2005), pp. 681-694. ISSN: 0896-6273.

Tepavcevic, V. & Blakemore, W.F. (2005). Glial grafting for demyelinating disease. *Philosophical Transactions of the Royal Society of London. Series B, Biological Sciences*, Vol.360, No.1461 (September 2005), pp. 1775-1795. ISSN: 0962-8436.

Thurnherr, T.; Benninger, Y.; Wu, X.; Chrostek, A.; Krause, S.M.; Nave, K.A.; Franklin, R.J.; Brakebusch, C.; Suter, U. & Relvas, J.B. (2006). Cdc42 and Rac1 signaling are both required for and act synergistically in the correct formation of myelin sheaths in the CNS. *Journal of Neuroscience*, Vol.26, No.40, pp. 10110-10119. ISSN: 0270-6474.

Trajkovic, K.; Dhaunchak, A.S.; Goncalves, J.T.; Wenzel, D.; Schneider, A.; Bunt, G.; Nave, K.A. & Simons, M. (2006). Neuron to glia signaling triggers myelin membrane exocytosis from endosomal storage sites. *Journal of Cell Biology*, Vol.172, No.6 (March 2006), pp.937-948. ISSN: 0021-9525.

Tsai, H.H.; Frost, E.; To,V.; Robinson, S.; ffrench-Cosntant, C.; Geertman, R.; Ransohoff, R.M & Miller, R.H. (2002). The chemokine receptor CXCR2 controls positioning of oligodendrocyte precursors in developing spinal cord by arresting their migration. *Cell*, Vol.110, No.3 (August 2002), pp. 373-383. ISSN: 0092-8674.

Wake, H.; Lee, P.R. & Fields, R.D. (2011). Control of local protein synthesis and initial events in myelination by action potentials. *Science*, Vol.333, No.6049 (September 2011), pp. 1647-1651. ISSN 0036-8075.

Wang, S.; Sdrulla, A.D.; diSibio, G.; Bush, G.; Nofziger, D.; Hicks, C.; Weinmaster, G. & Barres, B.A. (1998). Notch receptor activation inhibits oligodendrocyte differentiation. *Neuron*, Vol.21, No.1 (July 1998), pp. 63-75. ISSN: 0896-6273.

Wang, Z.; Colognato, H. & ffrench-Constant, C. (2007). Contrasting effects of mitogenic growth factors on myelination in neuron- oligodendrocyte co-cultures. *Glia*, Vol.55, No.5 (April 2007), pp. 537-545. ISSN: 0894-1491.

Watkins, T.A.; Emery, B.; Mulinyawe, S. & Barres, B.A. (2008). Distinct stages of myelination regulated by γ-secretase and astrocytes in a rapidly myelinating CNS coculture system. *Neuron*, Vol. 26, No.4 (November 2008), pp. 555-569. ISSN: 0896-6273.

Wenger, D.A.; Rafi, M.A.; Luzi, P.; Datto, J. & Costantino-Ceccarini, E. (2000). Krabbe disease: genetic aspects and progress toward therapy. *Molecular Genetics and Metabolism*, Vol.70, No.1 (May 2000), pp. 1-9. ISSN: 1096-7192.

Williams, A.; Piaton, G. & Lubetzki, C. (2007). Astrocytes - friends or foes in multiple sclerosis? *Glia*, Vol.55, No.13 (October 2007), pp. 1300-1312. ISSN: 0894-1491.

Windrem, M.S.; Nunes, M.C.; Rashbaum, W.K.; Schwartz, T.H.; Goodman, R.A.; McKhann, G. 2nd; Roy, N.S. & Goldman, S.A. (2004). Fetal and adult human oligodendrocyte progenitor cell isolates myelinate the congenitally dysmyelinated brain. *Nature Medicine*, Vol.10, No.1 (January 2004), pp. 93-97. ISSN: 1078-8956.

Wolswijk, G. (1998). Chronic stage multiple sclerosis lesions contain a relatively quiescent population of oligodendrocyte precursor cells. *Journal of Neuroscience*, Vol.18, No. 2 (January 1998), pp. 601-609. ISSN: 0270-6474.

Yang, J.; Rostami, A. & Zhang, G.X. (2009). Cellular remyelination therapy in multiple sclerosis. *Journal of the Neurological Sciences*, Vol.276, No. 1-2 (January 2009), pp. 1-5. ISSN: 0022-510X.

Yang, L.J.; Zeller, C.B.; Shaper, N.L.; Kiso, M.; Hasegawa, A.; Shapiro, R.E. & Schnaar, R.L. (1996). Gangliosides are neuronal ligands for myelin-associated glycoprotein. *Proceedings of the National Academy of Sciences of the USA*, Vol.93, No.2 (January 1996), pp. 814-818. ISSN: 0027-8424.

Zhao, C.; Fancy, S.P.; Magy, L.; Urwin, J.E. & Franklin, R.J. (2005). Stem cells, progenitors and myelin repair. *Journal of Anatomy*, Vol.207, No. 3 (September 2005), pp. 251-258. ISSN: 1469-7580.

Zhao, X.; Han, X.; Yu, Y.; Ye, F.; Chen, Y.; Hoang, T.; Xu, X.; Mi, Q.S.; Xin, M.; Wang, F.; Appel, B. & Lu, Q.R. (2010). MicroRNA-mediated control of oligodendrocyte differentiation. *Neuron*, Vol.65, No.5 (March 2010), pp. 612-626. ISSN: 0896-6273.

Zhou, Q.; Choi, G. & Anderson, D.J. (2001). The bHLH transcription factor Olig2 promotes oligodendrocyte differentiation in collaboration with Nkx2.2. *Neuron*, Vol. 31, No.5 (September 2001), pp. 791-807. ISSN: 0896-6273.

Section 3

Nutrition and Immunology

12

Innate Immune Responses in the Geriatric Population

Nathalie Compté and Stanislas Goriely
Institute for Medical Immunology,
Université Libre de Bruxelles
Belgium

1. Introduction

Demographic evolution represents a challenge for public health. Global population, especially in the developed countries is aging. The proportion of the population above 60 years has increased from 8% in 1950 to 10% in 2000 and is expected to reach 21% by 2050. Older people suffer from more frequent and more severe community-acquired and nosocomial infections than younger people. The clinical presentation is often atypical making diagnostic more difficult. "Latent" intracellular pathogens such as viruses (Herpesviridae) or Mycobacteriae are more prone to reactivate while opportunistic infections (such as Candida) manifest at increased rates (Ongradi & Kovesdi, 2010). Older individuals suffer from reactivation of mycobacterium tuberculosis that counts for 15 percent of all geriatric pulmonary infections. There is also an age-related decline in the magnitude of the responses to vaccination. Low-level chronic inflammation, a process referred to as "inflamm-aging", is commonly observed in older people. It results in both decreased immunity to exogenous antigens and increased autoreactivity. It is well documented that a significant fraction of older people are positive for low affinity autoantibodies without clinical significance. Rheumatoid factors are present in up to 5% of young healthy individuals, a proportion that increases up to five times in older persons. Similarly, the prevalence of antinuclear antibodies is higher in healthy individuals over 70 years of age compared to healthy young adults (Grolleau-Julius et al., 2010). Furthermore, older persons are more susceptible to develop cancer, probably because of accumulation of cell damages and reduced "immunosurveillance"(Malaguarnera et al., 2010; Fulop et al., 2010).

There is clear evidence of an age-related decline in effectiveness of the immune system in humans; it is common to most if not all vertebrates and to some invertebrates. For example, drosophilae display pro-inflammatory status with increasing age and have reduced capacity to produce antimicrobial peptides in response to infection. There is also substantial body of evidence reporting immunosenescence in wild birds (decline of T- and B-cell functions and altered innate immune responses) and mice (thymic atrophy and reduced recent thymic emigrants) (Shanley et al., 2009). Immunosenescence is characterized by the deleterious "filling" of the immunological space with memory and effector cells as a consequence of exposure to a variety of antigens. The continuous attrition caused by clinical and subclinical infections as well as the continuous exposure to other types of antigens (food, allergens) is likely to be responsible for the chronic activation of the immune system and inflammation. Immunosenescence process along with morbidity and mortality will be accelerated in those subjects who are exposed to an extra-burden of antigenic load. The phenomenology of HIV+ patients after several years of infection shows striking similarities (regarding T cell subset rearrangement, T cell clonal expansion, and telomere shortening) with that observed in the context of aging. It is tempting to speculate that chronic infections with other micro-organisms could also lead to this process (De Martinis et al., 2005).

Many studies have tried to collect immune data in older people to establish reliable "biomarkers of aging". However, the literature is full of confusing and conflicting data. There are many difficulties in interpreting immunogerontological observations. The major concern is the way "young" and "old" populations are defined in these studies. On one hand, restricting selection to only "healthy" older people might introduce a bias and not be representative of the general population. On the other hand, comorbidities that are encountered in the geriatric population will certainly affect many parameters of the immune responses. Some studies try to restrict inclusion criteria to better characterize age-associated alterations of immunity such as the SENIEUR protocol (Wikby, 2008; Chen et al., 2009; Ligthart et al., 1984). Unfortunately, it does not represent our geriatric population (only 10% of older people meet the criteria) (Chen et al., 2009). OCTO study was less restrictive for inclusion criteria, admitted 400 octogenarians that were not institutionalized, had no or only mild cognitive dysfunction and were not on drug regimen that might have influenced the immune system. This study predicts the same **immune risk profile (IRP)** of subsequent 2 year-mortality than SENIEUR protocols characterized by high level of CD8 T cells, inversion of the CD4+/CD8+ T cell ratio, poor mitogen stimulated lymphoproliferative responses and loss of CD28 costimulatory molecule (table 1).

Immune Risk Phenotype (IRP)
- Low levels of B cells
- Inversion of the CD4+/CD8+ ratio
- Poor mitogen stimulated lymphoproliferative response
- Increased levels of CD8+ CD28- CD57+ T cells
- Positive serology for Cytomegalovirus

Table 1. The "immune risk phenotype".

Finally, the NONA study did not exclude individuals because of compromised health to place immune risk phenotype in a broader context of health and cognitive dysfunctioning. It confirmed the OCTO study and demonstrated that the immune risk phenotype concept could be generalized to a sample of nonagenarians not specifically selected for good health at baseline (Pawelec et al., 2005; Wikby, 2008). Both studies demonstrated that aging is associated with low-grade inflammation and that inflammatory markers like increase of IL-6, C-reactive protein (CRP) and decrease of albumin are significant predictors of mortality in very old humans independently of disease and comorbidity (Wikby, 2008). The new HEXA study examined the IRP profile in hexagenarians and shows the same characteristics than in the very old. The study has now to examine the impact of the IRP on morbidity and mortality in this age group (Wills et al., 2011).

Herein, we will first review the major changes in adaptive immune responses observed in the geriatric population. We will then focus on what is known about innate immune responses in this age group. Finally, we will discuss the links between the specific clinical context of aging and alterations of immune responses.

2. Adaptative immune responses: thymic involution, T cell exhaustion and persistent infections

2.1 Thymic involution

The thymus is the site of T cells differentiation and maturation and is often referred to as the "immunologic clock" of aging. Age-associated thymic involution is a well-recognized factor associated with immunosenescence, and in particular with reduced vaccine efficacy. The thymus undergoes a progressive involution and the output of new cells falls significantly. Thymic functions already start decreasing after one year of life but the process becomes significant after 40 years of age. The expansion of perivascular space (adipocytes, peripheral lymphocytes, stroma) with age is such that thymic epithelial space represents less than 10% of the total thymic tissue by 70 years of age. When extrapolated, data suggest that the thymus would cease to produce new T cells by 105 years of age (Boren & Gershwin, 2004; Ongradi & Kovesdi, 2010; Gruver et al., 2007). There might be a benefit for the organism to reduce cell proliferation within the thymus, once a T-cell repertoire is established, so that energy can be devoted to other physiological processes (Shanley et al., 2009). Both intrinsic and extrinsic factors are thought to be involved in this process (Boren & Gershwin, 2004). Thymic epithelial cells produce a number of factors that can be thymosuppressive (Interleukin (IL)-6, LIF, OSM) or thymostimulatory (interleukin (IL)-7, Keratinocyte growth factor, Thymic stromal lymphopoïetin, growth hormone, leptin). Thymic atrophy is mediated by upregulation of thymosuppressive and decrease of thymostimulatory cytokines such as IL-7. This cytokine plays an important role for thymus function maintenance; it promotes thymopoiesis by maintaining anti-apoptotic protein Bcl-2 and inducing V-DJ recombination (Ongradi & Kovesdi, 2010; Gruver et al., 2007). Extrathymic factors including zinc, thymulin, cathepsin L, melatonin, thyroid hormone, growth hormone also contribute to thymus function. Stressful events, such as infections, septic shock, malnutrition, pregnancy, chemotherapy or irradiation have been associated with reversible thymic involution. Exogenous administration of leptin prevents this stress-induced thymic involution in mice, suggesting possible therapeutic intervention in aged humans (McElhaney & Effros, 2009; Boren & Gershwin, 2004; Gruver et al., 2007; Gruver et al., 2009; Hick et al., 2006). However, it is unclear whether age-associated and stress-induced thymic involutions result from the same mechanisms (McElhaney & Effros, 2009; Boren & Gershwin, 2004; Gruver et al., 2007). "Thymic rejuvenation" techniques have been sought for many years. Keratinocyte growth factor, IL-7 and ghrelin are interesting candidates (McElhaney & Effros, 2009; Aspinall et al., 2007). Keratinocyte growth factor enhances IL-7 production in the thymus, promoting development and maintenance of T cells following vaccination. IL-7 treatment has been shown to increase thymic output and number of central memory T cells and improve the antibody response to influenza vaccination in aged rhesus macaques (McElhaney & Effros, 2009). Intrathymic infection with IL-10-expressing adenovirus can prevent thymocyte apoptosis induced by sepsis in mice (Ongradi & Kovesdi, 2010; Gruver et al., 2007).

Thymic involution causes a continuous drop in the output of recent thymic emigrants while homeostatic mechanisms attempt to maintain constant peripheral T cell numbers. Consistent with greater proliferative history, naïve T cells from elderly have less T cell receptor excision circle (TREC) numbers and shorter telomere length (see below) (Ferrando-Martinez et al., 2011). However, the total number of T cells shows very little decline with advancing age, except in the very old. Furthermore, the proportion of naïve and memory T cells is well maintained up to the age of 65 years. It has been postulated that the majority of naïve T cells in the adult are generated by cell division of existing T cells, rather than thymic export. The repertoire of naïve CD4 T cells is also very well maintained up to the age of 65 years. It then dramatically dwindles and is found to be severely contracted and undistinguishable from the repertoire of memory T cells at 75-80 years of age. The same phenomenon is shown for naïve CD8 T cells. IL-7 plays an essential role in controlling homeostatic proliferation of naïve CD4+ and CD8+ T cells (Ferrando-Martinez et al., 2011; Arnold et al., 2011; Naylor et al., 2005; Kilpatrick et al., 2008).

Main lymphocyte subsets	
T lymphocytes cells (CD3+):	
	CD4+ helper T cells
	CD8+ cytotoxic T cells
	CD25+ Regulatory T cells
B lymphocytes cells (CD19+)	
	Naive B cells
	Memory B cells
	Plasmatocytes
Natural killer (NK) cells and NKT cells	
γδ T cells	

Table 2. Main lymphocyte subsets.

2.2 T lymphocytes

Memory and naïve human T cells are distinguished by their expression of members of the CD45 family surface antigens. CD45RA antigen is expressed primarily on naïve T lymphocytes and CD45RO is present on the cell surface of memory T lymphocytes (Figure 1). With normal aging, the slow turnover and long lifespan of naïve T cells are preserved but thymus output diminishes gradually and ultimately becomes insufficient to replace naïve T cells lost from the periphery. Conversely, cumulative chronic exposure to pathogens and environmental antigens promotes the accumulation of memory cells and eventually a state of "exhaustion". This phenomenon is associated with increased complication risk following viral illnesses such as influenza, respiratory syncytial virus and reactivation of herpes viruses (McElhaney & Effros, 2009; Desai et al., 2010).

In aged mice, formation of "immunological synapse" between CD4 T cells antigen presenting cells is hindered. This has been related to altered cholesterol/phospholipid ratio in lymphocyte membranes, leading to impaired T cell receptor (TCR)-dependent recruitment of signal molecules to the immunological synapse. In humans, alteration in the cholesterol/phospholipid ratio of lymphocyte membranes has also been documented and is associated with reduced proliferation rate (Arnold et al., 2011; Huber et al., 1991; Stulnig et al., 1995). With age, human and murine T cells tend to secrete less IL-2, an observation linked to important alterations in the proximal TCR signalling pathway (Boren & Gershwin, 2004; Fulop et al., 2007; Chakravarti & Abraham, 1999). Peripheral blood lymphocytes from aged individuals also display decreased NFAT expression, a key transcription factor implicated in IL-2 gene activation (Rink et al., 1998; Mysliwska et al., 1998; Wikby et al., 1994; Desai et al., 2010; DiPenta et al., 2007). However, when only "healthy older" people are considered (SENIEUR protocol), production of IL-2 was not different from that observed in younger individuals (Chen et al., 2009).

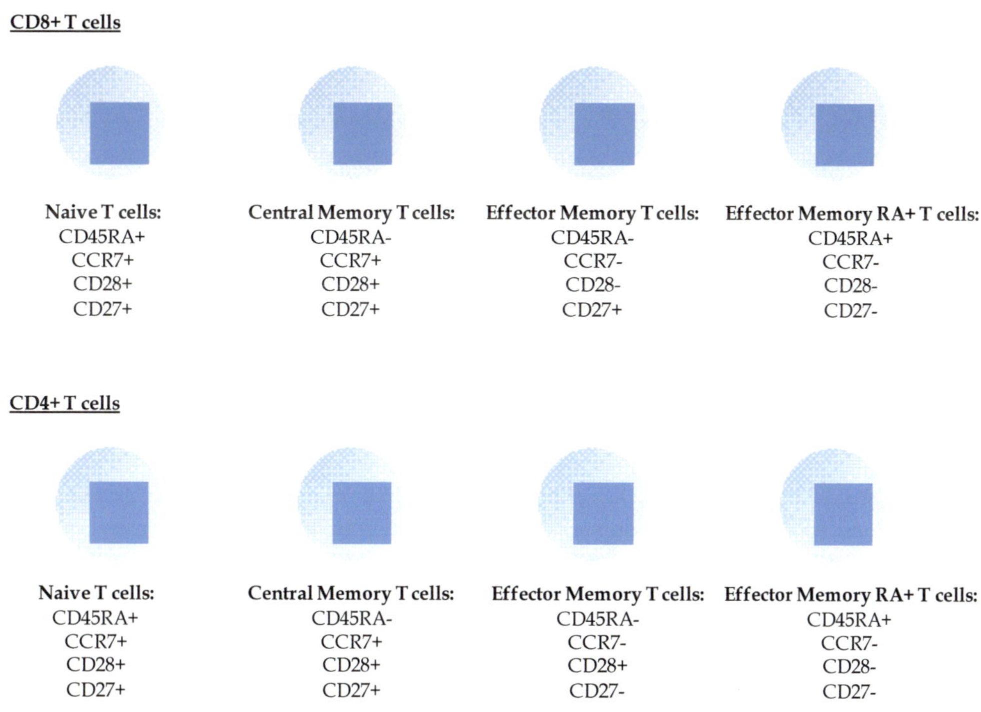

Fig. 1. Phenotype of different lymphocytes T cells subsets.

CD4 T lymphocytes from aged mice display decreased CD40L expression. In humans, CD40L expression is also reduced on peripheral blood CD4 T cells upon anti-CD3 stimulation in old people compared to younger individuals (Fernandez-Gutierrez et al., 1999). As this molecule is critical for B-T cell interactions, it could participate to the alteration of humoral responses observed in the old population. The function of "follicular helper T cells" in older people should be revisited in the light of the recent advances in the field (Ongradi & Kovesdi, 2010; Gruver et al., 2007; Crotty, 2011).

2.2.1 Naïve T cells

Naïve T cells from young and old adults differ significantly. Compared to young adults, 40% of human naïve CD8+ CD28+ T cells of older people do not express CD62L and CCR7, two receptors implicated in the migration to peripheral lymphoid tissues (Ongradi & Kovesdi, 2010; Aspinall et al., 2007). In humans, naïve CD8 T cells seem to be more susceptible to death receptor-mediated apoptosis and are more affected by age-related changes than the CD4+ T cell pool (Gupta & Gollapudi, 2006; Gupta & Gollapudi, 2008). CD45RA+CD28+CD8+ T cells from older people produce larger amounts of interferon (IFN)–γ upon polyclonal stimulation than those from young persons (Pfister & Savino, 2008).

As mentioned earlier, IL-7 plays an essential role in controlling homeostatic proliferation of naïve CD4+ and CD8+ T cells and supports the survival of naïve CD8+ T cells. IL-7 acts in conjunction with T cell receptor signals from contact with self-MHC/peptide that sustain the expression of anti-apoptotic molecules. However, this extended lifespan of naïve T cells could be associated with prolonged exposure to unfavourable environmental factors which cause DNA damage and contribute to decreased function in old age (Arnold et al., 2011).

2.2.2 Memory T cells

The three protocols (SENIEUR, OCTO and NONA) compared immune risk phenotype in older people with different state of comorbidities. Aging is associated with an increase of memory cells, a decrease of naïve T cells and a loss of CD28 molecules. Chronic cytomegalovirus (CMV) infection has been proposed as the main stimulus driving the *in vivo* process of "replicative senescence" (see section 4.3). CMV is associated with clonal expansion of CD8 T cells, increased numbers of CD8+ CD28- T cells, largely terminally differentiated effector memory T cells expressing CD45RA CCR7- (effector memory T cells, "EMRA") and inverted CD4:CD8 ratio (McElhaney & Effros, 2009; Pawelec & Derhovanessian, 2011; Pawelec et al., 2005; Derhovanessian et al., 2010). This will be further developed in this chapter.

Much effort has been dedicated to characterize cellular markers of immunosenescence. While T cell receptor repertoire contraction is a characteristic of the aging immune system, there is increasing evidence that clonal T cells of older persons may express a variety of receptors normally found on natural killer (NK) cells such as CD16, CD56, CD57, CD94, CD161, NKG2D and KIR family. NK receptors expression can have profound impact on immunity. Whereas, NK receptors diversity defines functional subsets of NK cells that contribute to normal innate antigen-independent responses, it is proposed that NK receptors expression on T cells from aged individuals is an adaptive mechanism of immunological diversity in the midst of a contracting T cell receptor repertoire. Studies with *in vitro* replicative senescence systems indicate stable NK receptors expression on T cells follows the loss of CD28 (Abedin et al., 2005; Alonso-Arias et al., 2011; Rajasekaran et al., 2010). Expression of CD57 is also found on T lymphocytes, where it is currently considered as a marker for "replicative senescence" (also termed "clonal exhaustion") i.e., a high susceptibility to activation-induced cell death and the inability to undergo new cell-division cycles despite preserved ability to secrete cytokines upon encounter with their cognate antigen. The phenotypes associated with replicative senescent CD8+ T lymphocytes are not well defined but are generally attributed to lack of CD28 or expression of CD57. CD8+CD57+ T lymphocytes have high cytotoxic effector potential including perforin, granzymes and granulysin. At the messenger and protein levels, CD8+CD57+T lymphocytes express more adhesion molecules and fewer chemokine receptors (CCR7 and CXCR4) than CD8+CD57– T lymphocytes but preferentially express CX3CR1. The lower expression level of genes involved in cell-cycle regulation supports the limited proliferation capacities of CD8+CD57+ T lymphocytes, even in response to polyclonal or cytokine stimulation (Focosi et al., 2010).

As detailed below, these CD8+CD57+T lymphocytes are commonly found in individuals with chronic immune activation and increase in frequency with age (from absence in newborns to 15–20% of circulating CD8 T cells), but the percentage of CD8+CD57+ cells increases in a series of clinical conditions whose common denominator is functional immune alteration, including HIV and CMV infections, common variable immunodeficiency, hematological cancers and autoimmune diseases (Pawelec & Derhovanessian, 2011; Focosi et al., 2010). OCTO, NONA and SENIEUR protocols conclude that the number of cells in the CD57+CD28-, CD45RACD27- and CD57+CD56+CD8+ T cells subsets in older people were independent of the individual's health status (disease interfering with immunity were excluded) (Nilsson et al., 2003). In older humans, CD4 T cells also express more NKG2D molecules and are associated with replicative senescence. NKG2D+ CD4+ T cells are mostly CD28- CD4+ T cells and also present cytotoxic properties (Alonso-Arias et al., 2011). These senescent cells resulting from permanent immune activation are potent producers of proinflammatory cytokines and have shorter telomeres than NKG2D- CD4+ T cells (Ongradi & Kovesdi, 2010; Gruver et al., 2007). Immune phenotype of T cells is correlated with individual "fitness" in individuals over 78 years. Unimpaired aged individuals display T cells expressing inhibitory NK receptors (CD158a, CD158e and NKG2a) and functionally impaired aged individuals display T cells expressing stimulatory NK receptors (CD56, CD16, NKG2D) (Vallejo et al., 2011).

It has been shown that high proportions of CD8+ CD25+ memory T cells are associated with healthy aging and are rare or absent in older people with latent CMV infection. The presence of CD8+CD25+ T cells is associated with the maintenance of intact humoral responses. They produce IL-2 and IL-4, assist B memory generation, induce MHC II upregulation on B cells, and promote antibody isotype switching to IgG1 and IgE. These T cells coexpress CD4 molecule and present a highly diverse TCR repertoire and longer telomere compared to the CD8+ CD25- subset (Herndler-Brandstetter et al., 2005).

Aged individuals (more than 65 years) have an increase in peripheral blood regulatory T cells expression. The increase of this population seems to be linked to the healthy state of elderly people. The *in vitro* function of this population is not altered with age (Ongradi & Kovesdi, 2010; Gruver et al., 2007; Gregg et al., 2005).

γδT cells represent a minor population of human peripheral lymphocytes (1-10%). They play a role in antiviral and antitumoral immunosurveillance. They produce high levels of cytokines, mainly TNFα and IFNγ. With increasing age, the absolute number of γδT cells and their proliferation rate is reduced while they express more TNFα. Inversely, they present no change in IFNγ expression and cytolytic activity with age (Argentati et al., 2002).

2.3 B lymphocytes and humoral responses

B cells also present alterations with increasing age. Decreased IL-7 production provokes a reduced ability to support B cell expansion by bone marrow stromal cells (Ongradi & Kovesdi, 2010). Bone marrow contains pluripotent stem cells that mature into bone tissue and cells that form peripheral blood cells, which further develop in specialized secondary compartments into functional immune cells. The stroma matrix of the bone marrow compartment is composed of accessory cells such as megakaryocytes, osteoblasts, osteoclasts, adipocytes, chondrocytes, myoblasts and fibroblasts. The hematopoietic compartment decreases with increasing age and is replaced by adipose tissue. Surprisingly, increased number of bone marrow resident macrophages is observed with age but these cells have decreased ability to secrete TNFα. Both TNFα and IL-1 are essential to promote secretion of other cytokines critical to stromal integrity, such as IL-6, IL-11, M-CSF or GM-CSF. There is no clear evidence that hematopoietic cells number (CD34+) decreases with age. Hematopoietic cells give rise into common lymphoid progenitors like pro-B cells. There are discrepancies about the evolution of pro-B cells with age. Conversely, pre-B cells decrease markedly with age (Gruver et al., 2007).

The proportion and numbers of total B cells (CD19+) decrease with age. Data on specific B cell subsets is less clear. Naïve B cells are defined as IgG- IgA- IgD+ CD27- whereas memory B cell population is very heterogeneous, comprising three subtypes (Figure2): "IgM memory" cells (that are IgD+ IgM+ CD27+, important against bacterial infections), "classical switched memory" (IgG+/IgA+ CD27+) and "double negative" B cells (IgG+/IgA+, IgD- CD27- B cells). This later group could emerge independently from T cell help.

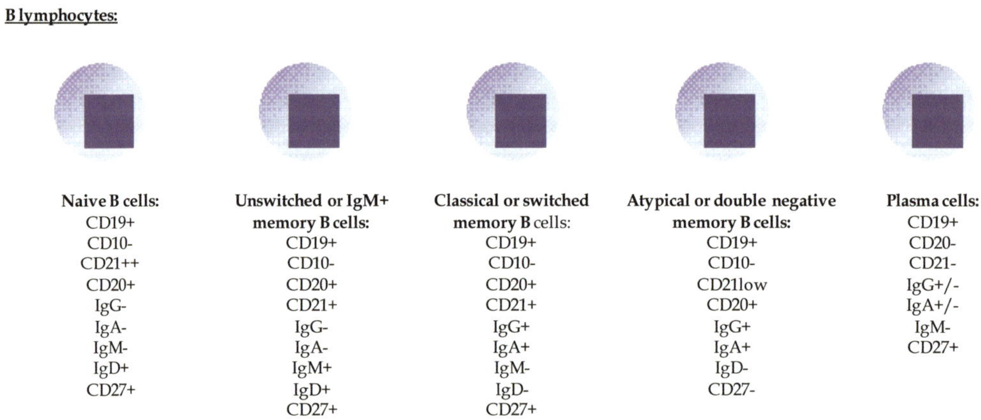

Fig. 2. Phenotype of different B lymphocyte cells subsets.

Proportion of naïve B cells decreases with age. Several reports indicate that the proportion and number of CD27+ (memory) B cells increase but other reports show the opposite (Bulati et al., 2011; Colonna-Romano et al., 2009). The discrepancy probably reflects differences in the subsets definition and study protocols. Naïve B cells exhibit a reduced susceptibility to apoptosis in aged individuals (Chong et al., 2005). B cells produce large amounts of proinflammatory cytokines upon CD40 and IL-4 activation and so could play a role in the generation or in the maintenance of the inflammatory environment of the older people (Buffa et al., 2011). The "IgM memory" subset decreases with age. Other reports indicate a decrease of "switched memory" B cells. Finally the proportion of "double negative" B cells seems to increase with age (Ademokun et al., 2010; Bulati et al., 2011; Colonna-Romano et al., 2003; Colonna-Romano et al., 2009; Chong et al., 2005). This "double negative" population in aged individuals presents reduced expression of CD40, HLA-DR and CD80 and shorter telomeres. These cells are also present in patients with systemic lupus erythematosus (Colonna-Romano et al., 2009). There is a significant increase of anergic, "exhausted" memory cells with CD27 downregulation (CD27-) in older people. In centenarians, naïve B cells (IgD+ CD27-) are more abundant whereas exhausted memory cells (IgD- CD27-) do not show the increase previously demonstrated in healthy older people. Authors conclude that the reservoir of naïve B cells might be one factor of "successfully aging" (Ongradi & Kovesdi, 2010; Fernandez-Gutierrez et al., 1999).

B cells progenitors undergo maturation and differentiation in secondary lymphoid tissue, such as spleen and lymph nodes. Spleen arteries are surrounded by T lymphocytes in the periarteriolar lymphoid sheath. Primary lymphoid follicules containing B cells are adjacent to the periarteriolar lymphoid sheath. Other cell types such as T cells, dendritic cells and macrophages make up the marginal zone. This constitutes the white pulp. Age-associated architectural changes have been documented. Spleen from aged humans demonstrates a decrease in arterial vessels and an increase in stromal cells over lymphocytes. Total splenic weight increases with age due to fibroblastic infiltration (Gruver et al., 2007).

The germinal centre reaction is essential for the generation of high affinity antibody in response to infectious agents. This process is accomplished by two distinct mechanisms: class switch recombination, which enables B cells to change antibody isotype, and somatic hypermutation, the process of introducing mutations into the B cell receptor to increase antigen affinity. Data indicate that there is no change in the fundamental mechanisms of somatic hypermutation with age in man but an impaired ability of class switch recombination has been described in aged mice (Ademokun et al., 2010).

There is also a collapse in B cell receptor repertoire diversity with age and an expansion of monoclonal cells. The incidence of "monoclonal gammopathy of undefined significance" (MGUS) has been shown to increase with age. Sensitive assays reveal that as many as 50% of old mice and 20% of elderly humans have serum monoclonal immunoglobulin. As half of serum monoclonal immunoglobulins reacts with autoantigens, it appears that cells producing monoclonal immunoglobulins are drawn preferentially from the population of "B1 cells" that expand with age in both humans and mice (Weksler & Szabo, 2000). These CD5+CD20+ cells are produced during fetal live and are T-independent (in contrast to CD5-CD20+ "B2 cells" that are produced post-natally and are T-dependent). In humans, approximately 1% of old subjects with serum monoclonal immunoglobulin develop multiple myeloma each year, derived probably from plasma cell clonal expansions. Chronic lymphocytic leukemia, another lymphoid malignancy that occurs late in life, may arise from malignant transformation of the large B-cell clonal expansions. Chronic lymphocytic leukemia is frequently associated with T-cell abnormalities, including an inversion of the normal CD4 to CD8 T cell ratio, expansions of large granular lymphocytes, and clonal expansions of CD4 and CD8 T cells. These T-cell clonal expansions may represent a clonotypic response to transformed B cells or their secreted immunoglobulins. This hypothesis is supported by the finding that T cells from myeloma patients can be activated by monoclonal Ig fragments (Ademokun et al., 2010; Bulati et al., 2011; Colonna-Romano et al., 2003; Weksler & Szabo, 2000). However, in humans, despite the reduced number of B cells and the defects in class-switching, serum IgG, IgA are increased with age; IgD levels decrease with age but IgE and IgM remain unchanged or are decreased. IgG1 and IgG3 (in men) subtypes are also increased with age (Ademokun et al., 2010; Bulati et al., 2011; Colonna-Romano et al., 2003).

The quality of the humoral response also declines with age, characterized by lower antibody responses and decreased production of high affinity antibodies. B cells from aged individuals can be directly activated by cytokine but are weakly activated by anti-CD3 activated PBMCs. This result suggests that poor B cell responses is a consequence of inadequate help from T cells (Ongradi & Kovesdi, 2010; Fernandez-Gutierrez et al., 1999). In mice, aged CD4+ T cells provide poor assistance in germinal centres and promote low-affinity antibody production. Furthermore, overproduction of Th2 cytokines could augment B cell-mediated autoimmune disorders by enhancing the production of autoreactive antibodies. The percentage of naïve follicular B cells declines whereas subsets of antigen-experienced mature B cells with longer life span increase including poly/self reactive subtypes. These cells may be reactivated due to age-associated reduced tolerance or loss of tissue integrity leading to the exposure of neo-self antigens that results in aberrant autoimmune response (Ongradi & Kovesdi, 2010). Taken together, these data indicate that in older people, B cell repertoire diversity is limited while there is an increase of polyspecific and auto-antibodies.

3. Innate immune responses and aging.

3.1 Monocytes and dendritic cells subsets, neutrophils

Monocytes represent about 5-10% of peripheral blood leukocytes in humans. They originate from a myeloid precursor in the bone marrow, circulate in the blood and spleen then enter tissues. Monocytes represent circulating precursors for tissue macrophages and dendritic cells. The differential expression of CD14 (part of the receptor for LPS) and CD16 (also known as FcγRIII) are commonly used to define two major subsets (Figure 3): "classical" $CD14^{++}$ $CD16^{-}$ cells, representing 95% of monocytes in healthy individuals and the "non-classical" $CD14^{+}$ $CD16^{+}$ comprising the remaining fraction. This later population is considered to represent activated cells that have undergone CD16 upregulation and CD14 downregulation and have been implicated in the pathogenesis of atherosclerosis. In healthy older volunteers, there is a shift of "classical" to "non-classical" monocytes. While "classical" monocytes express CCR2, "non-classical" monocytes preferentially express CX3CR1. Expression intensity of CXCR3 tends to decrease with age (Seidler et al., 2010; Sadeghi et al., 1999).

Dendritic cells (DCs) play a key role in the immune system since they orchestrate initiation, amplification and suppression of immune responses. In particular, maturation of DCs is crucial for the initiation of immunity. In fact, immature DCs are extremely efficient in capturing and processing antigens, but their unique ability to potently activate naïve T lymphocytes is acquired after maturation. This process is accompanied by the up-regulation of major histocompatibility complex molecules and the increased expression of membrane molecules that interact with T lymphocytes to enhance cell activation and adhesion. Furthermore, DC maturation leads to the release of high levels of cytokines that are

Main subsets of blood innate immune cells

Granulocytes:
- Neutrophils
- Eosinophils
- Basophils

Monocytes:
- « Classical » monocytes:
  - CD16- CD14++
- Inflammatory monocytes:
  - CD16++ CD14+
  - CD16++ CD14-

Dendritic cells:
- Plasmacytoid DC
  - CD123+ CD11c-
- Myeloid DC
  - CD123- CD11c+

Table 3. Blood innate immune cells.

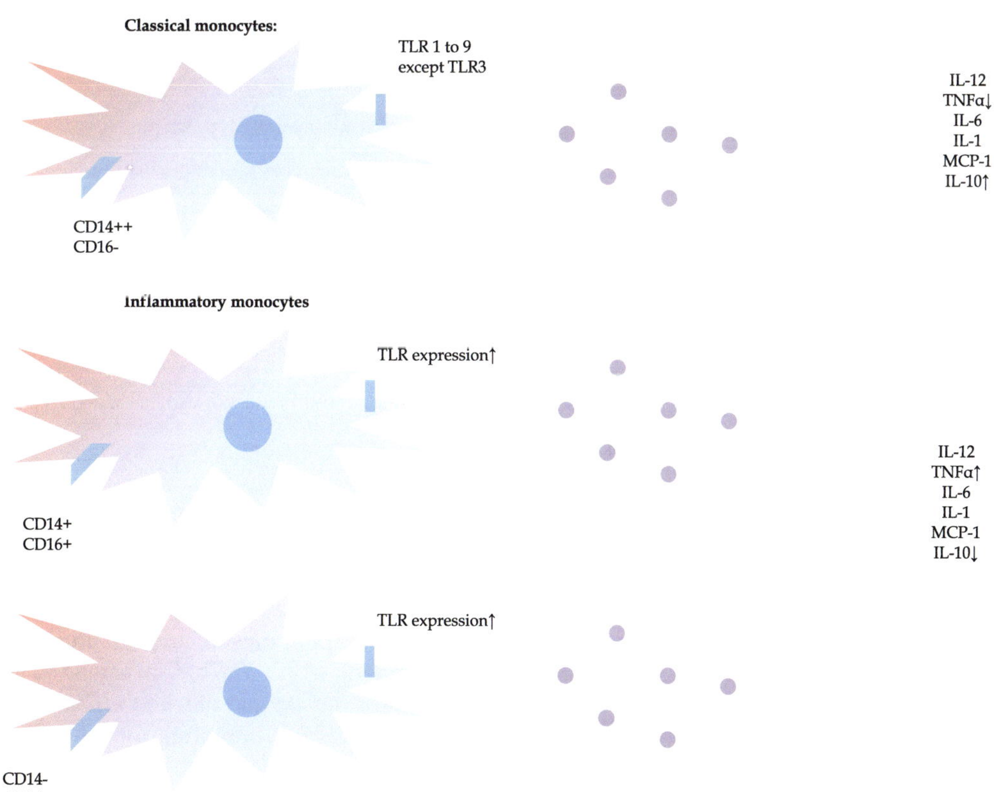

Fig. 3. Major subsets of monocytes.

responsible for the regulation and polarization of both innate and acquired immune responses (Ciaramella et al., 2011; Agrawal et al., 2007a). DCs are heterogeneous and are subdivided into two major categories: those that are present in peripheral blood (myeloid and plasmacytoid DCs) and those that are present in tissue/organs (Langerhans cells, interstitial and interdigitating DCs) (Agrawal et al., 2007b). Myeloid DCs express CD11c+ and low level of CD123 and can be subdivided into CD16+ (40-80%), CD1b/c+ (20-50%) and BDCA3+ (2-3%) subpopulations (Figure 4). Plasmacytoid DCs express low level of CD11c, high level of CD123, BDCA2 and BDCA4 and are specialized for production of type I IFNs in the context of viral infections (MacDonald et al., 2002; Dzionek et al., 2000).

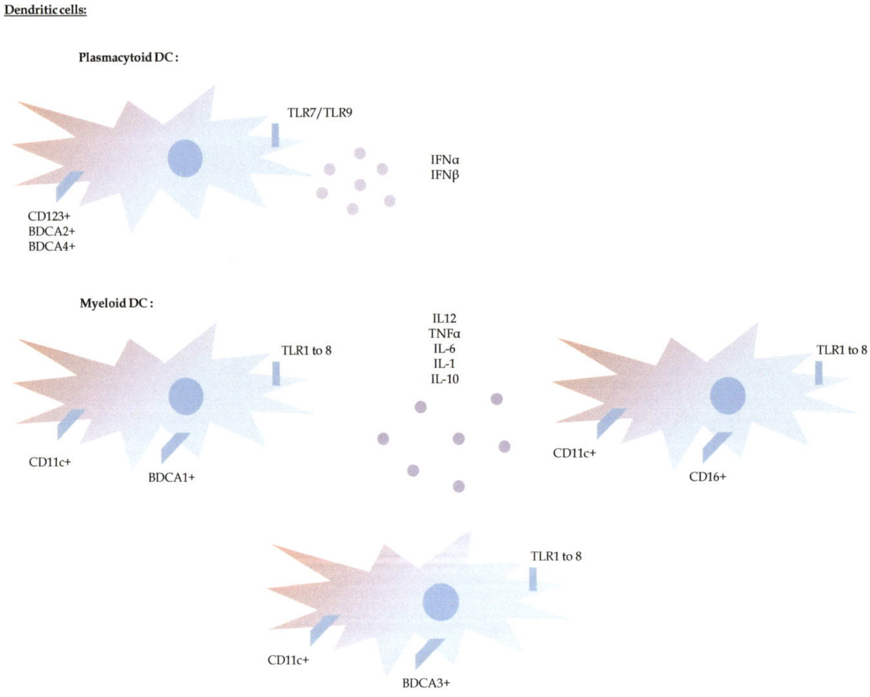

Fig. 4. Major subsets of dendritic cells.

In vitro monocyte-derived DCs, cultured with GM-CSF+IL-4, are closely related to interstitial or myeloid DCs (Agrawal et al., 2007b). Several studies used these *in vitro* cultured cells to assess the phenotype and functions of DCs in aged populations. Monocyte-derived DCs present no clear differences of costimulatory or activatory molecules (HLA-DR, CD80, CD86, CD40, CD83) except for CD25 and ICAM after lipopolysaccharide stimulation in healthy older individuals compared to younger (Agrawal et al., 2007b; Ciaramella et al., 2011; Agrawal et al., 2007a). Monocyte-derived DCs of older people are less efficient for micropinocytosis and phagocytosis of apoptotic cells and are impaired for migration (Agrawal et al., 2007b).

Several reports indicate that there are no significant differences in numbers of circulating myeloid and plasmacytoid DCs between older people and young subjects and that the expression of costimulatory molecules (CD86 and HLA DR) is similar (Agrawal et al., 2007a; Agrawal et al., 2007b; Pietschmann et al., 2000). In contrast, another study showed that numbers of myeloid DCs progressively declined with age while proportion of plasmacytoid DCs was unaffected. Peripheral blood DCs from healthy old subjects expressed CD86 and CD83, two markers of activation, on a higher percentage of cells, in comparison to young subjects. Maturation with lipopolysaccharide was unaffected with age (Della et al., 2007). Other studies showed reduced numbers of plasmacytoid DCs but not of myeloid DCs in healthy aged blood donors. Absolute numbers of circulating myeloid DCs is affected by declining health status (Perez-Cabezas et al., 2007; Panda et al., 2010; Shodell & Siegal, 2002; Jing et al., 2009). The use of Ficoll-enriched cells versus whole blood, differences in sample sizes, age groups, health status, genetic factors and subset definitions may contribute to the inconsistent findings with age in these studies. Taken together these data suggest that many factors, in addition to age itself, probably influence absolute/relative numbers or activation status of circulating DCs in geriatric populations.

Neutrophils are key players for early responses to bacterial infections. They rapidly produce reactive oxygen and nitrogen species when pathogens are encountered and produce many pro-inflammatory mediators. Several studies have shown alterations of neutrophil functions with age. Data remain conflicting in the literature concerning their number and phagocytic functions. One suggested alteration is their propensity to undergo apoptosis because of augmented cell oxidative load and perturbation of anti-apoptotic/proapoptotic mechanisms (Tortorella et al., 2006). Several reports indicate reduced chemotaxis (Fulop et al., 2004), phagocytosis and production of superoxide anion. Negative feedback mechanisms could also be perturbated (Fulop et al., 2004; Wessels et al., 2010). In contrast, centenarians do not present neutrophil defects compare to old people for adherence, chemotaxis, superanion production (Wessels et al., 2010; Alonso-Fernandez et al., 2008); (Crighton & Puppione, 2006).

3.2 Toll-like receptors

Toll-like receptors (TLR) are expressed on a variety of cells including macrophages, monocytes, natural killer cells, DCs, B and T lymphocytes. To date, 10 TLR are functional in humans. Pathogen associated molecular patterns serving as TLR ligands include lipopolysaccharide (LPS) on gram (-) bacteria (TLR4), diacetylated (TLR2/6) and triacetylated (TLR1/2) lipopeptides, peptidoglycan (TLR2), bacterial flagellin (TLR5), nucleic acid and double-stranded RNA (TLR3), single stranded RNA (TLR7 and TLR8) and unmethylated CpG oligodeoxynucleotides (TLR9). Recognition of microbial components by TLR initiates MYD88 and TRIF-dependent signal transduction pathways that culminate in both the elaboration of proinflammatory cytokine responses (via NFκB-dependent pathways) and the upregulation of type I IFNs and IFN-dependent genes. TLR-dependent activation of antigen presenting cells is a crucial step not only for the innate response but also for the ensuing initiation of the adaptive immune response. Inherited defects in TLR signaling are associated with a greater susceptibility to bacterial (especially Streptococcus pneumonia) and mycobacterial infection (Figure 5). Furthermore, TLR ligands as immunogens or adjuvants play an important role in mediating immune response to several human vaccines (Shaw et al., 2011; van Duin & Shaw, 2007).

Several studies in humans and mice have shown that TLR expression and functions tend to decline with age (van Duin & Shaw, 2007). Human monocytes from aged individuals present lower surface TLR1 expression than their younger counterparts (van Duin et al., 2007). These studies revealed an age-associated reduction in TNFα and IL-6 after stimulation of the TLR1/2 heterodimer. Similar observations were also noted for TLR7-induced IL-6 production. There is a significant decrease in TLR-induced upregulation of CD80 in older compared to young for all TLR ligands (van Duin & Shaw, 2007; Shaw et al., 2011). Myeloid DCs show decreased expression of TLR1, TLR3 and plasmacytoid DCs a decrease of TLR7 and TLR9 in older people compared to young individuals (Panda et al., 2010; Jing et al., 2009). DCs from older donors had diminished late phase responses such as the induction of transcription factors STAT1 and IRF7 and lower expression of IRF1,

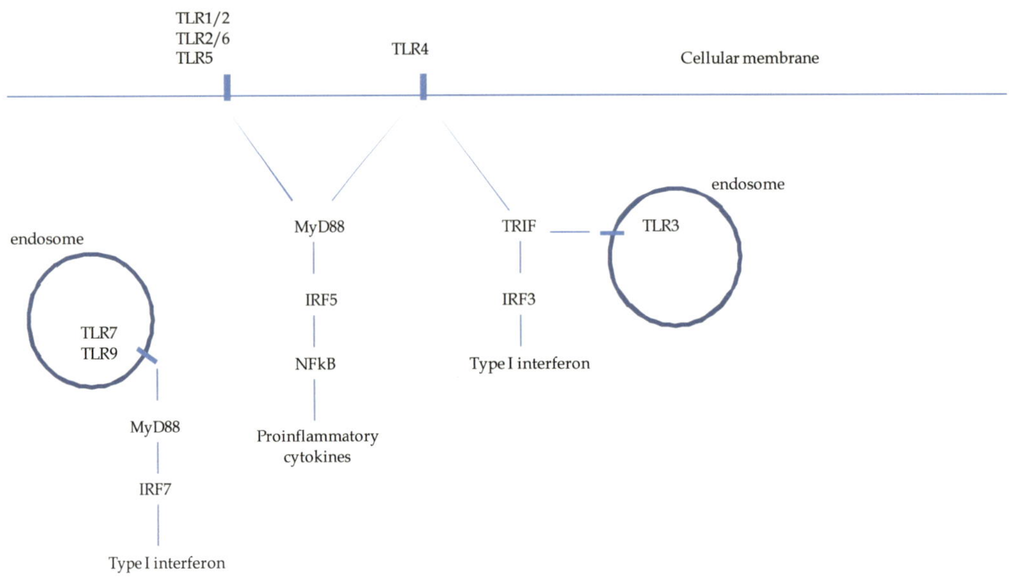

Fig. 5. Toll like receptor signaling.

suggesting a defective positive feedback regulation of type I IFN expression. Responses to TLR ligands may also be influenced by single nucleotide polymorphism within TLR genes. Authors report decreased IFNα, IL-6, IL-8 and TNFα in influenza virus-stimulated or HSV-2-stimulated plasmacytoid DCs from older compared to younger individuals (Shaw et al., 2011; Jing et al., 2009). IFNα production may be restored by zinc supplementation (Rink et al., 1998). Stimulated myeloid DCs and plasmacytoid DCs with different TLR ligands show a reduced expression of TNFα, IL-6, IL-12p40 and IFNα in healthy older people but an increased of the basal levels of this cytokine in older people (Panda et al., 2010). This decrease in TLR-induced cytokine production was strongly associated with the inability to mount protective antibody responses to the trivalent inactivated influenza vaccine currently recommended (Panda et al., 2010). LPS-stimulated monocytes from old people were reported to express less IL-12/23p40 levels in comparison to monocytes from young individuals (Della et al., 2007). However, their capacity to produce either bioactive IL-12 or IL-23 has not been addressed.

In contrast, analysis of monocyte-derived DCs from aged individuals revealed higher production of TNFα, IL-6 and IL-18 in response to LPS- and ssRNA but no difference in IL-

12p40/p70 (Ciaramella et al., 2011). There was no reduction of TLR4 expression with age but it was associated with decreased of phosphor-inositol 3(PI3) kinase, a negative regulator of TLR signalling. It manifested by decreased AKT phosphorylation and increased p38 mitogen activated protein kinase activation. They also present an increased expression of phosphatase and tensin homolog (PTEN), a negative regulator of PI3 kinase signalling pathway (Shaw et al., 2011; Agrawal et al., 2007a; Agrawal et al., 2007b).

Aging is generally associated with increased basal production of inflammatory cytokines but results of studies are often contradictory, depending on study designs and age groups (Beharka et al., 2001). Most studies report augmented plasma/serum levels of IL-6 and TNFα with increasing age, even in "selected" SENIEUR elderly over 85 years of age (Krabbe et al., 2004; Della et al., 2007). An elevated circulating IL-6 level is a strong predictor of thromboembolic complications while elevated TNFα levels are correlated with frailty (Krabbe et al., 2004). Another study shows that high basal IL-6 had a better predictive value for mortality than TNFα and that both cytokines were associated with classical risk factor like smoking, physical inactivity and body mass index (Bruunsgaard et al., 2003). A study confirmed increased serum IL-6, TGFβ and s-ICAM in the older people but IL-6 increased also with poor health status (comparing SENIEUR, OCTO and NONA elderly) (Forsey et al., 2003; Mysliwska et al., 1998). Serum IP-10 and CXCL9 levels have also been reported with increasing age, in contrast to IL-10 and IL-12p40. These chemokines display strong chemoattractant activity for Th1 lymphocytes and have been involved in the pathogenesis of autoimmune disorders, such as Grave's disease or Crohn's disease, and in metabolic disorders, such as diabetes mellitus or atherosclerosis (Shurin et al., 2007). A recent study confirms that "impaired" (poor functional status) older people express higher basal levels of IFNγ, IL-12p70, IL-6 and TNFα while "unimpaired" older people express higher basal levels of IL-5 and IL-13 when compared to each other (Vallejo et al., 2011).

High basal production of pro-inflammatory cytokines is generally associated with poor capacity to respond to TLR stimulation (Bruunsgaard et al., 1999a). Indeed, several studies indicate that reduced responsiveness to LPS stimulation (lower TNFα, IL-1β, IL-6, IL-10 and IL-1Ra production by whole blood cells) from 85-year olds is significantly associated with a worse survival and more risk factors like history of malignancies, chronic illness and elevated CRP levels (van den Biggelaar et al., 2004). Some whole blood studies however suggest that TNFα and IL-6 production upon TLR stimulation is increased in aged individuals, in particular for SENIEUR population under 85 years. This population probably does not display chronic low-grade inflammation (Gabriel et al., 2002). Zinc plasma levels could also represent an important factor to consider (Mariani et al., 2006).

IL-1 and TNFα are the earliest mediators of the acute phase response. Both cytokines induce a strong wave of cytokines including IL-6 and chemokines. In the course of S. *Pneumoniae* infection, inflammatory cytokines levels tend to persist for longer periods in older patients in contrast to younger ones (Bruunsgaard et al., 1999b). This observation could be related to increased pro-inflammatory environment in aged individuals but also to reduced clearing of the bacteria. It should also be interpreted in the light of possible alterations of renal function in the older people.

Taken together, low-grade chronic inflammation ("inflamm-aging") seems to be a cardinal feature of advanced "healthy" aging. The magnitude of this process at a given age is strongly influenced by multiple factors, including metabolic disorders and nutritional status. Indeed, poor health status and frailty will be associated with more intense inflammatory markers but poor responses to stimulation.

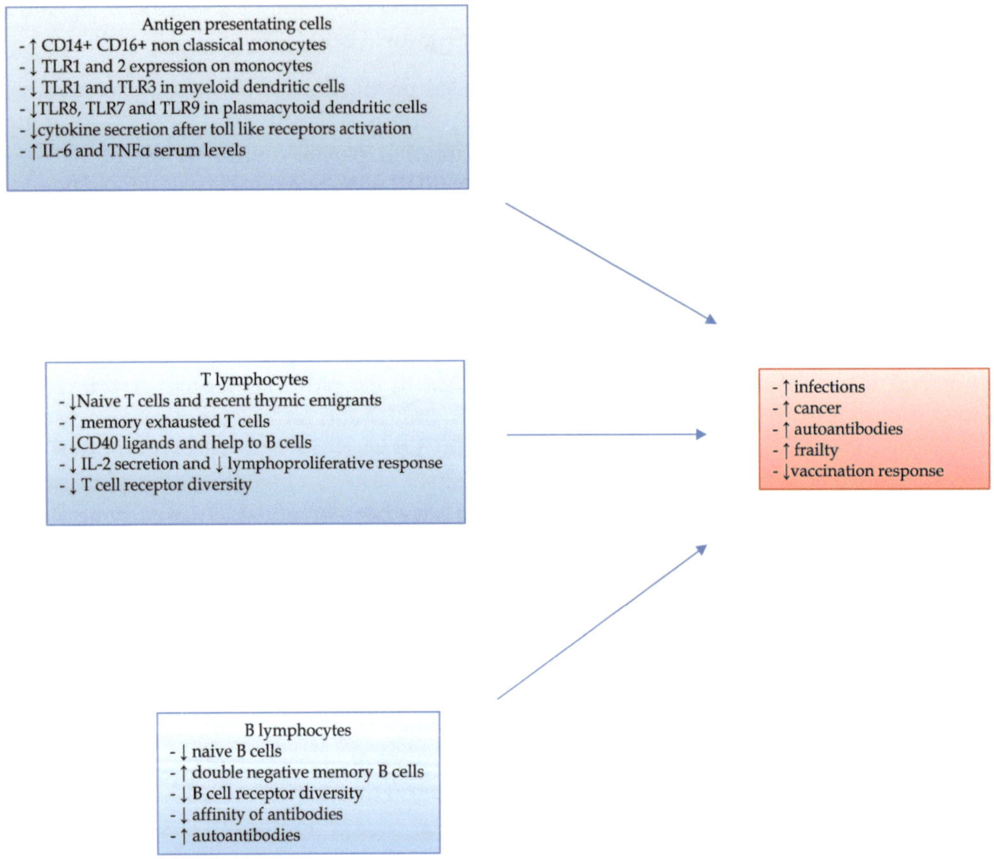

Fig. 6. Changes in immune responses observed in aged individuals.

4. Linking the characteristics of immune responses in the geriatric population to the clinical status.

"Normal" aging is determined genetically. At the cellular level, increased lifetime is associated with replicative-dependent shortening of chromosomal ends, also known as telomeres. In immune cells, this process is linked to immunosenescence. While this phenomenon is the normal destiny of dividing cells, it also reflects the global history of the organism. Here, we will discuss how the different immune parameters of the older people can be linked to the clinical characteristics encountered in the geriatric population.

4.1 Shortening of telomere length, genetic factors and hormonal changes

Telomeres consist of simple tandem DNA repeats (10-20kb) that do not encode for any gene products. The main function of telomeres is to cap the chromosome ends. Telomere capping is necessary to distinguish the chromosome ends from DNA breaks within the genome. DNA breaks within the genome lead to cell cycle arrest and DNA repair or to induction of apoptosis when the damage is too severe. In contrast to DNA breaks, chromosome ends do not provoke DNA damage responses (Ongradi & Kovesdi, 2010; Jiang et al., 2007). Telomeres are regarded as the molecular clock of aging, including that of the immune system, especially for lymphocytes. Telomere shortening is due to the end replication problem of DNA polymerase at each round of cell division and to diminished activity of telomerase that fails to add telomere repeat sequence to the end of chromosomes. Telomerase is active during embryogenesis but is suppressed postnataly in most somatic tissues. In adult humans, telomerase stays only active in germ cells, certain stem cells and progenitor compartment. Telomerase reactivation occurs in activated lymphocytes and human cancer cells (Jiang et al., 2007; Ongradi & Kovesdi, 2010). Regulation of the telomerase activity is complex and is limited by expression of the catalytic subunit hTERT. Many transcription factors act as activators (including c-Myc, SP1, USF1/2, Ets, HIF-1, hALP) or repressors (p53, AP1, Mad1, Wilm's tumor 1, Smad3,...). Oestrogens activate c-myc thereby influencing telomerase activity. Indeed, women present longer telomeres than men. Cortisol inhibits telomerase activity in CD4 and CD8 T cells, suggesting a mechanism by which stress can negatively affect immune response (Andrews et al., 2010; Balasubramanyam et al., 2007). Chronic psychological stress in caregivers of Alzheimer's patients or chronically ill children is associated with telomere loss in peripheral blood lymphocytes, possibly explained by increased cortisol levels. Another study shows reduced telomerase activity related to neuroendocrine and psychosocial data indicative of greater stress (cortisol, epinephrine, norepinephrine) in women but they failed to show an association between telomere shortening and negative mood or education (Andrews et al., 2010; Jiang et al., 2007; Epel et al., 2006). In humans, telomeres shorten by 50-100 base pairs with each cell division. Most human tissues and organs show significant telomere shortening during aging, including peripheral blood mononuclear cells (PBMCs), isolated lymphocytes, kidney epithelium, vascular endothelial cells, hepatocytes, intestinal and lung epithelial cells, muscle but not for brain. Telomere length in PBMCs also correlated inversely with the mortality rate in 60-75 year olds. Individuals with short telomeres have a 3.18-fold higher mortality rates from heart diseases and 8.54-fold higher mortality rates from infectious diseases compared to those with relatively long telomeres but it is not a significant prognostic factor for survival above 85 years. In addition to telomere shortening with aging, accelerated shortening observed in PBMCs occurs in various human diseases such as myelodysplasic syndrome (Jiang et al., 2007; Andrews et al., 2010; Ohyashiki et al., 1999), atherosclerosis and hypertension (Jiang et al., 2007; Andrews et al., 2010; Benetos et al., 2004), coronary artery disease, human immunodeficiency virus, rheumatoid arthritis (Jiang et al., 2007; Andrews et al., 2010; Steer et al., 2007) systemic lupus erythematosus, cognitive decline,... (Jiang et al., 2007; Andrews et al., 2010). Alzheimer patients present reduced telomere length in PBMCs compared to control. There was also a significant correlation between T cell telomere length and MMSE score, CD28 expression and an inverse correlation between serum TNFα production and telomere shortening in T cells (Panossian et al., 2003). Telomere shortening is also correlated with duration of type 1 and type 2 diabetes and systolic blood pressure but not with diabetes complications (Astrup et al., 2010; Sampson et al., 2006). Another study confirms the negative correlation between cardiovascular risk factor or coronary heart disease and telomere length (Spyridopoulos et al., 2009; Brouilette et al., 2007). This study also shows that treatment with statins in patients with high risk on the basis of telomere length results in substantial benefit effect (Brouilette et al., 2007). Oxidative stress is believed to be a major factor of accelerated aging, possible due to an increased pace of telomere shortening resulting from DNA damages observed upon smoking, obesity or cardiovascular diseases (Andrews et al., 2010; Balasubramanyam et al., 2007). The incidence of cancer sharply increases with aging. Telomere shortening appears to have a dual role in cancer formation. It was originally proposed that telomere shortening limits the lifespan of human cells thus acting as a tumor suppressor mechanism. The majority of human cancers exhibit very short telomeres, much shorter than the surrounding non-transformed tissue. However, more than 90% of human cancers show a strong reactivation of telomerase (Jiang et al., 2007).

Early studies showed that human somatic cells have a finite number of replicative cycles. The term "replicative senescence" is used to describe the stage at which telomeres are shortened to a critical length such that a proliferative response can no longer be elicited. One of the approaches to prevent or delay the generation of senescent CD8+ T cells is based on the well-documented link between telomere shortening and overall replicative potential and function of T lymphocytes. Although telomerase is capable of elongating telomeres and is upregulated in concert with T cell activation, the activity of this enzyme is completely turned off in CD8+ T cells that are chronically stimulated in cell culture. One suggested way to improve age-dependent decline of immune function would be to elicit strong cellular immunity by compounds that favour telomerase activity (McElhaney & Effros, 2009).

Other "genetic" factors have also been implicated in the process of immunosenescence. For example, IL-6 gene may be involved in the genetic regulation of longevity. IL-6 VNTR D/D genotypes were associated with increased levels in the blood and brain from Alzheimer's disease patients and IL6 VNTR allele B could be detrimental for reaching extreme longevity (Capurso et al., 2007; Krabbe et al., 2004). It was also reported that -1082 IL-10 promoter polymorphism was increased in male centenarians as compared to younger men and this genotype was associated with increased production of IL-10 (Krabbe et al., 2004).

Age is also characterized by hormone changes. It seems that oestrogens can have powerful immunomodulating effects, albeit mainly during stress. *In vitro* studies have shown that oestrogens deficiency leads to reduced IL-2 expression (Ku et al., 2009). Oestrogens seem to have important effects on B cells. A study shows that the percentage of conventional B cells (B-2, CD5- CD20+ cells) is significantly lower in late post menopause while B-1 cells (CD5+ CD20+) remain unchanged. It suggests that oestrogens may be involved in maintaining peripheral B-2 cell pool in women. Even if oestrogens seem to influence B cells, hormone replacement therapy does not influence the production of antinuclear antibodies or anti-IL-1 antibodies observed with aging (Kamada et al., 2001). Circulating oestradiol in late postmenopausal women without hormonal replacement therapy is positively correlated to CRP and serum level of IL-6 but the association for IL-6 was not significant anymore after adjustement for other clinical factors. Testosterone levels were also positively correlated with C-reactive protein, TNFα and IL-6 even after adjustement for confounders (Maggio et al., 2011).

Dehydroepiandrosterone (DHEA) has been considered for immunorestoration because serum levels dramatically decrease with age in both sexes. No DHEA-specific receptor has been identified in human T lymphocyte and it exerts probably its action indirectly via downstream conversion to other steroids, in particular sex steroid. Furthermore, DHEA exerts also anti-glucocorticoid action. *In vitro,* it increases IL-2 production, NK cell activity. Conversely, *in vivo,* it decreases circulating IL-6 levels. However, no consistent *in vivo* data on immune effect of DHEA supplementation in healthy older humans has been reported. Conversely, it shows a beneficial effect for patients treated in the context of systemic lupus erythematosus (Fulop et al., 2007; Arlt & Hewison, 2004). Other studies show that DHEA negatively correlates with basal IL-6 seric levels in older people but this relation is more complex in younger people. DHEA added in culture of PBMCs inhibits IL-6 secretion (Straub et al., 1998; James et al., 1997).

4.2 Comorbidities and medications

The main confounding factor that might impact on immune functions of the geriatric patient is the occurrence of multiple morbidities. These pathologies have potential direct effect on immune cells but the influence of pharmaceutical treatments should also be kept in mind. Recent research has attempted to identify risk factors for mortality and functional decline in older persons. A 7-year community based cohort study shows that 5% of "high functioning" aged individuals display three or four markers of inflammation (IL-6, cholesterol, albumin, CRP). This was associated with a more than 6-fold increased risk of 3-year mortality and a more than 3-fold risk of 7-year mortality independently of other measures of health status (Reuben et al., 2002). This indicates that innate immune parameters are strongly linked to clinical status.

4.2.1 Cardiovascular diseases and associated metabolic disorder

Atherosclerotic plaques contain smooth muscle cells, activated T lymphocytes and monocyte-derived macrophages. Several epidemiological studies have linked systemic low-grade inflammation in older populations to the prevalence and prognosis of cardiovascular disease. High IL-1β serum levels were associated with congestive heart failure, angina and dyslipidemia. High TNFα serum levels have been correlated with dyslipidemia and a higher prevalence of cardiovascular disease in 80 year olds and with high blood pressure, insulin resistance and common carotid intima media thickness in healthy middle-aged men. IL-6 acts as a marker of subclinical cardiovascular disease in older people and is a predictor of mortality related to cardiovascular disease (Krabbe et al., 2004). TNFα directly causes upregulation of cellular adhesion molecules at the surface of endothelial cells and causes insulin resistance. IL-6 induces procoagulant changes by increasing fibrinogen, tissue factor, factor VIII, von Willebrand factor and platelets. Moreover, both TNFα and IL-6 favour dyslipidemia (Bruunsgaard et al., 2003).

TLRs are expressed throughout the body and are mainly found on professional innate immune cells, including macrophages, dendritic cells and mast cells but also on non-professional immune cells such as endothelial cells and smooth muscle cells. All these cells are present in the atherosclerotic lesion and contribute to the inflammatory response. The expression of several TLRs is increased in atherosclerotic lesions. TLR4 is also increased on circulating monocytes from patients with coronary artery disease compared to controls. Several epidemiologic studies have reported elevated risk of atherosclerosis associated with a large number of infections (Chlamydia pneumonia, Helicobacter pylori, cytomegalovirus (CMV), Epstein-Barr virus (EBV), human immunodeficiency virus (HIV), herpes simplex virus (HSV) 1 and 2, Hepatitis virus A and B, influenza A virus). Studies have shown that vaccination above the age of 65 decreased the risk of acute coronary syndrome (Nichol et al., 2003; Lundberg & Hansson, 2010). The precise mechanism whereby pathogens are able to accelerate atherosclerosis is unclear but TLRs are probably involved in detection and initiation of a subsequent inflammatory response. TLRs also recognise endogenous ligands that are released during necrotic cell death or are derived from the degradation of extracellular matrix (Heat shock protein, oxidative Low density lipoprotein, endogenous mRNA, fibrinogens,...). While TLR signalling pathways activate the genes encoding IL-1β and IL-18, these mediators require a second signal resulting in cleavage of the pro-form to release the active molecules. This is regulated by a cytosolic protein complex (the "inflammasome") that leads to caspase-1 activation (Lundberg & Hansson, 2010). Various molecules can activate the inflammasome: ATP, crystalline structures (explaining the role of inflammasome in gout and pseudogout), aluminium salts (used as adjuvants), amyloid-B (playing important role in Alzheimer disease), fibers (silicosis, asbestosis) or the M2 channel from the influenza virus. Cholesterol crystals also directly activate the inflammasome, a process that is implicated in the pathogenesis of atherosclerosis (Duewell et al., 2010; McIntire et al., 2009). It would therefore be of interest to look at inflammasome activation/regulation in the context of aging. Other signalling pathways, such as those linked to the endoplasmic reticulum (ER) stress also participate to inflammation in the context of metabolic disorders (Hotamisligil, 2010). Whether perturbations in ER stress pathways could also contribute to age-related inflammation should also be further investigated (Naidoo, 2009).

Pravastatin, a 3-hydroxy-3-methylglutaryl coenzyme A reductase inhibitors or statin, has been recognize to have beneficial effects on atherosclerosis. Statins have pleiotropic effects, notably on immune system and dendritic cells. It has been shown that patients treated with pravastatin show decreased expression of CD86 on monocyte-derived dendritic cells, a reduced level of IFNα and IL-1β after four weeks of treatment and an increase of IL-10 and TGFβ in mixed lymphocyte reactions. It also reduces plasma levels of inflammation markers (IL-6, TNFα, CRP) and soluble CD40L without apparent link with the degree of lipid lowering achieved (Li et al., 2009; Schonbeck & Libby, 2004). Fenofibrate and simvastatine in type 2 diabetic patients with mixed dyslipidemia and in patients with hypercholesterolemia or impaired fasting glucose, reduce expression of TNFα, IL-1β, IL-6 and MCP-1 by LPS-stimulated monocytes. Both treatments significantly reduce high-sensitivity CRP levels (Krysiak et al., 2011b; Krysiak et al., 2011a) but there are conflicting results (Coen et al., 2010). Statin and aspirin decrease serum levels of IL-1β and C-reactive protein in hypercholesterolemic patients (Ferroni et al., 2003). Valsartan in hypertension patients also reduces the secretion of IL-1β by LPS-stimulated PBMCs. Angiotensin II is identified as the main mediator of vascular complications of hypertension. It stimulates the expression of vascular cell adhesion molecule-1 and induces IL-1β and MCP-1 production by vascular smooth cells (Li et al., 2005; Ferro et al., 2000).

Type 2 Diabetes mellitus is a serious chronic disease that is very prevalent in the developed world. Several studies have shown that IL-6 and IL-1β levels are independent predictors of type 2 diabetes development. The role of TNFα is more controversial, some studies show a relationship between TNFα and insulin resistance but this might be restricted to obese type 2 diabetic subjects. Higher serum IL-8 levels have also been found in diabetic patients

(DiPenta et al., 2007). Production of IL-6, IL-8, IL-1β upon LPS stimulation could also be influenced by glucose concentrations and insulin levels but *in vitro* results on PBMCs do not take into account the contribution of skeletal muscles, fibroblasts and vascular endothelial cells (Beitland et al., 2009).

Chronic heart failure is a major epidemiological burden in the industrialized world. Approximately 2% of the adult population is diagnosed with moderate or severe left ventricular systolic dysfunction with an incidence rate of 10 per 1000 population over the age of 65. Chronic inflammation interacting with increased oxidative stress, cytokine production, proteolytic matrix degradation and autoimmunity is implicated in heart failure pathophysiology by increasing cardiac injury, fibrosis and dysfunction. There are several sources of systemic inflammation in cardiac heart failure (TNFα, IL-1, IL-6, IL-18, MCP-1) due to release from leukocytes and blood platelets as well as the lungs, liver, endothelium and the failing heart itself. These cytokines are capable of modulating cardiovascular performance in an autocrine, paracrine or endocrine fashion. Inflammatory cytokines may enhance the expression of adhesion molecules and inflammatory chemokines in endothelial cells which in turn may further increase the inflammatory response within the vessel wall, representing a pathogenic loop leading to inappropriate endothelial activation in heart failure. TNF superfamily ligands may directly induce endothelial cell apoptosis (Picano et al., 2010). Aged patients with heart failure present higher IL-6 serum levels in the acute but also the recovery phase of cardiac failure compare to healthy aged controls (Vo et al., 2011).

In summary, these "metabolic disorders" are associated with chronic inflammation that contributes to the pathogenesis. Hence, "inflamm-aging" processes are likely to contribute to the development of these pathologies. Conversely, the increased prevalence of these diseases in the geriatric populations will affect innate immune parameters accordingly and favour the maintenance of low-grade inflammation.

4.2.2 The "Frailty" syndrome

Frailty has been defined as an age-related decline in lean body mass, decreased muscle strength, endurance, balance and walking performance, low activity, weight loss accompanied by a high risk of disability, incident falls, hospitalisation and mortality. Plasma levels of TNFα were strongly associated with impendent death independently of dementia and cardiovascular disease in centenarians. It supports the hypothesis that TNFα has specific biological effects and is a marker of the frailty syndrome in the oldest. Systemic low-grade inflammation has been associated with decreased muscle mass as well as the development of functional disability in older population. TNFα might directly contribute to sarcopenia. Indeed, *in vitro* experiments indicate that TNFα disrupts the differentiation process and promotes catabolism in muscle cells. It is also responsible for increased basal energy expenditure, anorexia, loss of muscle and bone mass *in vivo* and has been associated with cachexia in chronic inflammatory disorders such as rheumatoid arthritis, AIDS and cancer. His role in septic shock is well known. The potential role of IL-6 in sarcopenia is less clear. Age-related sarcopenia is partly reversed by exercise. Muscle contractions induce IL-6 production and release into the blood stream and it has been suggested that muscle-derived IL-6 contributes to the beneficial metabolic effect of exercise (Krabbe et al., 2004). Along the same line, another study shows that fatigue resistance and grip work correlate positively with IL-6 in older male participant. In contrast, the same group shows that older nursing home residents present a worse fatigue resistance and grip work related to high levels of IL-6, Heat shock protein 70 and TNFα (Bautmans et al., 2007; Bautmans et al., 2008). High levels of IL-6, C-reactive protein and TNFα predict an increased incidence of mobility limitation during a 30-month follow-up period in well functioning older people (Penninx et al., 2004).

4.2.3 Neurodegenerative disorders and depression

Cognitive impairment is an important problem with age. Epidemiological studies show an increasing body of evidence on the deleterious association between chronic peripheral cytokine elevation found in aged subjects and cognitive functions. Several studies show an association between serum levels of TNFα, IL-1β and Alzheimer disease. In contrast, IL-6 seems to be associated with vascular dementia (Krabbe et al., 2004; Ravaglia et al., 2007). Studies have suggested that inflamm-aging can be a prodrome for Alzheimer's disease. Alzheimer's disease is connected with a dysregulation in the metabolism of beta amyloid precursor protein with a consequent transient overproduction or a decreased degradation of β-amyloid in the brain. IFNγ and other pro-inflammatory cytokines interact with processing and production of β-amyloid peptides. Neopterin, a blood compound produced by monocyte-derived macrophages upon stimulation with IFNγ is increased in Alzheimer's disease patients compared to age-matched controls. 70% of these patients are seropositive for cytomegalovirus and it correlates with neopterin and C-reactive protein concentrations. It was suggested that elevated neopterin may be a vestigial result of serum immunity to cytomegalovirus (Giunta et al., 2008). IL-1, IL-6 and TNFα have been clearly involved in the local inflammatory process around amyloid plaques, might be cytotoxic when chronically produced and might stimulate the production of β-amyloid peptides (Krabbe et al., 2004; Ravaglia et al., 2007). As for atherosclerosis, inflammasome activation seems to be implicated in Alzheimer's disease. Amyloid β oligomers can disturb the function of K+ channels and decrease intracellular K+ concentration leading to activation of NALP-1 then caspase-1, production of IL-1β and IL-18, and cellular apoptosis through pyroptosis. Fibrillar amyloid β can also lead to the activation of NALP3 and lead to the same phenomenon (Cook et al., 2010). Plasma levels of IL-1β and TNFα are higher in patients with vascular dementia and late onset Alzheimer's disease when compared to control and after adjustment for confounding variables. IL-6 was only increased in patients with vascular dementia (Krabbe et al., 2004; Ravaglia et al., 2007) but not in Alzheimer's patients (Zuliani et al., 2007). Alzheimer's patients present a decrease of CD8+T lymphocytes, a slight increase of CD4+ T lymphocytes and CD19+ B lymphocytes compared to age-matched controls (Giunta et al., 2008). Once again, there is a strong link between this irreversible neurodegenerative process and general chronic inflammation.

Depression is also a cardinal feature of the geriatric population. Comorbidities, such as cardiovascular diseases, atherosclerosis, diabetes, osteoporosis, dementia, cancer or frailty can precipitate depressive states that are further enhanced by poor socioeconomic outcomes. Depression is a risk factor for low resistance to infection and insufficient response to vaccine. The pathogenesis and severity of depression are connected to chronic stress. Chronic diseases, stressfull life events, personal loss, decline in self concepts of efficacy may contribute to this process. Depression in older people is associated with increased exposure to cytomegalovirus in the past and a pro-inflammatory profile demonstrated by elevated

TNFα, IL-6, IFNα, C-reactive protein and deficiency of suppressive IL-10+cells. These changes negatively affect humoral and innate responses in depressed patients (Penninx et al., 2003; Bouhuys et al., 2004; Trzonkowski et al., 2004; Irwin & Miller, 2007). IL-6 and TNFα have the capacity to exert direct effects on the central nervous system by stimulating the hypothalamic-pituitary axis activity and the release of corticotrophin-releasing factor. These direct effects may lead to behavioural and neurochemical changes that may induce depression (Penninx et al., 2003). Depression has been associated with a decreased number of lymphocytes and NK and altered functions, which can be modulated by antidepressant treatment (Bouhuys et al., 2004; Irwin & Miller, 2007). Antidepressant therapy decreases LPS-induced IL-1β and IL-6 in whole blood from depressed patients. IL-1β has been shown to up-regulate hippocampus expression of serotonin transporters and proinflammatory cytokines might play a causative role in the depression-related activation of hypothalamic-pituitary-adrenal system (Himmerich et al., 2010).

4.2.4 Osteoporosis

Postmenopausal osteoporosis is a progressive disorder characterized by a decreased bone mass and increased susceptibility to fractures. It affects one out of three women after menopause (Breuil et al., 2010). Oestrogen deficiency leads to an uncoupling between activity of bone resorbing cells (osteoclasts) and bone forming cells (osteoblasts) responsible for accelerated bone loss. The concept of osteoimmunology recently emerged from increasing evidence of intimate links between bone tissue and the immune system. Indeed, recent studies have suggested that the increase in bone resorption induced by oestrogen deficiency is at least partly mediated by increased paracrine production of bone resorbing cytokines (Breuil et al., 2010). Multiple soluble mediators of immune cell function, including cytokines, chemokines and growth factors also regulate osteoblast and osteoclast activity. This is particularly true in pathological conditions such as rheumatoid arthritis and inflammatory bowel disease (Breuil et al., 2010). IL-1 is one of the most potent stimulators of bone resorption and IL-6 appears to be a potent osteotrophic factor that may play an important role in diseases characterized by increased bone resorption. Oestrogens inhibit IL-6 gene expression (Zheng et al., 1997; De Martinis et al., 2006). TNFα and IL-1 enhance bone resorption by stimulating development of osteoclast progenitors and increasing the activity of mature cells. IFNγ inhibits the process of IL-1 stimulated bone resorption. Some studies do not find any differences in the serum levels of IL-1β, IL-1α and IL-6 between osteoporotic and normal women. In contrast, Il-1β, IL-6, TNFα are significantly higher in whole blood after polyclonal activation in osteoporotic women than controls and negative correlation is found between lumbar bone mineral density and IL-1β, IL-6 or TNFα levels (De Martinis et al., 2005; Zheng et al., 1997). A study performed on osteoporotic women and controls without oestrogen or vitamin D deficiencies shows that osteoporotic women present a decrease in circulating B cells, decreased basal secretion of IFNγ by CD4+ T lymphocytes, a decreased in memory CD4+ T cells expressing RANK+ and CD28+ (Breuil et al., 2010). The TNF-family RANK-L and its receptor RANK are key regulator and essential for the development and activation of osteoclasts. RANK-L is expressed in osteoblasts and can be upregulated by bone resorbing factors such as glucocorticoids, 1,25(OH)2D3, IL-1, IL-6, IL-17, TNFα, PGE2, parathyroid hormone. RANK-L is produced by activated T cells and can directly induce osteoclastogenesis. Several factors can inhibit RANK-l such as osteoprotegerin, IFNγ, IL-12 and IL-18 (De Martinis et al., 2006).

Biphosphonates are currently widely used for the prevention and treatment of osteoporosis as well skeletal metastasis. It has been recently demonstrated that biphosphonates lead to the expansion and activation of $\gamma\delta$ T cells, these effects may represent potential novel anti-tumor mechanisms. Another study indicates that low dose zoledronate *in vitro* reduces TNFα production by monocytes, inhibits upregulation of typical maturation markers and NFκB activation in dendritic cells (CD83, CD86, CD40) (Wolf et al., 2006).

4.3 Chronic infections and immune "exhaustion"?

One of the hallmarks of the "immune risk phenotype" (see table 1) in the OCTA/NONA subjects is the accumulation of terminally-differentiated CD8 T cells, (lacking CD27 and CD28) leading to inversion of the CD4:CD8 ratio. An important fraction of these cells are specific for cytomegalovirus (CMV) antigens. These effector memory T cells contain large amount of cytotoxic effector molecules like granzyme and perforin and progressively acquire inhibitory receptors such as KLRG1, CD57 and PD-1 (Pawelec & Derhovanessian, 2011). Similarly, CMV-specific CD4 T cells are highly differentiated, have shorter telomeres and decreased telomerase induction after stimulation. These cells are thought to become dysfunctional and "exhausted" in old individuals (Hadrup et al., 2006). However, these cells are still capable of rapidly producing cytokines upon *in vitro* stimulation and display effector functions (Ouyang et al., 2003). Interestingly, a study performed on individuals genetically enriched for longevity, with a 30% decreased mortality risk, possess immune signatures different from those of the general population. Even if they are CMV-seropositive, they fail to show the CMV-(and age-) associated alterations of immune parameters that CMV-seropositive general population does show (Derhovanessian et al., 2010). As previously mentioned, it has been reported that IL-4 producing T cells with a CD25+ memory phenotype accumulate in a subgroup of healthy elderly people who have an intact humoral immune response after influenza vaccination. These apparently beneficial CD8+ CD25+ T cells are rare or even absent in older persons with latent CMV infection (Herndler-Brandstetter et al., 2005).

Could there be a direct link between this CMV-dependent immune signature and other parameters of immunosenescence? Conceptually, accumulation of these memory oligoclonal cells with age would occupy the "immunological space" and limit homeostatic proliferation of naïve T cells and response to new antigens. It has also been suggested that CMV infection could participate to the inflamm-aging process (Trzonkowski, 2003). Whether accumulation of CMV-specific T cells with age is actually detrimental remains to be established (Wills, 2011). Analysis of several recent cohorts does not support a relationship between CMV status, mortality or inflammatory markers (Wills 2011). Another recent study found a gradual increase in CMV antibody titers with deteriorating functional status in aged individuals (Moro-Garcia et al., 2011). CMV infection is also associated with atherosclerosis and the risk for heart diseases (Stranberg TE 2009). In longitudinal studies of CMV-seropositive patients, antibody levels have been reported to correlate inversely with survival in individuals with stable cardiovascular diseases, cardiovascular risk factors and in older women in their 70's. Furthermore, telomere shortening of CD8 CD28- T cells correlates with cardiac dysfunction in CMV+ patients with coronary heart diseases (Spyridopoulos et al., 2009).

In addition to these unresolved issues related to the association of CMV infection and disease states, the causality links are still unclear. Indeed, if CMV infection were directly implicated in age-dependent deterioration of immune functions and cardiovascular diseases, it would be highly beneficial to consider CMV eradication in the general population through vaccination (Pawelec, 2011).

4.4 How living habits and nutrition status impact on immune functions

Malnutrition is associated with a decrease in immunity and an increase in susceptibility to many infectious diseases, notably due to an inability to meet the energy demands associated with the immune response. Interventions on nutrition could have a large impact on immune functions (Ongradi & Kovesdi, 2010).

It seems that caloric restriction is the only known method to prolong median as well as maximal lifespan in all tested animals, from invertebrates to rodents and non-human primates. It is able to attenuate the natural shift from naive to memory phenotype T cells and maintain a higher number of naive T cells in aged animals. The increase of proinflammatory cytokines such as IL-6, TNFα and IFNγ can be reversed by caloric restriction. Caloric restriction is known to inhibit mTOR and thereby promoting autophagy mechanisms. It allows recycling of the cellular components to gain new building blocks for critical proteins by degrading momentarily unneeded proteins and even organelles (Arnold et al., 2011).

The dietary intake of essential macro and micronutrients is usually inadequate in the elderly and several factors contribute to this deficiency: poor socioeconomic status may lead to a greater consumption of inexpensive foods poor in micronutrients. Nutrient deficiency is exacerbated by loss of appetite, lack of teeth, intestinal malabsorption and decreased energy requirement. Many micronutrients contribute directly or indirectly to the biological activity of some antioxidant enzymes, to the efficiency of immune response and to the maintenance of metabolic functions (Mocchegiani et al., 2011).

Vitamin A contributes to the maintenance of epithelium integrity in the respiratory and gastrointestinal tracts. Pyridoxins, folic acid, vitamin E have been suggested to influence lymphocyte functions. Antioxidant vitamin supplements have been shown to enhance antibody titers upon influenza vaccination and to reduce incidence of infection over a 2-year study period (Lesourd, 2006).

Lipids are also important actors in immune system. High-density lipoprotein (HDL) has anti-inflammatory and anti-oxidative effects and influence proximal T cell signalling. Conjugated linoleic acid has been shown to have anticarcinogenic, antiatherogenic and antidiabetic properties correlating with increased lymphocyte proliferation and decreased proinflammatory cytokine secretion. The most important effect is a decrease of risk and severity of cardiovascular diseases originating from atherosclerosis, a chronic inflammatory condition. Living habits can serve as anti-aging process: aerobic exercise, weight loss and smoking cessation can raise HDL levels and physical activity tends to lower IL-6 and C-reactive protein serum levels (Fulop et al., 2007; Ongradi & Kovesdi, 2010).

The potential role for vitamin D and its active metabolite 1,25(OH)2vitD in modulating the immune response was first appreciated 25 years ago with three important discoveries: The ability of 1,25(OH)2vit D to inhibit T cell proliferation, the ability of disease-activated macrophages to produce 1,25 (OH)2vitD and the presence of vitamin D receptor in activated human inflammatory cells. 1,25(OH)2vitD suppresses proliferation and immunoglobulin production and delays the differentiation of B cell precursors into plasma cells. It shifts the balance to a Th2 cell phenotype and increased CD4/CD25 regulatory T cells. It inhibits Th17 development and appears beneficial for autoimmunity diseases. In innate immunity, vitamin D enhances activation of TLRs. It promotes innate immune responses to TLR activation by Mycobacterium tuberculosis. 1,25(OH)2vit D increases cathelicidin, a antimicrobial peptide after activation of TLR1/2 but inhibits the maturation of monocyte-derived dendritic cells (Bikle, 2009; Hewison, 2010; Schwalfenberg, 2011). By increasing cathelicidin, vitamin D supplementation improves the outcome of many diseases: it reduced dental caries and Helicobacter pylori infections. Vitamin D insufficiency is associated with Crohn's disease, pour outcome in severe pneumonia and urinary tract infections (Schwalfenberg, 2011). Vitamin D improves physical barrier by stimulating gap junctions genes, adherent genes and tight junction genes (Schwalfenberg, 2011). In contrast, a study failed to show influence of a short-term calcium and vitamin D treatment in healthy post menopausal woman on IL-6, TNFα and C-reactive protein serum levels (Gannage-Yared et al., 2003).

Vitamin C is an essential watersoluble nutrient, which primarily exerts its effect on host defence mechanisms and immune homeostasis, by being the most important physiological antioxidant. It has been implicated as having a preventative and therapeutic role in a variety of diseases including scurvy, viral infections and common cold, cancer and atherosclerosis. A study shows that *in vitro*, vitamin C inhibits IL-6 and TNFα production by monocytes after LPS stimulation and an inhibition of IL-2 production by lymphocytes after PMA ionomycin (Hartel et al., 2004).

Zinc is one of the most relevant nutritional factors in aging because it affects immune responses, metabolic harmony and antioxidant activity. The human body contains 2-3 g zinc most of which is bound to proteins. Plasma pool, which is required for the distribution of zinc represents less than one percent of the total body content. A multitude of factors is likely to influence zinc intake: malnutrition, socioeconomic factors, decreased intestinal absorption and medications like diuretics. The recommended daily allowance for zinc in adult in the United States is 11mg/day for men and 8 mg/day for women. In human, the most prominent example of the effect of zinc deficiency on the immune system is acrodermatitis enteropathica, a rare autosomal recessive inheritable disease that causes thymic atrophy and a high susceptibility to bacterial, fungal and viral infections. It is caused by zinc-specific malabsorption. The intracellular concentration of free zinc is regulated by three mechanisms: one is transport through the plasma membrane; another involves storage in zincosomes and finally zinc binding to metallothionein. Metallothioneins are a group of low molecular weight metal binding proteins with high affinity for zinc. It distributes intracellular zinc and has a protective role in transient and acute stress-like conditions. Elevated IL-6 levels observed in aged individual are also associated with increased and persistent metallothioneins expression in peripheral mononuclear cells, leading to an increased sequestration of zinc and immune impairment. Notably, centenarians display low levels of metallothioneins coupled with satisfactory zinc ion availability. *In vitro* studies show that many parameters are affected by zinc: caspases, reactive oxygen species production, NFκB and iNOS activity, superoxide dismutase, catalase, gluthatione peroxidase, telomere length, several cytokines and chemokines expression. The most prominent effect of zinc deficiency is a decline in T cell function, the shift of a Th1 toward Th2 responses. Effect of zinc on cytokine levels is concentration-dependent: it stimulates cytokine production in monocytes in response to lipopolysaccharide with moderated supplementation but higher concentrations can have an antagonistic effect. With regard to older people, inconsistent data exist on the beneficial effect of zinc supplementation upon the immune efficiency due to different doses and duration of treatment. The most important parameter affected by physiological dose (10-25 mg/day from 1 to 3 months) is the innate immunity represented by the natural killer cell cytotoxicity. Zinc treatment at the dose of 15mg a day for 1 month in older people and old infected patients restores thymic endocrine activity, lymphocyte mitogen proliferative response, CD4+ T cell number, peripheral immune efficiency and DNA repair. At clinical level, significant reduction of relapsing infections occurs in these patients (Mocchegiani et al., 2011; Haase & Rink, 2009; Mocchegiani, 2010). In hospitalized geriatric patients, poor zinc status has been associated with higher proportion of congestive cardiopathy, respiratory infections, gastrointestinal diseases and depression (Pepersack et al., 2001).

Protein energy malnutrition is common in elderly population. It is present in 2-4% of home-living self-sufficient older subjects and in more than 50% of institutionalized older subjects. During stress, the body reacts with acute phase responses associated with proinflammatory cytokine release from monocytes-macrophages. The cytokines induce the use of nutritional reserves which is particularly harmful in the older people for several reasons: 1) body reserves are already decreased in older individuals who exhibit osteoporosis and often sarcopenia 2) acute phase responses are long lasting in older people, so that more body reserves are used ; 3) nutritional reserves are never fully replaced in older individuals during recovery, since protein anabolism is decreased; 4) each acute phase response in the older people can therefore leads to lower nutritional reserves, mainly muscle protein reserves which can increase frailty (Lesourd, 2006).

In light of these observations, it is clear that addressing the specific nutritional requirements in advancing age could modulate immune functions. Whey proteins are a mixture of globular proteins isolated from milk. It is left when milk coagulates and contains everything that is soluble in milk. It has been shown that older people receiving whey proteins, in comparison to soy proteins, present greater antibody responses against four serotypes of S. *pneumoniae* (Freeman et al., 2010). Along the same line, Enprocal, a recently formulated supplementary food has been designed to meet the nutritional needs of frail older people. The ingredients of Enprocal are dairy-based proteins (Whey protein concentrate, skim milk powder, whole milk powder), vitamins and minerals (calcium, zinc, vitamins C, D, B and A), vegetable oils and inulin. An *in vitro* study suggested that Enprocal displays some immunomodulatory properties on immune cells (Kanwar & Kanwar, 2009). Lactoferrine has also important immune modulator protein. It belongs to the transferrin family and bind two irons ions reversibly. It is synthesized by glandular epithelia and found in milk, tears, bile, respiratory and gastrointestinal secretions. Protein antigens and bacteria within the digestive systems act as stimulating agents in the process. It has pleiotropic effects: bactericidal, anti-fungal and anti-viral effects, anti-oxidant activity, it reduces the production of proinflammatory cytokines, inhibits tumour growth by inhibiting angiogenesis, promoting apoptosis and finally, it promotes bone growth (Pierce et al., 2009).

Exercise has also been shown to have influence on immunological parameter. Studies have found that mitogen- or influenza- induced lymphocyte proliferation was increased, the number of natural killer cells was greater, antibody IgM and IgG response to influenza vaccine two weeks post immunization was greater in active old people. Greater levels of physical activity in terms of walking speed was also associated with lower serum levels of several inflammatory markers such as IL-6, TNFα, and C-reactive protein. In contrast, intervention trials involving frail older people were not promising suggesting that immune alterations in the frail state cannot be reversed (Senchina & Kohut, 2007). A study performed on older men shows that older people with long-term training present reduce levels of IL-6, IL-1ra, IL-10, sTNFRI but an increase of MCP-1 compared to sedentary older people. It was associated with increases of DHEA and IGF-1 levels (Gonzalo-Calvo et al., 2011). Another study shows also that exercise reduces inflammatory monocytes in hypercholesterolemic patients (Coen et al., 2010).

In summary, many different dietary factors are able to influence innate and adaptive immune parameters. It is very difficult from *in vitro* studies to draw hypothesis on how deficiency/supplementation of specific factors impact on the organism. However, clinical studies indicate that these factors should be taken into account and might be beneficial for healthy aging as a whole.

4.5 Erosion of epithelial barriers: susceptibility to infections and potential impact on chronic inflammatory status

Epithelial cells represent the first protective barrier towards invading pathogens. Aging is associated with alteration of these barriers, including the skin, lung, stomach, intestine and urinary tract. Bacteriemic pneumococcal pneumonia in persons older than 70 is associated with a death rate greater than 50 percent. It appears that oropharyngeal colonization with gram-negative bacilli plays an important predisposition role. With age, in the lung, there is a reduced function of the mucociliary tract, a reduced local immunity (T cells and reduced secreted immunoglobulin), and reduced cough reflex. All these factors but also deglutition trouble, reduced production of gastric acid secretion, antibiotics or antiacid treatment, favour the apparition of pneumonia in older people (Cretel et al., 2010; Yoshikawa, 1981).

Older people also present more urinary infections than young people. Urinary tract infection has an incidence of 5-35% in men and 15-50% in women. Poor emptying of the urinary bladder because of reduced muscle tonicity, prostatic hypertrophy, reduced oestrogen and increased pH level that lead to increased bacterial adherence, previous genitorurinary instrumentation and perineal contamination from fecal incontinence are possible reasons for the high incidence (Yoshikawa, 1981; Cretel et al., 2010).

Skin and soft tissue infection is a common complication in aged patients. Even minor trauma to the skin might result in serious skin and soft tissue infections because of skin changes (thinning of epidermis and subcutaneous tissues, decreased glandular secretions and atherosclerosis, pressure injuries). Skin also presents modifications of immune cells such as a decrease of Langerhan's cells (Cretel et al., 2010; Desai et al., 2010; Grewe, 2001; Yoshikawa, 1981).

Older patients are also at higher risk for bacterial meningitis (pneumococci, gram negative bacilli and listeria monocytogenes) and bacterial arthritis (Yoshikawa, 1981).

Gram-negative bacterial infections occur more frequently in patients older than 60 years. Intra-abdominal sepsis is of special importance to the older people. Complications like perforation, wound infection, abscess formation and pneumonia are more common in the older people following appendectomies. The risk of diverticulitis rapidly increases with aging and cholelithiasis is another disease of the aged.

With age, the capacity of the gastrointestinal tract to protect individuals from pathogens is lowered because of reduced gastric pH leading to pneumonia and malabsorption, mechanical trouble like diverticulitis and alteration of the mucosal immune system (Cretel et al., 2010). The mucosal immune system consists of an integrated network of tissues, lymphoid and mucous membrane-associated cells and innate effectors and acquired molecules. The IgA isotype is key players in mucosal immunity and seems to function in synergy with innate immune system. Mucosal inductive sites include the Peyer's patches; gut associated lymphoreticular tissues (GALT), waldeyer's ring of tonsil and adenoid. The mammalian lower intestine contains up to 10^{12} bacteria per gram of intestine. The normal microbiota is essential to maintain appropriate homeostatic conditions providing energy in the form of short chain fatty acids and nutrients and protection against colonization by pathogenic bacteriae. It also plays a role in maturation of the host immune system including intestinal secretory soluble IgA and intraepithelial lymphocyte development. There is some evidence in mice that there are alterations of the mucosal immune system with age. Reduced levels and quality of soluble IgA and alterations of mucosal dendritic cells functions have been reported. Qualitative change in the composition of the microbiota has also been reported (fewer total anaerobes bacteroides and bifidobacterium and higher levels of enterobacteriacea and endotoxin-producing, gram-negative bacteria like fusobacteria, clostridia, eubacteria species). As a direct result of these age-related changes in the microbiota, the quality of the secretary IgA response can be altered, although the absolute amount of these antibodies is generally unchanged (Fujihashi & Kiyono, 2009). Non-pathogenic bacteriae in the intestine play important role for protecting host from pathogens. It has been suggested that limited TLR stimulation will contribute to the physiological, low-level inflammation in healthy intestine. In contrast, true pathogens induce a rapid and more aggressive response that is initiated by microbial danger signals and tissue damage. It is now known that the innate and adaptive immune activation by the microbiota prevents other inflammatory responses and induces cytoprotective responses of the intestine epithelium that are critical for intestinal homeostasis. This is achieved by low expression of pattern recognition receptors on intestinal epithelial cells and limited gene activation via NF-κB. It promotes epithelial integrity through production of cytoprotective molecules such as heat shock proteins. Low-grade bowel inflammation is frequently present in the older population and may account for elevated systemic C-reactive protein and faecal calprotectin. Blood intestinal perfusions and oxygenation are also altered in the aged population. It is possible that the combination of a normally harmless bacterial signal, tissue injury and nutritional deficiency may trigger pathogenic inflammatory response. In the intestinal environment, a loss of barrier integrity may result in heightened exposure to exogenous components derived from the non-pathogenic intestinal microbiota and a breakdown in tolerance mechanisms. Impaired clearance of apoptotic cells by intestinal dendritic cells may lead to the accumulation of necrotic cells that release autoantigens such as nucleic acids, uric acid and the induction of an inflammatory dendritic cells phenotype. This might lead to autoimmune response and abnormal immune response to commensals.

Taken together, it seems that both endogenous signals (cell senescence and cumulative cell damage) and exogenous non-self signals (bacteria translocation through a leaky gut) may both contribute to chronic inflammation (Schiffrin et al., 2010).

5. Immunosenescence and cancer

Epidemiological studies indicate that about 55% of tumours are detected after the age of 65. The most frequent sites in men over 65 are represented by lung, colon, rectum, prostate and bladder; in women by breast, lung, colon-rectum, bladder and pancreas as well as non-Hodgkin lymphoma. The association between age and cancer can be explained by a multitude of factors, including a more prolonged exposure to carcinogens in older individuals and an increasingly favourable milieu for the induction of neoplasm in senescent cells. The immune system counteracts tumour cell growth through different ways:

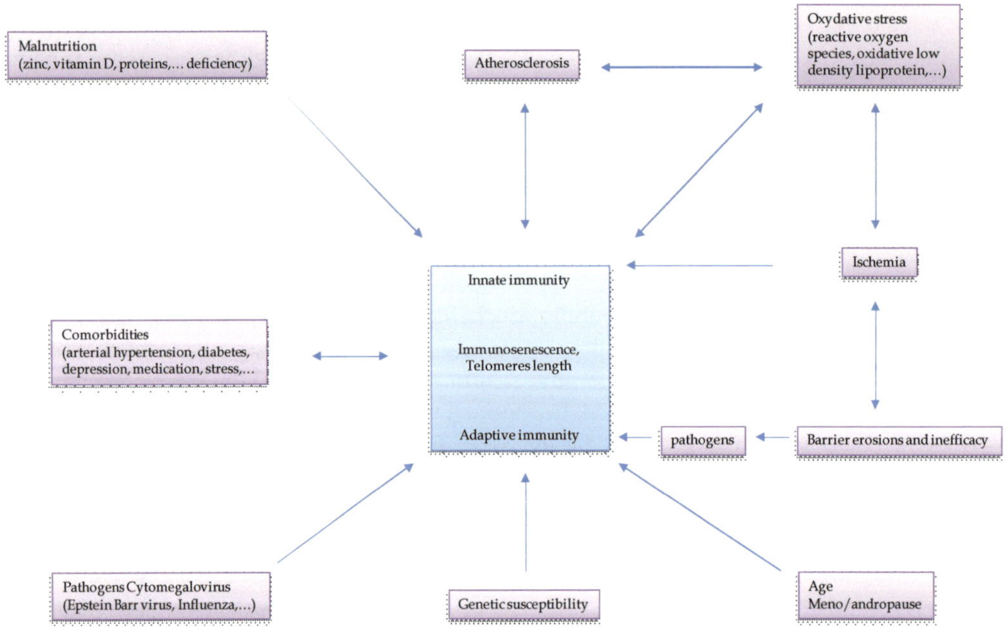

Fig. 7. External factors leading to immunosenescence.

1) protection of the host from virus-induced tumours by eliminating or suppressing viral infections 2) suitable eradication of pathogens and rapid resolution of inflammation thereby preventing the establishment of an inflammatory environment favourable to tumorigenesis 3) specific identification and elimination of tumour cells on the basis of their expression of tumour-specific antigens or molecules induced by cellular stress (a process known as "immunosurveillance"). Hence, reduction of T cell function and cellular immunity as seen in the older people could favour carcinoma development. In older people suffering from different types of cancer, there was a reduced number of CD3 T cells, CD4 T helper cells and

natural killer cells in peripheral blood compared to healthy older people (Malaguarnera et al., 2010; Fulop et al., 2010; Motta et al., 2003). "Inflamm-aging" processes could favour tumour development. For example, IL-1α plays a role in tumorigenesis (and promotes angiogenesis and chemoresistance). TNFα plays an important role in the initiation of tumour by stimulation the production of nitric oxide and reactive oxygen species which can lead to DNA damage. Enhanced TNFα levels are associated with increased risk of multiple myeloma, hepatocellular carcinoma, bladder, gastric and breast cancer. It also correlates with poor prognosis of haematological malignancies. The paracrine secretion of IL-6 acts as a growth factor for multiple myeloma, non-Hodgkin lymphoma, bladder, colorectal and renal cell carcinoma (Malaguarnera et al., 2010; Fulop et al., 2010).

Accumulation of memory CD8 T cells might also participate to cancer development. One of the most intriguing evidences about the role of CD57+ T lymphocytes in cancer comes from the fact that metastasis-free regional lymph nodes draining different human epithelial tumors present a reduction in almost all immune cells, except CD57+ lymphocytes (Kanwar & Kanwar, 2009). CD8+CD28–CD57+ T lymphocyte clones may be the result of persistent stimulation by tumor-associated antigens, combined with a reduced cellular death rate secondary to reduced expression of the apoptosis-related molecule CD95. A long-lived population of CD8+CD57+CD28– perforin+ T lymphocyte clones has been reported in the peripheral blood of patients with multiple myeloma. Despite being more commonly found in patients with progressive and advanced-stage disease, this population was associated with superior survival. In patients with relapsed/refractory multiple myeloma treated with thalidomide, multivariate analysis showed that inferior survival was associated with low pretreatment bone marrow CD57+ cells and overall, CD8+CD57+T lymphocytes account for up to 25% of the marrow T cell population. Such CD8+CD57+ T lymphocytes have been shown to suppress T cell functions in multiple myeloma (Focosi et al., 2010).

CD57+ lymphocytes in the lymph nodes of B-chronic lymphoid leukemia patients have abnormal orthogonal light-scattering signals and an abnormal density of CD57+ receptors in comparison with their peripheral blood CD57+lymphocytes or the CD57+ lymphocytes in the peripheral blood, bone marrow, and tonsils of hematological normal donors. It has been reported that these patients with neutropenia have higher numbers of peripheral blood CD8+CD57+ T lymphocytes than the non-neutropenic ones. An elevated frequency of CD4+CD57+ T cells was correlated with more advanced disease. The role of the CD4+perforin+ T cell population is at present uncertain. However, this potentially cytotoxic T cell population could contribute to enhancing survival of the B-chronic lymphoid leukemia cells through production of IL-4 and to the immunodeficient state seen frequently in patients with this tumor, independent of drug treatment. (Focosi et al., 2010).

Finally, few reports analyzed the impact of immunosenescence on the complications of patients with cancer. Neutropenia is a complication of patients treated by chemotherapy and responsible of infection called febrile neutropenia. In older patients, pyrexia can be absent and little is known about the consequence of neutrophil defect and other immune defects on the increased rate of infections in old cancer patients. It is well known that CSFs enhance bone marrow production and is used to counteract neutropenia. CSFs have proven to be beneficial in old people but they still suffer from increased infection rates compared to younger adults. Finally, the factors influencing immunity (such as malnutrition, alteration of intestinal barriers, depression...) can also negatively influence the outcome of cancer in geriatric patients. So, it will be important to reconsider guidelines and management of old patients suffering from cancer (Crighton & Puppione, 2006).

6. Immunosenescence and autoimmunity

"Inflamm-aging" results in both decreased immunity to exogenous antigens and increased autoreactivity. It is well documented that a significant fraction of older people has low affinity autoantibodies in their serum and the prevalence of autoantibodies associated with autoimmune disease increases with age without clinical significance. Rheumatoid factors are present in up to 5% of young healthy individuals and increase up to five times in older persons such as antinuclear antibodies. A number of hypotheses have been proposed to explain the relationship between aging and the development of autoimmunity: reduced thymic output has been postulated to induce compensatory autoproliferation of T cells which can lead to premature T cell senescence and contribute to autoimmunity; alteration in apoptosis in T cells, expansion of exhausted CD4 and CD8 T cells that have lost the expression of CD28 are associated with autoimmune disease like rheumatoid arthritis, reactivation of self-reactive memory B cells, a shift from Th1 to Th2 cytokine profile that enhances the production of autoreactive antibodies, elevated levels of circulating inflammatory cytokines such as IL-6, TNFα and C-reactive protein is related to age-related diseases such as coronary heart disease and stroke, diabetes mellitus, Alzheimer's disease, lupus, Sjogren's syndrome and rheumatoid arthritis (Grolleau-Julius et al., 2010).

7. Immunosenescence and vaccination

Influenza is the fifth leading cause of death in the developed world after 50 years of age. As such, this group is the major target of vaccination campaigns. While influenza vaccination has 70-90% efficacy in healthy adult in western countries, the success rate falls to 17-53% in older people when determined as specific immune responses. Nevertheless, vaccination campaigns in aged individuals result in 25% reduction of morbidity, 50% of pneumopathies, 20% of hospital care and 70% of mortality (Ongradi & Kovesdi, 2010; Gruver et al., 2007; Bouree, 2003; Nichol et al., 2003). Both humoral and cell-mediated influenza specific responses are lower than in young adults. Upon *in vitro* restimulation, peripheral blood mononuclear cells exhibit a decrease in the proportion of IFNγ+ T cells. Mortality is associated with coexistent bacterial infection in one third of case, which could be a consequence of altered innate immune responses (Ongradi & Kovesdi, 2010; Gruver et al., 2007; Bouree, 2003). In older people, low plasma level of DHEA, decreased TNFα in whole blood after lipopolysaccharide stimulation and increased IL-10 production in whole blood after PHA stimulation is correlated with lower antibody response to influenza vaccination. The increase of IL-10 is likely to inhibit the maturation of antigen presenting cells, together with decreased TNFα production, hampering their migration to draining lymph node, compromising the subsequent induction of the specific immune response. Furthermore, IL-10 can induce antigen-specific CD4 T cells anergy. Thus, it is intriguing that the possession of an anti-inflammatory genotype (high IL-10 and low TNFα production) is increased significantly in centenarians. It is tempting to speculate that the presence of "high IL-10/low TNFα" could be favorable in protecting against age-related diseases, particularly neurodegenerative diseases, but conversely it could hamper the immune response to infections and vaccine (Corsini et al., 2006). As said before, studies show a correlation between the cytomegalovirus seropositive status and non responsiveness to influenza vaccine. They show that majority of volunteers fulfilling the criteria of SENIEUR protocol belonged to responders generating protective titers of antibodies against antigens of the influenza vaccine. Proinflammatory status such as elevated serum IL-6, TNFα was also associated with non-responders. The increase of anti-inflammatory cytokines in non-responders may be seen as a compensation for the inflammatory activity of IL-6 and TNFα. The coexistence of high levels of IL-6 and anti-CMV IgG suggested to the authors that chronic infection may be one of the causes of the proinflammatory status in the non-responding group, shrinking the capacity of immune system (Trzonkowski et al., 2003). Decreased TLR responsiveness of dendritic cell subsets is also associated with the inability to mount protective antibody responses to the trivalent inactivated influenza vaccine currently recommended (Panda et al., 2010).

Infection caused by Streptococcus pneumonia account for 25-35% of bacterial pneumonia resulting in hospitalization, morbidities and mortality in the older people. The current pneumococcal polysaccharide vaccine is recommended for all individuals above 65 years of age and those between 18-65 years of age at risk. The data for efficacy in older people are not as persuasive. Antibodies levels are lower in the older people and in those with chronic disease, except for healthy older adults after the age of 75 (modified SENIEUR protocol) (Chen et al., 2009; Bouree, 2003). Antibody concentrations were found to be similar for six out of seven serotypes for streptococcus pneumonia after vaccination of older and young subjects while opsonization titers were significantly higher in six out of seven serotypes in the younger population. Antibody potency, as measured by the ratio of opsonization titer to antibody concentration was found to be significantly higher for the younger subjects for all serotypes. Effectiveness of antibodies seems to be reduced in the older adult population (Schenkein et al., 2008). Tetanus, diphtheria and pertussis vaccination coverage are low, persons aged of more than 60 years frequently do not have protective antibody. It is the same problem for hepatitis B virus vaccine (Chen et al., 2009; Bouree, 2003).

Widely used adjuvant formulations such as those containing alum are poorly effective in older people compared with young subjects (Fulop et al., 2007). Alteration of TLR function in older adults is particularly relevant in view of the increased development and use of TLR agonist in vaccine. Influenza vaccine formulation in clinical trials employs the TLR5 agonist flagellin that would not require yearly reformulation and administration. CpG-containing oligonucleotides are used as TLR9-dependent vaccine adjuvants in the 7-valent pneumococcal conjugate vaccine and significantly enhanced the proportion of vaccine responders amongst HIV-infected adults. MPL, a derivative of lipid A from lipopolysaccharide is already used as an adjuvant in vaccines against human papillomavirus (Cervarix) (Shaw et al., 2011).

8. Conclusion

The first obvious conclusion is that immunosenescence is a complex phenomenon, which does not only reflect the action of time on immune cells. As discussed herein, many other factors, such as genetics, infection history, nutritional status, co-morbidities, socio-economic factors are likely to contribute to this process and its clinical impact. Geriatric medicine has to take into account all these specific characteristics to provide better care to this age group.

Data from literature and our ongoing study tend to suggest that "inflammaging" appears not only with age but is associated with indicators of frailty and the occurrence of comorbidities. Frail geriatric individuals express higher seric levels of TNFα and IL-6. This persistent chronic inflammation could directly participate to dampened innate immune responses upon stimulation. Indeed, *ex vivo* whole blood response to molecules like LPS tends to be reduced in older people. In intensive care units, old people with high basal levels of TNFα and IL-6 show increased severity of sepsis after community-acquired pneumonia (Mira et al., 2008). Intriguingly, increased IL-6 levels in the course of community acquired-pneumonia, is also associated with more severe sepsis. This might reflect the fact that *ex vivo* blood experiments do not take into account cytokine production by stromal cells such as endothelial cells, adipocytes or muscle cells. Moreover, circulating cytokine levels are also influenced by kidney function that is generally altered in the course of sepsis (Gomez CMH, 2000). Finally, it is possible that in the earlier phase of infections, old people are less efficient to control infection, leading to increased late inflammatory response.

Epidemiological associations do not always reflect causality. It is possible to link altered immunological parameters with frailty and comorbidities (fig 3). Should we conclude that dampened immune responses and exacerbated inflammation contribute to the fragility of the organism or that specific pathologies lead to immunosenescence? It is likely that both hypothesis are valid and reinforce each other. It has important implications in terms of therapeutic interventions. Should we treat or prevent chlamydia, CMV or H. *pylori* that could be responsible for local inflammation within atherosclerotic plaques (Rosenfeld & Campbell, 2011)? Would treatment of metabolic disorders reduce "inflammaging" processes? Should we try to "rejuvenate" the immune system through cytokine or hormonal replacement (Dorshkind et al., 2009)? Is the CMV-associated immune phenotype responsible for increased mortality rate or is it possible that frail individuals undergo more frequent reactivation of CMV, leading to the skewing of the memory response? To answer these crucial questions, clear immunological and biological parameters will have to be used is well-defined populations to overcome the weight of confounding factors.

Finally, to improve geriatric health, it seems clear that one should take into account several features of older people. We cannot imagine improving vaccinal responses without correcting nutritional status, frailty, controlling comorbidities and evaluate the impact of drug treatments. So even in this specific field, geriatric medicine requires multidisciplinary approach.

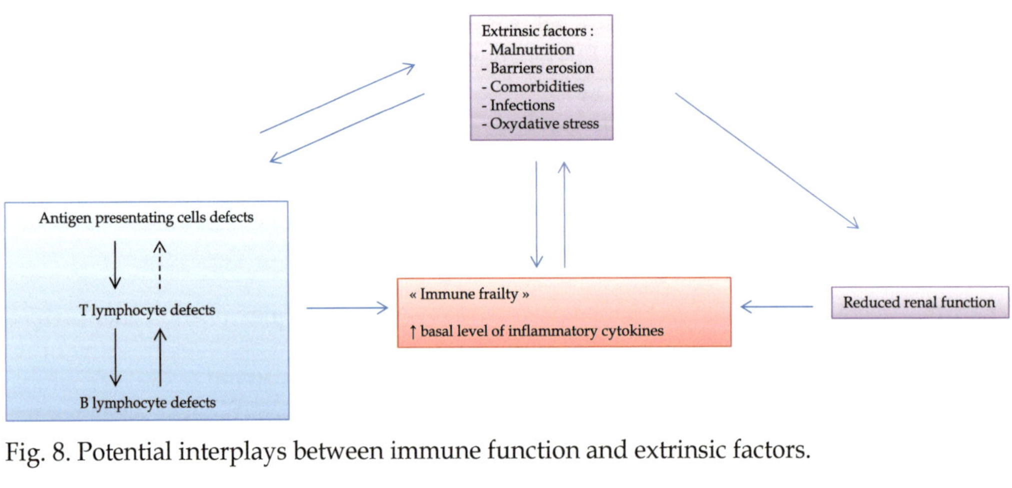

Fig. 8. Potential interplays between immune function and extrinsic factors.

9. References

Abedin,S., Michel, J. J., Lemster, B., & Vallejo, A. N. (2005). Diversity of NKR expression in aging T cells and in T cells of the aged: the new frontier into the exploration of protective immunity in the elderly. *Exp.Gerontol.* Vol.40, No.7, pp.537-548.

Ademokun,A., Wu, Y. C., & Dunn-Walters, D. (2010). The ageing B cell population: composition and function. *Biogerontology.* Vol.11, No.2, pp.125-137.

Agrawal,A., Agrawal, S., Cao, J. N., Su, H., Osann, K., & Gupta, S. (2007a). Altered innate immune functioning of dendritic cells in elderly humans: a role of phosphoinositide 3-kinase-signaling pathway. *J.Immunol.* Vol.178, No.11, pp.6912-6922.

Agrawal,A., Agrawal, S., & Gupta, S. (2007b). Dendritic cells in human aging. *Exp.Gerontol.* Vol.42, No.5, pp.421-426.

Alonso-Arias,R., Moro-Garcia, M. A., Lopez-Vazquez, A., Rodrigo, L., Baltar, J., Garcia, F. M., Jaurrieta, J. J., & Lopez-Larrea, C. (2011). NKG2D expression in CD4+ T lymphocytes as a marker of senescence in the aged immune system. *Age (Dordr.)* .

Alonso-Fernandez,P., Puerto, M., Mate, I., Ribera, J. M., & de la, F. M. (2008). Neutrophils of centenarians show function levels similar to those of young adults. *J.Am.Geriatr.Soc.* Vol.56, No.12, pp.2244-2251.

Andrews,N.P., Fujii, H., Goronzy, J. J., & Weyand, C. M. (2010). Telomeres and immunological diseases of aging. *Gerontology* Vol.56, No.4, pp.390-403.

Argentati,K., Re, F., Donnini, A., Tucci, M. G., Franceschi, C., Bartozzi, B., Bernardini, G., & Provinciali, M. (2002). Numerical and functional alterations of circulating gammadelta T lymphocytes in aged people and centenarians. *J.Leukoc.Biol.* Vol.72, No.1, pp.65-71.

Arlt,W. & Hewison, M. (2004). Hormones and immune function: implications of aging. *Aging Cell* Vol.3, No.4, pp.209-216.

Arnold,C.R., Wolf, J., Brunner, S., Herndler-Brandstetter, D., & Grubeck-Loebenstein, B. (2011). Gain and loss of T cell subsets in old age--age-related reshaping of the T cell repertoire. *J.Clin.Immunol.* Vol.31, No.2, pp.137-146.

Aspinall,R., Del Giudice, G., Effros, R. B., Grubeck-Loebenstein, B., & Sambhara, S. (2007). Challenges for vaccination in the elderly. *Immun.Ageing* Vol.4, pp.9.

Astrup,A.S., Tarnow, L., Jorsal, A., Lajer, M., Nzietchueng, R., Benetos, A., Rossing, P., & Parving, H. H. (2010). Telomere length predicts all-cause mortality in patients with type 1 diabetes. *Diabetologia* Vol.53, No.1, pp.45-48.

Balasubramanyam,M., Adaikalakoteswari, A., Monickaraj, S. F., & Mohan, V. (2007). Telomere shortening & metabolic/vascular diseases. *Indian J.Med.Res.* Vol.125, No.3, pp.441-450.

Bautmans,I., Gorus, E., Njemini, R., & Mets, T. (2007). Handgrip performance in relation to self-perceived fatigue, physical functioning and circulating IL-6 in elderly persons without inflammation. *BMC.Geriatr.* Vol.7, pp.5.

Bautmans,I., Njemini, R., Predom, H., Lemper, J. C., & Mets, T. (2008). Muscle endurance in elderly nursing home residents is related to fatigue perception, mobility, and circulating tumor necrosis factor-alpha, interleukin-6, and heat shock protein 70. *J.Am.Geriatr.Soc.* Vol.56, No.3, pp.389-396.

Beharka,A.A., Meydani, M., Wu, D., Leka, L. S., Meydani, A., & Meydani, S. N. (2001). Interleukin-6 production does not increase with age. *J.Gerontol.A Biol.Sci.Med.Sci.* Vol.56, No.2, pp.B81-B88.

Beitland,S., Opdahl, H., Aspelin, T., Saetre, L., & Lyberg, T. (2009). Blood leucocyte cytokine production after LPS stimulation at different concentrations of glucose and/or insulin. *Acta Anaesthesiol.Scand.* Vol.53, No.2, pp.183-189.

Benetos,A., Gardner, J. P., Zureik, M., Labat, C., Xiaobin, L., Adamopoulos, C., Temmar, M., Bean, K. E., Thomas, F., & Aviv, A. (2004). Short telomeres are associated with increased carotid atherosclerosis in hypertensive subjects. *Hypertension* Vol.43, No.2, pp.182-185.

Bikle,D. (2009). Nonclassic actions of vitamin D. *J.Clin.Endocrinol.Metab* Vol.94, No.1, pp.26-34.

Boren,E. & Gershwin, M. E. (2004). Inflamm-aging: autoimmunity, and the immune-risk phenotype. *Autoimmun.Rev.* Vol.3, No.5, pp.401-406.

Bouhuys,A.L., Flentge, F., Oldehinkel, A. J., & van, d. B. (2004). Potential psychosocial mechanisms linking depression to immune function in elderly subjects. *Psychiatry Res.* Vol.127, No.3, pp.237-245.

Bouree,P. (2003). Immunity and immunization in elderly. *Pathol.Biol.(Paris)* Vol.51, No.10, pp.581-585.

Breuil,V., Ticchioni, M., Testa, J., Roux, C. H., Ferrari, P., Breittmayer, J. P., Albert-Sabonnadiere, C., Durant, J., De Perreti, F., Bernard, A., Euller-Ziegler, L., & Carle, G. F. (2010). Immune changes in post-menopausal osteoporosis: the Immunos study. *Osteoporos.Int.* Vol.21, No.5, pp.805-814.

Brouilette,S.W., Moore, J. S., McMahon, A. D., Thompson, J. R., Ford, I., Shepherd, J., Packard, C. J., & Samani, N. J. (2007). Telomere length, risk of coronary heart disease, and statin treatment in the West of Scotland Primary Prevention Study: a nested case-control study. *Lancet* Vol.369, No.9556, pp.107-114.

Bruunsgaard,H., Ladelund, S., Pedersen, A. N., Schroll, M., Jorgensen, T., & Pedersen, B. K. (2003). Predicting death from tumour necrosis factor-alpha and interleukin-6 in 80-year-old people. *Clin.Exp.Immunol.* Vol.132, No.1, pp.24-31.

Bruunsgaard,H., Pedersen, A. N., Schroll, M., Skinhoj, P., & Pedersen, B. K. (1999a). Impaired production of proinflammatory cytokines in response to lipopolysaccharide (LPS) stimulation in elderly humans. *Clin.Exp.Immunol.* Vol.118, No.2, pp.235-241.

Bruunsgaard,H., Skinhoj, P., Qvist, J., & Pedersen, B. K. (1999b). Elderly humans show prolonged in vivo inflammatory activity during pneumococcal infections. *J.Infect.Dis.* Vol.180, No.2, pp.551-554.

Buffa,S., Bulati, M., Pellicano, M., Dunn-Walters, D. K., Wu, Y. C., Candore, G., Vitello, S., Caruso, C., & Colonna-Romano, G. (2011). B cell immunosenescence: different features of naive and memory B cells in elderly. *Biogerontology.* Vol.12, No.5, pp.473-483.

Bulati,M., Buffa, S., Candore, G., Caruso, C., Dunn-Walters, D. K., Pellicano, M., Wu, Y. C., & Colonna, R. G. (2011). B cells and immunosenescence: a focus on IgG+IgD-. *Ageing Res.Rev.* Vol.10, No.2, pp.274-284.

Capurso,C., Solfrizzi, V., D'Introno, A., Colacicco, A. M., Capurso, S. A., Semeraro, C., Capurso, A., & Panza, F. (2007). Interleukin 6 variable number of tandem repeats

(VNTR) gene polymorphism in centenarians. *Ann.Hum.Genet.* Vol.71, No.Pt 6, pp.843-848.

Chakravarti,B. & Abraham, G. N. (1999). Aging and T-cell-mediated immunity. *Mech.Ageing Dev.* Vol.108, No.3, pp.183-206.

Chen,W.H., Kozlovsky, B. F., Effros, R. B., Grubeck-Loebenstein, B., Edelman, R., & Sztein, M. B. (2009). Vaccination in the elderly: an immunological perspective. *Trends Immunol.* Vol.30, No.7, pp.351-359.

Chong,Y., Ikematsu, H., Yamaji, K., Nishimura, M., Nabeshima, S., Kashiwagi, S., & Hayashi, J. (2005). CD27(+) (memory) B cell decrease and apoptosis-resistant CD27(-) (naive) B cell increase in aged humans: implications for age-related peripheral B cell developmental disturbances. *Int.Immunol.* Vol.17, No.4, pp.383-390.

Ciaramella,A., Spalletta, G., Bizzoni, F., Salani, F., Caltagirone, C., & Bossu, P. (2011). Effect of age on surface molecules and cytokine expression in human dendritic cells. *Cell Immunol.* Vol.269, No.2, pp.82-89.

Coen,P.M., Flynn, M. G., Markofski, M. M., Pence, B. D., & Hannemann, R. E. (2010). Adding exercise to rosuvastatin treatment: influence on C-reactive protein, monocyte toll-like receptor 4 expression, and inflammatory monocyte (CD14+CD16+) population. *Metabolism* Vol.59, No.12, pp.1775-1783.

Colonna-Romano,G., Bulati, M., Aquino, A., Pellicano, M., Vitello, S., Lio, D., Candore, G., & Caruso, C. (2009). A double-negative (IgD-CD27-) B cell population is increased in the peripheral blood of elderly people. *Mech.Ageing Dev.* Vol.130, No.10, pp.681-690.

Colonna-Romano,G., Bulati, M., Aquino, A., Scialabba, G., Candore, G., Lio, D., Motta, M., Malaguarnera, M., & Caruso, C. (2003). B cells in the aged: CD27, CD5, and CD40 expression. *Mech.Ageing Dev.* Vol.124, No.4, pp.389-393.

Cook,G.P., Savic, S., Wittmann, M., & McDermott, M. F. (2010). The NLRP3 inflammasome, a target for therapy in diverse disease states. *Eur.J.Immunol.* Vol.40, No.3, pp.631-634.

Corsini,E., Vismara, L., Lucchi, L., Viviani, B., Govoni, S., Galli, C. L., Marinovich, M., & Racchi, M. (2006). High interleukin-10 production is associated with low antibody response to influenza vaccination in the elderly. *J.Leukoc.Biol.* Vol.80, No.2, pp.376-382.

Cretel,E., Veen, I., Pierres, A., Bongrand, P., & Gavazzi, G. (2010). [Immunosenescence and infections, myth or reality?]. *Med.Mal Infect.* Vol.40, No.6, pp.307-318.

Crighton,M.H. & Puppione, A. A. (2006). Geriatric neutrophils: implications for older adults. *Semin.Oncol.Nurs.* Vol.22, No.1, pp.3-9.

Crotty,S. (2011). Follicular helper CD4 T cells (TFH). *Annu.Rev.Immunol.* Vol.29, pp.621-663.

De Martinis,M., Di Benedetto, M. C., Mengoli, L. P., & Ginaldi, L. (2006). Senile osteoporosis: is it an immune-mediated disease? *Inflamm.Res.* Vol.55, No.10, pp.399-404.

De Martinis,M., Franceschi, C., Monti, D., & Ginaldi, L. (2005). Inflamm-ageing and lifelong antigenic load as major determinants of ageing rate and longevity. *FEBS Lett.* Vol.579, No.10, pp.2035-2039.

Della Bella S., Bierti, L., Presicce, P., Arienti, R., Valenti, M., Saresella, M., Vergani, C., & Villa, M. L. (2007). Peripheral blood dendritic cells and monocytes are differently regulated in the elderly. *Clin.Immunol.* Vol.122, No.2, pp.220-228.

Derhovanessian,E., Maier, A. B., Beck, R., Jahn, G., Hahnel, K., Slagboom, P. E., de Craen, A. J., Westendorp, R. G., & Pawelec, G. (2010). Hallmark features of immunosenescence are absent in familial longevity. *J.Immunol.* Vol.185, No.8, pp.4618-4624.

Desai,A., Grolleau-Julius, A., & Yung, R. (2010). Leukocyte function in the aging immune system. *J.Leukoc.Biol.* Vol.87, No.6, pp.1001-1009.

DiPenta,J.M., Green-Johnson, J. M., & Murphy, R. J. (2007). Type 2 diabetes mellitus, resistance training, and innate immunity: is there a common link? *Appl.Physiol Nutr.Metab* Vol.32, No.6, pp.1025-1035.

Dorshkind,K., Montecino-Rodriguez, E., & Signer, R. A. (2009). The ageing immune system: is it ever too old to become young again? *Nat.Rev.Immunol.* Vol.9, No.1, pp.57-62.

Duewell,P., Kono, H., Rayner, K. J., Sirois, C. M., Vladimer, G., Bauernfeind, F. G., Abela, G. S., Franchi, L., Nunez, G., Schnurr, M., Espevik, T., Lien, E., Fitzgerald, K. A., Rock, K. L., Moore, K. J., Wright, S. D., Hornung, V., Latz, E. (2010). NLRP3 inflammasomes are required for atherogenesis and activated by cholesterol crystals. *Nature* Vol.464, No.7293, pp.1357-1361.

Dzionek,A., Fuchs, A., Schmidt, P., Cremer, S., Zysk, M., Miltenyi, S., Buck, D. W., & Schmitz, J. (2000). BDCA-2, BDCA-3, and BDCA-4: three markers for distinct subsets of dendritic cells in human peripheral blood. *J.Immunol.* Vol.165, No.11, pp.6037-6046.

Epel,E.S., Lin, J., Wilhelm, F. H., Wolkowitz, O. M., Cawthon, R., Adler, N. E., Dolbier, C., Mendes, W. B., & Blackburn, E. H. (2006). Cell aging in relation to stress arousal and cardiovascular disease risk factors. *Psychoneuroendocrinology* Vol.31, No.3, pp.277-287.

Fernandez-Gutierrez,B., Jover, J. A., De Miguel, S., Hernandez-Garcia, C., Vidan, M. T., Ribera, J. M., Banares, A., & Serra, J. A. (1999). Early lymphocyte activation in elderly humans: impaired T and T-dependent B cell responses. *Exp.Gerontol.* Vol.34, No.2, pp.217-229.

Ferrando-Martinez,S., Ruiz-Mateos, E., Hernandez, A., Gutierrez, E., Rodriguez-Mendez, M. M., Ordonez, A., & Leal, M. (2011). Age-related deregulation of naive T cell homeostasis in elderly humans. *Age (Dordr.)* Vol.33, No.2, pp.197-207.

Ferro,D., Parrotto, S., Basili, S., Alessandri, C., & Violi, F. (2000). Simvastatin inhibits the monocyte expression of proinflammatory cytokines in patients with hypercholesterolemia. *J.Am.Coll.Cardiol.* Vol.36, No.2, pp.427-431.

Ferroni,P., Martini, F., Cardarello, C. M., Gazzaniga, P. P., Davi, G., & Basili, S. (2003). Enhanced interleukin-1beta in hypercholesterolemia: effects of simvastatin and low-dose aspirin. *Circulation* Vol.108, No.14, pp.1673-1675.

Focosi,D., Bestagno, M., Burrone, O., & Petrini, M. (2010). CD57+ T lymphocytes and functional immune deficiency. *J.Leukoc.Biol.* Vol.87, No.1, pp.107-116.

Forsey,R.J., Thompson, J. M., Ernerudh, J., Hurst, T. L., Strindhall, J., Johansson, B., Nilsson, B. O., & Wikby, A. (2003). Plasma cytokine profiles in elderly humans. *Mech.Ageing Dev.* Vol.124, No.4, pp.487-493.

Freeman,S.L., Fisher, L., German, J. B., Leung, P. S., Prince, H., Selmi, C., Naguwa, S. M., & Gershwin, M. E. (2010). Dairy proteins and the response to pneumovax in senior citizens: a randomized, double-blind, placebo-controlled pilot study. *Ann.N.Y.Acad.Sci.* Vol.1190, pp.97-103.

Fujihashi,K. & Kiyono, H. (2009). Mucosal immunosenescence: new developments and vaccines to control infectious diseases. *Trends Immunol.* Vol.30, No.7, pp.334-343.

Fulop,T., Kotb, R., Fortin, C. F., Pawelec, G., de Angelis, F., & Larbi, A. (2010). Potential role of immunosenescence in cancer development. *Ann.N.Y.Acad.Sci.* Vol.1197, pp.158-165.

Fulop,T., Larbi, A., Douziech, N., Fortin, C., Guerard, K. P., Lesur, O., Khalil, A., & Dupuis, G. (2004). Signal transduction and functional changes in neutrophils with aging. *Aging Cell* Vol.3, No.4, pp.217-226.

Fulop,T., Larbi, A., Hirokawa, K., Mocchegiani, E., Lesourds, B., Castle, S., Wikby, A., Franceschi, C., & Pawelec, G. (2007). Immunosupportive therapies in aging. *Clin.Interv.Aging* Vol.2, No.1, pp.33-54.

Gabriel,P., Cakman, I., & Rink, L. (2002). Overproduction of monokines by leukocytes after stimulation with lipopolysaccharide in the elderly. *Exp.Gerontol.* Vol.37, No.2-3, pp.235-247.

Gannage-Yared,M.H., Azoury, M., Mansour, I., Baddoura, R., Halaby, G., & Naaman, R. (2003). Effects of a short-term calcium and vitamin D treatment on serum cytokines, bone markers, insulin and lipid concentrations in healthy post-menopausal women. *J.Endocrinol.Invest* Vol.26, No.8, pp.748-753.

Giunta,B., Fernandez, F., Nikolic, W. V., Obregon, D., Rrapo, E., Town, T., & Tan, J. (2008). Inflammaging as a prodrome to Alzheimer's disease. *J.Neuroinflammation.* Vol.5, pp.51.

Gomez CMH. (2000). elimination of cytokines by the kidney: comparison between normal individuals and patients with severe sepsis or the systemic inflammatory response syndrome. *british journal of anesthesia* Vol.84, No.5. sheldon J, Riches P, and Palazo MGA.

Gonzalo-Calvo,D., Fernandez-Garcia, B., Luxan-Delgado, B., Rodriguez-Gonzalez, S., Garcia-Macia, M., Suarez, F. M., Solano, J. J., Rodriguez-Colunga, M. J., & Coto-Montes, A. (2011). Long-term training induces a healthy inflammatory and endocrine emergent biomarker profile in elderly men. *Age (Dordr.)* .

Gregg,R., Smith, C. M., Clark, F. J., Dunnion, D., Khan, N., Chakraverty, R., Nayak, L., & Moss, P. A. (2005). The number of human peripheral blood CD4+ CD25high regulatory T cells increases with age. *Clin.Exp.Immunol.* Vol.140, No.3, pp.540-546.

Grewe,M. (2001). Chronological ageing and photoageing of dendritic cells. *Clin.Exp.Dermatol.* Vol.26, No.7, pp.608-612.

Grolleau-Julius,A., Ray, D., & Yung, R. L. (2010). The role of epigenetics in aging and autoimmunity. *Clin.Rev.Allergy Immunol.* Vol.39, No.1, pp.42-50.

Gruver,A.L., Hudson, L. L., & Sempowski, G. D. (2007). Immunosenescence of ageing. *J.Pathol.* Vol.211, No.2, pp.144-156.

Gruver,A.L., Ventevogel, M. S., & Sempowski, G. D. (2009). Leptin receptor is expressed in thymus medulla and leptin protects against thymic remodeling during endotoxemia-induced thymus involution. *J.Endocrinol.* Vol.203, No.1, pp.75-85.

Gupta,S. & Gollapudi, S. (2006). TNF-alpha-induced apoptosis in human naive and memory CD8+ T cells in aged humans. *Exp.Gerontol.* Vol.41, No.1, pp.69-77.

Gupta,S. & Gollapudi, S. (2008). CD95-mediated apoptosis in naive, central and effector memory subsets of CD4+ and CD8+ T cells in aged humans. *Exp.Gerontol.* Vol.43, No.4, pp.266-274.

Haase,H. & Rink, L. (2009). The immune system and the impact of zinc during aging. *Immun.Ageing* Vol.6, pp.9.

Hadrup,S.R., Strindhall, J., Kollgaard, T., Seremet, T., Johansson, B., Pawelec, G., thor, S. P., & Wikby, A. (2006). Longitudinal studies of clonally expanded CD8 T cells reveal a repertoire shrinkage predicting mortality and an increased number of dysfunctional cytomegalovirus-specific T cells in the very elderly. *J.Immunol.* Vol.176, No.4, pp.2645-2653.

Hartel,C., Strunk, T., Bucsky, P., & Schultz, C. (2004). Effects of vitamin C on intracytoplasmic cytokine production in human whole blood monocytes and lymphocytes. *Cytokine* Vol.27, No.4-5, pp.101-106.

Herndler-Brandstetter,D., Schwaiger, S., Veel, E., Fehrer, C., Cioca, D. P., Almanzar, G., Keller, M., Pfister, G., Parson, W., Wurzner, R., Schonitzer, D., Henson, S. M., Aspinall, R., Lepperdinger, G., & Grubeck-Loebenstein, B. (2005). CD25-expressing CD8+ T cells are potent memory cells in old age. *J.Immunol.* Vol.175, No.3, pp.1566-1574.

Hewison,M. (2010). Vitamin D and the immune system: new perspectives on an old theme. *Endocrinol.Metab Clin.North Am.* Vol.39, No.2, pp.365-79, table.

Hick,R.W., Gruver, A. L., Ventevogel, M. S., Haynes, B. F., & Sempowski, G. D. (2006). Leptin selectively augments thymopoiesis in leptin deficiency and lipopolysaccharide-induced thymic atrophy. *J.Immunol.* Vol.177, No.1, pp.169-176.

Himmerich,H., Milenovic, S., Fulda, S., Plumakers, B., Sheldrick, A. J., Michel, T. M., Kircher, T., & Rink, L. (2010). Regulatory T cells increased while IL-1beta decreased during antidepressant therapy. *J.Psychiatr.Res.* Vol.44, No.15, pp.1052-1057.

Hotamisligil,G.S. (2010). Endoplasmic reticulum stress and atherosclerosis. *Nat.Med.* Vol.16, No.4, pp.396-399.

Huber,L.A., Xu, Q. B., Jurgens, G., Bock, G., Buhler, E., Gey, K. F., Schonitzer, D., Traill, K. N., & Wick, G. (1991). Correlation of lymphocyte lipid composition membrane microviscosity and mitogen response in the aged. *Eur.J.Immunol.* Vol.21, No.11, pp.2761-2765.

Irwin,M.R. & Miller, A. H. (2007). Depressive disorders and immunity: 20 years of progress and discovery. *Brain Behav.Immun.* Vol.21, No.4, pp.374-383.

James,K., Premchand, N., Skibinska, A., Skibinski, G., Nicol, M., & Mason, J. I. (1997). IL-6, DHEA and the ageing process. *Mech.Ageing Dev.* Vol.93, No.1-3, pp.15-24.

Jiang,H., Ju, Z., & Rudolph, K. L. (2007). Telomere shortening and ageing. *Z.Gerontol.Geriatr.* Vol.40, No.5, pp.314-324.

Jing,Y., Shaheen, E., Drake, R. R., Chen, N., Gravenstein, S., & Deng, Y. (2009). Aging is associated with a numerical and functional decline in plasmacytoid dendritic cells, whereas myeloid dendritic cells are relatively unaltered in human peripheral blood. *Hum.Immunol.* Vol.70, No.10, pp.777-784.

Kamada,M., Irahara, M., Maegawa, M., Yasui, T., Yamano, S., Yamada, M., Tezuka, M., Kasai, Y., Deguchi, K., Ohmoto, Y., & Aono, T. (2001). B cell subsets in postmenopausal women and the effect of hormone replacement therapy. *Maturitas* Vol.37, No.3, pp.173-179.

Kanwar,J.R. & Kanwar, R. K. (2009). Gut health immunomodulatory and anti-inflammatory functions of gut enzyme digested high protein micro-nutrient dietary supplement-Enprocal. *BMC.Immunol.* Vol.10, pp.7.

Kilpatrick,R.D., Rickabaugh, T., Hultin, L. E., Hultin, P., Hausner, M. A., Detels, R., Phair, J., & Jamieson, B. D. (2008). Homeostasis of the naive CD4+ T cell compartment during aging. *J.Immunol.* Vol.180, No.3, pp.1499-1507.

Krabbe,K.S., Pedersen, M., & Bruunsgaard, H. (2004). Inflammatory mediators in the elderly. *Exp.Gerontol.* Vol.39, No.5, pp.687-699.

Krysiak,R., Gdula-Dymek, A., & Okopien, B. (2011a). Effect of simvastatin and fenofibrate on cytokine release and systemic inflammation in type 2 diabetes mellitus with mixed dyslipidemia. *Am.J.Cardiol.* Vol.107, No.7, pp.1010-1018.

Krysiak,R., Gdula-Dymek, A., Scieszka, J., & Okopien, B. (2011b). Anti-inflammatory and monocyte-suppressing effects of simvastatin in patients with impaired fasting glucose. *Basic Clin.Pharmacol.Toxicol.* Vol.108, No.2, pp.131-137.

Ku,L.T., Gercel-Taylor, C., Nakajima, S. T., & Taylor, D. D. (2009). Alterations of T cell activation signalling and cytokine production by postmenopausal estrogen levels. *Immun.Ageing* Vol.6, pp.1.

Lesourd,B. (2006). Nutritional factors and immunological ageing. *Proc.Nutr.Soc.* Vol.65, No.3, pp.319-325.

Li,Q.Z., Deng, Q., Li, J. Q., Yi, G. H., & Zhao, S. P. (2005). Valsartan reduces interleukin-1beta secretion by peripheral blood mononuclear cells in patients with essential hypertension. *Clin.Chim.Acta* Vol.355, No.1-2, pp.131-136.

Li,X., Liu, C., Cui, J., Dong, M., Peng, C. H., Li, Q. S., Cheng, J. L., Jiang, S. L., & Tian, Y. (2009). Effects of pravastatin on the function of dendritic cells in patients with coronary heart disease. *Basic Clin.Pharmacol.Toxicol.* Vol.104, No.2, pp.101-106.

Ligthart,G.J., Corberand, J. X., Fournier, C., Galanaud, P., Hijmans, W., Kennes, B., Muller-Hermelink, H. K., & Steinmann, G. G. (1984). Admission criteria for immunogerontological studies in man: the SENIEUR protocol. *Mech.Ageing Dev.* Vol.28, No.1, pp.47-55.

Lundberg,A.M. & Hansson, G. K. (2010). Innate immune signals in atherosclerosis. *Clin.Immunol.* Vol.134, No.1, pp.5-24.

MacDonald,K.P., Munster, D. J., Clark, G. J., Dzionek, A., Schmitz, J., & Hart, D. N. (2002). Characterization of human blood dendritic cell subsets. *Blood* Vol.100, No.13, pp.4512-4520.

Maggio,M., Ceda, G. P., Lauretani, F., Bandinelli, S., Corsi, A. M., Giallauria, F., Guralnik, J. M., Zuliani, G., Cattabiani, C., Parrino, S., Ablondi, F., Dall'aglio, E., Ceresini, G., Basaria, S., & Ferrucci, L. (2011). SHBG, sex hormones, and inflammatory markers in older women. *J.Clin.Endocrinol.Metab* Vol.96, No.4, pp.1053-1059.

Malaguarnera,L., Cristaldi, E., & Malaguarnera, M. (2010). The role of immunity in elderly cancer. *Crit Rev.Oncol.Hematol.* Vol.74, No.1, pp.40-60.

Mariani,E., Cattini, L., Neri, S., Malavolta, M., Mocchegiani, E., Ravaglia, G., & Facchini, A. (2006). Simultaneous evaluation of circulating chemokine and cytokine profiles in elderly subjects by multiplex technology: relationship with zinc status. *Biogerontology.* Vol.7, No.5-6, pp.449-459.

McElhaney,J.E. & Effros, R. B. (2009). Immunosenescence: what does it mean to health outcomes in older adults? *Curr.Opin.Immunol.* Vol.21, No.4, pp.418-424.

McIntire,C.R., Yeretssian, G., & Saleh, M. (2009). Inflammasomes in infection and inflammation. *Apoptosis.* Vol.14, No.4, pp.522-535.

Mira,J.P., Max, A., & Burgel, P. R. (2008). The role of biomarkers in community-acquired pneumonia: predicting mortality and response to adjunctive therapy. *Crit Care* Vol.12 Suppl 6, pp.S5.

Mocchegiani,E. (2010). session 2 : micronutrients and the immune system : zinc, metallothioneins and immunosenescence. *Proc.Nutr.Soc.*

Mocchegiani,E., Costarelli, L., Giacconi, R., Piacenza, F., Basso, A., & Malavolta, M. (2011). Zinc, metallothioneins and immunosenescence: effect of zinc supply as nutrigenomic approach. *Biogerontology.*

Moro-Garcia,M.A., Alonso-Arias, R., Lopez-Vazquez, A., Suarez-Garcia, F. M., Solano-Jaurrieta, J. J., Baltar, J., & Lopez-Larrea, C. (2011). Relationship between functional ability in older people, immune system status, and intensity of response to CMV. *Age (Dordr.)* .

Motta,M., Ferlito, L., Malaguarnera, L., Vinci, E., Bosco, S., Maugeri, D., & Malaguarnera, M. (2003). Alterations of the lymphocytic set-up in elderly patients with cancer. *Arch.Gerontol.Geriatr.* Vol.36, No.1, pp.7-14.

Mysliwska,J., Bryl, E., Foerster, J., & Mysliwski, A. (1998). Increase of interleukin 6 and decrease of interleukin 2 production during the ageing process are influenced by the health status. *Mech.Ageing Dev.* Vol.100, No.3, pp.313-328.

Naidoo,N. (2009). ER and aging-Protein folding and the ER stress response. *Ageing Res.Rev.* Vol.8, No.3, pp.150-159.

Naylor,K., Li, G., Vallejo, A. N., Lee, W. W., Koetz, K., Bryl, E., Witkowski, J., Fulbright, J., Weyand, C. M., & Goronzy, J. J. (2005). The influence of age on T cell generation and TCR diversity. *J.Immunol.* Vol.174, No.11, pp.7446-7452.

Nichol,K.L., Nordin, J., Mullooly, J., Lask, R., Fillbrandt, K., & Iwane, M. (2003). Influenza vaccination and reduction in hospitalizations for cardiac disease and stroke among the elderly. *N.Engl.J.Med.* Vol.348, No.14, pp.1322-1332.

Nilsson,B.O., Ernerudh, J., Johansson, B., Evrin, P. E., Lofgren, S., Ferguson, F. G., & Wikby, A. (2003). Morbidity does not influence the T-cell immune risk phenotype in the elderly: findings in the Swedish NONA Immune Study using sample selection protocols. *Mech.Ageing Dev.* Vol.124, No.4, pp.469-476.

Ohyashiki,J.H., Iwama, H., Yahata, N., Ando, K., Hayashi, S., Shay, J. W., & Ohyashiki, K. (1999). Telomere stability is frequently impaired in high-risk groups of patients with myelodysplastic syndromes. *Clin.Cancer Res.* Vol.5, No.5, pp.1155-1160.

Ongradi,J. & Kovesdi, V. (2010). Factors that may impact on immunosenescence: an appraisal. *Immun.Ageing* Vol.7, pp.7.

Ouyang,Q., Wagner, W. M., Voehringer, D., Wikby, A., Klatt, T., Walter, S., Muller, C. A., Pircher, H., & Pawelec, G. (2003). Age-associated accumulation of CMV-specific CD8+ T cells expressing the inhibitory killer cell lectin-like receptor G1 (KLRG1). *Exp.Gerontol.* Vol.38, No.8, pp.911-920.

Panda,A., Qian, F., Mohanty, S., van Duin, D., Newman, F. K., Zhang, L., Chen, S., Towle, V., Belshe, R. B., Fikrig, E., Allore, H. G., Montgomery, R. R., & Shaw, A. C. (2010). Age-associated decrease in TLR function in primary human dendritic cells predicts influenza vaccine response. *J.Immunol.* Vol.184, No.5, pp.2518-2527.

Panossian,L.A., Porter, V. R., Valenzuela, H. F., Zhu, X., Reback, E., Masterman, D., Cummings, J. L., & Effros, R. B. (2003). Telomere shortening in T cells correlates with Alzheimer's disease status. *Neurobiol.Aging* Vol.24, No.1, pp.77-84.

Pawelec,G., Akbar, A., Caruso, C., Solana, R., Grubeck-Loebenstein, B., & Wikby, A. (2005). Human immunosenescence: is it infectious? *Immunol.Rev.* Vol.205, pp.257-268.

Pawelec,G. & Derhovanessian, E. (2011). Role of CMV in immune senescence. *Virus Res.* Vol.157, No.2, pp.175-179.

Penninx,B.W., Kritchevsky, S. B., Newman, A. B., Nicklas, B. J., Simonsick, E. M., Rubin, S., Nevitt, M., Visser, M., Harris, T., & Pahor, M. (2004). Inflammatory markers and incident mobility limitation in the elderly. *J.Am.Geriatr.Soc.* Vol.52, No.7, pp.1105-1113.

Penninx,B.W., Kritchevsky, S. B., Yaffe, K., Newman, A. B., Simonsick, E. M., Rubin, S., Ferrucci, L., Harris, T., & Pahor, M. (2003). Inflammatory markers and depressed mood in older persons: results from the Health, Aging and Body Composition study. *Biol.Psychiatry* Vol.54, No.5, pp.566-572.

Pepersack,T., Rotsaert, P., Benoit, F., Willems, D., Fuss, M., Bourdoux, P., & Duchateau, J. (2001). Prevalence of zinc deficiency and its clinical relevance among hospitalised elderly. *Arch.Gerontol.Geriatr.* Vol.33, No.3, pp.243-253.

Perez-Cabezas,B., Naranjo-Gomez, M., Fernandez, M. A., Grifols, J. R., Pujol-Borrell, R., & Borras, F. E. (2007). Reduced numbers of plasmacytoid dendritic cells in aged blood donors. *Exp.Gerontol.* Vol.42, No.10, pp.1033-1038.

Pfister,G. & Savino, W. (2008). Can the immune system still be efficient in the elderly? An immunological and immunoendocrine therapeutic perspective. *Neuroimmunomodulation.* Vol.15, No.4-6, pp.351-364.

Picano,E., Morales, M. A., del Ry, S., & Sicari, R. (2010). Innate inflammation in myocardial perfusion and its implication for heart failure. *Ann.N.Y.Acad.Sci.* Vol.1207, pp.107-115.

Pierce,A., Legrand, D., & Mazurier, J. (2009). [Lactoferrin: a multifunctional protein]. *Med.Sci.(Paris)* Vol.25, No.4, pp.361-369.

Pietschmann,P., Hahn, P., Kudlacek, S., Thomas, R., & Peterlik, M. (2000). Surface markers and transendothelial migration of dendritic cells from elderly subjects. *Exp.Gerontol.* Vol.35, No.2, pp.213-224.

Rajasekaran,K., Xiong, V., Fong, L., Gorski, J., & Malarkannan, S. (2010). Functional dichotomy between NKG2D and CD28-mediated co-stimulation in human CD8+ T cells. *PLoS.One.* Vol.5, No.9.

Ravaglia,G., Forti, P., Maioli, F., Chiappelli, M., Montesi, F., Tumini, E., Mariani, E., Licastro, F., & Patterson, C. (2007). Blood inflammatory markers and risk of dementia: The Conselice Study of Brain Aging. *Neurobiol.Aging* Vol.28, No.12, pp.1810-1820.

Reuben,D.B., Cheh, A. I., Harris, T. B., Ferrucci, L., Rowe, J. W., Tracy, R. P., & Seeman, T. E. (2002). Peripheral blood markers of inflammation predict mortality and functional decline in high-functioning community-dwelling older persons. *J.Am.Geriatr.Soc.* Vol.50, No.4, pp.638-644.

Rink,L., Cakman, I., & Kirchner, H. (1998). Altered cytokine production in the elderly. *Mech.Ageing Dev.* Vol.102, No.2-3, pp.199-209.

Rosenfeld,M.E. & Campbell, L. A. (2011). Pathogens and atherosclerosis: Update on the potential contribution of multiple infectious organisms to the pathogenesis of atherosclerosis. *Thromb.Haemost.* Vol.106, No.5, pp.858-867.

Sadeghi,H.M., Schnelle, J. F., Thoma, J. K., Nishanian, P., & Fahey, J. L. (1999). Phenotypic and functional characteristics of circulating monocytes of elderly persons. *Exp.Gerontol.* Vol.34, No.8, pp.959-970.

Sampson,M.J., Winterbone, M. S., Hughes, J. C., Dozio, N., & Hughes, D. A. (2006). Monocyte telomere shortening and oxidative DNA damage in type 2 diabetes. *Diabetes Care* Vol.29, No.2, pp.283-289.

Schenkein,J.G., Park, S., & Nahm, M. H. (2008). Pneumococcal vaccination in older adults induces antibodies with low opsonic capacity and reduced antibody potency. *Vaccine* Vol.26, No.43, pp.5521-5526.

Schiffrin,E.J., Morley, J. E., Donnet-Hughes, A., & Guigoz, Y. (2010). The inflammatory status of the elderly: the intestinal contribution. *Mutat.Res.* Vol.690, No.1-2, pp.50-56.

Schonbeck,U. & Libby, P. (2004). Inflammation, immunity, and HMG-CoA reductase inhibitors: statins as antiinflammatory agents? *Circulation* Vol.109, No.21 Suppl 1, pp.II18-II26.

Schwalfenberg,G.K. (2011). A review of the critical role of vitamin D in the functioning of the immune system and the clinical implications of vitamin D deficiency. *Mol.Nutr.Food Res.* Vol.55, No.1, pp.96-108.

Seidler,S., Zimmermann, H. W., Bartneck, M., Trautwein, C., & Tacke, F. (2010). Age-dependent alterations of monocyte subsets and monocyte-related chemokine pathways in healthy adults. *BMC.Immunol.* Vol.11, pp.30.

Senchina,D.S. & Kohut, M. L. (2007). Immunological outcomes of exercise in older adults. *Clin.Interv.Aging* Vol.2, No.1, pp.3-16.

Shanley,D.P., Aw, D., Manley, N. R., & Palmer, D. B. (2009). An evolutionary perspective on the mechanisms of immunosenescence. *Trends Immunol.* Vol.30, No.7, pp.374-381.

Shaw,A.C., Panda, A., Joshi, S. R., Qian, F., Allore, H. G., & Montgomery, R. R. (2011). Dysregulation of human Toll-like receptor function in aging. *Ageing Res.Rev.* Vol.10, No.3, pp.346-353.

Shodell,M. & Siegal, F. P. (2002). Circulating, interferon-producing plasmacytoid dendritic cells decline during human ageing. *Scand.J.Immunol.* Vol.56, No.5, pp.518-521.

Shurin,G.V., Yurkovetsky, Z. R., Chatta, G. S., Tourkova, I. L., Shurin, M. R., & Lokshin, A. E. (2007). Dynamic alteration of soluble serum biomarkers in healthy aging. *Cytokine* Vol.39, No.2, pp.123-129.

Spyridopoulos,I., Hoffmann, J., Aicher, A., Brummendorf, T. H., Doerr, H. W., Zeiher, A. M., & Dimmeler, S. (2009). Accelerated telomere shortening in leukocyte subpopulations of patients with coronary heart disease: role of cytomegalovirus seropositivity. *Circulation* Vol.120, No.14, pp.1364-1372.

Steer,S.E., Williams, F. M., Kato, B., Gardner, J. P., Norman, P. J., Hall, M. A., Kimura, M., Vaughan, R., Aviv, A., & Spector, T. D. (2007). Reduced telomere length in rheumatoid arthritis is independent of disease activity and duration. *Ann.Rheum.Dis.* Vol.66, No.4, pp.476-480.

Straub,R.H., Konecna, L., Hrach, S., Rothe, G., Kreutz, M., Scholmerich, J., Falk, W., & Lang, B. (1998). Serum dehydroepiandrosterone (DHEA) and DHEA sulfate are negatively correlated with serum interleukin-6 (IL-6), and DHEA inhibits IL-6 secretion from mononuclear cells in man in vitro: possible link between endocrinosenescence and immunosenescence. *J.Clin.Endocrinol.Metab* Vol.83, No.6, pp.2012-2017.

Stulnig,T.M., Buhler, E., Bock, G., Kirchebner, C., Schonitzer, D., & Wick, G. (1995). Altered switch in lipid composition during T-cell blast transformation in the healthy elderly. *J.Gerontol.A Biol.Sci.Med.Sci.* Vol.50, No.6, pp.B383-B390.

Tortorella,C., Simone, O., Piazzolla, G., Stella, I., Cappiello, V., & Antonaci, S. (2006). Role of phosphoinositide 3-kinase and extracellular signal-regulated kinase pathways in granulocyte macrophage-colony-stimulating factor failure to delay fas-induced neutrophil apoptosis in elderly humans. *J.Gerontol.A Biol.Sci.Med.Sci.* Vol.61, No.11, pp.1111-1118.

Trzonkowski,P., Mysliwska, J., Godlewska, B., Szmit, E., Lukaszuk, K., Wieckiewicz, J., Brydak, L., Machala, M., Landowski, J., & Mysliwski, A. (2004). Immune consequences of the spontaneous pro-inflammatory status in depressed elderly patients. *Brain Behav.Immun.* Vol.18, No.2, pp.135-148.

Trzonkowski,P., Mysliwska, J., Szmit, E., Wieckiewicz, J., Lukaszuk, K., Brydak, L. B., Machala, M., & Mysliwski, A. (2003). Association between cytomegalovirus infection, enhanced proinflammatory response and low level of anti-hemagglutinins during the anti-influenza vaccination--an impact of immunosenescence. *Vaccine* Vol.21, No.25-26, pp.3826-3836.

Vallejo,A.N., Hamel, D. L., Jr., Mueller, R. G., Ives, D. G., Michel, J. J., Boudreau, R. M., & Newman, A. B. (2011). NK-Like T Cells and Plasma Cytokines, but Not Anti-Viral Serology, Define Immune Fingerprints of Resilience and Mild Disability in Exceptional Aging. *PLoS.One.* Vol.6, No.10, pp.e26558.

van den Biggelaar,A.H., Huizinga, T. W., de Craen, A. J., Gussekloo, J., Heijmans, B. T., Frolich, M., & Westendorp, R. G. (2004). Impaired innate immunity predicts frailty in old age. The Leiden 85-plus study. *Exp.Gerontol.* Vol.39, No.9, pp.1407-1414.

van Duin,D., Mohanty, S., Thomas, V., Ginter, S., Montgomery, R. R., Fikrig, E., Allore, H. G., Medzhitov, R., & Shaw, A. C. (2007). Age-associated defect in human TLR-1/2 function. *J.Immunol.* Vol.178, No.2, pp.970-975.

van Duin,D. & Shaw, A. C. (2007). Toll-like receptors in older adults. *J.Am.Geriatr.Soc.* Vol.55, No.9, pp.1438-1444.

Vo,T.K., Saint-Hubert, M., Morrhaye, G., Godard, P., Geenen, V., Martens, H. J., Debacq-Chainiaux, F., Swine, C., & Toussaint, O. (2011). Transcriptomic biomarkers of the response of hospitalized geriatric patients admitted with heart failure. Comparison to hospitalized geriatric patients with infectious diseases or hip fracture. *Mech.Ageing Dev.* Vol.132, No.3, pp.131-139.

Weksler,M.E. & Szabo, P. (2000). The effect of age on the B-cell repertoire. *J.Clin.Immunol.* Vol.20, No.4, pp.240-249.

Wessels,I., Jansen, J., Rink, L., & Uciechowski, P. (2010). Immunosenescence of polymorphonuclear neutrophils. *ScientificWorldJournal.* Vol.10, pp.145-160.

Wikby,A. (2008). Immune risk phenotypes and associated parameters in very old humans. Ferguson, F., Strindhall, J., Forsey, R. J., Fulop, T., Hadrup S.R., Straten PT, Pawelec, G., and Johansson, B. *Immunosenescences, 2007* . landes biosciences and springer sciences.

Wikby,A., Johansson, B., Ferguson, F., & Olsson, J. (1994). Age-related changes in immune parameters in a very old population of Swedish people: a longitudinal study. *Exp.Gerontol.* Vol.29, No.5, pp.531-541.

Wills,M., Akbar, A., Beswick, M., Bosch, J. A., Caruso, C., Colonna-Romano, G., Dutta, A., Franceschi, C., Fulop, T., Gkrania-Klotsas, E., Goronzy, J., Griffiths, S. J., Henson, S., Herndler-Brandstetter, D., Hill, A., Kern, F., Klenerman, P., Macallan, D., Macualay, R., Maier, A. B., Mason, G., Melzer, D., Morgan, M., Moss, P., Nikolich-Zugich, J., Pachnio, A., Riddell, N., Roberts, R., Sansoni, P., Sauce, D., Sinclair, J., Solana, R., Strindhall, J., Trzonkowski, P., van Lier, R., Vescovini, R., Wang, G., Westendorp, R., & Pawelec, G. (2011). Report from the Second Cytomegalovirus and Immunosenescence Workshop. *Immun.Ageing* Vol.8, No.1, pp.10.

Wolf,A.M., Rumpold, H., Tilg, H., Gastl, G., Gunsilius, E., & Wolf, D. (2006). The effect of zoledronic acid on the function and differentiation of myeloid cells. *Haematologica* Vol.91, No.9, pp.1165-1171.

Yoshikawa,T.T. (1981). Important infections in elderly persons. *West J.Med.* Vol.135, No.6, pp.441-445. Zheng,S.X., Vrindts, Y., Lopez, M., De Groote, D., Zangerle, P. F., Collette, J., Franchimont, N., Geenen, V., Albert, A., & Reginster, J. Y. (1997). Increase in cytokine production (IL-1 beta, IL-6, TNF-alpha but not IFN-gamma, GM-CSF or LIF) by stimulated whole blood cells in postmenopausal osteoporosis. *Maturitas* Vol.26, No.1, pp.63-71.

Zuliani,G., Ranzini, M., Guerra, G., Rossi, L., Munari, M. R., Zurlo, A., Volpato, S., Atti, A. R., Ble, A., & Fellin, R. (2007). Plasma cytokines profile in older subjects with late onset Alzheimer's disease or vascular dementia. *J.Psychiatr.Res.* Vol.41, No.8, pp.686-693.

13

Development of the Immune System - Early Nutrition and Consequences for Later Life

JoAnn Kerperien[1], Bastiaan Schouten[2], Günther Boehm[2,3], Linette E.M. Willemsen[1], Johan Garssen[1,2], Léon M.J. Knippels[1,2] and Belinda van't Land[2,4]

[1]*Pharmacology, Utrecht Institute for Pharmaceutical Sciences (UIPS), University of Utrecht,*
[2]*Danone Research – Centre for Specialised Nutrition, Wageningen, The Netherlands and Friedrichsdorf,*
[3]*Sophia Children's Hospital, Erasmus University Rotterdam,*
[4]*Wilhelmina Children's Hospital, University Medical Center, Utrecht, The Netherlands*

1. Introduction

The immunological interaction between mother and fetus during pregnancy causes the fetal immune system to avoid excessive and destructive immunological reactions. This particular physiologic situation coexists with an immature immune system, which makes the infant very vulnerable for infections and susceptible to the development of immune system related disorders. At birth, the immune system of the infant is particularly characterized by a not fully developed non-specific immune system. In addition, a suppressed capacity of antigen-specific T cells, a deletion of activated T cells, and the presence of high amounts of regulatory T cells (Treg) hamper proper immune responsiveness. During the first months of life the antigen-specific immune response has to be developed in parallel to the maintenance of immune tolerance against compounds commonly found in the environment of mother and infant. There is evidence that disturbances of these complex developmental processes will have impact on the function of the immune system during lifetime causing immunological disorders such as allergy and autoimmunity.

Human milk contains several immunological active compounds which protect the infant from infection. Many of them such as antibodies are individually adapted to the maternal environment which is similar to the environment of the infant thus providing individual protection to the infant. Apart from this protection activated immediately after birth, human milk modulates also the described developmental processes. Although the mechanisms of this modulation are not fully understood there is evidence that human milk can transfer "immunological memory of the mother" to the infant. This concept of the role of human milk underlines the importance of quality of nutrition during first months of life for total development of the immune system. Individual human milk analyses will provide insight in components that are important modulators. Immunologic active peptides, long chain polyunsaturated fatty acids, several glycolipids and non-digestible oligosaccharides have already been identified as such modulators. The interaction of these active components with different parts of the immune system is very complex allowing a graduate and balanced development of the immune system.

One problem of studies in animals and humans is the fact that no single biomarker exists which describes completely the developmental status of the immune system. Although the question which biomarkers are of relevance is still a matter of intensive research there is evidence that many "classical" biomarkers are not useful. Many of these "classical" biomarkers are only sensitive in case the immune system is out of balance but not during a normal development. Consequently, research to identify relevant biomarkers characterizing healthy development is strongly required. There are many questions still open. However, first results are promising indicating that the quality of nutrition early in life might support development of the immune system for lifetime. Acceptance of such a concept might provide opportunities for new ways of primary prevention of immune related diseases later in life.

This chapter will summarise the newest and some specific insights of the mechanisms and impact of nutrition on the development of the immune system early in life.

2. Influences prior life

The nutritional status in early life has an important influence on human immune development, for example, a positive association is clearly observed between birth weight and antibody response to certain vaccines later in life (McDade, Beck et al. 2001). The precise relationship however between nutritional exposures during critical periods of development and later immune function warrants further investigation. The early postnatal environment is a vital determinant of adult health. An environmental exposure, like nutritional modulation of the evolving intestine during early infancy makes an impact on the development and function. A concept like this (as illustrated in *Figure 1*) will provide opportunities for primary prevention from immune related diseases later in life.

In order to understand the impact of nutrition on immune development early in life it is of key importance to know which steps in immune development are subjective to change and depend on specific nutrition. During embryogenesis, stem cells start to differentiate into specific progenitor stem cells, creating a pool of more specific and less totipotent stem cells. Hematopoietic stem cells (HSC) are the progenitor cells for our whole immune system (*Figure 2*). Identification of the first HSC is still difficult, because these regions don't contain many HSC and unique markers are lacking (Medvinsky, Rybtsov et al. 2011). After these few first HSC have colonized the human fetal liver, these cells expand and will relocate under influence of adhesion molecules and chemo-attractants to thymus, spleen and bone marrow (Mazo, Massberg et al. 2011). The bone marrow will start to produce immune cells from the hematopoietic lineage at four to five months of gestation in human pregnancy. Upon stimulation with 'early acting cytokines' a HSC will proliferate and differentiate into a myeloid or a lymphoid precursor cell depending on their surroundings (Grassinger, Haylock et al. 2010).

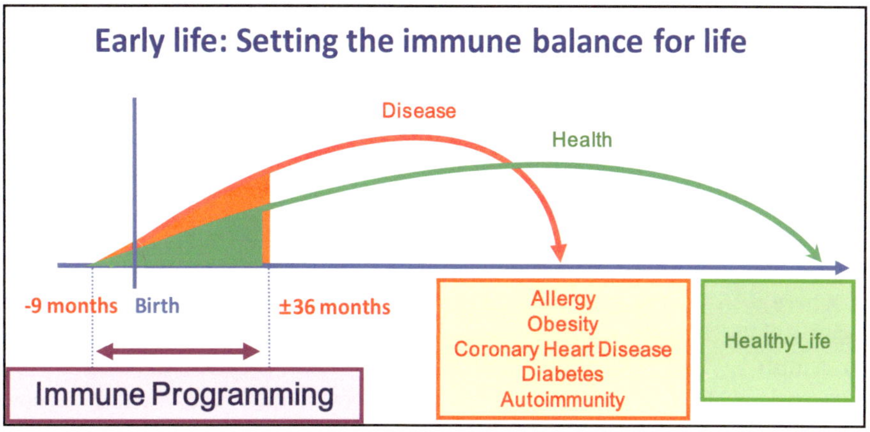

Fig. 1. Disturbances of immune developmental processes will have impact on the function of the immune system during life causing immunological disorders such as allergic disorders and autoimmunity. Although there are many questions still open first results are promising indicating that feeding early in life might support the development of the immune system for lifetime.

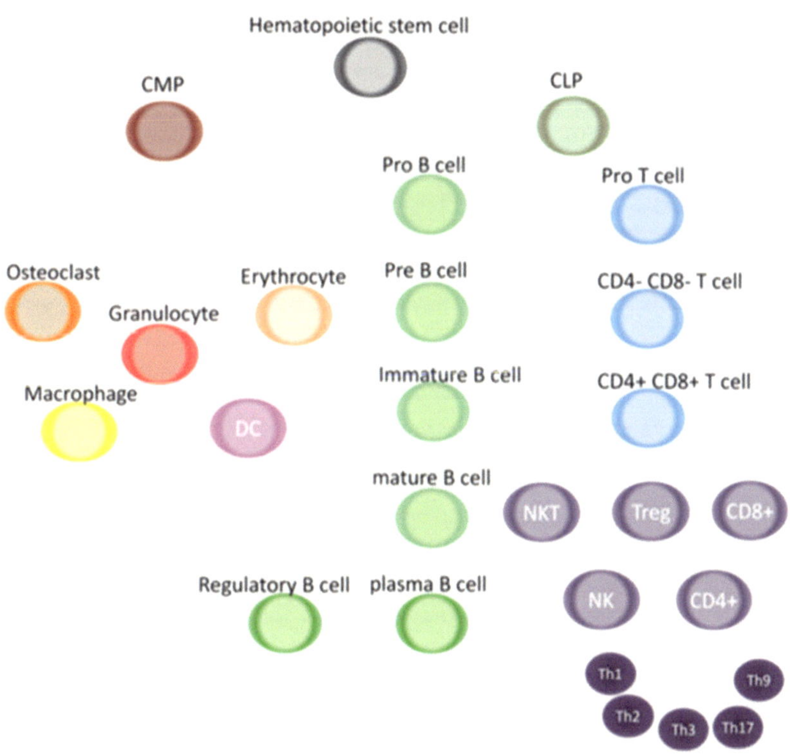

Fig. 2. Hematopoiesis/ immune cell development; From the hematopoetic stem cell the different immune cells develop, including; CMP, common myeloid precursor; CLP, common lymphoid precursor; DC, dendritic cell; NKT, natural killer T cell; NK, natural killer cell; Treg, regulatory T cell; CD8+, cytotoxic T cell; CD4+ Th, T helper cell.

2.1 Lymph node formation

Recent investigation showed that during lymph node development retinyl hydrogenase (RALDH) 2 is one of the enzymes essential in initial cross talk between different cell types (van de Pavert and Mebius 2010). RALDH-2 converts retinaldehyde to retinoic acid (RA). In absence of this enzyme proper lymphoid follicles are not developed. Retinoic acid is the active form of vitamin A and is important during embryogenesis, when axial patterning and organ formation take place (Campo-Paysaa, Marletaz et al. 2008). RA is involved in nerve development and expression of RALDH is found in nerve fibers near the lymph node anlagen, where RA can influence stromal cells to produce specific chemokines. Because RA is produced and used for different developmental processes, other factors should be present to direct lymph node development. One of these factors is CXC chemokine ligand 13 (CXCL13) produced by lymph node surrounding stromal cells. After a small cluster of pre-T- and -B cells is formed, more cells are attracted to this specific site for example via CC chemokine receptor (CCR) 7 and CC chemokine ligand (CCL) 19 and CCL21. When there are enough cells in the cluster, differentiation into lymph nodes occurs. Lymph nodes in the intestine are essential for priming of the whole immune system; therefore detailed development of the intestinal tract and intestinal immune tissues are described in *Box 1.* Peyers patches (PP) are the local small intestinal lymph nodes and mesenteric lymph nodes (MLN) are the collecting lymph nodes for small and large intestine. In essence these lymph structures develop very similar but there are some differences. For the development of PP the CD11c+ cells are required. In addition there are differences in essential transcription factors which are necessary to develop lymph nodes or PP, like interleukin (IL) 7 and RANK (Chappaz, Gartner et al. 2010). Using mice deficient for IL7 or Kit or both they showed that IL7 is important for lymph node anlagen but not for PP development whereas both Kit and Il7 are important for MLN anlagen (Chappaz, Gartner et al. 2010). But growth factors needed for lymph node development still remain poorly understood. The influence of vitamin A on the development of lymphoid structures is already a strong indication that nutritional components are of key importance at the base of infant's immune system.

> A human embryo consists two weeks after fertilisation of three layers, called ectoderm, endoderm and mesoderm. Ectoderm forms the nervous system and the exterior, endoderm forms among others the gastrointestinal tract and the mesoderm forms for example connective tissue and the cells of the immune system. In the fourth week of embryogenesis the flat tissue folds lateral and folds from head to toe, via which the endoderm is enclosed by the ectoderm and a foregut, midgut and a hindgut are being formed, surrounded by mesoderm. At the end of the fourth week the liver is also beginning to form. From one of the pouches in the forgut, thymus will be formed, between 3rd and fourth month during pregnancy.
>
> The loop of the midgut remains in contact with the yolk sac via the vitalline duct. In the same period that the definitive duodenum is formed, the midgut elongates and the hindgut becomes enlarged. When these changes in the pre-intestinal tract occur, the midgut migrates to the umbilical cord and returns in the embryo before the 4th month. During retraction the gut rotates to its final position. Throughout the whole gut enlargement of the surface is initiated via formation of crypts, villi and microvilli. The villi and microvilli start to develop after 9 to 10 weeks and at a later stage the colon loses it's villi. After birth the intestine needs approximately one week to organize it's lymph nodes with specific T- and B-cell regions and six months to acquire a tight epithelial barrier.

Box 1.

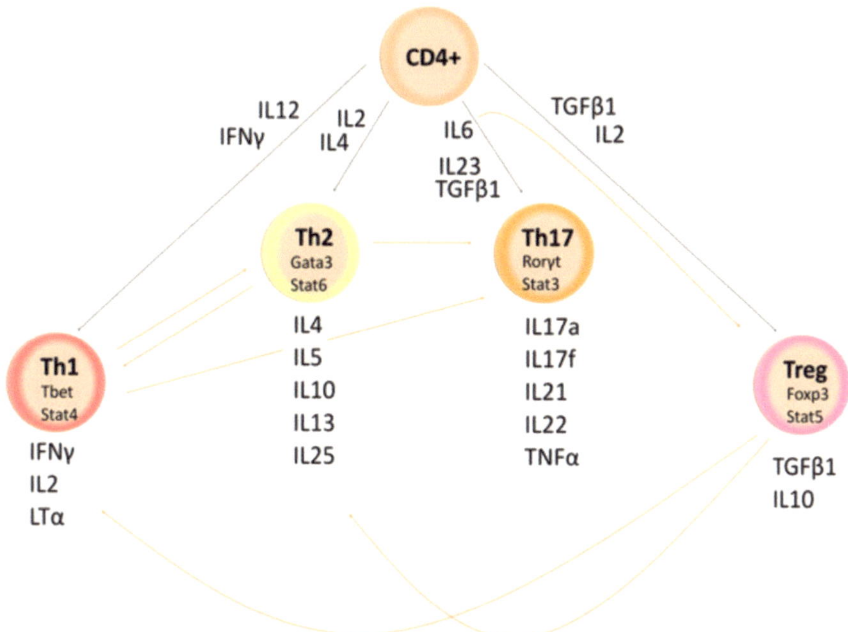

Fig. 3. Immune cell plasticity; Upon antigen encounter and T cell activation, naïve CD4+ T cells mature into several subsets. Several factors including cytokines, as described above determine the type of immune response, including Th1, Th2, Th17 and regulatory T cells. For example Th1 cell differentiation Interleukin (IL)12 and interferon gamma (IFNγ) is needed (blue arrow indicates stimulation). These cytokines help up regulate specific transcription factors like Tbet and Signal transducer and activator of transcription 4 (Stat4). These transcription factors activate certain genes to produce other cytokines like, IL2, LTα and IFNγ. When these cytokines are produced they help inhibit the differentiation of other Th-cells (red arrows indicate inhibition).

2.2 Immune cell development

The fetal common lymphoid progenitor cells (CLP) differ from the adult CLPs. The fetal CLPs have the ability not only to differentiate into all lymphoid cell types but also into macrophages. It is currently not known whether adult CLP are restricted to the division in myeloid and lymphoid progenitors or whether it is a gradual loss in lineage commitment (Chi, Bell et al. 2009). Via complex processes involving, a positive and negative selection, a lineage specific development in the thymus occurs. Only naïve T cells, intermediately recognizing the Major Histocompatibility Complex (MHC)-self-peptide and expressing CD4 or CD8, are allowed to migrate to their target organ (Singer, Adoro et al. 2008). CD4+ T cells form a subset of T cells called T helper (Th) cells and these cell types help to activate the B cells and CD8+ T cells. Th cells need binding of CD4 and CD28 to become activated Th cells and dependent on a specific set of cytokines, CD4+ T cells mature into different kinds of effector T cells, memory T cells or regulatory T (Treg) cells [*Box 2*]. Many factors are important for the development of both B and T cells, IL7 is of uttermost importance for both lymphocyte lineages (Kang, Der, et al. 2004). Recently it was shown that IL7 helps establish B cells, producing IgM, in the marginal zone of the spleen (Willems, Li, et al. 2011). Directly after birth maternal IL7 increases T cell production in the thymus and supports survival of T cells in other lymphoid structures in offspring, underlines the importance of IL7 during lymphogenesis (Aspinall, Prentice, et al. 2011).

The thymus is critically sensitive to malnutrition, with protein nutrition deficiency causing atrophy of the thymus (Savino and Dardenne 2010). This suggests that the thymus is a putative target for early-life programming effects. Most immune defence mechanisms are impaired in malnutrition, even in moderate nutritional deficiency. Protein-energy malnutrition is accompanied by deficiencies of micronutrients such as vitamin A, vitamin E, vitamin B6, vitamin C, folate, zinc, iron, copper, and selenium. Rapid proliferating T cells are especially affected by the lack of essential nutrients. Severe and chronic malnutrition may even lead to thymus atrophy affecting the basis of our immune system. The potential of adding certain nutrients, like vitamin C, D, or E, at levels above recommended dietary allowances (RDA) to the diet may improve immune function, is subject to increasing research.

Naïve CD4+ T cells are activated upon encountering an antigen presenting cell expressing MHC class II and the co-stimulatory signal CD28. They mature into effector, memory- of Treg dependent on which cytokines are produced by their APC. Already in 1986 two subsets were discovered by Mosmann and Cofmann (Zhu and Paul 2008) and now many more are well characterized. For Th1 Tbet and Signal transducer and Activator of transcription (Stat)1 are the initiating transcription factors , producing IFNγ, then Stat4 is amplifying the Th1 response. Th2 differentiation is activated by IL4, which induces Stat6. Stat6 in turn will activate the transcription factor Gata3. For Th17 RORγt is crucial, it is induced by transforming growth factor (TGF) β with IL6, then Stat3 and IRF4 are expressed. The transcription factors Foxp3 and Stat5 are needed, but without RA Tregs aren't formed. After the infection is cleared most cells die by apoptosis and some cells become memory cells to establish a faster response upon another infection (Zhu and Paul 2008; Zhu, Yamane et al. 2011).

Box 2.

The B cell lineage develops from HSC at the same sites as T cell development occurs. A major difference in lymphocyte development is that B cell development starts earlier, already in the pre-aorta gonad mesonephros region, which is also the most potent site for B cell development in the fetus (Dorshkind and Montecino-Rodriguez 2007). The HSC that migrate into the bone marrow are post natal responsible for B cell production. When B cells are activated they start to produce immunoglobulins, soluble and cell surface products to neutralize pathogens. Follicular B2 cells respond to microbial infections, they will present processed bacterial peptide to their CD4+ T cell partner. Because of this interaction B cells will undergo isotype switching and mature into plasma cells secreting antibodies to clear the infection. Some of these mature cells become memory B cells in peripheral lymphoid organs. Marginal B cells respond to bacterial polysaccharides without T cell stimulation. Recently it has been found that regulatory B cells can negatively influence the immune response via IL10 and transforming growth factor (TGF)β secretion (Vaughan, Roghanian et al. 2010). There are T cell independent B cell activators as mentioned above, but there is also T cell dependent B cell activation. Th1 type of CD4+ T cells are capable of helping B cells redirect to IgG2a in mice and IgG2 in humans. Th2 type of environment can induce switching towards IgE and IgG1 in mice and IgE and IgG4 in humans. At first the B cells will start with producing IgM and IgD. Upon stimulation they can switch towards an IgA,

IgE or IgG, depending on their surroundings and seem to be influenced by dietary components as discussed later. Neonatal B cells are capable of switching to IgG1 and IgG3 during the first 2 years of life, but the switch to IgG2 and IgG3 is inadequate during this period. To compensate the lack of protection in fetus and newborn, microbe-specific maternal IgG antibodies move across the placental barrier to provide some vital protection. During the last trimester of pregnancy IgGs are transferred intrauterine to the infant, because new-borns memory T cells capable of generating IgG and isotype switching aren't present yet. IgG1 and IgG4 are most effectively transported across the placenta compared to IgG3 and IgG2. Transfer of maternal antigen-specific IgG regulates the development of allergic airway inflammation early in life in a neonatal Fc region (FcRn)-dependent manner (Nakata, Kobayashi et al. 2010). This active transfer of IgGs from mother to child starts at week 17 and continues until birth. Moreover, just before birth, IgG levels of prenatal infants are even higher than levels present in the mother. The transfer and amount of pathogen specific IgGs is dependent on vaccinations and diseases the mother acquired during life. Many factors influence the IgG transportation processes which are described in a review by (Chucri, Monteiro et al. 2010). IgA IgD, IgM are the only known antibodies acquired after birth via breast feeding, covering the lack time during increasing antibody productions of infant's immune system itself. When the infant can produce the different B-cell antibodies, the activation, isotype switching and survival of B cells is for example under influence of B - cell activating factor (BAFF), TGFß1, IL-6, -7 and -10 produced by PP stromal cells (Finke, 2009). Not much is known about the involvement of Ig free light chains (IgfLC) in humoral immune response early in life. However the release of antigen specific IgfLC by B-cells/plasma cells like for example IgE may have implications for the health status of the newborn (Redegeld Nat Med 2003, Schouten JACI 2010). Furthermore compromised immune status may result in enhanced production and secretion of IgfLC at the cost of other immunoglobulins (van Esch CEA 2010).

Whereas T and B cell lineage experienced an in dept research into their origin, the origin and differentiation of dendritic cells (DC) is in its initial phase. One problem is to define specific precursor DC types (Liu and Nussenzweig 2010). Microbial exposure is one of the key developing factors for DCs (Plantinga, van Maren et al. 2011). The lamina propria (LP) contains mostly fractalkine positive DCs which sample the gut lumen with protrusions across the epithelial barrier, and are able to induce a Th17 response. Furthermore, in addition to the non-migrating DC population in PP there is a majority of DCs which will migrate to specific sites after encountering an antigen. For example the intestinal LP derived CD103+ DC subtype will migrate towards the MLN and is known for its capability to elicit a regulatory response, in the presence of RA and TGFβ. However if other factors are present a Th1 of a Th2 response can be induced. The activated T cell in the MLNs will migrate to the site of inflammation for instance in the intestine to initiate a proper immune response (*Figure* 4). Intestinal development is already influenced during pregnancy by the amniotic fluid as intestinal epithelial cells of the fetus can react to components in the amniotic fluid by different receptor expression (Drozdowski, Clandinin et al. 2010). So during gestation the gut can readily react to its micro-environment, but still much is unknown about the influence of maternal status on infantile gut development.

An increasing number of studies have identified interesting links between early nutrition, epigenetic processes and disease development later life (Boehm and Moro 2008). As the plasticity of growing and developing tissues shapes, the base of the responses to later

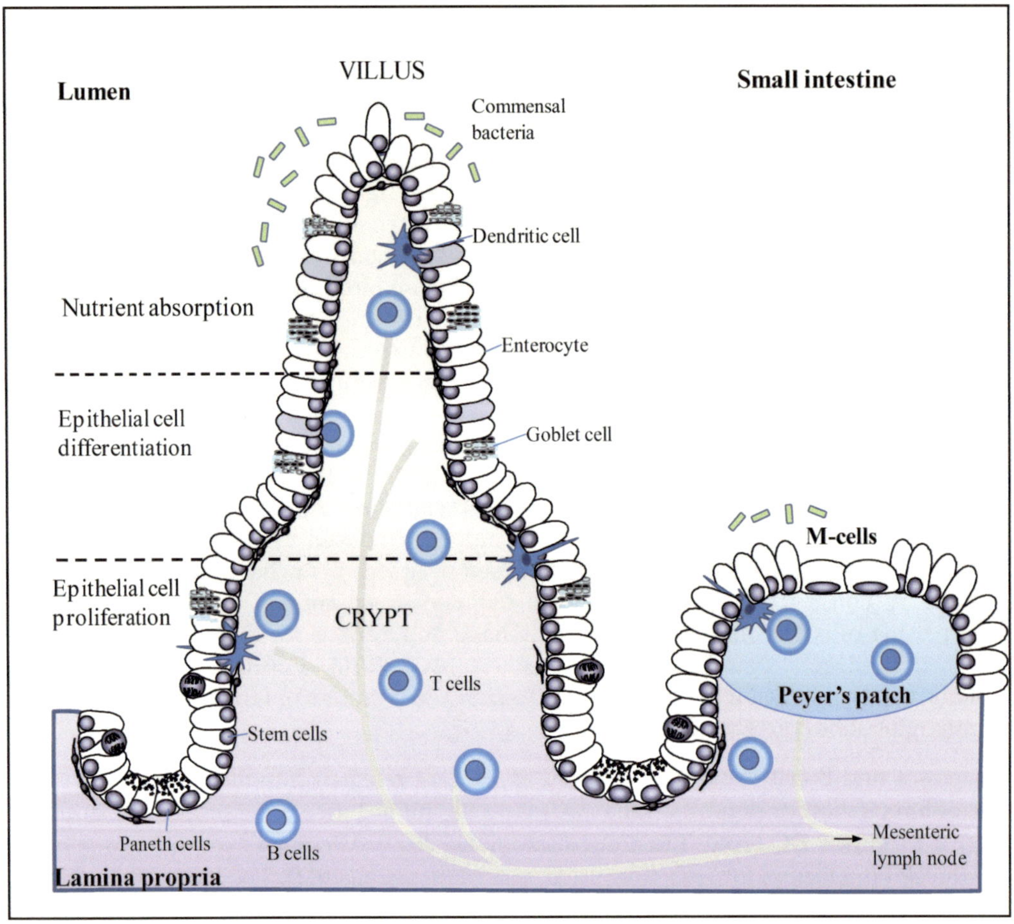

Fig. 4. Intestinal structure and development is already influenced during pregnancy and reacts to its micro-environment. The complex structure includes a variety of cross talk between different cells including epithelial cells, dendritic cells and lymphocytes. The lamina propria contains mostly dendritic cells which sample the lumen with protrusions across the epithelial barrier; in addition, the CD103+ DC subtype will migrate towards the mesenteric lymph nodes (MLN), after which the activated T cell in the MLNs will migrate back to the site of inflammation to initiate a proper immune response.

challenges is established, therefore the exposures during early life may be critical. Folate deficiency during pregnancy is associated with increased risk for aberrant reprogramming of DNA methylation inducing neural tube defects. Dietary folate intake can restore these deficiencies and neural tube defects. Folate is however not the only determinant of DNA methylation. Other methyl donor nutrients like betaine, vitamins B2, B6 and B12, and methionine, and choline, can also change DNA methylation status and therefore have an impact on development early in life (Niculescu and Lupu 2010).

3. Postnatal immune development in the gut

After birth a newborn changes from a sterile environment of the uterus into a world of constant challenges. In the first months of life newborns are more dependent on their innate immunity and immunoglobulins derived from the mother as described before. IgG is already acquired intrauterine but IgM and IgA are ingested via human milk to have an early defence against pathogens. Triggering the innate immunity repeatedly to microbial challenges after birth helps establishing a normal Th1 response postnatal. But the immune response is still less adequate compared to the adult response, possibly due to a general lower number of immune cells present. To build up an effective and balanced immune system interaction with germs and bacteria is needed (van't Land, Schijf et al. 2011). It is important that the immune balance is restored properly because a deregulation early in life could trigger an adverse reaction leading to an allergic reaction. The gut is the main processing site of food and, here immune tolerance against new food particles is established. But an improper chemical barrier and weak mucosal barrier integrity will complicate acquiring immune tolerance. There are some factors positively influencing development of the gut and immune system during pregnancy and after birth, of which only few of them will be discussed in detail below.

3.1 Influence of vitamins during and after pregnancy

Vitamin A has been recognized for its importance in lymphoid structure formation during embryogenesis. Sources of vitamin A are carrots, liver, sweet potatoes and butter. For example vitamin A supplementation before, during and after pregnancy using restricted dosages, results in long term positive effects on lung function which could be measured nine to thirteen years later.(Checkley, West et al. 2010). Shortly after the recognition of vitamin A essence during pregnancy, the teratogenic effect of excess vitamin A was shown. Malformations of the central nervous system, the eye and the thymus were found due to excessive use of vitamin A (Gutierrez-Mazariegos, Theodosiou et al. 2011). The teratogenic danger of vitamin A can also be induced via extra prolonged ingestion of this vitamin because it is stored in fat cells in the liver. It was already mentioned that RA could increase the progression from HSC into myeloid cell lineage. When RA is lacking from the diet CD4+ and CD8+ T cells and IgA+ B cells aren't found in the LP of the intestine, whereas CD4+ T cells were still present in lung tissue (Iwata 2009). Recently it was shown that stromal cells and DCs in the MLN induce high levels of RALDH expression postnatally, dependent on vitamin A and not on toll like receptor (TLR) signalling (Molenaar, Knippenberg et al. 2011). They compared MLN with other lymph nodes at different postnatal weeks and found an increased expression of RALDH only in the MLN residing DC, almost exclusively in CD103+ MHC-II+ CD11c+ DC cells. Vitamin A deficiency reduces this RALDH expression significantly. In addition, RA skews DC towards tolerance induction via instruction of Foxp3 Treg in the mother during pregnancy and in the infant just after birth (Coombes, Siddiqui et al. 2007; Duriancik, Lackey et al. 2010). Also vitamin A is necessary for the intestinal homing properties of activated T cells, Treg and certain B cells. *In vitro* it was shown that naïve CD4+ cells induce gut homing receptors when they are activated by CD3 and CD28 together with RA, this combination simultaneously down regulates skin homing receptors (Iwata 2009). In *vitro* DC from the gut associated lymphoid tissue could also induce activated IgA secreting B cells more effectively when RA was present in the medium, however the intracellular mechanism needs to be determined (Mora and von Andrian 2009). Not only RA is important for IgA secreting B cells, IL5 is essential for IgA production and TGFβ increases IgA secretion *in vitro*. There is also a positive feedback loop, IL6 stimulates IgA induction by DC and IL6 is induced by RA. Synergistic effect on IgA induction could be obtained by the aforementioned cytokines and therefore immune protection of the infant could be achieved (Mora and von Andrian 2009; Duriancik, Lackey et al. 2010). This indicates that also during early infancy the level of vitamin A is of importance for proper immune functioning, which may have profound consequences later in life.

An additional vitamin of interest for immune development is vitamin D. Worldwide there is no consensus on the healthy levels of vitamin D intake before and during pregnancy. Already during the first trimester of pregnancy vitamin D could be of importance for the development of the fetus. The 25-hydroxy vitamin D-1α-hydrolase CYP27B1), which converts vitamin D into its more active metabolite 1,25 $(OH)_2D$, can be detected in the placenta. There is some speculation about vitamin D deficiency and reduced fertility, this fertility problem may be caused by a reduced down regulation of the Th1 response by high levels of vitamin D as well as circumstantial evidence pointing at a relation between gestational diabetes and preeclampsia in correlation to circulating vitamin D levels (Dror and Allen 2010). In addition, vitamin D is important for the clearance of certain infections (Hoyer-Hansen, Nordbrandt et al. 2010).

Vitamin D is linked to monocyte activation via activation of TLR2 and TLR1(Lagishetty, Liu et al. 2011). Recently it was shown that IL4 and IFNγ are involved in the regulation of vitamin D expression (Edfeldt, Liu et al. 2010). IL4 promotes expression of CYP24A1, which down regulates active vitamin D, and IFNγ positively influences the expression of CYP24B1 in monocytes. Then it is suggested that vitamin D could skew the balance between Th1 and Th2 towards a Th2 phenotype directly or indirectly via monocyte activation, which however may be much more complex *in vivo* (Adams and Hewison 2008). Low vitamin D levels during pregnancy are suggested to be related in the development of food allergy (Nwaru, Ahonen et al. 2010). It was recently shown that active vitamin D can suppress DC maturation and inhibit T cell proliferation. Mature DC have high levels of vitamin D converting enzymes, suggesting that upon Vitamin D addition, mature DC can inhibit the development of immature DC. Suppression of DC maturation could then via vitamin D promote tolerance. Research with vitamin D receptor (VDR) and CYP27B1 knockout mice showed abnormal lymph node development due to the presence of more mature DC and increased DC trafficking (Hewison 2011).

There is still debate about the healthy amount of vitamin D intake during pregnancy (West, Videky et al. 2010). Indeed some studies show that vitamin D intake is associated with diminished wheeze, asthma and eczema in offspring (West, Videky et al. 2010). For vitamin D it is clear that lymphocytes are influenced, but to what extent this affects function later in life remains to be established. Increasing evidence from observational studies in infants at older ages, indicate that vitamin D insufficiency and deficiency might increase the risk of chronic diseases such as type 1 diabetes and multiple sclerosis. However, clear randomized trials on this association need to be conducted to confirm these findings. In the last decades, observations accumulate that vitamin D deficiency leads to more often and more serious respiratory infections than in individuals with sufficient vitamin D plasma levels. This illustrates the importance of the nutritional status early in life, to set the proper immune balance (Karatekin, Kaya et al. 2009).

3.2 Human milk

It is well established that breastfeeding reduces the incidence of gastrointestinal and non-enteric infections in infants, due to its antimicrobial activity against several viruses, bacteria, and protozoa (Chirico, Marzollo et al. 2008). In addition, it was shown that infants, breastfed for more than 4 months experienced significant reduced incidences of respiratory tract infection requiring hospitalization, as compared to infants who were not breastfed (Bachrach, Schwarz et al. 2003). Moreover, other studies showed that breastfeeding provides protection against urinary tract infections and otitis media and it reduces the development of inflammatory conditions like allergy (Fiocchi, Martelli et al. 2003), Crohn's disease and ulcerative colitis (Hanson 2007). This, moreover, emphasizes the diversity of activity and active components present in human breast milk. Although it is clear that allergy development is influenced by breast milk as well as atopy related disorders, still some controversy exists regarding the beneficial length of breastfeeding (van Odijk, Kull et al. 2003). These protective effects of human breast milk seem to persist at least during the first decade of life.

Fortunately prenatally the infant is supplied with maternal immunoglobulins, for the first protection against infections. It takes at least one year before an infant can produce about 60% of its IgG levels on its own. After birth the child can be supplied with essential IgG, IgM and IgA via human milk. For example, IgA is necessary as the first line of defence against microorganisms. This immunoglobulin also controls commensal (also called beneficial) bacteria all without activation of an inflammatory response. Because infants do not have an optimized Treg response and no memory cells, B cells cannot be directed to produce the right amount of Ig antibodies quickly as a first defence. IgM helps to eliminate the pathogen before IgGs are produced. As earlier mentioned IgM is normally produced by naive B cells before isotype switching occurs. The B cell response needs time after birth to be fully functional, so acquiring this component via human milk strengthens the first line of defence. Not only antibodies are factors present in human milk, other immune modulating components are present, including cytokines, non digestible oligosaccharides and poly unsaturated fatty acids (PUFA), which are discussed in more detail below.

3.3 Cytokines

TGFβ and IL10 are held responsible for the induction of oral tolerance in the intestine (du Pre and Samsom 2010). They educate the immune system locally not to respond to harmless antigens. In human milk TGFβ2 is the predominant isoform of the three existing mammalian isoforms. Addition of TGFβ2 to infant formula, can skew the Th2 allergic effector response towards Th1 in rat pups exposed to β-lactoglobulin, a cow's milk allergy protein (Penttila 2009). Not TGFβ2 but TGFβ1 is the major player to establish immune tolerance to food in the adult system. To guarantee the uptake of TGFβ, TGFβ receptors are abundantly expressed in the neonatal intestine, even the soluble TGFβ2 receptor is present in breast milk. But in addition it was found that TGFβ is not essential for tolerance induction when milk born-IgG antigen immune complexes are present (Verhasselt, Milcent et al. 2008). Moreover it is known that high levels of TGFβ together with RA skew the immune system towards a regulatory suppressive function, a low dose of TGFβ combined with IL6 or IL21 or IL23 will result in inflammatory Th17 activation instead of Treg upregulation (Konkel and Chen 2011). Recently Hering et al (2009) showed that *in vitro* TGFβ probably helps forming the intestinal epithelial barrier via exerting its effect on the reinforcement between the epithelial cells (van't Land, Meijer et al. 2002; Hering and Schulzke 2009). The production of IgA is also positively influenced by TGFβ (Cazac and Roes 2000; Borsutzky, Cazac et al. 2004). This indicates that the immune modulating components have their function alone, but this needs to be further investigated in combination.

3.4 Nondigestible oligosaccharides

There are different types of soluble dietary fibres e.g. (hemi)cellulose, lignin, β-glucans, pectins, gums, inulin and oligofructose. In addition different non-digestible oligosaccharides with specific properties are obtained or manufactured from natural sources (Calder, Krauss-Etschmann et al. 2006). Human milk contains approximately 7-12 g/L oligosaccharides (Hoppu, Kalliomaki et al. 2001). At least 130 different oligosaccharides have been isolated from human milk and the two main categories are neutral and acidic oligosaccharides (Lara-Villoslada, Olivares et al. 2007; Greer, Sicherer et al. 2008). These oligosaccharides are non-digestible carbohydrates that have many different properties and are believed to act on the microbiota in the gut (Host, Koletzko et al. 1999; Halken, Hansen et al. 2000; Hill, Murch et al. 2007; Niggemann and Beyer 2007). Due to physicochemical properties of non-digestible carbohydrates the absorption of minerals and fecal consistency improves. Some of these have specific properties and can be used as prebiotics as a dietary supplement. Prebiotics are defined as "a selectively fermented ingredient that allows specific changes, both in the composition and/or activity in the gastrointestinal microflora that confers benefits upon host wellbeing and health" (Host and Halken 2004). Prebiotics enhance defense mechanisms of the host by stimulation of growth of Bifidobacteria and Lactobacilli. As the intestinal microbiota plays a critical role in the establishment and maintenance of healthy immune responses, the delayed colonisation of the infant gut with commensal bacteria are suggested to be a risk factor for the development of immune mediated chronic disorders such as allergic and autoimmune diseases. Short-chain fatty acids, released by these bacteria upon fermentation of prebiotics, are essential nutrients for intestinal epithelial cells and support gut function (Gibson and Roberfroid 1995; Nakhla, Fu et al. 1999; Boehm and Stahl 2007). *In vivo* and *in vitro* studies have shown beneficial effects of prebiotics on the innate as well as the adaptive immune system (Boehm, Fanaro et al. 2003). Short-chain galacto-oligosaccharides (scGOS), long-chain fructo-oligosaccharides (lcFOS) and pectin-derived acidic oligosaccharides (pAOS) are some examples of non-digestible oligosaccharides that mimic the functionality and molecular size distribution of human milk oligosaccharides.

The effects of scGOS and lcFOS (9:1)(Immunofortis®) have been studied in a murine vaccination model (Vos, Haarman et al. 2006), in an allergic asthma model (Vos, van Esch et al. 2007) and a cow's milk allergy model (Schouten, van Esch et al. 2009). The response to vaccination of mice fed the scGOS/lcFOS diet was significant enhanced, as well as the fecal Bifidobacteria and Lactobacilli proportions. pAOS enhanced the murine vaccination response and the combination (scGOS/lcFOS/pAOS) was even more effective (Vos, Haarman et al. 2007). To stimulate the entire microbiota a great variation in the oligosaccharide structures will exert this effect, as human milk oligosaccharides comprise of many different oligosaccharides. The pAOS are not only another group of oligosaccharides, they act very specifically to their acidity. Based on this they are able to interact with surfaces and might prevent the adhesion of pathogens on the intestinal epithelium. In infants pAOS showed no difference in stool characteristics, pH, growth, crying, vomiting and regurgitation patterns as compared to control formula. In addition pAOS alone did not affect intestinal microecology (Fanaro, Jelinek et al. 2005). Furthermore, systemic Th1 dependent immune responses were enhanced using the prebiotics without inducing autoimmunity, as Th1 is low in newborn infants. In addition, in a murine model for cow's milk allergy dietary intervention with scGOS/lcFOS showed significant decrease of the allergic response and increased specific IgG2a levels (Meyer 2004; Schouten, van Esch et al. 2009).

Recently it was found in mice that dietary intervention with scGOS/lcFOS/pAOS reduces the development of an acute allergic response upon antigen challenge, although specific immunoglobulins levels remain high. *Ex vivo* depletion of $CD25^+$ Treg abrogated the diminished acute allergic response, combined with adoptive transfer studies, imply crucial involvement of antigen specific $CD25^+$ Treg cells in the suppression of the allergic effector response (Schouten, van Esch et al. 2010; van't Land, Schijf et al. 2010; Schouten, van Esch et al. 2011). Furthermore, clinical trials have been performed with the scGOS/lcFOS mixture in children at high risk for allergies. A reduction in the incidence of atopic dermatitis (AD) (Moro, Arslanoglu et al. 2006) and the incidence of allergic manifestations during the first 6 months of life (Arslanoglu, Moro et al. 2007) was observed, furthermore this reduction lasted at least until 2 years of age (Arslanoglu, Moro et al. 2008).

Recently, it was also shown, in a multicenter trial, that the scGOS/lcFOS/pAOS mixture could reduce the incidence of AD in healthy not at risk children (Gruber, van Stuijvenberg et al.). In another clinical study, using the scGOS/lcFOS mixture, fecal secretory IgA was increased in healthy infants (Bakker-Zierikzee, Tol et al. 2006). Also in healthy infants there is cumulative evidence that prebiotic mixtures might beneficially affect the host in both Th1 as well as Th2 prone settings as it might prevent food allergy (Th2) and enhances the vaccination response (Th1). Although it is believed that prebiotics exert their effect via stimulation of growth of selective bacterial species that beneficially improve host health, there is debate about this mechanism and there are potentially microbiota-independent mechanisms as well (Boehm, Fanaro et al. 2003; Vos, M'Rabet et al. 2007). As it was shown that epithelial cells can transport scGOS, lcFOS and pAOS across from apical to the basolateral side (Eiwegger, Stahl et al. 2010), this illustrates that besides a prebiotic immune modulating effect the oligosaccharides also come in direct contact with immune cells themselves, making it possible to act directly on the immune cells.

3.5 Poly unsaturated fatty acids

Omega-3 and omega-6 poly unsaturated fatty acids (PUFA) are essential for humans and have to be provided via the diet especially found in seafood. PUFA are incorporated into the cellular membrane and are eicosanoid precursors hereby affecting the immune response. In this regard in particular n-3 long chain (LC)-PUFA eicosapentaenoic acid (EPA) and docosahexaenoic acid (DHA) are regarded to be anti-inflammatory while n-6 LCPUFA, like linoleic and arachidonic acid, are able to boost inflammatory responses. Arachidonic acid, for example can be converted into 2 series prostaglandins, these are able to increase IL4 and decrease IFNγ, and 4 series of leukotrines, which are able to induce endothelial permeability and production of inflammatory cytokines (Moreno 2009).

In westernized countries the n-3 fatty acid ingestion is no longer favoured over n-6 PUFA which may have implications for immune homeostasis. It has been stated that the original diet of the human race had an n-6 : n-3 ratio of approximately 1:1 and that this has changed over the past decades to a ratio of at least 15:1 (Simopoulos 2008). This shift is suggested to be explanatory for the increased incidence of cardiovascular diseases, chronic inflammatory diseases, obesity and also allergic diseases. Therefore pre-clinical as well as clinical trials are performed in order to investigate this hypothesis. It has been reviewed that n-3 LCPUFA intake reduces the incidence of allergic disorders, e.g. AD, less sensitization to egg in the clinical trials (Blumer, Pfefferle et al. 2007). Two studies by Dunstan *et al.* show reduced sensitization to egg and less AD in offspring when pregnant woman were supplemented with fish oil, which contains EPA and DHA (Dunstan, Mori et al. 2003; Dunstan, Roper et al. 2004). They found a positive influence of n-3 LCPUFA on TGFβ mRNA levels in maternal peripheral blood and cord blood. This could imply a regulatory function of n-3 LCPUFA, but mRNA still needs to be processed towards an active component. Recently, it was shown that maternal n-3 LCPUFA intake decreased the risk of food allergy and IgE-associated eczema in children at risk for allergy (Furuhjelm, Warstedt et al. 2009). This shift in the decrease of allergy can be explained since n-3 LCPUFA is incorporated in the membrane of immune cells at the cost of n-6 LCPUFA as arachidonic acid, skewing towards a less inflammatory cytokine surrounding. In contrast, in a clinical study by Almqvist et al., (Almqvist, Garden et al. 2007) it is shown that supplementation of n-3 PUFA, starting at a maximum of six months of age, did not prevent children with a family history of asthma from developing atopy, eczema nor asthma at the age of 5 years. Hence discrepancy on effects of n-3 PUFA in prevention of allergic disease exists. There are also discrepancies between studies in the preparation of fish oil, influencing EPA and DHA content (Prescott and Calder 2004). Of concern is the dosage in human studies, this is often much lower than used in animal studies, which makes it difficult to extrapolate the outcome and could explain differences observed. However interventions using dietary factors like LCPUFAs are under-explored and that there is a need for additional research. One of the strategies that are proposed is the use of selected LCPUFA in the formula feeding of young children at high risk for allergies (Vanderhoof 2008). Another strategy could be to supplement a novel LCPUFA during pregnancy; LCPUFA maybe has its largest positive effect on an infant health status when primary immune responses are still developing. In addition novel synthetic LCPUFA may reveal to be potent in the reduction of the allergic burden (Prescott and Calder 2004).

4. Consequences later in life conclusion

During the different phases of life, several nutritional factors influence our immune system and immune responsiveness in collaboration with endogenous immune modulating mediators like humoral factors, lipids and oligosaccharides. A vast amount of literature is available on the role that nutrients and human milk (as reviewed in this article), have on the development of the immune system; a lot less is known about the exact requirements in the phases thereafter, in toddlers, during adolescence, and in the later stages of life. Moreover, as no single biomarker exists able to determine a proper functioning immune system, it is almost impossible to describe completely the developmental status of the immune system and the important influences of nutrition. Although it is clear that each phase in life puts specific requirements on nutrition, no clear statement can be made based on literature as to what the exact dietary requirements are in order to fully support the immune system during these stages in life. But food as a beneficial dietary component is currently under very active scientific investigation, so more information about nutrition will be available soon.

5. References

Adams, J. S. and M. Hewison (2008). "Unexpected actions of vitamin D: new perspectives on the regulation of innate and adaptive immunity." *Nat Clin Pract Endocrinol Metab* 4(2): 80-90.

Almqvist, C., F. Garden, et al. (2007). "Omega-3 and omega-6 fatty acid exposure from early life does not affect atopy and asthma at age 5 years." *J Allergy Clin Immunol* 119(6): 1438-44.

Arslanoglu, S., G. E. Moro, et al. (2007). "Early supplementation of prebiotic oligosaccharides protects formula-fed infants against infections during the first 6 months of life." *J Nutr* 137(11): 2420-4.

Arslanoglu, S., G. E. Moro, et al. (2008). "Early dietary intervention with a mixture of prebiotic oligosaccharides reduces the incidence of allergic manifestations and infections during the first two years of life." *J Nutr* 138(6): 1091-5.

Aspinall, R., Prentice, A.M., Ngom, P.T. Interleukin 7 from maternel milk crosses the intestinal barrier and modulates T-cell development in offspring. PloS One, 2011;6(6) e20812

Bachrach, V. R., E. Schwarz, et al. (2003). "Breastfeeding and the risk of hospitalization for respiratory disease in infancy: a meta-analysis." *Arch Pediatr Adolesc Med* 157(3): 237-43.

Bakker-Zierikzee, A. M., E. A. Tol, et al. (2006). "Faecal SIgA secretion in infants fed on pre- or probiotic infant formula." *Pediatr Allergy Immunol* 17(2): 134-40.

Blumer, N., P. I. Pfefferle, et al. (2007). "Development of mucosal immune function in the intrauterine and early postnatal environment." *Curr Opin Gastroenterol* 23(6): 655-60.

Boehm, G., S. Fanaro, et al. (2003). "Prebiotic concept for infant nutrition." *Acta Paediatr Suppl* 91(441): 64-7.

Boehm, G. and G. Moro (2008). "Structural and functional aspects of prebiotics used in infant nutrition." *J Nutr* 138(9): 1818S-1828S.

Boehm, G. and B. Stahl (2007). "Oligosaccharides from milk." *J Nutr* 137(3 Suppl 2): 847S-9S.

Borsutzky, S., B. B. Cazac, et al. (2004). "TGF-beta receptor signaling is critical for mucosal IgA responses." *J Immunol* 173(5): 3305-9.

Calder, P. C., S. Krauss-Etschmann, et al. (2006). "Early nutrition and immunity - progress and perspectives." *Br J Nutr* 96(4): 774-90.

Campo-Paysaa, F., F. Marletaz, et al. (2008). "Retinoic acid signaling in development: tissue-specific functions and evolutionary origins." *Genesis* 46(11): 640-56.

Cazac, B. B. and J. Roes (2000). "TGF-beta receptor controls B cell responsiveness and induction of IgA in vivo." *Immunity* 13(4): 443-51.

Chappaz, S., C. Gartner, et al. (2010). "Kit ligand and Il7 differentially regulate Peyer's patch and lymph node development." *J Immunol* 185(6): 3514-9.

Checkley, W., K. P. West, Jr., et al. (2010). "Maternal vitamin A supplementation and lung function in offspring." *N Engl J Med* 362(19): 1784-94.

Chi, A. W., J. J. Bell, et al. (2009). "Untangling the T branch of the hematopoiesis tree." *Curr Opin Immunol* 21(2): 121-6.

Chirico, G., R. Marzollo, et al. (2008). "Antiinfective properties of human milk." *J Nutr* 138(9): 1801S-1806S.

Chucri, T. M., J. M. Monteiro, et al. (2010). "A review of immune transfer by the placenta." *J Reprod Immunol* 87(1-2): 14-20.

Coombes, J. L., K. R. Siddiqui, et al. (2007). "A functionally specialized population of mucosal CD103+ DCs induces Foxp3+ regulatory T cells via a TGF-beta and retinoic acid-dependent mechanism." *J Exp Med* 204(8): 1757-64.

Dorshkind, K. and E. Montecino-Rodriguez (2007). "Fetal B-cell lymphopoiesis and the emergence of B-1-cell potential." *Nat Rev Immunol* 7(3): 213-9.

Dror, D. K. and L. H. Allen (2010). "Vitamin D inadequacy in pregnancy: biology, outcomes, and interventions." *Nutr Rev* 68(8): 465-77.

Drozdowski, L. A., T. Clandinin, et al. (2010). "Ontogeny, growth and development of the small intestine: Understanding pediatric gastroenterology." *World J Gastroenterol* 16(7): 787-99.

du Pre, M. F. and J. N. Samsom (2010). "Adaptive T-cell responses regulating oral tolerance to protein antigen." *Allergy* 66(4): 478-90.

Dunstan, J. A., T. A. Mori, et al. (2003). "Fish oil supplementation in pregnancy modifies neonatal allergen-specific immune responses and clinical outcomes in infants at high risk of atopy: a randomized, controlled trial." *J Allergy Clin Immunol* 112(6): 1178-84.

Dunstan, J. A., J. Roper, et al. (2004). "The effect of supplementation with fish oil during pregnancy on breast milk immunoglobulin A, soluble CD14, cytokine levels and fatty acid composition." *Clin Exp Allergy* 34(8): 1237-42.

Duriancik, D. M., D. E. Lackey, et al. (2010). "Vitamin A as a regulator of antigen presenting cells." *J Nutr* 140(8): 1395-9.

Edfeldt, K., P. T. Liu, et al. (2010). "T-cell cytokines differentially control human monocyte antimicrobial responses by regulating vitamin D metabolism." *Proc Natl Acad Sci U S A* 107(52): 22593-8.

Eiwegger, T., B. Stahl, et al. (2010). "Prebiotic oligosaccharides: in vitro evidence for gastrointestinal epithelial transfer and immunomodulatory properties." *Pediatr Allergy Immunol* 21(8): 1179-88.

Fanaro, S., J. Jelinek, et al. (2005). "Acidic oligosaccharides from pectin hydrolysate as new component for infant formulae: effect on intestinal flora, stool characteristics, and pH." *J Pediatr Gastroenterol Nutr* 41(2): 186-90.

Finke, D. Induction of intestinal lymphoid tissue formation by intrinsic and extrinsic signals. Semi. Immunopathol. 2009, july; 31(2) 151-169

Fiocchi, A., A. Martelli, et al. (2003). "Primary dietary prevention of food allergy." *Ann Allergy Asthma Immunol* 91(1): 3-12; quiz 12-5, 91.

Furuhjelm, C., K. Warstedt, et al. (2009). "Fish oil supplementation in pregnancy and lactation may decrease the risk of infant allergy." *Acta Paediatr* 98(9): 1461-7.

Gibson, G. R. and M. B. Roberfroid (1995). "Dietary modulation of the human colonic microbiota: introducing the concept of prebiotics." *J Nutr* 125(6): 1401-12.

Grassinger, J., D. N. Haylock, et al. (2010). "Phenotypically identical hemopoietic stem cells isolated from different regions of bone marrow have different biologic potential." *Blood* 116(17): 3185-96.

Greer, F. R., S. H. Sicherer, et al. (2008). "Effects of early nutritional interventions on the development of atopic disease in infants and children: the role of maternal dietary restriction, breastfeeding, timing of introduction of complementary foods, and hydrolyzed formulas." *Pediatrics* 121(1): 183-91.

Gruber, C., M. van Stuijvenberg, et al. "Reduced occurrence of early atopic dermatitis because of immunoactive prebiotics among low-atopy-risk infants." *J Allergy Clin Immunol* 126(4): 791-7.

Gutierrez-Mazariegos, J., M. Theodosiou, et al. (2011). "Vitamin A: A multifunctional tool for development." *Semin Cell Dev Biol* 22(6): 603-10.

Halken, S., K. S. Hansen, et al. (2000). "Comparison of a partially hydrolyzed infant formula with two extensively hydrolyzed formulas for allergy prevention: a prospective, randomized study." *Pediatr Allergy Immunol* 11(3): 149-61.

Hanson, L. A. (2007). "Session 1: Feeding and infant development breast-feeding and immune function." *Proc Nutr Soc* 66(3): 384-96.

Hering, N. A. and J. D. Schulzke (2009). "Therapeutic options to modulate barrier defects in inflammatory bowel disease." *Dig Dis* 27(4): 450-4.

Hewison, M. (2011). "Vitamin D and innate and adaptive immunity." *Vitam Horm* 86: 23-62.

Hill, D. J., S. H. Murch, et al. (2007). "The efficacy of amino acid-based formulas in relieving the symptoms of cow's milk allergy: a systematic review." *Clin Exp Allergy* 37(6): 808-22.

Hoppu, U., M. Kalliomaki, et al. (2001). "Breast milk--immunomodulatory signals against allergic diseases." *Allergy* 56 Suppl 67: 23-6.

Host, A. and S. Halken (2004). "Hypoallergenic formulas--when, to whom and how long: after more than 15 years we know the right indication!" *Allergy* 59 Suppl 78: 45-52.

Host, A., B. Koletzko, et al. (1999). "Dietary products used in infants for treatment and prevention of food allergy. Joint Statement of the European Society for Paediatric Allergology and Clinical Immunology (ESPACI) Committee on Hypoallergenic Formulas and the European Society for Paediatric Gastroenterology, Hepatology and Nutrition (ESPGHAN) Committee on Nutrition." *Arch Dis Child* 81(1): 80-4.

Hoyer-Hansen, M., S. P. Nordbrandt, et al. (2010). "Autophagy as a basis for the health-promoting effects of vitamin D." *Trends Mol Med* 16(7): 295-302.

Iwata, M. (2009). "Retinoic acid production by intestinal dendritic cells and its role in T-cell trafficking." *Semin Immunol* 21(1): 8-13.

Kang, J., Der, S.D. Cytokine functions in the formative stages of a lymphocyte's life. Current opinion in Immunology, April 2004, Vol. 16, issue 2, 180-190

Karatekin, G., A. Kaya, et al. (2009). "Association of subclinical vitamin D deficiency in newborns with acute lower respiratory infection and their mothers." *Eur J Clin Nutr* 63(4): 473-7.

Konkel, J. E. and W. Chen (2011). "Balancing acts: the role of TGF-beta in the mucosal immune system." *Trends Mol Med* 17(11): 668-76.

Lagishetty, V., N. Q. Liu, et al. (2011). "Vitamin D metabolism and innate immunity." *Mol Cell Endocrinol* 347(1-2): 97-105.

Lara-Villoslada, F., M. Olivares, et al. (2007). "Beneficial effects of probiotic bacteria isolated from breast milk." *Br J Nutr* 98 Suppl 1: S96-100.

Liu, K. and M. C. Nussenzweig (2010). "Development and homeostasis of dendritic cells." *Eur J Immunol* 40(8): 2099-102.

Mazo, I. B., S. Massberg, et al. (2011). "Hematopoietic stem and progenitor cell trafficking." *Trends Immunol* 32(10): 493-503.

McDade, T. W., M. A. Beck, et al. (2001). "Prenatal undernutrition, postnatal environments, and antibody response to vaccination in adolescence." *Am J Clin Nutr* 74(4): 543-8.

Medvinsky, A., S. Rybtsov, et al. (2011). "Embryonic origin of the adult hematopoietic system: advances and questions." *Development* 138(6): 1017-31.

Meyer, P. D. (2004). "Nondigestible oligosaccharides as dietary fiber." *J AOAC Int* 87(3): 718-26.

Molenaar, R., M. Knippenberg, et al. (2011). "Expression of retinaldehyde dehydrogenase enzymes in mucosal dendritic cells and gut-draining lymph node stromal cells is controlled by dietary vitamin A." *J Immunol* 186(4): 1934-42.

Mora, J. R. and U. H. von Andrian (2009). "Role of retinoic acid in the imprinting of gut-homing IgA-secreting cells." *Semin Immunol* 21(1): 28-35.

Moreno, J. J. (2009). "Differential effects of arachidonic and eicosapentaenoic Acid-derived eicosanoids on polymorphonuclear transmigration across endothelial cell cultures." *J Pharmacol Exp Ther* 331(3): 1111-7.

Moro, G., S. Arslanoglu, et al. (2006). "A mixture of prebiotic oligosaccharides reduces the incidence of atopic dermatitis during the first six months of age." *Arch Dis Child* 91(10): 814-9.

Nakata, K., K. Kobayashi, et al. (2010). "The transfer of maternal antigen-specific IgG regulates the development of allergic airway inflammation early in life in an FcRn-dependent manner." *Biochem Biophys Res Commun* 395(2): 238-43.

Nakhla, T., D. Fu, et al. (1999). "Neutral oligosaccharide content of preterm human milk." *Br J Nutr* 82(5): 361-7.

Niculescu, M. D. and D. S. Lupu (2010). "Nutritional influence on epigenetics and effects on longevity." *Curr Opin Clin Nutr Metab Care* 14(1): 35-40.

Niggemann, B. and K. Beyer (2007). "Diagnosis of food allergy in children: toward a standardization of food challenge." *J Pediatr Gastroenterol Nutr* 45(4): 399-404.

Nwaru, B. I., S. Ahonen, et al. (2010). "Maternal diet during pregnancy and allergic sensitization in the offspring by 5 yrs of age: a prospective cohort study." *Pediatr Allergy Immunol* 21(1 Pt 1): 29-37.

Penttila, I. A. (2009). "Milk-derived transforming growth factor-beta and the infant immune response." *J Pediatr* 156(2 Suppl): S21-5.

Plantinga, T. S., W. W. van Maren, et al. (2011). "Differential Toll-like receptor recognition and induction of cytokine profile by Bifidobacterium breve and Lactobacillus strains of probiotics." *Clin Vaccine Immunol* 18(4): 621-8.

Prescott, S. L. and P. C. Calder (2004). "N-3 polyunsaturated fatty acids and allergic disease." *Curr Opin Clin Nutr Metab Care* 7(2): 123-9.

Savino, W. and M. Dardenne (2010). "Nutritional imbalances and infections affect the thymus: consequences on T-cell-mediated immune responses." *Proc Nutr Soc* 69(4): 636-43.

Schouten, B., B. C. van Esch, et al. (2010). "Oligosaccharide-induced whey-specific CD25(+) regulatory T-cells are involved in the suppression of cow milk allergy in mice." *J Nutr* 140(4): 835-41.

Schouten, B., B. C. van Esch, et al. (2011). "A potential role for CD25+ regulatory T-cells in the protection against casein allergy by dietary non-digestible carbohydrates." *Br J Nutr*: 1-10.

Schouten, B., B. C. van Esch, et al. (2009). "Cow milk allergy symptoms are reduced in mice fed dietary synbiotics during oral sensitization with whey." *J Nutr* 139(7): 1398-403.

Simopoulos, A. P. (2008). "The importance of the omega-6/omega-3 fatty acid ratio in cardiovascular disease and other chronic diseases." *Exp Biol Med (Maywood)* 233(6): 674-88.

Singer, A., S. Adoro, et al. (2008). "Lineage fate and intense debate: myths, models and mechanisms of CD4- versus CD8-lineage choice." *Nat Rev Immunol* 8(10): 788-801.

van't Land, B., H. P. Meijer, et al. (2002). "Transforming Growth Factor-beta2 protects the small intestine during methotrexate treatment in rats possibly by reducing stem cell cycling." *Br J Cancer* 87(1): 113-8.

van't Land, B., M. Schijf, et al. (2010). "Regulatory T-cells have a prominent role in the immune modulated vaccine response by specific oligosaccharides." *Vaccine* 28(35): 5711-7.

van't Land, B., M. A. Schijf, et al. (2011). "Influencing mucosal homeostasis and immune responsiveness: The impact of nutrition and pharmaceuticals." *Eur J Pharmacol* 668 Suppl 1: S101-7.

van de Pavert, S. A. and R. E. Mebius (2010). "New insights into the development of lymphoid tissues." *Nat Rev Immunol* 10(9): 664-74.

van Odijk, J., I. Kull, et al. (2003). "Breastfeeding and allergic disease: a multidisciplinary review of the literature (1966-2001) on the mode of early feeding in infancy and its impact on later atopic manifestations." *Allergy* 58(9): 833-43.

Vanderhoof, J. A. (2008). "Hypoallergenicity and effects on growth and tolerance of a new amino acid-based formula with DHA and ARA." *J Pediatr Gastroenterol Nutr* 47 Suppl 2: S60-1.

Vaughan, A. T., A. Roghanian, et al. (2010). "B cells--masters of the immunoverse." *Int J Biochem Cell Biol* 43(3): 280-5.

Verhasselt, V., V. Milcent, et al. (2008). "Breast milk-mediated transfer of an antigen induces tolerance and protection from allergic asthma." *Nat Med* 14(2): 170-5.

Vos, A. P., M. Haarman, et al. (2006). "A specific prebiotic oligosaccharide mixture stimulates delayed-type hypersensitivity in a murine influenza vaccination model." *Int Immunopharmacol* 6(8): 1277-86.

Vos, A. P., M. Haarman, et al. (2007). "Dietary supplementation of neutral and acidic oligosaccharides enhances Th1-dependent vaccination responses in mice." *Pediatr Allergy Immunol* 18(4): 304-12.

Vos, A. P., L. M'Rabet, et al. (2007). "Immune-modulatory effects and potential working mechanisms of orally applied nondigestible carbohydrates." *Crit Rev Immunol* 27(2): 97-140.

Vos, A. P., B. C. van Esch, et al. (2007). "Dietary supplementation with specific oligosaccharide mixtures decreases parameters of allergic asthma in mice." *Int Immunopharmacol* 7(12): 1582-7.

West, C. E., D. J. Videky, et al. (2010). "Role of diet in the development of immune tolerance in the context of allergic disease." *Curr Opin Pediatr* 22(5): 635-41.

Willems, L., Li, S., Rutgeerts, O., Lenaerts, C., Waer, M., Billiau, A.D. IL-7 is required for the development of the intrinsic function of marginal zone B cells and the marginal zone microenvirnment. J. Immunol., October 2011; 187 (7); 3587-3594

Zhu, J. and W. E. Paul (2008). "CD4 T cells: fates, functions, and faults." *Blood* 112(5): 1557-69.

Zhu, J., H. Yamane, et al. (2011). "Differentiation of effector CD4 T cell populations (*)." *Annu Rev Immunol* 28: 445-89.

14

Immune System and Environmental Xenobiotics - The Effect of Selected Mineral Fibers and Particles on the Immune Response

Miroslava Kuricova et al.*
Slovak Medical University, Bratislava
Slovak Republic

1. Introduction

Mineral fibers and particles are finding growing applications in industry and thus entering into the human environment. The utility of using such products for various purposes is promising but detailed information related to immune safety is needed. Immunotoxic effects may be displayed as immunosuppression, immunostimulation, hypersensitivity and autoimmunity. Humans may be exposed to fibers and particles from a variety of sources, including occupational settings, ambient air, consumer products, drinking water and food. This chapter is dedicated to the effect of inhalation exposure to asbestos, rock wool, glass wool, ceramic fibers and nickel oxide particles on the immune system.

Findings of *in vitro* studies, *in vivo* animal experiments and molecular epidemiological studies conducted during the period of several years are summarized. *In vitro* studies comprised studies on alveolar macrophages and alveolar epithelial type II cells. Refractory ceramic fibers, asbestos and stone wool fibers were tested *in vitro*. *In vivo* testing involved both inhalation and intratracheal instillation studies using amosite, wollastonite, rock wool and glass fibers. Moreover, three population based studies in workers occupationally exposed to asbestos, rock wool and glass fibers were performed.

Finally, options and pitfalls to the use of immune assays as sensitive biomarkers of possible immunotoxic effects are discussed. Since, in human studies, specimens from living people used to examine the effects of particles and fibers on the immune response are typically limited to minimally invasive (whole blood, plasma or serum by venipuncture, sputum) or moderately invasive techniques (bronchoalveolar lavage or nasal lavage), human blood

* Jana Tulinska[1], Aurelia Liskova[1], Mira Horvathova[1], Silvia Ilavska[1], Zuzana Kovacikova[1], Elizabeth Tatrai[2], Marta Hurbankova[1], Silvia Cerna[1], Eva Jahnova[1], Eva Neubauerova[1], Ladislava Wsolova[1], Sona Wimmerova[1], Laurence Fuortes[3], Soterios A. Kyrtopoulos[4] and Maria Dusinska[1,5]

[1] *Slovak Medical University, Bratislava, Slovak Republic*
[2] *Department of Pathology, National Institute of Occupational Health, Budapest, Hungary*
[3] *University of Iowa, College of Public Health, Iowa City, Iowa, USA*
[4] *National Hellenic Research Foundation, Institute of Biological Research and Biotechnology, Athens, Greece*
[5] *NILU Norwegian Institute for Air Research, Kjeller, Norway*

leukocytes are the most appropriate specimens for *in vitro* cellular assays. Macrophages and lymphocytes are appropriate models for examining the effects of xenobiotics on cell functions. Serum cytokines, chemokines or soluble adhesion molecules have potential to contribute to the panel of biomarkers used to assess immunotoxicity.

1.1 Immunotoxicology

Immune dysregulation resulting from inhalation, skin exposure or ingestion of chemicals in the workplace and general environment is an important health problem in industrialized an industrializing societies (National Research Council, 1992). Immunotoxicity is an important aspect of the safety evaluation of drugs and chemicals (Descotes, 2005). It has been generally accepted that all new chemicals require safety evaluation before marketing and sale. This is a difficult task due to the large number of chemicals directly consumed by man, such as drugs and food additives, and those that are widely used such as pesticides, household chemicals, and industrial products (De Rosa et al., 2002; IPCS/WHO, 1999).

Immunotoxicity refers to any adverse effect on the structure or function of innate and adaptive immunity. It can be divided into immunosuppression, immunostimulation, hypersensitivity and autoimmunity (Duramad & Holland, 2011; Descotes, 2005; Fig. 1). The outcome of immunotoxicity is influenced by the dose of the immunotoxicant as well as mechanism of action of exposure to other agents, such as bacteria, viruses, parasites, or chemicals normally harmless. Direct immunotoxic effects of xenobiotics including particles and fibers can lead to the suppression or stimulation of immune response. Immunosuppression can result in increased occurrence of infectious diseases or and neoplasias, in particular lymphomas, as shown in both transplant and cancer patients treated with potent immunosuppressive drugs (Descotes, 2000; Vial & Descotes, 1996). Immunosuppression caused by chemicals, may make the course of infections more severe, atypical and or likely to relapse. The target organ systems affected could be the respiratory, gastrointestinal tracts, CNS or the skin (Descotes, 2005). Flu-like reactions, autoimmune diseases and hypersensitivity reactions to unrelated allergens are among the adverse effects related to immunostimulation (Descotes, 2005). Hypersensitivity reactions are the most frequently detected immunotoxic effects of chemicals. They include immune-mediated ('allergic') and non immune-mediated ('pseudoallergic') reactions. Particles and mineral fibers are recognized causes of hypersensitivy reactions provoked mostly within respiratory tract and skin (D'Amato et al., 2005; Di Giampaolo et al., 2011). A large number of drugs and an increasing number of environmental agents can result in the appearance of a number of autoantibodies or even autoimmune diseases. Systemic lupus erythematosus, scleroderma or dermal vasculitis have been associated with exposure to a variety of chemical agents (Hess, 2002; Van Loveren et al., 2001).

1.2 Models and methods in immunotoxicology

The immune system is a complex network comprised of several cell types (i.e., lymphocytes, macrophages, granulocytes, and natural killer cells) whose diversity of functions includes maintaining homeostasis and health (Luster et al., 1989). Scientists use immunocompetent cells as models for studying the toxic mechanisms of xenobiotics at the cellular and

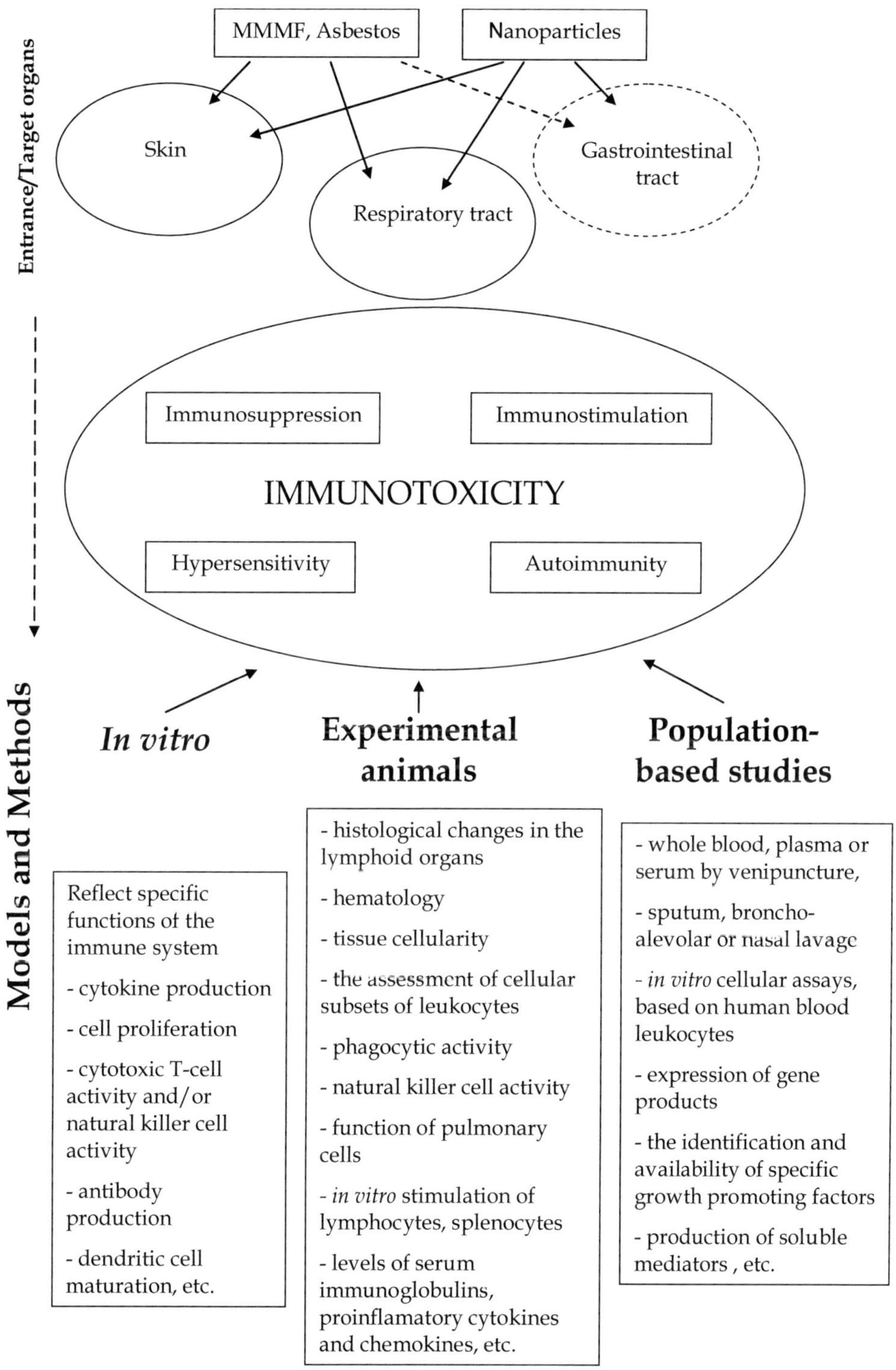

Fig. 1. Strategy for immunotoxicity testing in particle and fiber toxicology. Options for *in vitro, in vivo* and population studies.

molecular levels. In general, biological effects of xenobiotics (including particles and fibers) depend on several factors, e.g., chemical composition and physico-chemical properties such as solubility, chemical reactivity, size, length:width ratio, persistence in the organism, surface properties, dose, duration of exposure, the ability of a material to interact with body proteins etc. Host factors such as underlying health status, individual susceptibility to xenobiotics, metabolism, age, nutrition status, life style (smoking, etc.), presence of immune disease (asthma, allergic rhinitis, immunosuppression etc.) and other factors are also important determinants of immunotoxicity.

Increasing evidence that the immune system is a frequent target of xenobiotics following chronic, subchronic, or acute exposure underlines the need for development of models and immune assays suitable for use in screening potential immunotoxic compounds. For hazard assessment of xenobiotics, *in vitro* studies, experimental studies in laboratory animals, as well as epidemiological studies may provide necessary information (Fig. 1). Recently, several review papers have been published on design and methods used in immunotoxicological studies (Dietert & Holsapple, 2007; Lankveld et al., 2010; Oostingh et al., 2011). Haley published best practice guidelines for routine pathology evaluation of the immune system (Haley et al., 2005). Study methods of immunotoxicology have been reviewed and guidance documents developed by United States and European regulatory agencies (Committee for Proprietary Medicinal Products, 2000; Food and Drug Administration, 2004; Gopinath, 1996; ICICIS 1998; Kuper et al., 2002; Schuurman et al., 1994). In addition, harmonization of immunotoxicity guidelines in the ICH (International Conference on Harmonisation) process has been discussed by Ruehl-Fehlert (2005). One of the first steps in planning and conducting immunotoxicity studies is the identification and characterization of fibers/particles of interest. Secondly, attention must be paid to choosing proper *in vitro* immune cell models, sensitive animal models or occupationally or environmentally exposed human populations to assess the effect of xenobiotics on the immune system. Furthermore the selection of suitable immune assays as sensitive biomarkers of immunotoxic effect is also important.

In vitro assessment of immunotoxicity

In vitro testing has several advantages over *in vivo* animal testing. Among others, 3R requirements - reduction, refinement, and replacement of animal experiments are fulfilled, detailed mechanistic understanding of target immune cell/molecule is a clear benefit to consider and costs are lower. Most assays that are currently used to analyze immunotoxicity were originally designed for diagnostic purposes to examine hereditary or acquired immune disease in humans. Subsequently, these methods have been adapted for analysis of immunotoxicity of xenobiotics. *In vitro* assays may reflect specific functions of the immune system (cytokine production, cell proliferation, cytotoxic T-cell activity, natural killer cell activity, antibody production, and dendritic cell maturation). To avoid inter-species extrapolation, assays should preferably use human primary cells. They reproduce the response of normal cells of normal individuals. However, the use of primary cells is not always feasible (e.g., in the case of primary lung epithelial cells). As an alternative, the use of animal primary cells or human cell lines (transformed or tumor cells with unrestrained proliferative capacity) is applicable to first line screening of immunomodulatory effects. Furthermore, whole blood has the advantage of comprising multiple cell types in their natural proportion and environment (Lankveld et al., 2010).

In vivo models in experimental animals

In investigating potential effects of compounds on the immune system in experimental animals, a tiered approach is recommended. Studies aimed on the identification of histologic changes in the lymphoid organs and functional immune alterations in laboratory animals are useful for detecting probable immunotoxicants and may play an important role as a first indicator of direct immunotoxicity, i.e. immunosuppression (De Jong & Van Loveren, 2007). First tier, general toxicity studies may include parameters for detection of relatively gross toxic effects on the immune system. Hematology, tissue cellularity and the assessment of cellular subsets of T- and B-leukocytes by flow cytometry as non-functional assay are common initial tests. Some authors consider such bioeffects as insensitive indicators of immunotoxicity.

Second tier consists of studies of immune function. Phagocytic activity and determination of Natural Killer (NK) cell activity may be used in evaluation of direct immunotoxicity. In animal models, there is no limitation to obtain cell suspensions from lung tissue or bronchoalveolar lavage to look at function of pulmonary cells affected by particles and fibers. Several other possibilities are presented by thymus, bone marrow or spleen tissues for *in vitro* stimulation of lymphocytes by potential mitogens. These methods may indicate effects of xenobiotics on the functionality of splenic cell populations. Concanavalin A (Con A) and phytohemagglutinin (PHA) activate T-cells, while lipopolysaccharide (LPS) activates primarily B-cell populations. In addition, serum can be obtained for determination of serum immunoglobulins or proinflamatory cytokines and chemokines. Comparison of treated and control groups may give a first indication of possible direct immunotoxic effects (De Jong & Van Loveren, 2007).

Population-based studies

Biological endpoints used in molecular epidemiology are called biomarkers. Several definitions of biomarkers as tools used in human or animal studies to assess exposure and disease risks have been published (Benford et al., 2000). Bottrill defined biomarkers as "parameters which can be evaluated quantitatively, semi-quantitatively or qualitatively and which provide information on exposure to a xenobiotic or on the actual or potential effects of that exposure in an individual or in a group" (Bottrill, 1998). There is a high degree of complexity of the immune system and an enormous variety of responses and mechanisms involved in immunotoxic injury. Therefore it is a challenge to identify a key parameter to develop as a biomarker. The inclusion of several immune endpoints applicable to man is thus essential. Specimens from living people to examine the effects of particles and fibers on the immune response are typically limited to minimally invasive (whole blood, plasma or serum by venipuncture, sputum) or moderately invasive techniques (bronchoalveolar or nasal lavage). *In vitro* cellular assays are typically based on human blood leukocytes. In particular, macrophages and lymphocytes are appropriate models for examining the effects of various agents on cell maturation and function. The expression of gene products can be used as markers of differentiation, the identification and availability of specific growth promoting factors (e.g., interleukins), and their potential to undergo terminal differentiation resulting in production of soluble mediators (e.g., monokines, lymphokines, or antibodies) or indicating effector function (e.g., tumor target cell killing) (Luster et al., 1989).

1.3 Immunotoxicity studies of mineral fibers

The adverse effects that arise from exposure to asbestos have stimulated the development of substitute materials, man-made mineral fibers. However, little is known about the health effects of these fibers. The potentially harmful effects of all types of respirable fibers are at present one of the most important fields of interest in industrial toxicology. The production, sale and use of asbestos are no longer permitted in Europe. Some of the properties of asbestos (e.g. as an insulation material) can be substituted by alternative man-made fibers. In view of the importance of the possible biological effects of fibers we have conducted *in vitro*, animal and a molecular epidemiology studies to examine the relationship between relevant biomarkers and exposure to asbestos, mineral wool and glass fibers. We have measured a range of biomarkers of exposure, effects and individual susceptibility. In this chapter, biomarkers of immunotoxicity will be presented.

1.3.1 Asbestos

Asbestos has long been recognized as a cause of both benign and malignant lung disease (interstitial and pleural fibrosis, lung cancer and mesothelioma). Asbestos refers to a group of naturally occurring mineral fibers with a ≥ 3:1 length to diameter ratio. These fibers once inhaled and displaced by various means to lung tissues, can cause a spectrum of diseases including cancer and disorders related to inflammation and fibrosis (American Thoracic Society, 2004; Mossman et al., 1996). Mechanisms of asbestos-induced carcinogenesis are thought to be multiple, including generation of reactive oxygen (ROS) and nitrogen species (RNS), alteration of mitochondrial function, physical disturbance of cell cycle progression, and activation of several signal transduction pathways (Jaurand, 1997; Nymark et al., 2008). Asbestos fibers having iron (or even chrysotile) and producing ROS/RNS can cause DNA damage to nearby cells, and fibers are sometimes directly inserted into the cells and injure chromosomes, while retained fibers may adsorb other carcinogens on their surface (known asbestos bodies) (Toyokuni, 2009a, 2009b).

The extrapulmonary consequences of asbestos exposure were discussed in Bunderson-Schelvan et al., (2011). Authors used several hundred epidemiological, *in vivo* and *in vitro* studies and finally they supported a strong association between asbestos exposure and peritoneal neoplasm. On the other hand, the correlations between asbestos exposure and immune-related disease were less conclusive and effects of asbestos exposure to the GIT (gastrointestinal tract) appeared to be minimal. Immunomodulatory effects of asbestos have been well established in patients with asbestosis and mesothelioma (American Thoracic Society, 2004; Corsini et al., 1994; Mascagni et al., 2003; Rosenthal et al., 1999) however there is limited information on effects in individuals with minimal evidence for asbestos related lung disease or exposure only. Our study offered an opportunity to assess biomarkers which may represent individual susceptibility to and/or early evidence for asbestos related health effects.

1.3.2 Man made fibers

Rock wool, glass fibers and ceramic fibers

The evidence for adverse health effects following exposure to asbestos has prompted a drastic reduction in the use of asbestos, resulting in the increased use of substitutes composed of both naturally occurring and synthetic materials which are thought to have lower toxicity. Man-made mineral fibers include glass fibers (used in glass wool and continuous glass filament), rock (stone)/slag wool and refractory ceramic fibers. Rock (stone) wool, slag wool and glass wool are used extensively in thermal and acoustic insulation, typically in buildings, vehicles and appliances. Refractory ceramic fibers are designed for high-temperature applications, mainly in industrial settings. Continuous glass filament is used primarily in reinforced composite materials for the insulation, electronics and construction industries (IARC, 2002; National Toxicology Program, 2009). Man-made vitreous fibers have some physical similarities to asbestos, in particular, their fibrous character which gives them the same aerodynamic properties and leads to their deposition throughout the respiratory tract. Unlike amphibole asbestos, however, they are synthetic and amorphous, and generally have a lower biopersistence in lung tissues. Also, unlike serpentine asbestos, they tend to break transversely rather than cleaving along the fiber axis (IARC, 2002).

Data on respiratory cancer of man-made mineral (MMMFs) and vitreous fibers (MMVFs) are not consistent. Statistically significant increases in respiratory cancer mortality were observed among glass wool-exposed workers in unadjusted analyses in the United States (Marsh et al., 2001), European (Boffetta et al., 1997), and Canadian cohorts (Shannon et al., 2005). Excesses of lung cancer incidence were observed among the European workers (Boffetta et al., 1997) and Canadian workers (Shannon et al., 2005), but not among French workers (Moulin et al., 1986). Marsh et al., (2001) concluded that the US cohort study of man-made vitreous fiber workers has not provided consistent evidence of a relationship between man-made vitreous fiber exposure and mortality from malignant or non-malignant respiratory disease. Gillissen et al. (2006) stated that MMMFs or MMVFs including glass wool, rock wool, slag wool, glass filaments, microfibers, refractory ceramic fibers are bioactive under certain experimental conditions. Although it has been shown that MMMFs may cause malignancies when injected intraperitoneally in high quantities in rodents, inhalation trials and human studies have not shown such effects. The amorphous structure of synthetic vitreous fibers facilitates designing fibers with low biopersistence. In 2001, IARC reclassified these fibers from Category 2b to Category 3 (with RCF and special purpose fibers remaining in 2b) based on epidemiological data and the animal studies database indicating that there is little if any health risk associated with the use of SVFs of low biopersistence (Bernstein, 2007).

Occupational or environmental exposures to many inhaled particles and fibers have been linked with immunotoxicity. First of all, silica and silicates have been associated with the development of lung inflammation, interstitial fibrosis, bronchitis, small airway disease, emphysema, and vascular diseases as well as immunologic reactions (Song & Tang, 2011). Recent studies showed that Th1 and Th2 cytokines may be involved in silicosis and regulatory T-cells (Treg cells) have crucial role in modulation of immune homeostasis by regulating Th1/Th2 polarization. Studies in animals provided knowledge that depletion of Tregs may attenuate the progress of silica-induced lung fibrosis and enhance Th1 response and decelerate Th1/Th2 balance toward a Th2 phenotype in silica-induced lung fibrosis (Liu et al., 2010). Exposure to diesel exhaust particles (Inoue & Takano, 2011), coal dust (Ates et al., 2011), soil dust (Schenker et al., 2009), beryllium (Martin et al., 2011; Mikulski et al., 2011; Sood, 2009), heavy metal fumes (Montero et al., 2010) can evoke new or facilitate existing immune-mediated pulmonary inflammation.

1.3.3 NiO nanoparticles

Nickel and nickel compounds are widely used in industry. In occupational settings, exposure to nickel and nickel compounds occurs primarily during nickel refining, electroplating, and welding. In addition to nickel, workers in metal mining and processing are exposed to diesel emissions, oil mists, blasting agents and also to various other substances prevalent in the mine or industry (Lightfoot et al., 2010). Some of them, such as silica (Costantini et al., 2011; Huaux, 2007), radon (Chauhan et al., 2011) or arsenic (Burchiel at al. 2009) are known to be potent immunotoxic agents thus implicating possible synergistic effects on the immune response. The most common airborne exposures to nickel in the workplace are to insoluble nickel species, such as metallic nickel, nickel sulfide, and nickel oxides from dusts and fumes. The chemical and physical properties of nickel and nickel compounds strongly influence their bioavailability and toxicity. The lung and the skin are the principal routes of entry and target organs of occupational exposure. The most serious adverse health effects due to occupational exposure to nickel and its compounds are lung fibrosis and lung cancer, nickel is also hematotoxic, hepatotoxic and nephrotoxic. Allergic skin reactions are relatively common in individuals who are exposed to nickel (Brüske-Hohlfeld, 2009; Das & Buchner, 2007; Panizza, 2011; Zhao, 2009).

Recently, nickel nanoparticles are increasingly used in modern industries such as catalysts, sensors and electronic applications (Ahamed, 2011). Due to known toxic effects of "bulk" nickel products, caution in industrial applications of new nickel nanoproducts is important. Several *in vivo* studies in rats demonstrated that nickel oxide nanoparticles (NiO NP) have inflammatory effects in lungs by transient increase in cytokine expression (IL-1alpha, IL-1beta in lung and monocyte chemotactic protein-1 in bronchoalveolar lavage fluid) and persistent increase in CC chemokine (macrophage inflammatory protein-1alpha in lung and bronchoalveolar lavage fluid - BALF) (Morimoto et al., 2010). Cytokine-induced neutrophil chemoattractant-1 (CINC-1), CINC-2 alpha, beta, and CINC-3 were involved in the persistent pulmonary inflammation by NiO NP (Nishi et al., 2009) but NiO NP did not induce the gene expression of MMP-2 and TIMP-2 mRNA in rat lungs (Morimoto et al., 2011). *In vitro* assessment of the toxic effect of nickel nanoparticles in human lung epithelial A549 cells showed reduced mitochondrial function, induction of the leakage of lactate dehydrogenase (LDH) and induction of oxidative stress in dose and time-dependent manner (Ahamed, 2011).

Other airborne and engineered nanoparticles in addition to nickel, such as carbon nanotubes (He et al., 2011), titanium dioxide (Morimoto et al., 2011), cobalt - Co_3O_4 (Cho et al., 2011a) or quantum dots (Jacobsen et al., 2009) has been reported to induce lung inflammation. Anoher example is ZnO nanoparticles (ZnO NP) discovered to induce eosinophilia, proliferation of airway epithelial cells, goblet cell hyperplasia, and pulmonary fibrosis. Fibrosis was associated with increased myofibroblast accumulation and transforming growth factor-beta positivity. Serum IgE levels were up-regulated by ZnO NP along with the eosinophilia whilst serum IgA levels were down-regulated by ZnO NP (Cho et al., 2011b).

1.4 Hazard assessment of mineral fibers and particles

Humans may be exposed to fibrous particles from a variety of sources, including occupational settings, ambient air, consumer products, drinking water and food (De Vuyst et al., 1995). Potential effects of airborne fibers in humans can only occur after a complex process of inhalation, deposition, elimination, retention and translocation. The biological effects of inhaled fibers are highly dependent on dose (fiber exposure concentration - numbers of long fibers), fiber size (diameter/length), (Donaldson & Tran, 2004; Kohyama et al., 1997; Yamato et al., 1998), durability of material in the organism (biopersistence) (Mossman et al., (2011), duration of exposure, chemical composition and properties, solubility, chemical reactivity, surface properties of the material, ability of a material to interact with body proteins etc. Host factors such as efficiency of defense mechanisms of the respiratory tract between the initial deposition and the ultimate contact of the fibers with the target cell, individual susceptibility to xenobiotics, metabolism, age, nutrition status, life style (smoking), presence of immune disease (asthma, allergic rhinitis, immunosuppression etc.) and other factors influence the development of immunotoxicity.

2. *In vitro* studies on lung cells

The lung consists of more than 40 different cell types; each type has its special function, localization and morphology. From the toxicological point of view, the most important cell types being alveolar macrophages (AM - free living cells, whose function is to phagocyte the inhaled particles and maintain the alveoli clean and sterile) and alveolar epithelial type II cells (TII - localized on the inner surface of lung alveoli and which play an important role in tissue renewal). For this reason we focused on these cell types, isolated them from rats and maintained them in cell culture (Hoet et al., 1994; Richards et al., 1987). After 20 h cultivation the cells were exposed to different dose (1, 5, 10 $\mu g.ml^{-1}$) of mineral fibers and the cultivation was prolonged for another 20 h period when the experiment was terminated and the analyses were done.

2.1 Lectin histochemistry

Bandeiraea simplicifolia agglutinin (BSA) and *Maclura pomifera* agglutinin (MPA) are able to bind to the terminal N-acetyl-α-galactosaminyl or α-D-galactose/galactosamine residues in the membranes of AM and TII cells which makes them suitable for detection of cell membrane injuries (Tatrai et al., 1994). Control cells showed regular, linear staining with BSA or MPA. Stone wool at the concentration 5 $\mu g.ml^{-1}$ caused moderate injury to membranes of AM and incomplete phagocytosis in a small fraction of AM. Alveolar epithelial type II cells did not develop detectable membrane damage at any tested fiber dose. Refractory ceramic fibers (RCF) evoked changes in both cell types only at the highest dose: the membranes were not continuous and reduplicated. Wollastonite caused a decreased reaction in the membranes only at the highest dose. After exposure to the lowest dose of crocidolite the membranes of both cell types were fragmented irregularly and frustrated phagocytosis could be found in AM (Tátrai et al., 2004; 2006a; 2006b).

2.2 Effect of mineral fibers on cells using TEM

The control cells and those exposed to fibers at a dose of 1 $\mu g.ml^{-1}$ were examined. TII cells did not show any alterations after RCF or stone wool exposure. AM cells phagocyted RCF fibers without injuries of cell organelles, intact organelles remained also after exposure to stone wool. In both cell types crocidolite evoked severe damage in the organelles and necrobiosis of whole cells (Tátrai et al., 2004; 2006a; 2006b).

2.3 Immunological studies

Production of proinflammatory peptides MCP-1 and MIP-1α was assayed in growth media after termination of cell cultivation. Exposure to wollastonite did not change production of MCP-1 and MIP-1α in TII cells, but in AM the production was significantly enhanced: MCP-1 at the concentration 10 μg.ml^{-1}, MIP-1α at the concentration 5 μg.ml^{-1}. The results after exposure to stone wool were different: in TII cells the production of MCP-1 was enhanced at all concentrations, MIP-1α at doses of 5 and 10 μg.ml^{-1}; in AM the production of both cytokines was statistically significantly enhanced after doses of 5 and 10 μg.ml^{-1}. Crocidolite evoked statistically significant dose dependent enhancement of the production of MCP-1 in AM, for MIP-1α and both cytokines in TII at doses of 5 and 10 μg.ml^{-1} in all cases (Tátrai et al., 2004; 2006a; 2006b). Comparing the results from different fibers on 2 various primary cell types the following differences are clearly seen: crocidolite (asbestos) evoked the greatest changes, both morphologically and functionally. Effects of wollastonite were seen more significant comparing to stone wool. AM cells are more sensitive to the fibers exposure than TII cells.

3. Animal model

3.1 Intratracheal instillation studies in rat model

Four types of fibers: asbestos and three types of ASMF fibers (asbestos substitute mineral fibers): wollastonite, rock wool and glass fibers were intratracheally instilled at 2 doses (2 mg or 8 mg of fibers) to Fisher 344 rats. Dose of 2 mg was suspended in 0.2 ml of saline solution per animal or control group with 0.2 ml saline only. A dose of 8 mg was divided and instilled 4 times (weekly 2 mg/0.2 ml saline solution). The assays were performed 4 or 16 weeks after last instillation of the fibers. After sacrifice, markers of immune response and hematology were analyzed. Immunotoxic effects were examined using a panel of immune and hematological assays. Phenotypic analysis of leukocytes (T-lymphocytes, activated T-cells, B-lymphocytes, NK-cells, T-helpers, T-cytotoxic cells) and expression of adhesion molecules (CD11b, CD54) were performed by flow cytometry. Immune functions were evaluated by proliferative activity of T and B-lymphocytes *in vitro* stimulated with mitogens and antigen and phagocytic activity of leukocytes.

Our findings demonstrate the immunomodulatory effect of mineral fibers in the rat animal model 4 and 16 weeks after intratracheal exposure to amosite, wollastonite, rock wool and glass fibers. Significant changes were observed in total white blood cell count and percentages neutrophils in all fiber-treated, especially high-dosed, animals after 4 weeks of exposure. The percentage of lymphocytes was altered in rock wool fiber-treated especially in high-dosed animals after 4 weeks of exposure (Table 3.1-1).

Analysis of lymphocyte subsets showed significantly increased percentage of T-lymphocytes, mainly cytotoxic cells and decreased percentage of B-lymphocytes in peripheral blood of animals exposed to amosite. Rats exposed to wollastonite had increased percentage of T-helper cells. Exposure to mineral fibers decreased expression of adhesion molecule CD54 (ICAM-1) on granulocytes (amosite, glass fibers) and monocytes (rockwool). Suppressed expression of adhesion molecules CD11b was found on granulocytes (wollastonite, glass fibers) and monocytes (glass fibers) (data not shown).

		Amosite	Wolastonite	Rock wool	Glass Fibers
White blood cells (10^9/l)	4 weeks, 2mg				
	4 weeks, 8mg	↓ *	↓ *		↑ *
	16 weeks, 2mg			↓ *	
	16 weeks, 8mg	↓ *			
Neutrophils (%)	4 weeks, 2mg				
	4 weeks, 8mg	↑ *	↑ *	↑ *	↑ *
	16 weeks, 2mg		↑ *		
	16 weeks, 8mg				
Lymphocytes (%)	4 weeks, 2mg				
	4 weeks, 8mg			↓ *	
	16 weeks, 2mg				
	16 weeks, 8mg				

* $p<0.05$; ** $p<0.01$; *** $p<0.001$; ↓ - decrease ↑ - increase in comparison with relevant control;

Table 3.1-1. White blood cell (WBC) count and differential WBC in Fisher 344 rats administered with 2 mg or 8 mg of amosite, wollastonite, rock wool or glass fibers.

Although amosite seems to be most potent suppressor of T- and B-lymphocyte proliferation, especially in high-dosed animals, wollastonite and rock wool also interfered with lymphocyte proliferation and suppressed the response of T-lymphocytes. The opposite stimulative effect on proliferative capacity of B-cells was found in animals exposed to glass fibers (Table 3.1-2). Phagocytic activity was dramatically affected by exposure to rock wool and glass fibers. A highly significant dose-dependent suppression was found in neutrophils and monocytes. Rats exposed to wollastonite fibers also had decreased phagocytic activity of peripheral blood phagocytes 4 weeks after instillation of either dose. Surprisingly, the phagocytic activity of animals exposed to amosite was affected only in high dosed rats (Table 3.1 2).

In conclusion, animal exposure to mineral fibers leads to alterations in systemic immune response. Immune dysregulation consisted of changes of the main lymphocyte subsets. Moreover, the function of immunocompetent cells that are responsible for the specific immune response (T- and B-lymphocytes) and phagocytic cells was impaired. Our results correspond with the hypothesis of Hurbánková (1994), who observed that the phagocytic activity of granulocytes and monocytes is altered in asbestos-treated rats up to one year following treatment, displaying a two-phase progress: an initial increase (phase I) followed by a decrease below the average values of the control animals (phase II).

3.2 Inhalation studies in rat model

The effects of industrial fibrous dusts on the respiratory system represent a potential environmental and occupational health hazard for humans. Chronic asbestos exposure can cause pleural plaques, asbestosis and cancer diseases. These effects stimulated research activities aiming at the study of the health effects of fibrous substitutes as well as combined effects with other noxious materials respectively (Boor et al., 2009; Donald & Gardner, 2006; IARC, 2002; 2004). This study gives information about the dose-response relationships after

Function of lymphocytes		Amosite	Wolastonite	Rock wool	Glass Fibers
Proliferative activity of T-lymphocytes	4 weeks, 2mg	↑ Con A *		↓ PHA **	
	4 weeks, 8mg	↓ Con A *** ↓ PHA **	↓ Con A *** ↓ PHA ***		
	16 weeks, 2mg			↓ CD3 *	
	16 weeks, 8mg	↓ Con A **			
Proliferative activity of B-lymphocytes	4 weeks, 2mg				↑ PWM ***
	4 weeks, 8mg	↓ PWM *			↑ STM *
	16 weeks, 2mg				
	16 weeks, 8mg	↓ PWM ***			
Function of phagocytes					
Phagocytic activity of neutrophils	4 weeks, 2mg		↓ *	↓ ***	↓ ***
	4 weeks, 8mg	↓ ***	↓ **	↓ **	↓ ***
	16 weeks, 2mg			↓ *	↓ *
	16 weeks, 8mg			↓ **	↓ *
Phagocytic activity of monocytes	4 weeks, 2mg		↓ *	↓ ***	↓ ***
	4 weeks, 8mg	↓ ***	↓ *	↓ ***	↓ ***
	16 weeks, 2mg			↓ *	
	16 weeks, 8mg			↓ **	↓ *

* $p<0.05$; ** $p<0.01$; *** $p<0.001$; ↓ - decrease in comparison with relevant control; ↑ - increase in comparison with relevant control

Table 3.1-2. Activity of immune cells measured via lymphocyte proliferation test and phagocytic test in Fisher 344 rats administered with 2 mg or 8 mg of amosite, wollastonite, rock wool or glass fibers.

inhalation of two concentration levels of amosite asbestos and wollastonite alone or combined with daily exposure to cigarette smoke together with the basic lung inflammation and cytotoxic parameters. Male Fisher 344 rats were exposed for 6 months. Animals inhaled amosite asbestos or wollastonite fibers in a nose-only inhalation device (In-Tox, USA). Amphibole asbestos - amosite and wollastonite fibers belong to naturally occurring silicate inorganic fibers. Wollastonite is used as a substitute of asbestos. Dust aerosol was produced at two dosages: 30 mg/m^3 air and 60 mg/m^3 air for one hour per exposure. Exposure of animal groups to dusts proceeded every second day, 5 days per week. Six groups, each of 11 animals were exposed to:

- 60 mg/m^3 amosite fibers for one hour every two days; combined with exposure to mainstream smoke from three cigarettes daily;

- 60 mg/m^3 amosite fibers for one hour every two days;
- 30 mg/m^3 amosite fibers for one hour every two days, combined with exposure to mainstream smoke from three cigarettes daily;
- 30 mg/m^3 amosite fibers for one hour every two days;
- exposure to mainstream smoke from three cigarettes daily plus immobilization stress as for animals exposed to dust;
- immobilization stress as for animals exposed to dust.

Cigarette smoke exposure: Standard research cigarettes of the 1R1 type (Tobacco and Health Research Institute - THRI, Lexington, KY, USA) were used in all experiments. A whole-body actively ventilated exposure chamber was used, with a cigarette smoke generator and pumps (THRI, Lexington, KY, USA) allowing all smoker animal groups to breathe at the same time diluted main-stream tobacco smoke at the target concentration 30 mg of total particulate matter (TPM)/m^3 air for one hour daily (an exposure requiring to burn three cigarettes).

Length [μm]	%	Diameter [μm]
< 20	5	
20 - 30	75	0.71
>30	20	

Diameter [μm]	%
= 1	47
<1	22
<3	21
=3	6
>3	4
Length [μm]	%
1 - 10	48
11 - 30	40
>30	12

Tables 3.2-1. and 3.2-2. Length, diameter and percentage of wollastonite fibers (top) and amosite fibers (bottom).

The aim of our study was to find and compare the combined effect of amosite or wollastonite (asbestos substitute) with cigarette smoke on the selected immune, inflammatory and cytotoxic parameters. The rats inhaled two doses: 30 and 60 mg/m^3 of amosite (asbestos) and wollastonite fibers (mineral asbestos substitute) for 1 hour every 2 days and cigarette smoke from 3 cigarettes/day. They were sacrificed after 6 months exposure.

3.2.1 Combined effect of mineral fibers and tobacco smoke on respiratory tract

Six months after the beginning of the inhalation exposures, the animals were anesthetized and BAL was performed.

The following BAL parameters were examined:

Inflammatory response biomarkers

- Total cell count/ml BAL (bronchoalveolar lavage) fluid
- AM count/ml BAL fluid
- Differential cell count (alveolar macrophages - AM, lymphocytes - Ly, granulocytes - Gr)

Cytotoxic parameters

- Phagocytic activity of AM
- Viability of AM
- Lactate dehydrogenase activity (in the cell - free lavage fluid)
- Acid phosphatase activity (in the cell- free lavage fluid and in the BAL cell suspension)
- The cathepsin D activity (in the cell - free lavage fluid and in the BAL suspension)

Methods are described in papers of Hurbánková & Kaiglová (1999) and Černá et al. (2004). The results were statistically evaluated using Mann-Whitney test.

	Fibers alone			Fibers/Tobacco smoke		
	Control	30 mg/m³	60 mg/m³	Tobacco smoke alone	Tobacco smoke + fibers 30 mg/m³	Tobacco smoke + fibers 60 mg/m³
N	7	7	7	7	7	6
Total cell count/ml BALF ($10^3 \cdot ml^{-1}$)						Am ↑ **
AM count/ml BALF ($10^3 \cdot ml^{-1}$)						Am ↓ **
Ly %		Am ↑ *	Am ↑**			Am ↑ ***
AM %		Am ↓ *	Am ↓ *	Am ↓ *	Am ↓ **	Am ↓ ***
PMN %			Am ↑ *		Am ↑ *	Am ↑ **
Immature forms of AM (%)		Am ↑ *		Am ↑ **	Am ↑ *	Am ↑ **
Multinucleated cells (%)			Am ↑**			

Comparison of exposed group with the control group; *p<0.05, **p<0.01, ***p<0.001; ↑ - increase against compared group; ↓ - decrease against compared group; abbreviations: Le - leukocytes; AM - alveolar macrophages; PMN – polymophonuclear leukocytes, BAL - bronchoalveolar lavage

Table 3.2-3. Amosite – inhalation exposure - with/without tobacco smoke; inflammatory response parameters in BAL.

Increased numbers of bronchoalveolar lavage fluid (BALF) cells after asbestos or other fiber-exposure as a result of inflammatory response have been described by numerous authors (Hurbankova & Kaiglova, 1999; Greim et al., 2001; Morimoto & Tanaka, 2001; Osinubi et al., 2000). In our study, a significantly increased number of BALF cells after exposure to amosite in comparison with the control group was observed in the smoker plus 60 mg/m³ fiber group (by 11.4 %) as well as in the corresponding-dose, non-smoker group (by about 16%). This increase could be ascribed to the increase of lymphocyte population proportions. These changes were accompanied by an inverse change in the AM count in BALF, which significantly decreased in the same group exposed to combined higher dust plus cigarette smoke. A very similar but shorter exposure only to cigarette smoke has been reported to lead to a higher (35%) difference of BALF cell counts in comparison with the control values (Hurbánková et al., 2010; Ishihara et al., 1997; Nelson & Kelsey, 2002). The higher

	Fibers alone			Fibers/tobacco smoke		
	Control	30 mg/m^3	60 mg/m^3	Tobacco smoke alone	Tobacco smoke + fibers 30 mg/m^3	Tobacco smoke + fibers 60 mg/m^3
N	7	7	7	7	7	6
Phagocytic activity of AM (%)				Am ↓** Woll ↓**	Am ↓**	Am ↓*
Viability of living AM (%)			Am ↓*			Am ↓*
LDH μkat.g prot.$^{-1}$						
ACP nkat.g prot.$^{-1}$					Woll ↑*	
ACP nkat.10^{-6} cells						
Cathepsin D U_{tyr}.mg prot.$^{-1}$					Am ↑* Woll ↑*	Woll ↑*
Cathepsin D U_{tyr}.10^{-6} cells		Woll ↑*	Am ↑* Woll ↑*	Am ↑ **	Am ↑ **	Am ↑ **

Comparison of exposed groups with the control group: *$p<0.05$, **$p<0.01$, ***$p<0.001$; ↑ - increase against compared group, ↓ - decrease against compared group; (1) enzyme activity expressed as μmol of p-nitrophenol.hour^{-1} mg protein^{-1}; abbreviations: LDH: lactate dehydrogenase; ACP: acid phosphatase; U_{tyr} : μg of thyrosine released in an hour time

Table 3.2-4. Amosite and wollastonite - inhalation exposure - with/without tobacco smoke; cytotoxic parameters in BAL.

proportions of PMN and lymphocytes in the BALF than control values indicate the presence of inflammation in the lungs at sacrifice. The magnitude of the increase of these parameters was dose-dependent. AM are the predominant cells present in BALF and changes in their number or function are important factors determining the lung inflammatory response and characterizing the pathogenesis of such response. A decrease in macrophage number or phagocytic capacity may result in the reduction of the clearance of inhaled materials and thus can lead to an increase of the effective dose of the potentially injurious agent (Aoshiba et al., 2001; Dziedzic et al., 1993). A significant reduction in the number of AM after intratracheal instillation of amosite has been observed also in our previous experiments (Hurbankova & Kaiglova, 1999). Associated with inflammatory changes, a dose-dependent increase in multinuclear cells (MNC) proportions was found in the BALF as well as in the lung tissue suspensions. MNC were increased after exposure (separate or in combination) to tobacco smoke as well as both fiber concentrations but significantly only after higher dose without smoking. Similarly, immature forms of AM in all exposed groups were increased in comparison with control (Beňo et al., 2005). Strongly dose dependent decrease of AM viability (higher dose with and without smoking) as well as phagocytic activity of AM (all group with smoking) was found in this experiment. That is in accordance with previously described effect of asbestos (Hurbánková & Kaiglová, 1999).

Increased LDH and ACP activity in extracellular fluids are generally accepted as good markers of cell or tissue injury and used for evaluation of the cytotoxic effect. We did not find significant changes in activities of measured enzymes in our experiment. Cathepsin D activity was significantly changed after amosite inhalation. These results are in good accordance with study of Sjörstrand et al. (1989). Wollastonite inhalation confirmed the lower cytotoxicity in comparison with asbestos. Significant changes were found only by measurement of cathepsin D activity in BAL cells (increased levels), decreased percentage of phagocytic activity of AM in "tobacco smoke alone" group and increased levels of ACP in "tobacco smoke + wollastonite fibers 30mg/m^3" group.

Amosite

- Inflammatory parameters were mostly changed after 60mg/m^3 in combined group (amosite exposure and tobacco smoke).
- Tobacco smoke alone induced changes in inflammatory parameters. It confirms that smoking alone might play an important role in inflammatory processes.
- Smoking alone caused some changes of cytotoxic parameters and intensified the harmful effect of amosite exposure.
- Mild dose dependence between 30mg/m^3 and 60mg/m^3 in groups without tobacco smoke was seen.

Wollastonite

- No dose dependence of inflammatory parameter changes in this study was recorded in groups without smoking and very weak in combined exposure groups.
- Mild dose dependence of cytotoxic parameters changes in groups without or with tobacco smoke was observed.
- Influence of tobacco smoke on cytotoxic parameters was not explicit.

3.2.2 Combined effect of mineral fibers and tobacco smoke on immune parameters

Cellular immunity was examined by phenotypic analysis of leukocytes (CD3$^+$, MHC II, CD4$^+$, CD8$^+$, CD161$^+$, B-lymphocytes) and by expression of adhesion molecules (CD11b, CD54) on leukocytes (Table 3.2-5). Inhalation of high dose of amosite fibrous dust resulted in a significantly increased percentage of B-lymphocytes and elevated expression of adhesion molecule CD11b on lymphocytes of peripheral blood in non-smoking rats. Similarly, inhalation of high dose of wollastonite increased the percentage of B-lymphocytes, and this elevation was reinforced with combined exposure to lower dose of wollastonite and tobacco smoke. Moreover, the combined exposure to wollastonite and smoking caused a significant, dose-dependent increase of the percentage of cytotoxic cells and enhanced expression of adhesion molecule CD11b on granulocytes in peripheral blood. On the other hand, cigarette smoke and higher dose of wollastonite resulted in decrease of T-cells (CD3$^+$). The stimulative effect of exclusive exposure to smoking on the immune system was shown as significantly elevated percentage of some lymphocyte subsets (T-cytotoxic, T-helper lymphocytes, B-lymphocytes) and elevated expression of adhesion molecule CD11b in comparison with non-smoking animals.

Immune function assays included proliferative response of T- and B-lymphocytes and phagocytic activity of blood leukocytes (Table 3.2-6). The proliferative activity of T-lymphocytes stimulated with CD3 antigen and T-dependent B-cell response in rats exposed to amosite was significantly decreased. The immunosuppressive effect was more pronounced

Proportion of lymphocyte subsets in peripheral blood	30 mg/m³	60 mg/m³	Tobacco smoke alone	Tobacco smoke + fibers 30 mg/m³	Tobacco smoke + fibers 60 mg/m³
CD3⁺ – T-lymphocytes (%)					Woll ↓ [a]
CD3⁺/MHC II – activated T-lymphocytes (%)					
CD4⁺ – T-helper lymphocytes (%)			↑ **		
CD8⁺ – T-cytotoxic lymphocytes (%)			↑ *	Woll ↑ *	Woll ↑ *
CD161⁺- Natural killer cells (%)					
B-Lymphocytes (%)		Am ↑ * Woll ↑ *	↑ *	Woll ↑ *	
Adhesion molecules on leukocytes					
Expression of CD11b on lymphocytes (%)		Am ↑ * Woll ↑ **	↑ *		
Expression of CD11b on monocytes (%)					
Expression of CD11b on granulocytes (%)		Am ↑ *			Woll ↑ *
Expression of CD54 on lymphocytes (%)					
Expression of CD54 on monocytes (%)					
Expression of CD54 on granulocytes (%)					

Ly – lymphocytes; Mono – monocytes; Gr – granulocytes; */[a] $p<0.05$; **/[aa]$p<0.01$; ***/[aaa]$p<0.001$; *– significant level calculated in exposed rats in comparison with control rats without tobacco smoke exposure; [a] – significant level calculated in exposed rats in comparison with control rats with tobacco smoke exposure; ↓ - decrease in comparison with relevant control; ↑ - increase in comparison with relevant control; Am – amosite; Woll – wollastonite

Table 3.2-5. Cellular immunity of rats treated via inhalation exposure with two doses of amosite/wollastonite fibers and with/without tobacco smoke.

in low-dosed rats. No effect of exposure to amosite fibers alone on proliferative activity of B-cells stimulated with STM (lipopolysacharide from *Salmonella typhimurium*) was seen in non-smoking rats, while a moderate enhancement was recorded in animals exposed to amosite and tobacco smoke. A marked suppressive effect of amosite on phagocytic activity of leukocytes was also found. Stimulation of the immune system was observed as increased phagocytic activity of leukocytes in animals exposed to cigarette smoke. Animals exposed to wollastonite or cigarette smoke alone caused enhancement of proliferative activity of T-lymphocytes stimulated with concanavalin A. All animals exposed to wollastonite fibers had suppressed phagocytic activity of monocytes and granulocytes. Moreover, decrease of phagocytosis was recorded also in combined exposure to wollastonite and cigarette smoke. In conclusion, inhalation of amosite and wollastonite mineral fibers resulted in marked changes in specific and non-specific immunity. Moreover, findings indicate mutual

Function of lymphocytes	30 mg/m³	60 mg/m³	Tobacco smoke alone	Tobacco Smoke + fibers 30 mg/m³	Tobacco smoke + fibers 60 mg/m³
Proliferative activity of T-lymphocytes stimulated with Con A (cpm)		Woll ↑ *	↑ *		
Proliferative activity of T-lymphocytes stimulated with PHA (cpm)					Am ↓ [a]
Proliferative activity of T-dependent B-lymphocytes stimulated with PWM (cpm)	Am ↓ *				
Proliferative activity of B-lymphocytes stimulated with STM (cpm)					Am ↑ *
Proliferative activity of T-lymphocytes stimulated with CD3 (cpm)	Am ↓ *	Am ↓ *			
Function of phagocytes					
Phagocytic activity of neutrophils (%)	Woll ↓ *	Am ↓ ** Woll ↓ *	↑ *	Am ↓ [a]	Am ↓ [aaa]
Phagocytic activity of monocytes (%)	Am ↓ ** Woll ↓ *	Am ↓ *** Woll ↓ **		Am ↓ [aaa] Woll ↓ *	Am ↓ [aaa] Woll ↓ *

*/a $p<0.05$; **/aa $p<0.01$; ***/aaa $p<0.001$; *– significant level calculated in exposed rats in comparison with control rats without tobacco smoke exposure; a– significant level calculated in exposed rats in comparison with control rats with tobacco smoke exposure; ↓ - decrease in comparison with relevant control; ↑ - increase in comparison with relevant control; Woll – wollastonite; Am – amosite; Con A-concanavalin A; PHA-phytohemmagglutinin; PWM-pokeweed mitogen; STM-lipopolysaccharide from *Salmonella typhimurium*; CD3-alloantigen

Table 3.2-6. Proliferative activity of lymphocytes and phagocytic activity in rats treated via inhalation exposure with two doses of amosite/wollastonite fibers and with/without tobacco smoke.

interference of mineral fibers and smoking in the modulation of the systemic immune response during combined exposure.

3.3 Assessment of Immunotoxicity of ceramic fibers and NiO nanoparticles

The aim of the study was the assessment of immune effects of exposure to ceramic fibers and/or NiO nanoparticles in experimental animals - male Sprague-Dawley rats. Rats were treated by intratracheal instillation with 1 mg of refractory ceramic fibers and/or 1mg NiO nanoparticles. Controls were treated with 1 ml physiological saline (1ml per animal). One and six months after instillation, the animals were killed. The blood samples were taken and the spleen was aseptically removed and placed into RPMI medium. Panel of immune assays was performed. The phagocytic activity of blood monocytes and granulocytes was assessed by ability to ingest bacteria *Staphylococcus aureus* (Tulinska et. al., 2005). One month after exposure of animals to ceramic fibers and/or NiO nanoparticles no alterations in phagocytic activity and respiratory burst was shown. However 6 months after exposure, situation was different. Exposure to NiO nanoparticles and combined exposure to ceramic fibers and NiO nanoparticles caused significantly increased phagocytic activity of granulocytes, as well as percentage of cells with respiratory burst (Table 3.3-1). NiO nanoparticles and combined exposure of ceramic fibers and NiO nanoparticles stimulated this important function of nonspecific immune response.

Function of phagocytes	Ceramic fibers 1 month	NiO nanoparticles 1 month	Ceramic fibers and NiO nanoparticles 1 month
Phagocytic activity of monocyes (%)			
Phagocytic activity of granulocytes (%)			
% of phagocytic cells with respiratory burst			
	Ceramic fibers 6 months	NiO nanoparticles 6 months	Ceramic fibers and NiO nanoparticles 6 months
Phagocytic activity of monocyes (%)			
Phagocytic activity of granulocytes (%)		↑ *	↑ ***
% of phagocytic cells with respiratory burst		↑ *	↑ **

* $p<0.05$, ***$p<0.001$; ↑ - increase in comparison with relevant control

Table 3.3-1. Phagocytic activity and respiratory burst of peripheral blood cells in male Sprague-Dawley rats administered with 1 mg refractory ceramic fibers, NiO nanoparticles and combined exposure to both elements.

Function of T- and B-lymphocytes was studied using lymphoproliferation assay in spleen cells derived from rats exposed to ceramic fibers and/or NiO nanoparticles. Cells were *in vitro* stimulated with mitogens - concanavalin A (Con A), phytohemagglutin (PHA) and pokeweed (PWM) mitogen. One month after exposure, significant decrease of proliferative activity of lymphocytes stimulated with all three mitogens was found in animals exposed to ceramic fibers. To the contrary, 6 months after exposure, significant increase of lymphocyte proliferation stimulated with phytohemagglutin and pokeweed mitogen was recorded. The effect of combined exposure to ceramic fibers and NiO nanoparticles on spleen cells was manifested as significant increase of proliferative activity of T-lymphocytes after stimulation with Con A. Moreover, significant increase of basal proliferative response of spleen cells derived from rats 1 month after exposure to NiO nanoparticles alone and combined exposure to fibers and nanoparticles was seen. (Table 3.3-2).

Immunophenotypic analysis of leukocytes was examined using panel of surface markers: CD3, CD4, CD8, CD161 and MHC II. Six months after exposure, immunophenotypic analysis of leukocytes performed by flow cytometry revealed statistically significant decrease of expression of marker for T-lymphocyte subpopulations (CD4, CD8) in rats administered with ceramic fibers. On the other hand, increase of expression of CD4 marker after combined exposure was observed. 6 months after exposure to NiO nanoparticles, significant increase of expression of molecule MHC II on lymphocytes, monocytes and granulocytes was shown. Similar effect of combined exposure on expression MHC II on monocytes and granulocytes was found (Table 3.3-3).

Function of lymphocytes	Ceramic fibers 1 month	NiO nanoparticles 1 month	Ceramic fibers and NiO nanoparticles 1 month
Proliferative activity of T-lymphocytes stimulated with Conncanavalin A – Con A (cpm)	↓ *		↑ *
Proliferative activity of T- lymphocytes stimulated with Phytohemmagglutinin - PHA (cpm)	↓ ***		
Proliferative activity of T-dependent B-lymphocytes stimulated with Pokeweed mitogen - PWM (cpm)	↓ *		
Basal proliferative activity (cpm)		↑ ***	↑ ***
	Ceramic fibers 6 months	NiO nanoparticles 6 months	Ceramic fibers and NiO nanoparticles 6 months
Proliferative activity of T- lymphocytes stimulated with Con A (cpm)			
Proliferative activity of T- lymphocytes stimulated with PHA (cpm)	↑ *		
Proliferative activity of T- dependent B-lymphocytes stimulated with PWM (cpm)	↑ *		
Basal proliferative activity of lymphocytes (cpm)			

* $p<0.05$, *** $p<0.001$; cpm-counts per minutes after ^3H incorporation into lymphocytes, ↓ - decrease in comparison with relevant control; ↑ - increase in comparison with relevant control

Table 3.3-2. Proliferative response of lymphocytes in male Sprague-Dawley rats administered with 1 mg refractory ceramic fibers, NiO nanoparticles and combined exposure to both elements.

Proportion of leukocyte subsets in peripheral blood	Ceramic fibers 6 months	NiO nanoparticles 6 months	Ceramic fibers and NiO nanoparticles 6 months
$CD3^+$ – T-lymphocytes (%)			
$CD4^+$ – T-helper lymphocytes (%)	↓ *		↑ **
$CD8^+$ – T-cytotoxic lymphocytes (%)	↓ *		
$CD4^+/CD8^+$ lymphocytes (%)	↓ *		
Expression of MHCII marker on lymphocytes (%)		↑ *	
Expression of MHCII marker on monocytes (%)		↑ **	↑ *
Expression of MHCII marker on granulocytes (%)		↑ **	↑ ***

* $p<0.05$; ** $p<0.01$; *** $p<0.001$; ↓ - decrease in comparison with relevant control; ↑ - increase in comparison with relevant control

Table 3.3-3. Proportion of leukocyte subsets in peripheral blood in male Sprague-Dawley rats administered with 1 mg refractory ceramic fibers, NiO nanoparticles and combined exposure to both elements.

Phagocytosis is a major host defense mechanism of the innate immune system. The specific molecular pathways that direct the process of ingestion depend on the size of the particle (Hazenbos & Brown, 2006). Several other mechanisms, such as release of inflammatory mediators, antigen presentation (Garcia-Garcia & Rosales, 2005; Rabinovitch, 1995) and expression of different membrane receptors (Garcia-Garcia, 2005; Johansson et. al., 1997) are also involved. It is known that different pulmonary macrophages (airway, alveolar, interstitial, pleural, intravascular) are an important part of the lung's defenses against particles deposited by inhalation (Oberdorster, 1994). After phagocytic stimulation, macrophages release various chemotactic factors for neutrophils and other inflammatory cells including TNF, neutrophil chemotactic factor and many proinflammatory mediators such as prostaglandins, leukotrienes, thromboxane. Apart from that, macrophages produce free radical oxygen and release lysosome enzymes which may cause lung tissue injury. Published literature, studying influence ceramic and metal nanoparticles *in vitro,* showed that ceramic nanoparticles had effect on production of cytokines in monocytes. This effect resulted to the shift of cytokine balance towards inflammation. Moreover, obtained results showed that nanoparticles have significant effects on the expression of some TLR molecules, suggesting that they could affect cell reactivity to infections by altering the expression of innate receptors. Particularly interesting is the finding that ceramic nanoparticles can enhance expression of TLR chains important for viral-dependent stimulation (Lucarelli et al., 2004). Another study (Yagil-Kelmer et al., 2004) compared influence of ceramic particles on monocytes of peripheral human blood and human monocytes cell line U937. They found out the higher variability of expression of cytokines of primary human blood monocytes from donors in compared with cell line. Importantly, studies consistently demonstrated that smaller, sub-micrometer ceramic particles provoke relatively larger amounts of the cytokines IL-l alpha, IL-I beta, IL-8, TNF-alpha and IL-10 when compared to 1.5 um particles. The variation in the reactivity of different human individuals to particle stimulation may have highlighted another major contributory factor - genetic capacity of an individual to express related cytokines with their susceptibility to, and subsequently, the severity of, a particular disease (Matthews et al., 2000). Nkamgueu et al., (2000) recorded suppression of phagocytic activity and respiratory burst after *in vitro* exposure of cells to ceramic particles. The results of another study indicated that refractory ceramic fibers 6 months after intratracheal instillation significantly changed the majority of examined BAL parameters. The presence of inflammatory and cytotoxic response in lung may signalize beginning or developing disease process (Hurbankova et al., 2005).

Observations that nickel oxide-induced changes may contribute to significant immunodysfunction are known from immunotoxicity studies examining "bulk" nickel oxide aerosols. 65-day inhalation study in mice showed, that exposure to nickel oxide resulted in increased numbers of lung-associated lymph nodes (LALN), enhanced numbers of nucleated cells in lavage samples, increased antibody-forming cells (AFC) in LALN, but decreased AFC/10^6 spleen cells and suppressed alveolar macrophage phagocytic activity (Haley et al., 1990). Significant alterations of humoral immune system and alveolar macrophages were found also in rats after 4 weeks or 4 months of exposure to nickel oxide aerosols, respectively (Spiegelberg et al., 1984). Nanoform might have substantial impact on toxic effects including immunotoxicity. *In vitro* studies demonstrated that ultrafine NiO particles showed higher cytotoxicities toward human keratinocyte HaCaT cells and human lung carcinoma A549 cells *in vitro* than fine NiO particles (Horie et al., 2009). Transmission electron microscope observations revealed uptake of both ultrafine and fine NiO particles into HaCaT cells. Cellular uptake of NiO nanoparticles (NiO NP) was found to be associated with the release of Ni^{2+} ions after 24-48 h (Pietruska et al., 2011). The intracellular Ni^{2+} release could be an important factor that determines the cytotoxicity of NiO. Pathological features of different sizes of nickel oxide following intratracheal instillation in rats were studied by Ogami et al. (2009). Submicrometer nano-nickel oxide was associated with greater toxicity, as for crystalline silica, than micrometer-sized nickel oxide. Biological effects of factors of particle size reduction, when dealing with finer particles such as nanoparticles, were reconfirmed to be important in the evaluation of respirable particle toxicity.

In vivo studies in experimental animals showed persistent high level of inflammation in lungs even at low doses of NiO NP. Cho et al. (2010) described chronic neutrophilic/lymphocytic cytotoxic inflammation in rats 4 weeks after instillation NiO NP accompanied by increased MIP-2, IFN-γ, and LDH in BALF. The alveolar lipoproteinosis evident in NiO NP-exposed lungs was reflected in very high protein and LDH levels in the BALF. Increased levels of neutrophils and macrophages have been observed from 3 days to 3 months after instillation of agglomerated NiO NP suspended in distilled water in Wistar rats (Nishi et al., 2009; Ogami et al., 2009). Gene expression profiling of the rat lung after whole-body inhalation exposure to ultrafine NiO particles induced high expression of genes associated with chemokines, oxidative stress, and matrix metalloproteinase 12 (Mmp12), suggesting that Uf-NiO particles lead to acute inflammation (Fujita et al., 2009). *In vitro* studies conducted to test the possible toxic effects (Ada et al., 2010) bring evidence that one of the contributing underlying mechanisms is oxidative stress. The levels of intracellular reactive oxygen species and lipid peroxidation in A549 cells enhanced with increasing exposure to NiO nanoparticles and growth in gene expressions of HO-1 and SP-D were observed in A549 cells (Horie et al., 2011).

Our data of suppressed proliferative activity of T-lymphocytes and decreased T-dependent B-cell response indicate fiber-induced changes in systemic immune response. The hypothesis that inhaled particles or fibers can exert adverse effects outside of the lung is supported by several studies. Although, most of findings refer to systemic effect of particles, similar influence of fibers can be assumed. For example, ultrafine particles were found to decrease the number of blood PMNs and increase the intracellular oxidation of a fluorescent dye (DCFD) in blood PMNs (Elder et al., 2004). Diesel exhaust particles and carbon black particles had significant adjuvant effect on the local immune-mediated inflammatory response in the draining popliteal lymph node and on the systemic specific IgE response to model allergen ovalbumin in BALB/c mice (Lovik et al., 2003). The data of van Eeden (van Eeden et al., 2002) showed the effects of particulate air pollution on bone-marrow stimulation in animals. Acute exposure to ambient particles accelerates the transit of polymorphonuclear leukocytes (PMN) through the marrow whereas chronic exposure expands the size of the bone marrow pool of PMN. A communication between the fiber-induced processes in the pulmonary compartment and peripheral tissues can be mediated by: 1) leakage of reactive oxygen species and stress-induced cytokines directly into the peripheral blood, 2) (pre)activation of peripheral blood leukocytes that can result in aberrant homing and activation of inflammatory cells in distant tissues, and 3) the liberation of proinflammatory mediators by leukocytes and/or stromal cells present in the pulmonary tissues (Oudijk et al., 2003).

4. Molecular epidemiological studies in human population

The possible immunomodulatory effects of mineral fibers, in workers occupationally exposed to asbestos, rock wool and glass fibers, were examined in the context of a large-scale molecular epidemiology study (Ilavska et al., 2005; Tulinska et al., 2004). In addition to biomarkers of immunotoxicity, biomarkers of genotoxicity (Beňo et al., 2005; Dusinska et al., 2004; Horská et al., 2006; Topinka et al., 2004; 2006), oxidative damage and antioxidant defense (Staruchova et al., 2008) were also examined in the same cohorts. The studies involved workers with at least 5 years' exposure to asbestos, rock wool and glass fibers, respectively, at 3 industrial plants in Slovakia. A control group of clerical workers, matched for sex, age, smoking habits and alcohol use were also studied. All workers underwent clinical examination, including functional spirometry testing, and radiological examination.

Exposure: Fiber samples were used for asbestos fiber and ASMF identification, fiber morphology and quantification, using a microscope with phase contrast (Nikon, Japan) according to the Reference Method for the Determination of Airborne Asbestos Fiber Concentration at Workplaces by Light Microscopy (Membrane Filter Method), AIA 1979, London, UK. Exposure assessment had been based on personal and environmental monitoring.

Subjects and health status: In each plant, 61, 98 and 80 exposed workers and 21, 43 or 36 control clerical subjects, respectively, were recruited. In the case of the asbestos-exposed subjects, an additional town-control group of 49 people was included. Evidence of pulmonary fibrosis was found in 42% of the asbestos-exposed workers, while evidence of pleural fibrosis was found in 24%. The asbestos-exposed cohort had significantly decreased forced vital capacity of lungs as well as forced expiratory volume per first second.

Immune parameters: Markers of lymphocyte function were found to differ significantly between fiber-exposed cohorts and corresponding controls. Workers from the former asbestos cement plant had significantly decreased proliferative capacity of lymphocytes stimulated by T-cell mitogen PHA. In contrast, the proliferative activity of T-lymphocytes in subjects from the rock wool and glass fiber factories was stimulated (Table 4). A significant *in vitro* stimulatory effect was observed in cultured B-lymphocytes stimulated with PWM from peripheral blood obtained from the glass fiber workers, while no such effect was found in workers from the asbestos and rock wool plants in comparison with the corresponding controls (Table 4). Although no other published data on functional changes of lymphocytes has been published in rock wool and glass fiber workers, depression of cell mediated immune response with a clear relationship between defective T-cell function and pulmonary fibrosis was seen in asbestos-exposed individuals. *In vitro* studies have clarified that asbestos fibers inhibit proliferation at an early stage (G_0 phase) of the cell cycle of PHA-stimulated cells. Besides the evidence for an important role of specific immunity in chemically induced pulmonary disease, including asbestosis, and published results on the protective role of T-lymphocytes especially in asbestos-induced pulmonary inflammation, our data also suggest immunomodulatory effects for two man-made fibers. We propose that the different patterns of T-cell proliferative activity found in workers exposed to asbestos versus rock wool and glass fibers may be due to differences in the duration of exposure to the different fibers as well as differences in the underlying health status of the populations studied. In contrast to the relatively good clinical status, shorter duration and low level of fiber exposure in rock wool and glass fiber workers, the former asbestos cement workers had historically high levels of exposure to fibrogenic dust and showed clinical evidence of asbestosis and a high prevalence of low forced vital capacity. It is notable that a biphasic immune response has been reported with silica exposure. In a rat model two distinct phases were noted in development of silicosis: in early stages, silica activates both humoral and cellular immunity; however, in late phases no activated adaptive immune system effects were observed.

The phagocytic activity of polymorphonuclear leukocytes and monocytes as well as respiratory bursts of cells did not differ significantly between the exposed and control groups. Similarly, the results of the natural killer cell assays indicated no significant differences in cytotoxic activity of NK-cells between exposed and controls in the cohort exposed to asbestos and rock wool (cytotoxicity assays were not done in the glass fiber workers). Phenotypic analysis of peripheral blood leukocytes was performed to assess the proportions of the main lymphocyte subsets. Flow cytometry analysis revealed significantly decreased expression of markers $CD16^{+}56^{+}$ (natural killer cells) in exposed workers from the glass fiber plant in comparison with the corresponding controls (Table 4). No significant alterations between workers exposed to asbestos, rock wool and glass fibers exposed and controls have been found in proportion of $CD3^{+}$, $CD4^{+}$, $CD8^{+}$, $CD19^{+}$ cells in peripheral blood.

Table 4	**Parameters**	**Asbestos**	**Rock wool**	**Glass Fibers**
Hematology	White blood cell count ($x10^{9}/l$)			↓ *
	Lymphocytes (%)			
	Basophils and eosinophils (%)			
	Neutrophils (%)			
	Lymphocyte count ($x10^{9}/l$)			↑ **
	Basophil and eosinophil count ($x10^{9}/l$)			↑ *
	Neutrophil count ($x10^{9}/l$)			
	Erythrocyte count ($x10^{12}/l$)			
	Hemoglobin (g/l), hematocrit (%)			
	Mean cell volume (fl)			↓ *
	Platelets ($x10^{9}/l$)			
Function of lymphocytes	Proliferative activity of T-lymphocytes stimulated with Concanavalin A – ConA (cpm)		↑ *	↑ **
	Index Con A		↑ **	↑ **
	Proliferative activity of T-lymphocytes stimulated with Phytohemagglutinin - PHA (cpm)			↑ *
	Index PHA	↓ *	↑ **	↑ **
	Proliferative activity of T-dependent B-lymphocytes stimulated with Pokewed mitogen - PWM (cpm)			↑ *
	Index PWM			

Table 4	Parameters	Asbestos	Rock wool	Glass Fibers
	Proliferative activity of T-lymphocytes stimulated with CD3 antigen (cpm), Index CD3			
	Proliferative activity of lymphocytes stimulated with Tetanus antigen - TET (cpm), Index TET			
	Basal proliferative activity of lymphocytes (cpm)			↑ **
Function of phagocytes	Phagocytic activity of monocytes and granulocytes (%)			
	Respiratory burst of granulocytes (%)			
Function of NK cells	Natural killer cell activity (%)			not done
Proportion of lymphocyte subsets in peripheral blood	$CD3^+$ – T-lymphocytes (%) $CD3^+$/HLA DR – activated T-cells (%)			
	$CD4^+$ - T-helper lymphocytes (%)			
	$CD8^+$ - T-cytotoxic lymphocytes (%)			
	$CD16^+56^+$ - Natural killer cells (%)			↓ *
	CD 19^+ - B-lymphocytes (%)			
	CD25, CD81 – activated T-lymphocytes (%)			
Adhesion molecules on leukocytes	Expression of CD62L on lymphocytes (%)	↑ **		
	Expression of CD62L on granulocytes (%)	↑ ***		
	Expression of CD62L on monocytes (%)	↑ ***		
	Expression of adhesion molecules CD11b, CD11c, CD18, CD49d and CD54 – ICAM on lymphocytes, granulocytes and monocytes (%)			
Activation markers on eosinophils	Expression of CD66b on eosinophils (%)	↑ ***		↑ *
	Expression of CD69 on eosinophils (%)	↑ ***		
Soluble adhesion molecules	E-Selectin (ng/ml)			↑ ***
	Intercellular Adhesion Molecule - ICAM (ng/ml)	↑ *	↑ ***	
Immunoglobulins	Immunoglobulin A – IgA (mg/dl)	↑ **		
	Immunoglobulin E – IgE (U/ml)	↑ **	↑ *	
	Immunoglobulin G – IgG (mg/dl)			
	Immunoglobulin M - IgM (mg/dl)		↓ **	
Complement	C3 and C4 Components of Complement (mg/dl)			
Proinflammatory cytokines	Interleukin 1 beta – IL1β (pg/ml)			
	Interleukin 6 – IL6 (pg/ml)	↑ **		
	Interleukin 8 - IL-8 (pg/ml)	↑ ***	↑ ***	↑ ***

* $p<0.05$; ** $p<0.01$; *** $p<0.001$; ↓ - decrease ↑ - increase in comparison with relevant control;

Table 4. Immune parameters measured in population study- humans occupationally exposed to asbestos and two man-made mineral fibers (rock wool and glass fibers).

The expression of adhesion molecules on blood leukocytes was analyzed using flow cytometry. In workers from the former asbestos cement plant, expression of adhesion molecule CD62L (L-selectin) on monocytes and granulocytes was significantly increased (Table 4). Increased levels of soluble adhesion molecules ICAM-1 were found in sera from the cohorts who worked with asbestos and rock wool (Table 4). The chi square test confirmed a significantly increased proportion of people with high levels of soluble ICAM-1 (>306 ng/ml) not only among the asbestos cohort but also in glass fiber workers (asbestos $p<0.02$, glass fibers $p<0.03$) compared with the controls. Exposure to glass fibers enhanced the level of soluble E-selectin in workers' sera (Table 4). Pathologically relevant increases in the expression and function of adhesion molecules have been observed in humans with such pulmonary disease/conditions as bronchial hyperreactivity, allergic rhinitis, idiopathic pulmonary fibrosis or neoplasia.

Analysis of serum levels of proinflammatory cytokines revealed increased serum concentrations of interleukin 6 (IL-6) in former asbestos workers. Significantly elevated serum concentrations of IL-8 were found in workers exposed to all three types of fibers, while no changes in IL-1β were recorded in exposed populations. Inflammatory cytokines are rapidly induced and expressed early in a disease or injury process. They mediate and modulate the healing processes but, if overexpressed, may exacerbate the severity of a disease condition as well as give rise to oxidative stress. Up-regulation of IL-8 secretion has been found in patients with fibrosing lung disease and, because IL-8 is the main chemotactic and activation factor for neutrophils, secretion of IL-8 was associated with neutrophil accumulation in the lower respiratory tract. Since the presence of neutrophils in BAL fluid is frequently reported in humans with asbestosis changes in levels of inflammatory cytokines were examined in the context of the present study.

Exposure to asbestos and rock wool was associated with significantly increased levels of immunoglobulin E. The results of the analysis of expression of markers CD66b and CD69 on eosinophils are summarized in Table 4, where it can be seen that workers from the former asbestos cement plant and glass fiber factory had significantly elevated expression of marker CD66b, while significantly increased expression of CD69 on eosinophils was found only in asbestos workers. Immunoglobulin E is well known as being involved in the mechanisms of development of allergic diseases. The observation of significantly increased levels of total immunoglobulin E in asbestos workers is in agreement with published results of Rosenthal et al., (1999) who concluded that asbestos appears to produce a hyperresponsive state, with chronically exposed individuals manifesting an elevation in circulating immunoglobulins (IgG, IgM, IgE). No data are available on populations occupationally exposed to rock wool for comparison.

5. Biomarkers

5.1 Proliferative activity of lymphocytes (lymphocyte transformation test)

Lymphocytes are important cells of the adaptive immune response. T-cells are involved in cell-mediated immunity whereas B-cells are primarily responsible for humoral immunity (relating to antibodies). The function of T-cells and B-cells is to recognize specific "non-self" antigens, during a process known as antigen presentation. Our study revealed high sensitivity of T-lymphocyte response to exposure to mineral fibers. Meanwhile in workers exposed to asbestos, significant suppression of proliferative response of T-cells *in vitro* stimulated with phytohemagglutinin was found, stimulative effect of rock wool and glass fibers on activity of T-lymphocytes in peripheral blood of exposed population were recorded. Our findings indicate that one of the immune targets of mineral fiber exposure seems to be specific cellular immunity. Proliferative activity of lymphocytes might be a sensitive indicator of immunomodulatory effects of mineral fibers; however the limitations of use it as a biomarker of individual susceptibility are interindividual differences.

5.2 Phagocytic activity of leukocytes

Pulmonary macrophages are crucial cells in contact with mineral fibers and nanoparticles representing the first line of defense in the lung alveoli. Expansion of macrophages in the lung is a typical characteristic of that type of exposure in both humans and experimental animals. Total macrophage numbers in the lung may increase by migration of blood monocytes, local proliferation of the alveolar macrophages or induced generation of chemotaxins (Rosenthal et al., 1998). Phagocytosis of asbestos fibers has been shown to be accompanied by the activation of macrophages, which results in the generation of ROS as well as a variety of chemical mediators and cytokines. These mediators amplify the local inflammatory reaction. Persistence of asbestos fibers in the lung interstitium or in the sub-pleural connective tissue may lead to a sustained chronic inflammatory reaction accompanied by fibrosis and proliferation of epithelial and mesenchymal cells (Branche, 2009). Surprisingly, in contrast to a marked suppressive effect of mineral fibers on the activity of phagocytes observed in our animal studies, no dramatic influence was found in worker populations. A statistically significant deterioration of phagocytic activity of monocytes was observed only among smoking workers exposed to asbestos, in comparison with exposed non-smokers (Tulinska et al., 2004).

5.3 Percentage of $CD16^{+}56^{+}$ cells (natural killer cells – NK cells) and cytotoxic activity of NK cells

Natural killer cells (NK cells) are crucial members of innate immunity responsible for killing of virus infected cells, overseeing of mutated or other way transformed cells and as a first defense line toward cancer cells. They kill cells by releasing small cytoplasmic granules of proteins called perforin and granzyme that cause the target cell to die by apoptosis (programmed cell death). Several authors have reported increased numbers of circulating NK cells and their reduced activity in asbestos exposed humans (Froom et al., 2000; Rosenthal et al., 1999). The results from our study do not confirm these findings. Neither asbestos cement nor rock wool workers were noted to have significant changes in NK-cell activity or the percentage of cells with NK phenotype. However, significantly decreased expression of marker $CD16^{+}56$ was found in glass fiber-exposed workers in comparison with controls. Although the effect was not dramatic, this observation suggests that exposed workers need to be screened preventively for this marker. This finding is surprising because glass fiber exposure has not as yet been connected with malignant tumors as has asbestos. Synthetic vitreous fibers (that include insulation glass wool and continuous glass filament) were reclassified by International Agency for Research on Cancer (IARC) commission from category 2b (*possibly carcinogenic to humans*) to category 3 (*not classifiable as to their carcinogenicity to humans*) in 2001 (Bernstein, 2007; IARC, 2002). Regardless, that in our study population no significant differences in cytotoxic activity of natural killer cells were found between workers exposed to asbestos and rock wool and corresponding controls (assay in glass fiber workers not done), the assay is considered an important member of a panel to assess antitumor immunity in workers exposed to probable, possible or susceptible carcinogens. We assume that both numbers and activity of NK cells are important in individual health surveys of workers exposed to mineral fibers.

5.4 The phenotypical analysis of peripheral blood leukocytes

T-lymphocytes, CD3, CD4, CD8, HLA DR markers

Published data suggest that asbestos may affect immunocompetent cells such as $CD4^+$ responder T-cells, $CD4^+$ regulatory T-cells, Th17 T-cells, $CD8^+$ cytotoxic T-cells (CTL) or dendritic cells (DC). Continuous exposure to chrysotile produces a stronger Treg function, at least with the capacity to produce soluble functional factors (i.e., IL-10 and TGF-β) (Kumagai-Takei et al., 2011). Recent research indicates that asbestos is able to act as a superantigen (Otsuki et al., 2007). The increased expression of T-cell receptor Vβ without a clonal expansion of T-lymphocytes has been demonstrated after asbestos exposure. This is in line with our results. We did not detect changes either in absolute or relative number of T-lymphocytes and activated T-lymphocytes in the asbestos exposed workers in comparison to controls. Previous papers referred changes in Th/Ts ratio as well as decreased relative and absolute number of circulating T-lymphocytes (Kagan et al., 1977; Tsang et al., 1988). These parameters were without change also in case of rock wool or glass fiber exposure.

Expression of CD81 and CD25 on activated T-lymphocytes

In spite of inhibition of T-cell proliferation observed in the case of asbestos or stimulation in case of glass fibers and rock wool we did not find changes in expression of early activation markers CD81 and CD25 on $CD4^+$ and $CD8^+$ T-cells after PHA stimulation (data not published). Their spontaneous stimulation was not damaged either. Chronic exposure to all of three fibers had no effect on these tested parameters. Similar results were recorded by Wu et al. (2000). The marker CD81 was not expressed on peripheral T-lymphocytes after *in vitro* cultivation with chrysotile asbestos. Dysregulation and long-term T-cell activation can lead to survival of self-recognizing cells, and consecutively to initiation of autoimmune responses. We assume that synthetic mineral fibers do not impact the human organism in the same manner as in the case of asbestos. The expression of T-cells activation markers was not changed after glass fibers and rock wool exposure.

B- lymphocytes, CD19 marker, and immunoglobulins IgG, IgA, IgM, IgE

An increased number of B-cells have been reported in patients with asbestosis, fibrosis or malignant diseases after asbestos exposure (Gaumer et al., 1981; Ozesmi et al., 1988). We did not detect this change after asbestos, glass fiber or rock wool exposure. However, among those with asbestos exposure we confirmed a hyperresponsive B-lymphocytes as seen by Rosenthal et al., (1999) with increased levels of immunogloulins IgE and IgA. Exposure to rock wool was also associated with increased IgE levels and in contrast with decreased levels of IgM. Exposure to glass fibers did not affect these parameters. An elevation in serum immunoglobulins (IgA, IgG, IgM, IgE) and mucosal (salivary) IgA and the presence of autoantibodies, antinuclear antibody and rheumatoid factor is one of the most consistent findings in individuals chronically exposed to asbestos (Doll, 1983). IgE is well known for being a central regulator in the allergic reactions. The increased level of IgE and a higher production of proinflammatory interleukins, IL-6 and IL-8, suggest inflammation with a shift from Th1 to Th2 immune response. Our findings correspond to other studies which confirm a shift towards a Th2 mediated immune response in BAL fluid after asbestos exposure (elevated levels of cytokines IL-1b, Il-4, Il-5, IL-6, Il-13) (Sabo-Attwood et al., 2005; Shukla et al., 2007).

Activation markers on eosinophils

Eosinophils are known for their participation on allergic reactions. Pulmonary diseases as asthma or allergic rhinitis are associated with elevated number of circulating eosinophils (Venarske & deShazo, 2003). The expression of activation markers on eosinophils can indicate a growing allergic status. Workers from the World Trade Center crash (with high exposure to asbestos and synthetic mineral fibers) had enormously increased numbers of eosinophils in BAL fluid but circulating eosinophils were not changed (Rom et al., 2002). Also in our study, we did not detect increased number of peripheral blood eosinophils after mineral fibers exposure, but we observed evidence of their activation. The expression of CD69 and CD66b markers was associated primarily with asbestos exposure, and glass fibers enhanced only CD66b. Rock wool did not have impact on these parameters.

Expression of adhesion molecules CD11b, CD11c, CD18, CD54, CD62L, and CD49d on lymphocytes, monocytes and granulocytes

Transendothelial migration of leukocytes into tissues is a multistep process. Leukocytes express adhesion molecules as mediators. We evaluated the expression of adhesion molecules CD11b, CD11c, CD18, CD54, CD62L and CD49d on leucocytes and detected the increased expression of L-selectin (CD62-L) on monocytes and granulocytes in workers exposed to asbestos. Selectins mediate the rolling of leukocytes on the stimulated endothelium. Increased numbers of alveolar macrophages in the lower human airways is a typical finding after asbestos exposure (Rosenthal et al., 1999). Circulating monocytes transmigrate to tissue in response to chemotactic factors and become tissue macrophages. The over-expression of CD62L as well as IL-8, a chemotactic factor for neutrophils, may be an important part of this process.

5.5 The assessment of soluble markers

Complement components C3 and C4

Sabo-Attwood et al., (2005) showed changes in the gene expression of C1 complement component in a mouse model. The incubation of human plasma with asbestos fibers induced production of C5a fragment of C5 component of complement (Governa et al., 2000). We did not detect any changes of C3 and C4 complement components in human serum of workers exposed to mineral fibers (data not published).

Interleukins IL-1β, IL-6, and IL-8

Asbestosis is accompanied by persistent inflammation and by production of mediators of inflammation. Certain asbestos substitute fibers, e.g. wollastonite fibers are potential angiogenic agents that can induce regenerative cytokine (IL-6, IL-8) and angiogenic factor production (VEGF-A) resulting in the formation of new blood vessels (Carbonari et al., 2011). Many *in vitro* studies showed that measurement of interleukin levels is equally sensitive for testing of cell activation after air-transmitted particles exposure *in vitro*

(Mitschik et al., 2008). In connection with asbestosis, there are cytokines, mainly IL-1β, IL-6, IL-8, which appear to have a role in pathology of this disease (Mossman & Churg, 1998; Tsuda et al., 1997). In spite of the fact that IL-1β is a proinflammatory cytokine required for the synthesis of others cytokines (e.g. IL-8), we did not detect differences in exposed groups in comparison to controls. Our findings were in accordance to observations of Simeonova and Luster (Simeonova & Luster et al., 1996) who noted an enhancement of IL-8 without IL-1β stimuli. IL-6 was previously known as a factor for B-cell differentiation and immunoglobulin production. The increased level of IL-6 may be associated with the increased IgE and IgA levels seen in asbestos exposed individuals. Monitoring of IL-8 in peripheral blood could serve as an early and sensitive marker of developing pulmonary inflammation in consequence of asbestos, glass fibers and rock wool exposure. Across all three exposed groups we observed an increase of cytokine IL-8. Despite the highly significant ($p<0.001$) differences in IL-8 between exposed workers and human control subjects, these interleukin levels were still in normal reference range.

Soluble adhesion molecules sICAM-1, sVCAM-1 and sE-selectin

The soluble adhesion molecules are products of activated endothelial cells. They are known for their involvement in processes of inflammation. Ciebiada et al., (2011) declared that concentrations of sICAM-1 are significantly higher in patients with asthma, and are dependent on a seriousness of disease. Our observations of increased adhesion molecules are in agreement with findings of Kristovich who stated that in the context of the pulmonary microenvironment, TNF-α elaborated by particulate-laden alveolar monocytes could act upon proximal septal capillary endothelial cells, inducing their expression of endothelial leukocyte adhesion molecules ICAM-1, vascular cell adhesion molecule (VCAM -1 and E-selectin (Kristovich et al., 2004). Based on this fact we can speculate that levels of sICAM-1 corresponded with inflammation of the airways. Levels of sICAM-1 were increased in the asbestos exposed group. This was not surprising because asbestos fibers are persistent and insoluble in the lungs and are known as causative factor of inflammation. Although in the case of rock wool was a rather disturbing finding for a reason of better elimination of these inhaled synthetic mineral fibers from organism. Usually they have a high solubility and short-term durability in the airways. Among others, there was a shorter duration and lower concentration of fiber in the case of rock wool than asbestos exposure. We noted a statistically significantly higher elevation of sICAM-1 levels in individuals exposed to rock wool compared to the group exposed to asbestos. Glass fibers were not associated with differences in sICAM-1 levels. Adhesion molecules seem to be a sensitive indicator of activation of the immune system and inflammatory response in humans exposed to mineral fibers. Oxidative stress and production of ROS is an important component of the multiple effects of asbestos on human airways (Manning et al., 2002; van Helden et al., 2009). ROS modulate receptor signals and immune responses under physiological conditions, but their overproduction mediates endothelial damage through growth and migration of inflammatory cells, over-expression of inflammatory cytokines and adhesion molecules such as ICAM-1, VCAM-1, and E-selectin (Urso et al., 2011). The elevated production of IL-8, sICAM-1 (rock wool exposure) and sE-selectin (glass fibers exposure) signify immunotoxic effects of synthetic fibers from the airways and increased production of ROS.

6. Summary

This chapter addresses the effects of asbestos, man made mineral fibers (rock wool, glass wool, ceramic fibers) and nickel oxide nanoparticles on the immune system using *in vitro* model, animal model and molecular-epidemiological studies. Data from *in vitro* studies contained results of experiments on alveolar macrophages (AM) and alveolar epithelial type II cells (TII). Stone wool, refractory ceramic fibers (RCF), asbestos (crocidolite) and wollastonite have been tested by lectin histochemistry. Stone wool caused moderate membrane injury of AM and incomplete phagocytosis in a small fraction of AM. RCF caused gaps and reduplicated changes in membranes of both cell types (high dose). Wollastonite caused a decreased reaction in the membranes (high dose). After exposure to the lowest dose of asbestos (crocidolite), the membranes of both cell types were fragmented irregularly and frustrated phagocytosis could be found in AM. Analysis using transmission electron microscopy found severe damage in the organelles and cell death of both cell types exposed to crocidolite. No alterations were found after RCF or stone wool exposure. Analysis of proinflammatory peptides showed that exposure to wollastonite did not change production MCP-1 and MIP-1α in TII cells but in AM the production was significantly enhanced. Different doses of stone wool enhanced production of both peptides in TII cells and AM cells. Crocidolite evoked statistically significant dose dependent enhancement of the production of MCP-1 in AM, for MIP-1α; and both cytokines in TII cells. Comparing the results from different fibers on 2 various primary cell types the following differences are clearly seen: crocidolite (asbestos) evoked the greatest changes, both morphologically and functionally. Increased effects in wollastonite were seen when compared to stone wool. AM cells are more sensitive to the fiber exposure than TII cells.

Intratracheal instillation studies in rat model

Four types of mineral fibers were administered intratracheally to rats. Four (4w) and 16 weeks (16w) later, immune parameters were examined. Amosite, wollastonite (4w) and rock wool (16w) significantly decreased number of white blood cells; while opposite effect of glass fibers was seen (4w). A consistent increase in percentage of neutrophils was found in animals exposed to all fibers (4w) while decreased percentage of lymphocytes was observed only in rock wool fiber-treated rats (4w). Analysis of lymphocyte subsets in amosite exposed rats showed significantly increased percentage of T-lymphocytes (4w, 16w), mainly cytotoxic cells (4w) and decreased percentage of B-lymphocytes (4w). An increased percentage of T-helper cells was seen in wollastonite group (4w). Exposure to mineral fibers decreased expression of adhesion molecule CD54 (ICAM-1) on peripheral blood leukocytes (amosite, glass fibers and rockwool; all 4w) and CD11b (glass fibers, wollastonite; 4w). Although amosite (4w, 16w) seems to be most potent suppressor of T- and B-lymphocyte proliferation, especially in high-dosed animals, wollastonite (4w) and rock wool (4w, 16w) also interfered with lymphocyte proliferation and suppressed the response of T-lymphocytes. The opposite, stimulative, effect on proliferative capacity of B-cells was found in animals exposed to glass fibers (4w). A highly significant dose-dependent suppression of phagocytic activity of neutrophils and monocytes was found mainly in rock wool and glass fiber exposed animals (4w, 16w), but present also in wollastonite and amosite group (4w).

Inhalation studies in rat model - combined effect of mineral fibers and tobacco smoke on inflammatory response and cytotoxicity

In rats administered with amosite, weak dose-dependence was seen in simple exposure to fibers without smoking but inflammatory parameters were mostly changed in animals with combined exposure to high dose of fibers and tobacco smoke. In case of wollastonite exposure, no clear dose-dependence in changes of inflammatory parameters was recorded in those administered with fibers alone and very weak in combined exposure groups (fibers and tobacco smoke). Additionally, mild dose dependence of cytotoxic parameters changes in groups without or with tobacco smoke was observed. Tobacco smoke alone induced changes predominantly in inflammatory parameters; alterations in cytotoxic parameters were not explicit.

Combined effect of mineral fibers and tobacco smoke on immune parameters

Inhalation of high dose of both fibers (amosite and wollastonite) resulted in a significantly increased percentage of B-lymphocytes in peripheral blood of exposed rats. Except the percentage the B-cells, the combined exposure to wollastonite and smoking caused a significant, dose-dependent increase of cytotoxic cells, but total T-lympocytes were decreased. Exposure to amosite and wollastonite increased expression of adhesion molecule CD11b on peripheral blood leukocytes. The proliferative activity of T-lymphocytes and T-dependent B-cell response in animals exposed to amosite in simple or combined exposure with smoking was mostly suppressed. The only exception was combined exposure to amosite fibers and smoking resulting in significant increase of proliferative activity of B-cells. Enhanced proliferative reponse of T-cells was found in animals given high dose of wollastonite. A marked suppressive effect of amosite and wollastonite on phagocytic activity of leukocytes was observed. Moreover, decrease of phagocytosis was recorded in combined exposure to wollastonite and cigarette smoke.

Assessment of immunotoxicity of ceramic fibers and NiO nanoparticles

Immunophenotypic analysis of leukocytes was examined only 6 months after exposure to fibers and nanoparticles. Analysis revealed statistically significant decreased expression of marker for T-lymphocyte subpopulations ($CD4^+$, $CD8^+$) in rats administered with ceramic fibers. On the other hand, increased expression of $CD4^+$ marker after combined exposure was observed. Exposure to NiO nanoparticles significantly increased expression of MHC II on leukocytes. A similar effect was found on expression of MHC II with combined exposure. A significant decrease of proliferative activity of lymphocytes stimulated with all three mitogens was found in animals exposed to ceramic fibers one month after exposure. To the contrary, 6 months after exposure, opposite effect was seen. Moreover, significant increase of basal proliferative response of spleen cells derived from rats was seen 1 month after exposure to NiO nanoparticles alone and combined exposure to fibers and nanoparticles. Combined exposure to nickel oxide nanoparticles manifested a significant increase of proliferative activity of T-lymphocytes after stimulation with Con A. No alterations in phagocytic activity and respiratory burst were shown one month after exposure of animals to ceramic fibers and/or NiO nanoparticles. However 6 months after exposure, situation was different. Exposure to NiO nanoparticles and combined exposure to ceramic fibers and NiO nanoparticles caused significantly increased phagocytic activity of granulocytes, as well as percentage of cells with respiratory burst.

Molecular epidemiological studies in human population

In the context of a large-scale molecular epidemiology study, the possible immunomodulatory effects of mineral fibers, in workers occupationally exposed to asbestos, rockwool and glass fibers, were examined. Results of hematological evaluation shown decreased white blood cell count and increased number of lymphocytes and (common) eosinophil and basophil count in glass fiber exposed population. Our findings indicate that exposure to all three types of fibers examined the modulation of immune response to a different degrees. Suppression of T-cell immunity was found in the workers from a former asbestos cement plant, while stimulation of T-cell response was observed in rockwool workers. In addition to an elevated T- lymphocyte response, stimulated T-dependent B-cell response and basal proliferative activity of lymphocytes was seen in workers from glass fiber factory. Changes in lymphocyte subpopulation of CD $16^{+}56$ (natural killer cells) in peripheral blood may indicate negative effects of glass fibers on natural cellular immunity. No significant alterations between workers exposed to asbestos, rock wool and glass fibers and controls were found in proportion of $CD3^{+}$, $CD4^{+}$, $CD8^{+}$, $CD19^{+}$ cells in peripheral blood. Significantly increased serum levels of immunoglobulins IgA (asbestos), IgE (asbestos, rockwool) and decreased levels of IgM (rockwool) were recorded in people exposed to fibers. Increased levels of proinflammatory cytokines (IL-6 asbestos; IL-8 all three fibers), expression of adhesion molecule L-selectin on granulocytes and monocytes (asbestos), levels of soluble adhesion molecules in sera (ICAM-1 asbestos, rockwool; E-selectin glass fibers), increased levels of immunoglobulin E (asbestos and rockwool) and elevated expression of activation markers on eosinophils (CD66b asbestos, glass fibers; CD69 asbestos) may indicate hypersensitivity and an elevated inflammatory status in workers exposed to mineral fibers.

7. Conclusions

With the increasing commercial needs for substitutes of asbestos fibers, a number of man-made and other naturally occurring mineral fibers will appear as a part of living and occupational environments. Fibers discussed in this chapter can enter the human body mainly via the lungs, significance of exposure through digestive tract is less clear. Asbestos has long been recognized as a cause of both benign and malignant lung disease. Man made mineral fibers, once inhaled and displaced to lung tissues, can cause respiratory diseases related to inflammation and fibrosis. Skin diseases have been also reported. In reference to nanoparticles besides the lung and digestive tract, penetration via the skin also occurs (Fig. 1). Knowledge from air pollution showing increased risk of cardiopulmonary, respiratory, hypersensitivity disease and cancer requires specific assessments to be performed for newly produced nanoparticles. The assays currently used to test the safety of materials might be applicable to identify hazards of nanoparticles. Special attention is needed for nanoparticles designed for drug delivery or food components.

To optimize risk assessment for immune system toxicity, it is still necessary to increase our understanding of the underlying immunomodulatory mechanisms which cause negative effects and the quantitative relationships between the immunological tests conducted in the laboratory and manifestation of disease in human populations. There is no universal "consequence of exposure", each type of immunotoxicant should be treated individually when health risks are expected. As mentioned throughout this chapter, the immune system has been identified as a potential target organ for chemicals including particles and fibers. The immune system plays a critical role in host defense from disease as well as in normal homeostasis; thus identification of immunotoxic risk is important in the protection of human, animal and wildlife health. Clear understanding of normal development of cellular components of the immune system, the means by which they interact, and the known parameters by which their structure and function can be modified is necessary for designing investigations into how environmental agents may affect health through the immune system.

A growth of knowledge in immunology and cell biology connected with an explosion in methodologic and technologic capabilities is very promising for the science of immunotoxicology. There are several challenges yet to be solved within the discipline of immunotoxicology: (1) to improve traditional tests and establish a new tests, which reflect the variety of potential impacts of immunotoxicity; (2) to identify valid, sensitive human biomarkers of immunotoxicity; (3) to interpret minor, moderate, or significant immunotoxic effects in animal models in relation to human risk assessment; (4) better integration of methods of exposure assessment and immunotoxicological risk assessment, especially for simultaneous exposure to multiple agents ; (5) to design better human studies to assess the impact on the immune system in the species of the greatest interest in the context of risk assessment and (6) the better understanding of the role of genetic predisposition and susceptibility in identifying sensitive subpopulations to immune-altering agents (Kaminiski et al., 2008). These challenges are not unique to immunotoxicology, but they are critical, and need to be addressed through intensive and systematic efforts to improve human immune testing strategies.

8. Acknowledgment

The work was supported by EU grant, contract No. QLK4-CT-1999-01629-FIBRETOX; NIEHS grants of University of Iowa, Iowa, USA: IMUGENFIB, US NIH # 2 D43 TW00621-006 and NIEHS # 510 20 5240 00000 1 15010 9220; Hungarian-Slovak grants: NKFP-1/B-047/2004, OTKA 046733, ETT 154/2003-6 (Hungarian Medical Research Council), NILU internal grant 106170, EC FP7 [Health-2007-1.3-4, Contract no: 201335].

We would like to express our gratitude to Viera Vachalkova, Helena Turazova, Maria Valentova, Edita Mrvikova, Olga Liskova, Mikulas Krnac, Adriana Paulikova, Darina Cepcova, Jarmila Jantoskova and Lubica Mikloskova and for their excellent technical help.

This article was created by the realization of the project ITMS No.24240120033, based on the supporting Operational research and development program financed from the European Regional Development Fund.

9. References

Ada, K.; Turk, M.; Oguztuzun, S.; Kilic, M.; Demirel, M.; Tandogan, N.; Ersayar, E. & Latif, O. (2010). Cytotoxicity and apoptotic effects of nickel oxide nanoparticles in cultured HeLa cells. *Folia Histochem Cytobiol.* 2010 Dec;48(4):524-9, ISSN (printed): 0239-8508. ISSN (electronic): 1897-5631

Ahamed, M. (2011). Toxic response of nickel nanoparticles in human lung epithelial A549 cells. *Toxicol In Vitro.* 2011 Jun;25(4):930-6. Epub 2011 Mar 3, ISSN: 0887-2333

American Thoracic Society. (2004). Diagnosis and initial management of nonmalignant diseases related to asbestos. *Am J Respir Crit Care Med.* 2004, Vol.170, pp. 691-715, ISSN: 1073-449X

Aoshiba, K.; Tamaoki, J. & Nagai, A. (2001). Acute cigarette smoke exposure induces apoptosis of alveolar macrophages, *Am J Physiol Lung Cell Mol Physiol*, Vol.281, pp. 1392–1401, ISSN: 1040-0605

Ates, I.; Yucesoy, B.; Yucel, A.; Suzen, SH.; Karakas, Y. & Karakaya, A. (2011). Possible effect of gene polymorphisms on the release of TNFα and IL1 cytokines in coal workers' pneumoconiosis. *Exp Toxicol Pathol.* 2011 Jan;63(1-2):175-9. Epub 2009 Dec 11, ISSN: 0940-2993

Benford, DJ.; Hanley, AB.; Bottrill, K.; Oehlschlager, S.; Balls, M.; Branca, F.; Castegnaro, JJ.; Descotes, J.; Hemminiki, K.; Lindsay, D. & Schilter, B. (2000). Biomakers as predictive tools in toxicity testing. The report and recommendations of ECVAM Workshop 40, *ATLA*, pp. 119–131, ISSN: 0261-1929

Beňo, M.; Hurbánková, M.; Černá, S.; Dušinská, M.; Volkovová, M.; Staruchová, M.; Barančoková, M.; Kažimírová, A.; Kováčiková, Z.; Mikulecký, M. & Kyrtopoulos, AS. (2005). Multinucleate cells (MNC) as sensitive semiquantitative biomarkers of the toxic effect after experimental fibrous dust and cigarette smoke inhalation by rats, *Exp Toxicol Pathol.* Vol.57, No.1, pp. 77-87, ISSN: 0940-2993

Bernstein, DM. (2007). Synthetic vitreous fibers: a review toxicology, epidemiology and regulations, *Crit. Rev. Toxicol.*, Vol.37, No.10, pp. 839-86, ISSN: 1547-6898

Boffetta, P.; Saracci, R.; Andersen, A.; Bertazzi, PA.; Chang-Claude, J.; Cherrie, J.; Ferro, G.; Frentzel-Beyme, R.; Hansen, J.; Olsen, JH.; Plato, N.; Teppo, L.; Westerholm, P.; Winter, PD. & Zocchetti, C. (1997) Cancer mortality among man-made vitreous fibre production workers. *Epidemiology*, 8, 259–268, ISSN (printed): 1044-3983. ISSN (electronic): 1531-5487

Boor, P.; Casper, S.; Cele, P.; Hurbánková, M.; Beňo, M.; Heidland, A.; Amann, K. & Šebeková, K. (2009). Renal, vascular and cardiac fibrosis in rats exposed to passive smoking and industrial dust fibre amosite. *J. Cell. Mol. Med.* Vol Vol. 13, No 11-12, pp. 4484-4491, ISSN (printed): 1582-1838. ISSN (electronic): 1582-4934

Bottrill, K. (1998). The use of biomarkers as alternatives to current animal tests on food chemicals, *ATLA*, Vol.26 pp. 421–480, ISSN: 0261-1929

Branche, Ch. (2009). Asbestos fibers and other elongated mineral particles: State of the science and roadmap for research, *NIOSH Current Intelligence Bulletin*, pp. 1-129,

Brüske-Hohlfeld, I. (2009). Environmental and occupational risk factors for lung cancer. *Methods Mol Biol.* 2009;472:3-23, ISSN: 1064-3745

Bunderson-Schelvan, M.; Pfau, JC.; Crouch, R. & Holian, A. (2011). Non-pulmonary outcomes of asbestos exposure. *J Toxicol Environ Health B Crit Rev* 14:122–152, ISSN (printed): 1093-7404. ISSN (electronic): 1521-6950

Burchiel, SW.; Mitchell, LA.; Lauer, FT.; Sun, X.; McDonald, JD.; Hudson, LG. & Liu, KJ. (2009). Immunotoxicity and biodistribution analysis of arsenic trioxide in C57B1/6 mice following a two-week inhalation exposure. *Toxicol Appl Pharmacol.* 2009 December 15; 241(3): 253–259, ISSN (printed): 0041-008X. ISSN (electronic): 1096-0333

Carbonari, D.; Campopiano, A.; Ramires, D.; Strafella, E.; Staffolani, S.; Tomasetti, M.; Curini, R.; Valentino, M.; Santarelli, L. & Amati, M. (2011). Angiogenic effect induced by mineral fibres, *Toxicology*, Vol.288 No.1-3, pp. 34-42, ISSN: 0300-483X

Ciebiada, M.; Gorska-Ciebiada, M. & Gorski, P. (2011). sICAM and TNF-α in asthma and rhinitis: relationship with the presence of atopy. *J. Asthma*, Vol.48, No.7, pp. 660-666, ISSN 0022-1899

Černá, S.; Beňo, M.; Hurbánková, M.; Kováčiková, Z.; Bobek, P. & Kyrtopoulos, SA. (2004). Evaluation of Bronchoalveolar lavage fluid cytotoxic parameters after inhalation exposure to amosite and wollastonite fibrous dusts combined with cigarette smoke, *Cent Eur J Health.* 12 Suppl.: pp. 20-23, ISSN: 1210-7778.

Chauhan, V.; Howland, M.; Kutzner, B.; McNamee, JP.; Bellier, PV. & Wilkins, RC. (2011). Biological effects of alpha particle radiation exposure on human monocytic cells. *Int J Hyg Environ Health.* 2011 Dec 6. Epub ahead of print, ISSN: 1438-4639

Cho, WS.; Duffn, R.; Poland, CA.; Howie, SAM.; MacNee, W.; Bradley, M.; Megson, JL. & Ken Donaldson, K. (2010). Metal Oxide Nanoparticles Induce Unique Infammatory Footprints in the Lung: Important Implications for Nanoparticle Testing, *Environmental Health Perspectives*, 118, 12, December 2010, Epub 2008 Sep 17, ISSN: 0091-6765

Cho, WS.; Duffin, R.; Bradley, M.; Megson, IL.; Macnee, W.; Howie, SE. & Donaldson, K. (2011a). NiO and Co3O4 Nanoparticles Induce Lung DTH-Like Responses and Alveolar Lipoproteinosis. *Eur Respir J.* 2011 Aug 4. Epub ahead of print, ISSN (printed): 0903-1936. ISSN (electronic): 1399-3003

Cho, WS.; Duffin, R.; Howie, SEM.; Scotton, ChJ.; Wallace, WAH.; MacNee, W.; Bradley, M.; Megson, IL. & Donaldson, K. (2011b). Progressive severe lung injury by zinc oxide nanoparticles; the role of Zn2+ dissolution inside lysosomes, *Particle and Fibre Toxicology* 2011, 8:27, ISSN: 1743-8977

Committee for Proprietary Medicinal Products (2000) http://www.emea.eu.int/pdfs/human/swp/104299en.pdf

Corsini, E.; Luster, MI.; Mahler, J.; Craig, WA.; Blazka, ME. & Rosenthal, GJ. (1994). A protective role for T lymphocytes in asbestos-induced pulmonary inflammation and collagen deposition. *Am J Respir Cell Mol Biol.* 1994 Nov;11(5):531-9, ISSN: 1044-1549.

Costantini, LM.; Gilberti, RM. & Knecht, DA. (2011). The phagocytosis and toxicity of amorphous silica. *PLoS One.* 2011 Feb 2;6(2):e14647, ISSN: 1932-6203

D'Amato, G.; Liccardi, G.; D'Amato, M. & Holgate, S. (2005). Environmental risk factors and allergic bronchial asthma. *Clin Exp Allergy.* 2005 Sep;35(9):1113-24, ISSN: 0954-7894 (Print) 1365-2222 (Electronic) 0954-7894 (Linking)

Das, KK. & Buchner, V. (2007). Effect of nickel exposure on peripheral tissues: role of oxidative stress in toxicity and possible protection by ascorbic acid. *Rev Environ Health.* 2007 Apr-Jun;22(2):157-73. ISSN (printed): 0048-7554. ISSN (electronic): 2191-0308

De Rosa, CT.; Smith, LS.; Hicks, H.; Nickle, R. & Williams-Johnson M. (2002). The impact of toxicology on public health policy and service. In: Impact of Hazardous Chemicals on Public Health, Policy and Service, 556pp. De Rosa, CT; Holler, JS & Mehlman,

MA.(eds). In: *Advances in modern environmental toxicology*, vol. XXVI International Toxicology Books, Inc Princeton, New Jersey, ISSN:0748-2337 vol:19 issue:2

Descotes, J.; Choquet-Kastylevsky, G.; Van Ganse, E.; & Vial, T. (2000). Responses of the Immune System to Injury, *Toxicol. Pathol.*, Vol.28, pp. 479-481, ISSN (printed): 0192-6233; ISSN (electronic): 1533- 1601.

Descotes J. (2005). Immunotoxicology: role in the safety assessment of drugs. *Drug Saf.*, Vol.28, No.2, pp. 127-36, ISSN: 0114-5916

De Jong, W.H. & Van Loveren, H. (2007). Screening of xenobiotics for direct immunotoxicity in an animal study, *Methods*, Vol.41, Issue 1, pp. 3-8, ISSN (printed): 1046-2023. ISSN (electronic): 1095-9130

De Vuyst, P.; Dumortier, P.; Swaen, G.M.H.; Pairon, J.C. & Brochard, P. (1995). Respiratory health effects of man-made vitreous (mineral) fibres, *Eur Respir J*, Vol.8, pp. 2149–2173, ISSN 0903 - 1936

Dietert, RR. & Holsapple, MP. (2007). Methodologies for developmental immunotoxicity (DIT) testing. *Methods* 41:123-131, ISSN: 1046-2023

Di Giampaolo, L.; Quecchia, C.; Schiavone, C.; Cavallucci, E.; Renzetti, A.; Braga, M. & Di Gioacchino, M. (2011) Environmental pollution and asthma. *Int J Immunopathol Pharmacol.* 2011 Jan-Mar;24(1 Suppl):31S-38S. Review, ISSN: 0394-6320 (Print) 0394-6320 (Linking)

Doll, NJ.; Diem, JE.; Jones, RN.; Rodriguez, M.; Bozelka, BE.; Stankus, RP.; Weill, H. & Salvaggio JE. (1983). Humoral immunological abnormalities in workers exposed to asbestos cement dust, *J Allergy Clin Immunol*, Vol.72, pp. 509-512, ISSN: 0091- 6749

Donald, E.; & Gardner, I. (2006). Toxicology of the Lung., Taylor & Francis Group, USA, 2006: 681 s., ISBN 0-8493-2835-7

Donaldson, K & Tran, L. (2004). An introduction to the short-term toxicology of respirable industrial fibres, *Mutation Research/Fundamental and Molecular Mechanisms of Mutagenesis*, Volume 553, Issues 1-2, 3 September 2004, Pages 5-9, ISSN 1386-1964

Duramad, P. & Holland, N.T. (2011). Biomarkers of Immunotoxicity for Environmental and Public Health Research, *Int. J. Environ. Res. Public Health*, Vol.8, pp. 1388-1401, ISSN 1660-4601

Dusinska, M.; Collins, A.; Kazimírová, A.; Barancoková, M.; Harrington, V.; Volkovová, K,.; Staruchová, M.; Horská, A.; Wsólová, L.; Kocan, A.; Petrík, J.; Machata, M.; Ratcliffe, B. & Kyrtopoulos, S. (2004). Genotoxic effects of asbestos in humans. *Mutat Res.* 2004 Sep 3;553(1-2):91-102, ISSN: 0027-5107

Dziedzic, D.; Wheeler, C.S. & Gross, K.B., (1993). Bronchoalveolar lavage: detecting markers of lung injury, in: *Handbook of Hazardous Materials.* New York: Academic Press. pp. 99-111, ISBN: 012189410X 9780121894108

Elder, AC.; Gelein, R.; Azadniv, M.; Frampton, M.; Finkelstein, J. & Oberdorster G. (2004) Systemic effects of inhaled ultrafine particles in two compromised, aged rat strains. *Inhal Toxicol.* 16, 461-71, ISSN: 8750-7587

Food and Drug Administration, Washington, USA (2004). http://www.fda.gov/cder/guidance/6636dft.htm

Froom, P.; Lahat, N.; Kristal-Boneh, E.; Cohen, C.; Lerman, Y. & Ribak, J. (2000). Circulating natural killer cells in retired asbestos cement workers, *J. Occup. Environ. Med.*, Vol.2, No.1, pp. 19-24, ISSN 1076-2752

Fujita, K.; Morimoto, Y.; Ogami, A.; Myojyo, T.; Tanaka, I.; Shimada, M.; Wang, WN.; Endoh, S.; Uchida, K.; Nakazato, T.; Yamamoto, K.; Fukui, H.; Horie, M.; Yoshida, Y.; Iwahashi, H. & Nakanishi, J. (2009). Gene expression profiles in rat lung after inhalation exposure to C60 fullerene particles. *Toxicology*. 2009 Apr 5;258(1):47-55. Epub 2009 Jan 9, ISSN: 0300-483X (Print), 1879-3185 (Electronic)

Gillissen, A.; Gessner, C.; Hammerschmidt, S.; Hoheisel, G & Wirtz, H. (2006). [Health significance of inhaled particles] *Dtsch Med Wochenschr*. 2006 Mar 24;131(12):639-44, ISSN: 0012-0472

Garcia-Garcia, E. (2005). Diversity in PhagocyticSignaling: A Story of Greed, Sharing and Exploitation, In book: *Molecular mechanisms of phagocytosis*, pp.1-154, Springer, ISBN: 1423724070 9781423724070

Garcia-Garcia, E. & Rosales, C. (2005). Adding Complexity to Phagocytic Signaling: Phagocytosis-Associated Cell Response and Phagocytic Efficiency, In book: *Molecular mechanisms of phagocytosis*, pp.1-154, Springer, ISBN:1423724070 9781423724070,

Gaumer, HR.; Doll, NJ.; Kaima, J.; Schuyler, M. & Salvaggio, JE. (1981). Diminished suppressor cell function in patients with asbestosis. *Clin. Exp. Immunol.*, Vol.44, No.1, pp. 108-116, ISSN 0009-9104

Gopinath, C. (1996). Pathology of toxic effects on the immune system. *Inflamm Res* 45(suppl 2): S74-S78, ISSN: 1023-3830

Governa, M.; Amati, M.; Valentino, M.; Visona, I.; Fubini, B ; Botta, GC. ; Volpe, AR. & Carmignani, M. (2000). *In vitro* cleavage by asbestos fibers of the fifth component of human complement through free-radical generation and kallikrein activation, *J. Toxicol. Environ. Health A.*, Vol.59, No.7, pp. 539-52, ISSN:1528-7394

Greim, H.; Borm, P.; Schins, R.; Donaldson, K.; Driscoll, K.; Hartwig, A.; Kuempel, E.; Oberdorster, G. & Speit, G. (2001). Toxicity of fibers and particles. Report of the workshop held in Munich, Germany, 26–27 October, 2000. *Inhal Toxicol* 2001;13:737–54, ISSN: 0895-8378 print

Haley, PJ.; Shopp, GM.; Benson, JM.; Cheng, YS.; Bice, DE.; Luster, MI.; Dunnick, JK. & Hobbs, CH. (1990). The immunotoxicity of three nickel compounds following 13-week inhalation exposure in the mouse. *Fundam Appl Toxicol*. 1990 Oct;15(3):476-87, ISSN: 0272-0590

Haley, P.; Perry, R.; Ennulat, D.; Frame, S.; Johnson, C.; Lapointe, J.M.; Nyska, A.; Snyder, P.W.; Walker, D. & Walter, G. (2005). *Toxicol. Pathol.*, Vol.33, pp. 404–407, ISSN: 0192-6233 print

Hazenbos, WLW. & Brown, EJ. (2006). Phagocytosis: receptors and biology, in book Phagocytosis of Bacteria and Bacterial Pathogenicity, *Ernst JD. & Stendahl O., (September 2006), Cambridge University Press, New York, ISBN 9780511242977*

He, X.; Young, SH.; Schwegler-Berry, D.; Chisholm, WP.; Fernback, JE. & Ma, Q. (2011). Multiwalled Carbon Nanotubes Induce a Fibrogenic Response by Stimulating Reactive Oxygen Species Production, Activating NF-κB Signaling, and Promoting Fibroblast-to-Myofibroblast Transformation. *Chem Res Toxicol*. 2011 Nov 22. Epub ahead of print, ISSN (printed): 0893-228X. ISSN (electronic): 1520-5010

Hess, E.V. (2002). Environmental chemicals and autoimmune disease: cause and effect, *Toxicology* Vol.181–182, pp. 65–70, ISSN: 0300-483X.

Hoet, P.H.M.; Lewis, C.P.L.; Demedts, M. & Nemery, B. (1994). Putrescine and paraquast uptake in human slices and isolated type II pneumocytes, *Biochem. Pharmacol.*, Vol.48, pp. 517-524, ISSN 0006-2952

Horie, M.; Nishio, K.; Fujita, K.; Kato, H.; Nakamura, A.; Kinugasa, S.; Endoh, S.; Miyauchi, A.; Yamamoto, K.; Murayama, H.; Niki, E.; Iwahashi, H.; Yoshida, Y. & Nakanishi, J. (2009). Ultrafine NiO particles induce cytotoxicity *in vitro* by cellular uptake and subsequent Ni(II) release. *Chem Res Toxicol.* 2009 Aug;22(8):1415-26, ISSN (printed): 0893-228X. ISSN (electronic): 1520-5010

Horie, M.; Fukui, H.; Nishio, K.; Endoh, S.; Kato, H.; Fujita, K.; Miyauchi, A.; Nakamura, A.; Shichiri, M.; Ishida, N.; Kinugasa, S.; Morimoto, Y.; Niki, E.; Yoshida, Y. & Iwahashi, H. (2011). Evaluation of acute oxidative stress induced by NiO nanoparticles *in vivo* and *in vitro*. *J Occup Health.* 2011;53(2):64-74. Epub 2011 Jan 11, ISSN: 1341-0725

Horská, A.; Kazimírová, A.; Barancoková, M.; Wsólová.; L, Tulinská, J. & Dusinská, M. (2006). Genetic predisposition and health effect of occupational exposure to asbestos. *Neuro Endocrinol Lett.* 2006 Dec;27 Suppl 2:100-3, ISSN: 1478-4491

Huaux, F. (2007). New developments in the understanding of immunology in silicosis. *Curr Opin Allergy Clin Immunol.* 2007 Apr;7(2):168-73, ISSN (printed): 1528-4050. ISSN (electronic): 1473-6322

Hurbánková, M. & Kaiglová, A. (1999). Compared effects of asbestos and wollastonite fibrous dusts on various biological parameters measured in bronchoalveolar lavage fluid, *J Trace Microprobe Techn.*, 17, pp. 233-43, ISSN: 0272-9172

Hurbánková, M.; Cerná, S.; Gergelová, P. & Wimmerová, S. (2005). Influence of refractory ceramic fibres - asbestos substitute - on the selected parameters of bronchoalveolar lavage 6 months after intratracheal instillation to W-rats, *Biomed Pap Med Fac, Univ Palacky Olomouc Czech Repub.*, Vol.149, No.2, pp. 367-71, ISSN: 2005-6745

Hurbánková, M.; Cerna, S.; Beno, M.; Tatrai, E.; Wimmerova, S. & Kovacikova, Z. (2010). The combined effect of refractory ceramic fibers and smoking in terms of selected inflammatory and cytotoxic parameters of bronchoalveolar lavage and histological findings in the experiment [Kombinovaný účinok keramických vlákien a fajčenia z hľadiska vybraných zápalových a cytotoxických parametrov bronchoalveolárnej laváže a histologických nálezov v experimente]. *Pracovní Lékařství.*, Vol. 62, 2010, No. 3, p. 102–108. ISSN: 0032-6291

IARC. (2002). Man-made Vitreous Fibres, Summary of Data Reported and Evaluation; *IARC Monographs on the Evaluation of Carcinogenic Risks to Humans*, WHO, Lyon, France, Vol.81: pp. 403, ISBN 92-832-1281-9, http://monographs.iarc.fr/ENG/Monographs/vol81/volume81.pdf

IARC. (2004). Tobacco Smoke and Involuntary Smoking. *IARC Monographs on the Evaluation of Carcinogenic Risks to Humans*, WHO, Lyon, France, Vol.83: pp. 1452, ISBN 92-832-1283-5, http://monographs.iarc.fr/ENG/Monographs/vol83/mono83.pdf

ICICIS (1998). *Toxicology*, Vol.125, pp. 183–201. ISSN: 0300-483X.

Ilavska, S.; Jahnova, E.; Tulinska, J.; Horvathova, M.; Dusinska, M.; Wsolova, L.; Kyrtopoulos, S.A. & Fuortes, L. (2005). Immunological monitoring in workers occupationally exposed to asbestos, *Toxicol.*, Vol.206, pp. 299-308, ISSN: 0300-483X

Inoue, KI. & Takano, H. (2011). Aggravating Impact of Nanoparticles on Immune-Mediated Pulmonary Inflammation, *TheScientificWorldJOURNAL* (2011) 11, 382–390 Special Issue: Nanoparticles and Inflammation, ISSN: 1537-744X

IPCS/WHO, 1999 IPCS/WHO, Environmental health criteria, No. 210. Principles for the Assessment of Risks to Human Health from Exposure to Chemicals, (1999), pp. 7–10, ISSN 0250-863X

Ishihara, Y.; Nagai, A. & Kagawa, J. (1997). Comparison of the effect of exposure to filter cigarette and nonfilter cigarette smoke in rat bronchoalveolar lavage fluid and blood: the antioxidant balance and protease-antiprotease balance *in vivo, Inhal Toxicol.* Vol.9, pp. 273-86, ISSN (printed): 0895-8378.

Jacobsen, NR.; Møller, P.; Jensen, KA.; Vogel, U.; Ladefoged, O.; Loft, S. & Wallin, H. (2009). Lung inflammation and genotoxicity following pulmonary exposure to nanoparticles in ApoE-/- mice. *Part Fibre Toxicol.* 2009 Jan 12;6:2, 1-17, ISSN: 1743-8977

Jaurand, M.C. (1997). Mechanisms of fiber-induced genotoxicity, *Environmental Health Perspectives*, Vol.105, suppl. 5, pp. 1073–1084, ISSN: 1082-6076

Johansson, A.; Lundborg, M.; Sköld, C.M.; Lundahl, J.; Tornling, G.; Eklund, A. & Camner, P. (1997). Functional, morphological, and phenotypical differences between rat alveolar and interstitial macrophages, *Am. J. Respir. Cell Mol. Biol.*, Vol.16, pp. 582–588, Print ISSN: 0741-5400; Online ISSN: 1938-3673.

Kagan, E.; Solomon, A.; Cochrane, JC.; Kuba, P.; Rocks, PH. & Webster, I. (1977). Immunological studies of patients with asbestosis. II. Studies of circulating lymphoid cell numbers and humoral immunity. Clin. Exp. Immunol., Vol.28, No.2, pp. 268-275 ISSN 0271-9142

Kaminski, NE.; Kaplan, BLFK. & Holsapple, MP. (2008). Toxic response of the immune system, pp.485-555, In: Klaassen, CD. *Casarett and Doull's Toxicology - The Basic Science of Poisons* (7th Edition). 2008 McGraw-Hill, USA, ISBN-13: 978-0-07-147051-3, ISBN-10: 0-07-147051-4

Kohyama, N.; Tanaka, I.; Tomita, M.; Kudo, M. & Shinohara, Y. (1997). Preparation and characteristics of standard reference samples of fibrous minerals for biological experiments. *Ind Health* 35, 415–32, ISSN: 0895-8378 print 11091-7691

Kristovich, R.; Knight, DA.; Long, JF.; Williams, MV.; Dutta, PK. & Waldman WJ. (2004). Macrophage-Mediated Endothelial Inflammatory Responses to Airborne Particulates: Impact of Particulate Physicochemical Properties, *Chem. Res. Toxicol.*, Vol.17, No.10, pp. 1303-1312, ISSN: 0893-228X (Print) 1520-5010 (Electronic) 0893-228X (Linking)

Kumagai-Takei, N.; Maeda, M.; Chen, Y.; Matsuzaki, H.; Lee, S.; Nishimura, Y.; Hiratsuka, J. & Otsuki, T. (2011). Asbestos Induces Reduction of Tumor Immunity, *Clinical and Developmental Immunology*, Volume 2011, Article ID 481439, 9 pages, doi:10.1155/2011/481439, ISSN: 17402522

Kuper, C.F.; De Heer, E.; Van Loveren, H.; Vos, J.G.; Haschek, W.; Rousseaux, C.G. & Wallig, M.A. (2002). Editors Handbook of Toxicologic Pathology, vol. 2 (2nd ed.), *Academic Press*, San Diego pp. 585–646. ISSN: 0192-6233

Lankveld, DP.; Van Loveren, H.; Baken, KA. & Vandebriel, RJ. (2010). *In vitro* testing for direct immunotoxicity: state of the art. *Methods Mol Biol.* 2010;598:401-23, ISSN: 0022-3042

Lightfoot, NE.; Pacey, MA. & Darling, S. (2010). Gold, nickel and copper mining and processing. *Chronic Dis Can.* 2010;29(Suppl 2):101-24, ISSN: 0228-8699 (Print), 1481-8523 (Electronic)

Liu, F.; Liu, L.; Weng, D.; Chen, Y.; Song, L.; He, Q. & Chen, J. (2010). CD4+CD25+Foxp3+ Regulatory T Cells Depletion May Attenuate the Development of Silica-Induced Lung Fibrosis in Mice, *PLoS One.* 2010; 5(11): e15404, Published online 2010 November 3, ISSN: 1932-6203

Lovik, M.; Hogseth, AK.; Gaarder, PI.; Hagemann, R. & Eide, I. (2003). Diesel exhaust particles and carbon black have adjuvant activity on the local lymph node response and systemic IgE production to ovalbumin. *Eur Respir J* Suppl. 46, 5s-13s, ISSN 1529-7322

Lucarelli, M.; Gatti, A.M.; Savarino, G.; Quattroni, P.; Martinelli, L.; Monari, E. & Boraschi, D. (2004). Innate defence functions of macrophages can be biased by nano-sized ceramic and metallic particles. *Eur Cytokine Netw.*, Vol.15, No. 4,pp. 339-46, ISBN 10 : 2-89631-027-4, ISSN : 0820-8395

Luster,M.; Ackermann, M.F.; Germolec, D.R. & Rosenthal G.J. (1989). Perturbations of the Immune System by Xenobiotics, Environmental Health Perspectives, Vol.81, pp. 157-162, ISSN: 0091-6765.

Manning, CB.; Vallyathan, V. & Mossman, BT. (2002). Diseases caused by asbestos: mechanisms of injury and disease development. *Int. Immunopharmacol*, Vol.2, No.2-3, 191-200, ISSN: 1567-5769.

Marsh, GM.; Buchanich, JM. & Youk, AO. (2001). Historical cohort study of US man-made vitreous fiber production workers: VI. Respiratory system cancer standardized mortality ratios adjusted for the confounding effect of cigarette smoking. *J Occup Environ Med.* 2001 Sep;43(9):803-8, ISSN: 1076-2752

Martin, AK.; Mack, DG.; Falta, MT., Mroz, MM.; Newman, LS.; Maier, LA. & Fontenot, AP. (2011). Beryllium-specific CD4+ T cells in blood as a biomarker of disease progression. *J Allergy Clin Immunol.* 2011 Nov;128(5):1100-6.e1-5. Epub 2011 Sep 23, ISSN (printed): 0091-6749. ISSN (electronic): 1097-6825

Mascagni, P.; Corsini, E;. Pettazzoni, M.; Baj, A.; Feltrin, G.; Ferraioli, E. & Toffoletto, F. (2003). [Determination of interleukin-8 in induced sputum of workers exposed to low concentrations of asbestos]. *G Ital Med Lav Ergon.* 2003 Jul-Sep;25 Suppl(3):137, ISSN 0022-3166

Matthews, JB.; Green, TR.; Stone, MH.; Wroblewski, BM.; Fisher, J. & Inghani E. (2000). Comparison of the response of primary human peripheral blood mononuclear phagocytes from different donors to challenge with model polyethylene particles of known size and dose. *Biomaterials*, Vol.21, pp. 2033-44, ISSN: 0142-9612.

Mikulski, MA.; Leonard, SA.; Sanderson, WT.; Hartley, PG.; Sprince, NL. & Fuortes, LJ. (2011). Risk of beryllium sensitization in a low-exposed former nuclear weapons cohort from the Cold War era. *Am J Ind Med.* 2011 Mar;54(3):194-204. Epub 2010 Oct 28, ISSN (printed): 0271-3586. ISSN (electronic): 1097-0274

Mitschik, S.; Schierl, R.; Nowak, D. & Jörres, RA. (2008).Effects of particulate matter on cytokine production *in vitro*: a comparative analysis of published studies. Inhal. Toxicol., Vol.20, No.4, pp. 399- 414, ISSN (printed): 0895-8378

Montero, MA.; de Gracia, J. & Morell, F. (2010). Hard Metal Interstitial Lung Disease, *Arch Bronconeumol.* 2010;46(9):489-491, ISSN: 0300-2896 (Print), 1579-2129 (Electronic)

Morimoto, Y. & Tanaka, I. (2001). *In vivo* studies of man-made mineral fibers -fibrosis-related factors, *Ind Health.*, Vol.39, pp. 106-13, ISSN (printed): 0019-8366.

Morimoto, Y.; Ogami, A.; Todoroki, M.; Yamamoto, M.; Murakami, M.; Hirohashi, M.; Oyabu, T.; Myojo, T.; Nishi, K.; Kadoya, C, Yamasaki, S, Nagatomo, H, Fujita, K, Endoh, S, Uchida, K, Yamamoto, K, Kobayashi, N, Nakanishi, J. & Tanaka, I. (2010). Expression of inflammation-related cytokines following intratracheal instillation of nickel oxide nanoparticles. *Nanotoxicology.* 2010 Jun;4(2):161-76, ISSN (printed): 1743-5390. ISSN (electronic): 1743-5404

Morimoto, Y.; Oyabu, T.; Ogami, A.; Myojo, T.; Kuroda, E.; Hirohashi, M.; Shimada, M.; Lenggoro, W.; Okuyama, K. & Tanaka, I. (2011). Investigation of gene expression of MMP-2 and TIMP-2 mRNA in rat lung in inhaled nickel oxide and titanium dioxide nanoparticles. *Ind Health.* 2011;49(3):344-52, Epub 2011 Mar 1, ISSN (printed): 0019-8366. ISSN (electronic): 1880-8026

Mossman, BT.; Kamp, DW. & Weitzman, SA. (1996). Mechanisms of carcinogenesis and clinical features of asbestos-associated cancers, *Cancer Investigation*, Vol.14, No.5, pp. 466–480, ISSN (printed): 0735-7907.

Mossman, BT. & Churg, A. (1998). Mechanisms in the pathogenesis of asbetosis and silicosis. *Am. J. Respir. Crit. Care Med.*, Vol.157, pp. 1666–1680, ISSN (printed): 1073-449X

Mossman, BT.; Lippmann, M.; Hesterberg, TW.; Kelsey, KT.; Barchowsky, A. & Bonner, JC. (2011). Pulmonary endpoints (lung carcinomas and asbestosis) following inhalation exposure to asbestos. *J Toxicol Environ Health B Crit Rev* 14:76–121, ISSN (printed): 1093-7404. ISSN (electronic): 1521-6950

Moulin, JJ.; Mur, JM.; Wild, P.; Perreaux, JP. & Pham, QT. (1986) Oral cavity and laryngeal cancers among man-made mineral fiber production workers. *Scand. J. Work Environ. Health*, 12, 27–31, ISSN: 0355-3140

National Research Council. (1992) Subcommittee on Immunotoxicology, Committee on Biologic Markers, Board on Environmental Studies and Toxicology, National Research Council, Biologic Markers in Immunotoxicology, NATIONAL ACADEMY PRESS, Washington, D.C., 1992, ISBN-13: 978-0-309-04389-2

National Toxicology Program. (2009). Final report on carcinogens background document for glass wool fibers. *Rep Carcinog Backgr Doc.* 2009 Sep;(9-5980):i-280, ISSN: 2151-7746 (Print); 2151-3805 (Electronic); 2151-3805 (Linking)

Nelson, HH. & Kelsey, KT. (2002). The molecular epidemiology of asbestos and tobacco in lung cancer, *Oncogene*, Vol.21, 48, pp. 7284-7288, ISSN: 0950-9232.

Nishi, K.; Morimoto, Y.; Ogami, A.; Murakami, M.; Myojo, T.; Oyabu, T.; Kadoya, C.; Yamamoto, M.; Todoroki, M.; Hirohashi, M.; Yamasaki, S.; Fujita, K.; Endo, S.; Uchida, K.; Yamamoto, K.; Nakanishi, J. & Tanaka, I. (2009). Expression of cytokine-induced neutrophil chemoattractant in rat lungs by intratracheal instillation of nickel oxide nanoparticles. *Inhal Toxicol.* 2009 Oct;21(12):1030-9, ISSN (printed): 0895-8378, ISSN (electronic): 1091-7691

Nkamgueu, EM.; Adnet, JJ.; Bernard, J.; Zierold, K.; Kilian, L.; Jallot, E.; Benhayoune, H.; Bonhomme, P. (2000). *In vitro* effects of zirconia and alumina particles on human blood monocyte-derived macrophages: X-ray microanalysis and flow cytometric studies. *J Biomed Mater Res.* 2000 Dec 15;52(4):587-94, ISSN (printed): 0021-9304.

Nymark, P.; Wikman, H.; Hienonen-Kempas, T. & Anttila, S. (2008). Molecular and genetic changes in asbestos-related lung cancer, *Cancer Letters*, Vol. 265, No. 1, pp. 1–15, ISSN: 0304-3835.

Oberdorster, G. (1994). Macrophage-associated responses to chrysotile, *Ann Occup Hyg.*, Vol.38, No.4, pp. 601-15, 421-2, ISSN (printed): 0003-4878.

Ogami, A.; Morimoto, Y.; Myojo, T.; Oyabu, T.; Murakami, M.; Todoroki, M.; Nishi, K.; Kadoya, C.; Yamamoto, M. & Tanaka I. (2009). Pathological features of different sizes of nickel oxide following intratracheal instillation in rats. *Inhal Toxicol.* 2009 Aug;21(10):812-8, ISSN (printed): 0895-8378.

Oostingh, GJ.; Casals, E.; Italiani, P.; Colognato, R.; Stritzinger, R.; Ponti, J.; Pfaller, T.; Kohl, Y.; Ooms, D.; Favilli, F.; Leppens, H.; Lucchesi, D.; Rossi, F.; Nelissen, I.; Thielecke, H.; Puntes, VF.; Dusch A. & Boraschi, D. (2011). Problems and challenges in the development and validation of human cell-based assays to determine nanoparticle-induced immunomodulatory effects. *Particle and Fibre Toxicology* (9 February 2011), 8:8, pp. 1-21, ISSN:1743-8977

Osinubi, OYO.; Gochfeld, M. & Kipen, HM., (2000). Health effects of asbestos and nonasbestos fibers. *Environ Health Perspect*, Vol.108, (Supp.4), pp. 665-674, ISSN: 1078-0475.

Otsuki, T.; Maeda, M.; Murakami, S.; Hayashi, H.; Miura, Y.; Kusaka, M.; Nakano,T.; Fukuoka,K ; Kishimoto, T.; Hyodoh, F.; Ueki, A. & Nishimura, Y. (2007). Immunological effects of silica and asbestos. *Cell. Mol. Immunology*, Vol.4, No.4, pp. 261-268, ISSN: 1672-7681.

Oudijk, EJ.; Lammers, JW. & Koenderman, L. (2003). Systemic inflammation in chronic obstructive pulmonary disease. *Eur Respir J Suppl.* 46, 5s-13s, ISSN: 0904-1850.

Ozesmi, M.; Hillerdal, G.; Karlsson-parra, A. & Forsum, U. (1988). Phenotypes of peripheral blood lymphoid cells in patients with asbestos-related pleural lesions. *Eur. Respir J.*, Vol.1, No.10, pp. 938-942, ISSN (printed): 0903-1936.

Panizza, C.; Bai, E.; Oddone, E.; Scaburri, A.; Massari, S.; Modonesi, C.; Contiero, P.; Marinaccio, A. & Crosignani, P. (2011). Lung cancer risk in the electroplating industry in Lombardy, Italy, using the Italian occupational cancer monitoring (OCCAM) information system. *Am J Ind Med.* 2011 Sep 14. doi: 10.1002/ajim.21004. [Epub ahead of print], ISSN (printed): 0271-3586. ISSN (electronic): 1097-0274

Pietruska, JR.; Liu, X.; Smith, A.; McNeil, K.; Weston, P.; Zhitkovich, A.; Hurt, R. & Kane, AB. (2011). Bioavailability, intracellular mobilization of nickel, and HIF-1α activation in human lung epithelial cells exposed to metallic nickel and nickel oxide nanoparticles. *Toxicol Sci.* 2011 Nov;124(1):138-48. Epub 2011 Aug 9, ISSN:1096-6080 (Print)1096-0929 (Electronic)

Rabinovitch, M. (1995). Professional and non-professional phagocytes: an introduction, *Trends in Cell Biology*, 5, 85-87, ISSN: 0962-8924

Richards, RJ.; Davies, N.; Atkins, J. & Oreffo, VIC. (1987). Isolation, biochemical characterization and culture of lung epithelial cell of the rat. *Lung*, Vol.165, pp. 143-158, ISSN (printed): 0341-2040.

Rom, WN.; Weiden, M.; Garcia, R.; Yie, TA.; Vathesatogkit, P.; Tse, DB.; McGuinness, G.; Roggli, V. & Prezant, D. (2002). Acute eosinophilic pneumonia in a New York City firefighter exposed to World Trade Center dust. *Am. J. Respir. Crit. Care Med.*, Vol.166, No.6, pp. 797-800, ISSN (printed): 1073-449X.

Rosenthal, GJ.; Corsini, E. & Simeonova, E. (1998). Selected New Developments in Asbestos Immunotoxicity, *Environ Health Perspect*, Vol.106 (Suppl 1), pp. 159-169, Available from http://ehpnetl.niehs.nih.gov/docs/1998/Suppl-1/159-169rosenthal/abstract.html ISSN: 1078-0475.

Rosenthal, G.J.; Simeonova, P. & Corsini, E. (1999) Asbestos toxicity: An immunologic perspective, *Rev. Environ. Health*, Vol.14, No.1, pp. 11-20, ISSN (printed): 0048-7554.

Ruehl-Fehlert, C.; Bradley, A.; George, C.; Germann, P.G.; Bolliger, A.P. & Schulte, A. (2005). Harmonization of immunotoxicity guidelines in the ICH process--pathology considerations from the guideline Committee of the European Society of Toxicological Pathology (ESTP) . *Exp. Toxicol. Pathol.*, Vol.57, pp. 1–5, ISSN: 0940-2993.

Sabo-Attwood, T.; Ramos-Nino, M.; Bond, J.; Butnor, KJ.; Heintz, N.; Gruber, AD.; Steele, C.; Taatjes, DJ.; Vacek, P. & Mossman, BT. (2005). Gene expression profiles reveal increased mClca3 (Gob5) expression and mucin production in a murine model of asbestos-induced fibrogenesis. *Am. J. Pathol.*, Vol.167, No.5, pp. 1243-56, ISSN (printed): 0002-9440.

Schenker, MB; Pinkerton, KE.; Mitchell, D.; Vallyathan, V.; Elvine-Kreis, B. & Green, FHY. (2009). Pneumoconiosis from Agricultural Dust Exposure among Young California Farmworkers. *Environmental Health Perspectives* 117, 6, June 2009, ISSN: 0091-6765

Shannon, H.; Muir, A.; Haines, T. & Verma, D. (2005). Mortality and cancer incidence in Ontario glass fiber workers. *Occup Med (Lond).* 2005 Oct;55(7):528-34, ISSN (printed): 0962-7480. ISSN (electronic): 1471-8405

Shukla, A.; Lounsbury, KM.; Barrett, TF.; Gell, J.; Rincon, M.; Butnor, KJ.; Taatjes, DJ.; Davis, GS.; Vacek, P.; Nakayama, KI.; Nakayama, K.; Steele, C. & Mossman, BT. (2007). Asbestos-induced peribronchiolar cell proliferation and cytokine production are attenuated -oslabene-in lungs of protein kinase C-delta knockout mice. *Am. J. Pathol.*, Vol.170, No.1, pp. 140-51, ISSN (printed): 0002-9440.

Schuurman, HJ; Kuper CF. & Vos JG. (1994). Histopathology of the immune system as a tool to assess immunotoxicity. *Toxicology* 86:187–212, ISSN: 0300-483X.

Simeonova, PP. & Luster, MI. (1996). Asbestos induction of nuclear transcription factors and interleukin 8 gene regulation. *Am. J. Respir. Cell. Mol. Biol.* Vol.15, No.6, pp. 787–795, ISSN: 1044-1549.

Sjörstrand, M.; Rylander, R. & Bergström, R. (1989). Lung cell reactions in guinea pigs after inhalation of asbestos (amosite), *Toxicology*, Vol.57. pp. 1-14, ISSN: 0300-483X.

Song, Y. & Tang, S. (2011). Nanoexposure, Unusual Diseases, and New Health and Safety Concerns, *TheScientificWorldJOURNAL* (2011) 11, 1821–1828, ISSN: 1537-744X

Sood, A. (2009). Current Treatment of Chronic Beryllium Disease, *J Occup Environ Hyg*. 2009 December ; 6(12): 762–765, ISSN (printed): 1545-9624. ISSN (electronic): 1545-9632

Spiegelberg, T.; Kördel, W. & Hochrainer, D. (1984). Effects of NiO inhalation on alveolar macrophages and the humoral immune systems of rats. *Ecotoxicol Environ Saf*. 1984 Dec;8(6):516-25, ISSN: 0147-6513

Staruchova, M.; Collins, AR.; Volkovova, K.; Mislanová, C.; Kovacikova, Z.; Tulinska, J.; Kocan.; A, Staruch, L.; Wsolova, L. & Dusinska, M. (2008). Occupational exposure to mineral fibres. Biomarkers of oxidative damage and antioxidant defence and associations with DNA damage and repair. *Mutagenesis*. 2008 Jul;23(4):249-60, Epub 2008 Feb 14, ISSN (printed): 0267-8357

Tátrai, E.; Ungváry, G. & Adamis, Z. (1994). On the structural differences in the membranes between ciliated bronchial and non-ciliated lymphoepithelium in rats. *Eur. J. Histochem*. Vol.38, pp. 59-64, ISSN (printed): 1121-760X.

Tátrai, E.; Kováčiková, Z.; Brózik, M. & Six, E. (2004). Pulomary toxicity of wollastonite *in vivo* and *in vitro*. *J. Appl. Toxicol.*, Vol.24, pp. 147-154, ISSN: 1099-1263

Tátrai, E.; Brózik, M.; Drahos, A.; Kováčiková, Z.; Six, E.; Csík, M. & Dam, A. (2006a). The effect of stone-wool on rat lungs and on the primary culture of rat alveolar macrophages and type II pneumocytes. *J. Appl. Toxicol*. Vol.26, pp. 16-24, ISSN: 1099-1263

Tátrai, E.; Kováčiková, Z.; Brózik, M.; Six, E.; Csík, M.; Drahos, A. & Dam, A. (2006b). The influence of refractory ceramic fibres on pulmonary morphology, redox and immune system in rats, *J. Appl. Toxicol*, Vol.26, pp. 500-508, ISSN: 1099-1263

Topinka, J.; Loli, P.; Georgiadis, P.; Dusinská, M.; Hurbánková, M.; Kovácikovà, Z.; Volkovová, K.; Kazimírová, A.; Barancokovà, M.; Tatrai, E.; Oesterle, D.; Wolff, T. & Kyrtopoulos, SA. (2004). Mutagenesis by asbestos in the lung of lambda-lacI transgenic rats. *Mutat Res*. 2004 Sep 3;553(1-2):67-78, ISSN: 1383-5718

Topinka, J.; Loli, P.; Dusinská, M.; Hurbánková, M.; Kovácikovà, Z.; Volkovová, K.; Kazimírová, A.; Barancokovà, M.; Tatrai, E.; Wolff, T.; Oesterle, D.; Kyrtopoulos, SA. & Georgiadis, P. (2006). Mutagenesis by man-made mineral fibres in the lung of rats. *Mutat Res*. 2006 Mar 20;595(1-2):174-83, ISSN: 1383-5718

Toyokuni, S. (2009a). Mechanisms of asbestos-induced carcinogenesis, *Nagoya Journal of Medical Science*, Vol.71, No.1-2, pp. 1- 10. ISSN: 0027-7622.

Toyokuni, S. (2009b). Role of iron in carcinogenesis: cancer as a ferrotoxic disease, *Cancer Science*, Vol.100, No.1, pp. 9–16, ISSN (printed): 1347-9032.

Tsuda, T.; Morimoto, Y.; Yamato, H.; Nakamura, H.; Hori, H.; Nagata, N.; Kido, M.; Higashi, T. & Tanaka, I. (1997). Effects of Mineral Fibers on the Expression of Genes Whose Product May Play a Role in Fiber Pathogenesis, *Environ Health Perspect*, Vol.105(Suppl 5), pp.1173-1178, ISSN: 1078-0475.

Tsang, PH.; Chu, FN.; Fischbein, A. & Bekesi, JG. (1988). Impairments in functional subsets of T-suppressor (CD8) lymphocytes, monocytes, and natural killer cells among asbestos-exposed workers. *Clin. Immunol. Immunopathol.*, Vol.47. No.3, pp. 323-32, ISSN: 0090-1229.

Tulinska, J.; Jahnova, E.; Dusinska, M.; Kuricova, M.; Liskova, A.; Ilavska, S.; Horvathova, M.; Wsolova, L.; Kyrtopoulos, S.A.; Collins, A.; Harrington, V. & Fuortes, L. (2004).

Immunomodulatory effects of mineral fibres in occupationally exposed workers. *Mutat. Res.*, Vol.553, No.1-2, pp. 111-24, ISSN: 1383-5718

Tulinska, J.; Kuricova, M.; Liskova, A.; Kovacikova, Z. Tatrai E, (2005). The effect of ceramic fibres on the immune system, *Biomed Pap Med Fac Univ Palacky Olomouc Czech Repub.* 2005, 149(2):397–9, ISSN:1213-8118

Urso, C. & Caimi, G. (2011). Oxidative stress and endothelial dysfunction, *Minerva Med.*, Vol.102, No.1, pp. 59-77, ISSN: 0026-4806

van Eeden, SF. & Hogg, JC. (2002). Systemic inflammatory response induced by particulate matter air pollution: the importance of bone-marrow stimulation. *J Toxicol Environ Health* A. 65, 1597-613, ISSN (printed): 1528-7394.

van Helden, YG.; Keijer, J.; Knaapen, AM.; Heil, SG.; Briede, JJ.; van Schooten, FJ. & Godschalk, RW. (2009). Bete-carotene metabolites enhance inflammation-induced oxidative DNA damage in lung epithelial cells. *Free Radic. Biol. Med.*, Vol.46, No.2, pp. 299-304, ISSN: 0891-5849.

Van Loveren, H.; Vos, J.G.; Germolec, D.; Simeonova, P.P.; Eijkemanns, G. & McMichael, A.J. (2001). Meeting report. Epidemiologic associations between occupational and environmental exposures and autoimmune disease: Report of a meeting to explore current evidence and identify research needs, *Int. J. Hyg. Environ. Health,* Vol.203, pp. 483-495, ISSN: 1438-4639.

Venarske, D. & deShazo, RD. (2003). Molecular mechanisms of allergic disease, *South Med. J.*, Vol.96, No.11, pp. 1049–1054, ISSN: 0038-4348.

Vial, T. & Descotes, J. (1996). Drugs affecting the immune system. In: *Meyler's Side-Effects of Drugs*, 13th ed, Dukes MNG (ed). Elsevier, Amsterdam, pp 1090-1165, ISBN: 0 85369 460 5.

Wu, J.; Liu, W.; Koenig, K.; Idell, S. & Broaddus, VC. (2000). Vitronectin adsorption to chrysotile asbestos increases fiber phagocytosis and toxicity for mesothelial cells. *Am. J. Physiol. Lung Cell. Mol. Physiol.*, Vol.279. No. 5, pp. 916-23, ISSN:1040-0605.

Yamato, H.; Morimoto, Y.; Tsuda, T.; Ohgami, A.; Kohyama, S. & Tanaka, I (1998) Fiber numbers per unit weight of JFM standard reference samples determined with scanning electron microscope. *Ind Health* 36, 384–7, ISSN: 1549-3199.

Yagil-Kelmer, E.; Kazmier, P.; Rahaman, MN.; Bal, BS.; Tessman, RK.; Estes, DM. (2004). Comparison of the response of primary human blood monocytes and the U937 human monocytic cell line to two different sizes of alumina ceramic particles, *Journal of Orthopaedic Research* 22 (2004) pp.832-838, ISSN: 1554-527X

Zhao, J.; Shi, X.; Castranova, V. & Ding M. (2009). Occupational toxicology of nickel and nickel compounds, *J Environ Pathol Toxicol Oncol.* 2009;28(3):177-208, ISSN: 0731-8898

Section 4

Basic of Immunology and Parasite Immunology

15

Molecular Aspects of Neutrophils as Pivotal Circulating Cellular Innate Immune Systems to Protect Mammary Gland from Pathogens

Jalil Mehrzad[1,2]
[1]*Sections Immunology and Biotechnology, Department of Pathobiology, Faculty of Veterinary Medicine,*
[2]*Institute of Biotechnology, Ferdowsi University of Mashhad, Mashhad, Iran*

1. Introduction

As a pivotally cellular and molecular arms of circulating innate immune system, polymorphonuclear cells (PMNs) are the most vital primary mobile phagocytes in the body of mammals; their appropriate function is very essential to enhance animals' and humans' health performance. As the first type of innate immune cells arriving at the site of infection, neutrophils play a key role in initiating an innate, inflammatory, and specific immune responses; their importance for protection of organs in the body from pathogens has long been a crucial concern (Burvenich et al., 1994; Paape et al., 1996; Reeves et al., 2002; Burvenich et al., 2003; Mehrzad et al., 2004; 2005a; Letiember, et al., 2005; Liu et al., 2005; Borregaard et al., 2007; Stevens, et al., 2011a; 2011b; Bruhn et al., 2011). The proof of vital roles of neutrophils is that the neutropenic animals/humans are always highly susceptible to many pathogens. Clearly, the complex phenomenon of PMN chemotaxis, diapedesis, phagocytosis, and eventually microbicidal activity each contributes to the ability of PMN to provide an effective first line defense for the body and organs like udder (Burvenich et al., 2003; Mehrzad et al., 2000; 2001a; 2001b; 2002a; 2002b; 2004; 2005a; 2007; 2008a; 2008b; 2009; Mayadas & Cullere, 2005; Borregaard et al., 2008). In this concept many powerful afferent (sensing) and efferent (effector) arms of the neutrophils inside and outside of the cytoplasm are involved; the most common arms are enzymes, granules, free radicals or reactive oxygen species (ROS) and reactive nitrogen species (RNS) and in phagolysosome, into which microbicidal agents are released, neutrophil extracellular traps (NETs), neutrophils' membrane receptors like pattern recognition receptors (PRRs), opsonin receptors etc. that sense, bind and efficiently kill invading microbes, destroy virulence factors, or prevent them from spreading.

Oscillation and/or impairment of neutrophils' functions, originating from the bone marrow, is a peculiar feature during the physiological and environmental stresses; this impairment might be cumulative upon diapedesis/extravasation of neutrophils (Mehrzad et al., 2001a; 2002a; 2005a, 2004; 2007; 2008a; 2008b; Van Oostveldt et al., 2002a; 2002b; Burvenich et al., 2003). Generalised PMN impairment can be multifactorial, e.g. due to metabolic (Suriyasathaporn et al., 1999) and hormonal (Gray et al., 1982; Alexandrova, 2009; Lai &

Gallo, 2009) changes. The inevitable occurring of general and local immunocompromised conditions in biologically pivotal organ, mammals' udder, (Burvenich et al., 1994; Hoeben et al., 2000a; Burvenich et al., 2003; Mehrzad et al., 2001a; 2004; 2005a; 2008a; 2009) leads to udder infection and/or inflammation and breast disorders, affecting adult mammals, especially high yielding dairy cows, thereby causing neonatal infections, critical public health damage and economic losses to bovine, meat, dairy and food industries and overall human food chains.

Most researchers see the immunocompromised condition in animals and human as a result of neutrophils' dysfunction; this neutrophils' dysfunctional status can be cumulative upon neutrophils' influx into the udder (Mehrzad et al., 2001a; 2004; 2005a; 2008a; 2009). Despite all progresses and advances in the efferent and afferent branches of molecular aspects of neutrophils, the molecular basis of neutrophils interactions with other immune and non-immune cells in the udder is incompletely understood.

This chapter presents the cellular and acellular branches of neutrophils-pathogens interactions and factors affecting the effectiveness of particularly neutrophils' efferent arms of innate molecules in bovine. I chose bovine as a model to update our knowledge and to incorporate new observations that broaden our understanding of 1) overall neutrophils' involvement in innate immunity 2) how neutrophils engulf and kill invading pathogens and 3) how some key mechanisms of neutrophil's oscillatory events occur in bovine model. I discuss various aspects of bovine neutrophils that are absolutely relevant to their pivotal roles in an efficient innate immune response against pathogens. Aspects such as cellular and molecular innate immunity and host-pathogen interactions, biology, biochemistry and biophysics of bovine neutrophils as well as immunotoxicology, especially environmental immunotoxins (Mehrzad et al., 2011) and some nutritional immunology (Ibeagha et al., 2009), applying basic techniques like luminometry and flow cytometry will be schematically addressed to gain more insight into the static and dynamics branches of circulating and post-diapedetic neutrophils' functions. Although it is hardly possible in this chapter to address the breadth of information available on efferent arms of neutrophils in healthy and diseased animals and humans, our readers are therefore referred to many more recent detailed references of the many aspects of neutrophils in healthy and diseased hosts and their impacts on udders' health and performance as well.

2. Fine structure of neutrophils

As the primary and pivotal cells providing innate host defence against pathogens, neutrophils are characterized by their multi-lobed or sometimes picnotic dark-bluish stained nuclei (see figure 1) with the plenty of membrane receptors. The fine structure of bovine PMN has been exclusively demonstrated in classic studies (Paape et al., 2002; Mehrzad et al., 2001a; 2005b). The cell is delineated by a plasma membrane that has a number of functionally important receptors. These include L-selectin and β_2-integrin adhesion molecules associated with the binding of PMN to endothelial cells that are important for migration into sites of infection (Stevens et al., 2011a; 2011b; Pezeshki et al., 2011). Membrane receptors for the Fc component of the IgG_2 and IgM classes of immunoglobulins and C3b are necessary for mediating effective phagocytosis of invading microbes (Paape et al., 1996). Dying or apoptotic PMN express receptors that mark them for quick disposal by macrophages.

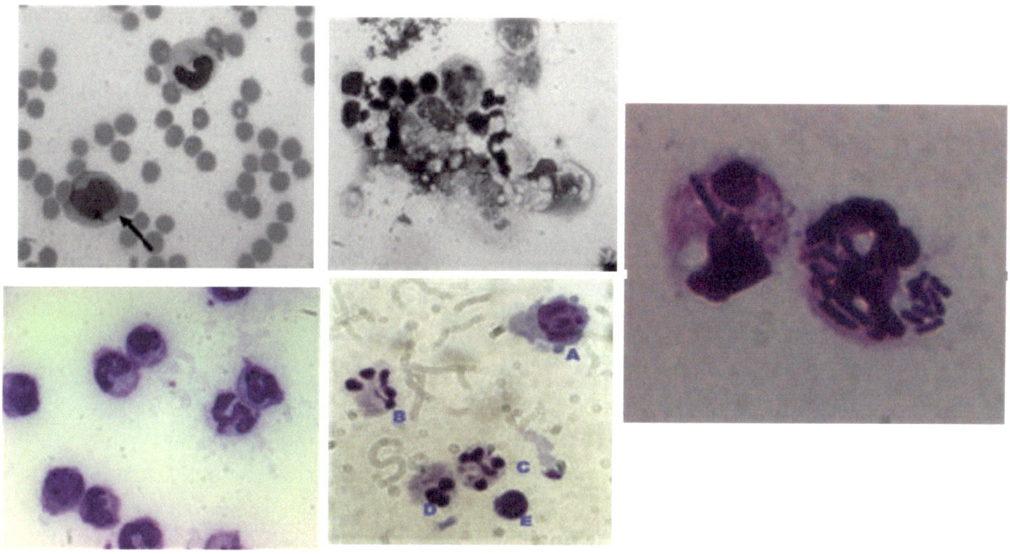

Fig. 1. Upper: Whole blood smear (left), immature neutrophil (arrow); milk neutrohils after first step of centrifugation (right), which is almost indistinguishable, with the techniques established in routine laboratories they can easily be distinguishable. A typical phagocytosed microbes by milk neutrophils (far right); these engulfed microbes must be destroyed effectively to limit infection. Lower: Isolated bovine blood neutrohils from healthy animal (left), which is pure, and postdiapedetic udder (right) neutrohils (B, C and D) macrophage (A) and lymphocyte (E).

The most prominent characteristic of the PMN is the multilobulated nucleus (see figures 1 and 2). The multilobulated nucleus is important because it allows the PMN to line up its nuclear lobes in a thin line, permitting rapid migration between endothelial cells. Macrophages on the other hand have a large horseshoe shaped nucleus that makes migration between endothelial cells more difficult. Thus, the PMN is the first newly migrated phagocytic cell to arrive at an infection site. Their surface microvilli are also pivotal for their functionality (see figures 2 and 3). Within the cytoplasm there are isles of glycogen that make up 20% of the cell on a dry weight basis and numerous bactericidal granules that are used by the cell for bactericidal activity. Generally, human neutrophils have two predominantly distinct granule populations; azurophilic (primary) granules which are large and appear as electron dense granules on electron microscopy, and specific (secondary) granules which are small and appear as light staining granules on electron microscopy. Azurophilic granules are more abundant in immature lineage of neutrophils than specific granules (Borregaard et al., 2007). Similarly, bovine PMN contains azurophilic and specific granules (figure 2). They also contain a third novel granule that is larger, denser and more numerous than the other two granules. These granules contain lactoferrin, which is also found in secondary granules, but they do not contain constituents common to azurophilic granules. Instead, they contain a group of highly cationic proteins and are the exclusive store of powerful oxygen-independent bactericidal compounds (Gennaro et al., 1983). The most important antibacterial mechanism derived from azurophilic granules is the MPO-H_2O_2-halide system (Heyneman et al., 1990; Heyneman & Burvenich, 1992; Mehrzad et al., 2001a; 2002a; 2009). MPO in the presence of hydrogen peroxide (H_2O_2) and halide ions kills bacteria. The functionality of these ROS producing granules might be altered during physiological and pathological conditions of animals, and should therefore be further investigated.

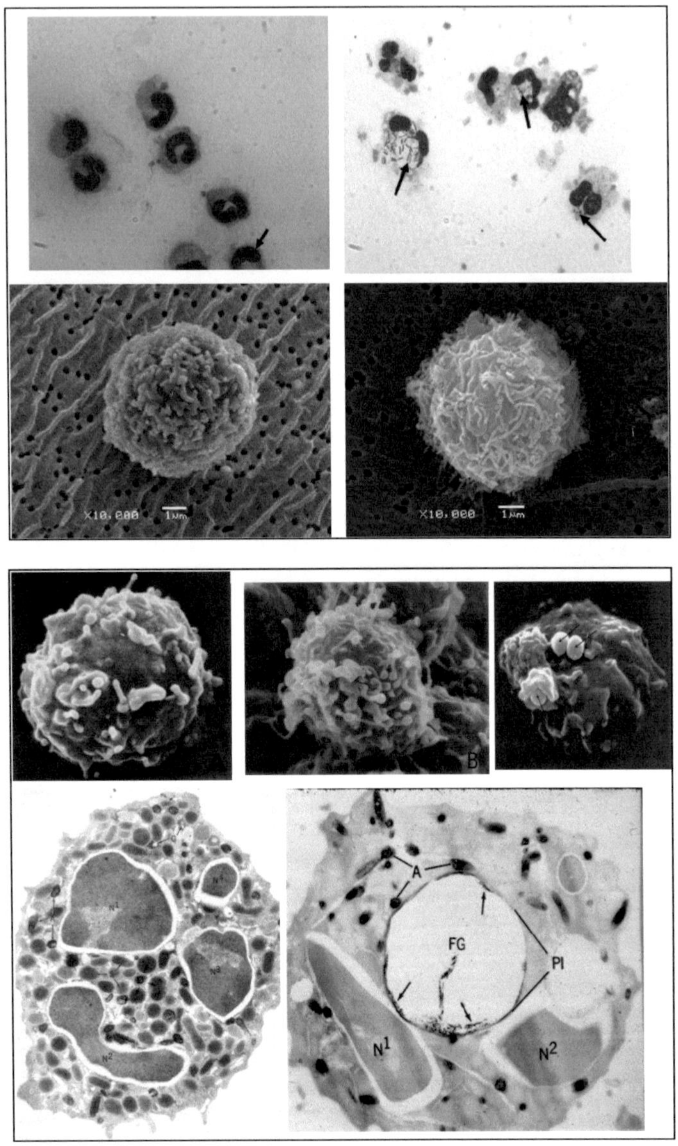

Fig. 2. Upper panel: upper: Isolated neutrophils from blood (left), in which the presence of immature neutrophil (arrow) is distinguishable and post-diapedetic neutrophils in lactating udder (right), in which phagocytosed bacteria (arrows) are visible. Lower: Scanning electron micrograph of PMN isolated from blood (left) and milk (right). Protruding pseudopods needed for phagocytosis in PMN, which is distinguishable in blood and post-diapedetic neutrophils. The blood PMN has higher convulsed cell membrane that forms protruding pseudopods. This might be due to phagocytosis of milk fat globules and casein miscelles. Samples were taken from cows suffering from *E. coli* mastitis. Lower panel: (A) Scanning

electron micrograph of a neutrohil isolated from post-diapedesis in udder. As a result of the cell ingesting its membrane material during phagocytosis of milk fat globules and casein miscelles, the neutrophils lost the protruding pseudopods required for phagocytosis (×20,000). (B) Scanning electron micrograph of a neutrohil isolated from blood. It has a highly convoluted cell membrane that forms protruding pseudopods (×15,000). Far right: Scanning electron micrograph of a PMN isolated from milk with three Staphylococcus aureus (arrows) are present on the surface of the neutrophil; the bacterium at lower left is partially engulfed by a pseudopod (×20,000). Lower left, transmission electron micrograph of bovine neutrophils isolated from blood. The neutrohil, which is limited by the plasma membrane, contains portions of a multilobed nucleus (N1 to N4), glycogen granules (G), specific granules (S), azurophilic granules (A), and large electron dense granules (D). Azurophilic granules are stained more intensely than the specific and large electron dense granules because the neutrophils were incubated with diaminobenzidine and hydrogen peroxide. As a result, an electron-dense product, indicative of peroxidatic activity, has formed in azurophilic granules (×22,000). Lower right, transmission electron micrograph of bovine neutrophils isolated from lactating udder. Deposition of an electron-dense product performed on neutrophils, which was not stained, electron dense product corresponds to areas that are high in peroxidatic activity. These areas represent the azurophilic granules and periphery (arrows) of phagolysosomes containing a milk fat globule. Nuclear lobes (N1, N2), azurophilic granules (A), phagolysosome (Pl), fat globule (FG) (×25,000). Partially adapted from (Paape M., Mehrzad j., et al., 2002).

3. Movement of neutrophils from bone marrow to the mammary glands

The issue of life span, mechanomics and biophysics of this dynamically mobile cell, neutrophil, is very pivotal issue in biomedical research. The neutrophilic PMN leukocytes of the blood circulation are specialized terminally differenciated with a short life-span. All blood and immune cells originate from a self-renewing small population of pluripotent stem cells (CFU-S) that can replicate themselves, or can become committed to a particular development pathway. Neutrophils are the major class of leukocytes in peripheral blood of human and domestic animals. The circulation of a healthy human adult contains 4,500-10,000 leucocytes/µl with approximately 60% or more being neutrophils (Nathan, 2006). A healthy adult human produces ~10^{11} neutrophils each day each of which survives about 6-8 hours in the circulation. Almost similar pattern on leukocyte and neutrophils quantities existed in bovine leukocyte and neutrophils (see e.g., Mehrzad et al., 2001a; 200ab; 2001c; 2002a; 2004; 2005a and plenty more). These vital circulating innate immune cells, neutrophils, are formed through the multi-step process of granulopoiesis, from the colony-forming unit of granulocytes (CFU-G) through myeloblasts, promyelocytes, myelocytes, metamyelocytes, and band cells. Precursor cells undergo substantial morphologic, biochemical and functional changes during granulocytic maturation. These changes are associated with significant changes in cell size and nuclear shape, and with the development of stage-specific proteins essential for phagocytosis and microbial killing (Smit et al., 1996; Van Merris et al., 2001a; 2001b; 2002; Burvenich et al., 2003; Mehrzad et al., 2001a; 2001c).

The efficiency of PMN against invading pathogens was previously shown to be highly dependent on the rate of diapedesis into the infection site (Heyneman et al., 1990; Heyneman & Burvenich, 1992; Mehrzad et al., 2001b; 2004; 2005a; 2005b) and on the ability of these PMN to generate ROS (Heyneman & Burvenich, 1992) and Mehrzad et al., 2001a;

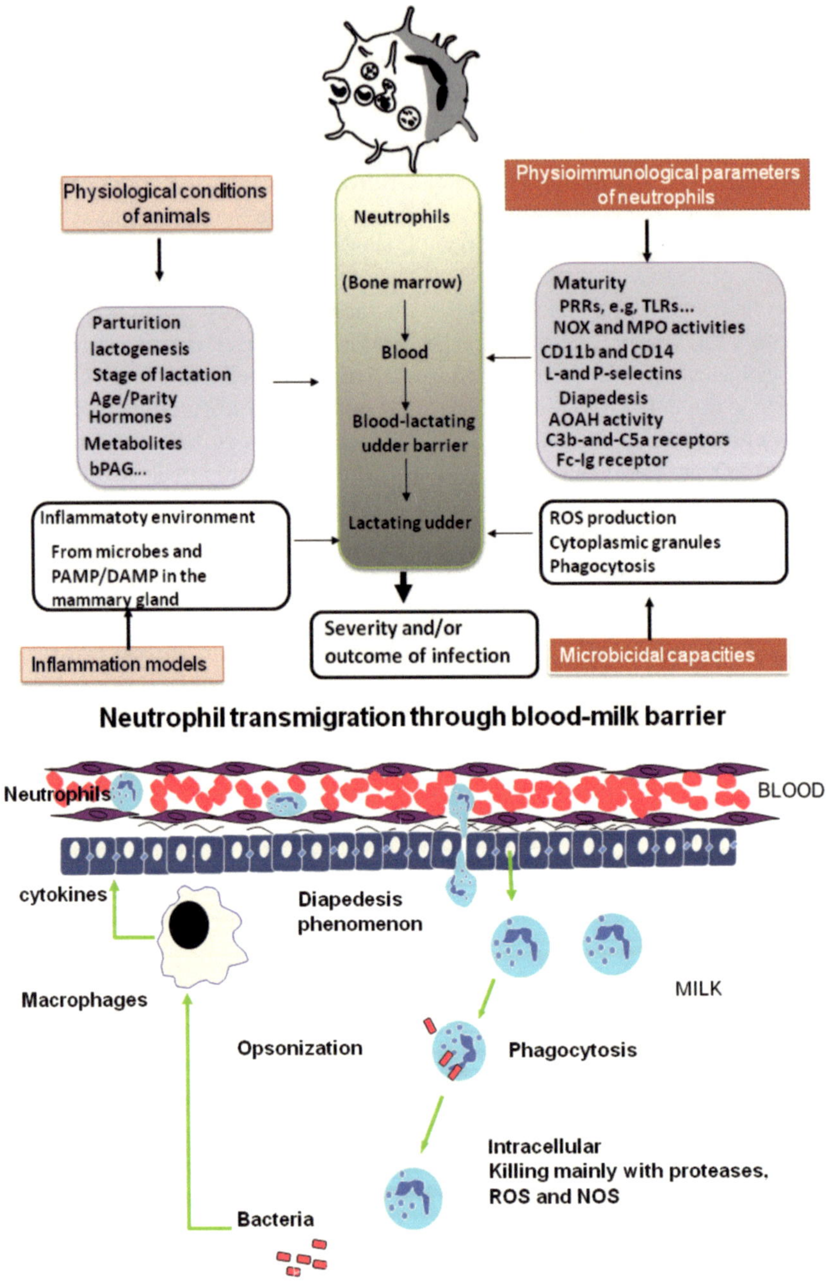

Fig. 3. Upper panel: A schematic representation of the major contributing factors such as some physiological conditions (lactation, parity or age and status of inflammation) to microbicidal capacity of neutrophils in the blood and mammary gland, and the strong link of these conditions to some key immunophysiological parameters of innate host defence in bovine model. This interrelated link happens not only in the blood, but also in the bone marrow, affecting on the most pivotal efferent branches of neutrophil functions in the organs and body, thereby contributing to the outcome or severity of infection. Because

neutrophils are the first cells recruited to the site of infection, their capacity and functionality make this pivotal cell of the circulating innate immune system as one of the cornerstones of the induction and shaping of adaptive immunity in body and organs. Microbicidal activity of neutrophils occurs mainly intracellularly during phagocytosis, with the contribution of many soluble and insoluble proteins, enzymes and ROS produced both inside and outside of the neutrophils. Neutrophils are activated by a wide array of compounds, such as inflammatory mediators, cytokines and ligands for many receptors like pattern recognition receptors (PRRs) (e.g. via Toll-like receptors or TLRs). The activation elicits classic neutrophil functions such as chemotaxis, adherence, ingestion and eventually killing of phagocytosed microbes. Some mediators, cytokines, hormones and metabolites suppress neutrophils' functions throughout the body. Like blood PMN, post-diapedetic PMN functional impairment occurs immediately around parturition; this is coincided with oscillatory events in the cellular and molecular parts of post-diapedetic PMN like viability and killing capacity in the udder. These impairments are more pronounced immediately after parturition and beginning of lactogenesis, which is far more pronounced in older animals. This diagram is based on the author's own studies on bovine PMN functions (see some references appeared in the reference section). The scheme observed in animal model of innate immune system is a fundamental consideration in human, and many molecular aspects of this diagram remains to be further studied in the area of innate immunology in animals and human. Lower panel: Simple scheme of the complex blood-milk barrier showing enterance of invading microbes, which is almost always ascendingly, via teat canal, in the udder cisterna. When microbes enter the gland the triger of innate immune cells in the gland, mainly macrophages and neutrophils, producing veriety of cytokines, chemokins and plenty more immunogenic molecules, creating cell-cell signaling, activating epithelial and endothelial cells, thereby resulting in a masive recruitment of neutrophils in the mammary gland. When real professional phagocytes, neutrophils, reach the site of infection they capture and ingest microbes by phagocytosis and eventually destroy the pathogenic microbes with their microbicidal arsenal, mainly ROS and proteases and RNS (reactive nitrogen species). This final step of first line defence mechanism is the main focus of the future resaerch in the area of molecular immunobiology.

2001c; 2005a; 2005b; 2009). Although the immature neutrophils expressed already the membrane adhesion molecule CD (cluster of differentiation) 11b, they were not capable of rapidly migrating to the infected organs to efficiently ingest and kill the invading pathogens. The impairment of ROS production was attributed to the absence of membrane-bound NADPH-oxidase activity, as myeloperoxidase was already present in the rare azurophilic granules at the promyelocytic stage (Van Merris et al., 2002). Thus, when maturation is impaired due to an increased proliferation rate, a higher number of immature neutrophils will appear in the blood circulation. These findings support the hypothesis postulated by (Heyneman & Burvenich, 1992; Mehrzad et al, 2001a; 2005a; 2005b; 2009) namely that the presence of myelocytes, metamyelocytes and band cells (shift to the left) observed during acute inflammation and sepsis may compromise the animals' resistance by supplying more cells that are morphologically immature and functionally insufficient. Van Werven et al. (1997) and Mehrzad et al. (2001a; 2002a; 2004; 2005a; 2007) demonstrated that the increase of neutrophil functionality was a result of increased enzyme activity per neutrophil, rather than an increase of the number of neutrophils. Therefore, the enhanced enzymatic activity in neutrophils after onset of infection/inflammation was believed to be induced by granulocyte-moncyte colony-stimulating factors (GM-CSF), reflecting an increased proliferation and differentiation of bone marrow granulocytes (Heyneman et al., 1990; Heyneman & Burvenich, 1992; Mehrzad et al., 2001a; 2001b; 2004; 2005a). It has been postulated that myeloid stem cells leave the bone marrow almost by a pipeline mechanism, the older cells being released first (Heyneman & Burvenich, et al., 1992). The molecular mechanisms that control the release of mature PMN from the bone marrow into the circulating pool and then extravasation are very complex and poorly understood (see figures 3 and 4).

Neutrophils circulate in the blood until recruited to sites of infection by chemical signals. This migration begins when neutrophils interact with activated endothelial cells. Inflammatory cytokines like tumor necrosis factor-α (TNF-α), interleukin-1 (IL-1), and interferon-γ (IFN-γ) produced by activated macrophages at sites of infection activate endothelial cells and induce expression of receptors like E-selectin (CD62E) and P-selectin (CD62P) and ligands like Sialyl-Lewis X on glycan-bearing cell adhesion molecule-1 (GlyCAM-1) and P-selectin glycoprotein ligand-1 [PSGL-1]) which interact with neutrophil receptors like L-selectin (CD62L) (Diez-Fraille et al., 2004; Sohn et al., 2007a; 2007b ; Zarbock A & Ley, 2008). Selectin-ligand interactions are of low affinity leading to only "rolling" and slowing of neutrophils on the endothelial cell surface in post capillary venules to enable stronger associations.

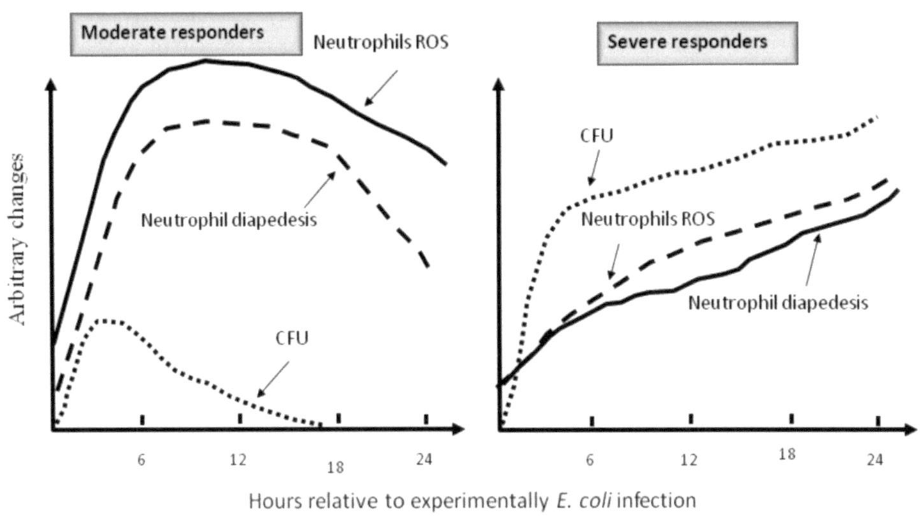

Fig. 4. This figure shows the overall disparities of neutrophils' diapedesis rate, post-diapedetic neutrophil ROS production capacity and *E. coli* CFU dynamics in modertate and severe responders of animal infection model; it is based on the study of the kinetics of chemiluminescence and intramammary infection/inflammation (Mehrzad et al., 2001b, 2004; 2005a). Moderate responders' neutrophils are functioning much more appropriately than severs'. The fast increase in neutrophils' diapedesis rate and post-diapedetic neutrophil ROS production capacity during acute infection of mammary gland lags exponential growth of *E. coli* in the gland. Compared with severe responders, the fast-strong local response in moderate responders facilitated recovery of acute infection and inflammation. The bacterial growth in the lactating udder is exceeded to the neutrophils' diapedesis and ROS

production rates in sever responders. This is very important and basic cellular part of innate immunity of mammary gland. This different response is mainly due to the far stronger pre-infection blood and post-daipedetic neutrophils' functions, especially, ROS production as well as the neutrophils' ROS production during the "early phase" of infection/inflammation. So, the capacity of PMN ROS production (especially intracellular) and quality of pos-diapedetic neutrophils both before and during early infection, is crucial for the severity of the diseases, and leads to a faster elimination of pathogens, becuae the fast-strong local response in moderate responders facilitated recovery of infection/inflammation.

Besides increased expression of selectins, TNF- α and IL-1 also enhance endothelial cell expression of vascular cell adhesion moledule-1 (VCAM-1) and intracellular adhesion molecule-1 (ICAM-1) and ICAM-2, which are ligands for the neutrophil integrins very late antigen-4 (VLA-4) and leukocyte function antigen-1 (LFA-1 or CD11a/18 or $\alpha_L\beta_2$) and macrophage-1 antigen (Mac-1, CD11b/18 or $\alpha_m\beta_2$), respectively. Interactions of neutrophils with these molecules results in firm attachment to the endothelium, followed by their activation, and spreading. Interactions of neutrophil receptors CXCR1 and CXCR2 down a concentration gradient of their ligand chemokine CXCL8 result in transmigration of neutrophils between endothelial cell spaces to the infectious site (Paulsson et al., 2010). Neutrophil LFA-1-endothelial ICAM-1 and CD177-CD31 (platelet endothelial cell adhesion molecule-1 [PECAM-1]) interactions facilitate this migration (Sachs et al., 2007).

A potential role of adhesion molecules like L-selectin in the release of neutrophils from the bone marrow is very critical, because L-selectin is highly expressed on mature PMN in the post-mitotic pool in the bone marrow and in the circulation (Diez-Fraile et al., 2004). The process of granulopoiesis is strictly controlled by regulatory growth factors, comprising cytokines and colony-stimulating factors, which have pleiotropic effects on proliferation, differentiation and functional activation of precursor cells (Burvenich et al., 2003). Using an optimised cell culture assay for the bovine (Smit et al., 1996; Van Merris et al., 2001a; 2001b), it was demonstrated that physiological concentrations of β-hydroxybutyric acid and acetoacetic acid induced remarkable suppression on the proliferation of hematopoietic cells (van Werven et al., 1997; Hoeben et al., 1999). Bovine pregnancy-associated glycoprotein also reduced the proliferative activity of bovine progenitor cells (Hoeben et al., 1999). Therefore, the neutrophil circulating pool is largely depending on the proliferative capacity of the bone marrow. After having exerted their role in immune function, PMN die by senescence (Mehrzad et al., 2001a; Van Merris et al., 2002; Burvenich et al., 2003). Aged PMN undergo spontaneous apoptosis in the absence of pro-inflammatory agents prior to their removal by macrophages (Paape et al., 2002; Burvenich et al., 2003), thus preventing the release of their cytotoxic content. Inflammation and infection hugely increase the rate of PMN production, shortening the maturation time, thereby leading to the release of immature neutrophils in the circulation pool.

Advances in mammary gland immunology of recent decades have provided insights into the mechanisms responsible for the defense of the mammary gland against infection. PMN has a pivotal role in the protection of the gland from infections (Paape et al., 2002; Burvenich et al., 2003; Mehrzad et al., 2001a; 2001b; 2001c; 2002; 2004; 2005a; 2005b; 2009). The life cycle of the bovine PMN is short. Formed in the bone marrow, PMN require 10 to 14 days to mature (Bainton et al., 1971; Burvenich et al., 2003). After maturation, PMN may be stored for a few additional days. Mature PMN leave the hematopoietic compartment of the bone marrow and enters the vascular sinus by travelling in migration channels through endothelial cells. Normally, mature neutrophils circulate in the blood stream briefly (half-life of ~9 hours), then leave the blood stream by diapedesis and enter tissues where they function as strong phagocytes for 1 to 2 days. In healthy animals, production and destruction of PMN is tightly regulated, which keeps their number in blood, milk, and tissue almost constant (Heyneman et al., 1990; Heyneman & Burvenich, 1992; Paape et al., 2002; Burvenich et al., 2003; Mehrzad et al., 2002a) and this is an essential element of their role in the first line of immune defense. Continuous influx of PMN is orchestrated by the local accumulation of chemotactic factors, which may be of endogenous or exogenous origin. Examples of the former include complement derived factors (e.g., C5a), lipid-derived mediators (e.g., leukotriene B4, platelet-activating factor or PAF) and tissue-derived chemokines (in particular IL-8). The dynamic of PMN diapedesis through blood/milk barrier helps to explain the observed PMN activity fluctuations in milk (Smits et al., 1999; Mayadas & Cullere 2005; Pezeshki et al., 2011).

Transendothelial/epithelial concentrations of neutrophils is very critical to effectively kill invading microbes (Li et al., 2002; Mehrzad et al., 2005a; 2005b). The issue of blood and post-diapedetic PMN functions and concentrations in different physiological and pathological conditions remains the focus of most concern. Although the presence of strong chemotactic factors in non-inflamed udder is the subject of debate, their presence in inflammatory environment of udder and milk is indisputable (Manlongat et al., 1998; Rainard, 2002; Stevens et al., 2011a; 2011b; Pezeshki et al., 2011). Most inflammatory chemoattractants are only induced and released during acute infection. However, a restricted number of chemoattractants can be constitutively present in normal plasma at high concentrations, e.g. Regakine-1 (Struyf et al., 2001). During mastitis, inflammatory chemoattractants simply guide PMN toward infection foci. Potent bovine PMN chemoattractants include C5a, an active cleavage product of the C5 in the complement system, various lipopolysaccharides (LPS), IL-1, IL-2 and IL-8 (Gray et al., 1982). These chemoattractants bind to specific receptors on the PMN plasma membrane.

When the completely equipped neutrophils reach the site of infection/inflammation, they with macrophages capture and ingest microbes by phagocytosis and destroy them with their microbicidal arsenal. Neutrophils engage microorganisms through extracellular membrane receptors like PRRs, e.g., TLRs, C-type lectins (mannose receptor), scavenger receptors like CD36, Nod-like receptors (NLRs), and N-formyl Met-Leu-Phe (f- MLP) receptors (Nathan., 2006; Diez-Fraille et al., 2004; Bellocchio et al., 2004; Sohn et al., 2007a; 2007b ; Zarbock A & Ley, 2008; Rainard, 2002; Stevens et al., 2011a; 2011b). Neutrophils also bind to pathogens coated with various opsonins like IgG, complement components (e.g. iC3b), and lectins. Activated neutrophils express the high affinity Fc-receptor, FcγR1, which binds to IgG-Fc of antibody-coated microbes, and β_2 integrins on the neutrophil surface can capture pathogens coated with the iC3b. Bound pathogens are then surrounded by neutrophil membrane projections and engulfed in the cellular cytoplasm inside a phagosome. The phagosome fuses with a lysosome to produce a phagolysosome where the captured pathogens are destroyed.

One of the critically hottest topics in the molecular aspects of inflammation, infection and sepsis in relation to neutrophils in animals and human would be the cross-talk between C5a and neutrophils' surface receptors, e.g., C5a-C5aR, C5aR-TLR4 interactions. Normally, C5aR is up-regulated in inflammatory environment (Bruhn et al., 2011; Stevens et al., 2011a; 2011b). There is considerable evidence for the participation of C5aR in the harmful consequences of experimental infection, sepsis and cancer in human and animals. Therefore, interception of either C5a or C5aR dramatically improves the exaggerated inflammatory reactions which can be good direction to treat and remodel tissue injuries and damages. This evidence would open a new door to the molecular aspects of controlling and treating of inflammation, infection and sepsis. For example, *in vivo* blockade of C5aR resulted in greatly improved survival of animals after sepsis. Similar phenamena could be observed and would be applied for other key molecules like IL-1-IL-1R interactions as well as TLRs antagonists/agonists in the inflammatory environment.

Extravasation of activated PMN occurs after their adhesion to the endothelial surface. This is accomplished by the expression of specific membrane adhesion molecules. The essential role of the CD11/CD18 family of adhesion molecules in bovine PMN-surface adhesion is well-documented (Diez-Fraille et al., 2004). These molecules bind to ICAM-1, ICAM-2 and endothelial leukocyte adhesion molecules (ELAM-1) on the endothelial surface. After binding to these molecules, PMN leave the circulation and are ready to function at the infection site. Down-regulated CD11/CD18 in circulating PMN can cause a harder and slower PMN recruitment into the mammary gland (Burvenich et al., 2003; Diez-Fraille et al., 2004). Inflammatory environment of the udder induces adherence of circulating PMN to the endothelium by up-regulation of CD11b/CD18 (Diez-Fraille et al., 2004), of which activity is crucial to bovine PMN diapedesis across the blood/milk barrier (Smits et al., 2000); in such an environment, blood PMN number, and effective adhesion, migration, opsonization, phagocytosis and killing are of crucial importance to the outcome of the infection and the severity of the disease (Gray et al., 1982; Burvenich et al., 1999; 2003; Mehrzad et al., 2001a; 2001b; 2005a; 2005b; 2009). The impact of fast PMN diapedesis during udder infection/inflammation on PMN quality and their ROS production capability could cause dissimilarities between post-diapedetic PMN from inflamed and non-inflamed quarters (Mehrzad et al., 2001b; 2005a; 2005b; 2009) (see later figures of this chapter). The underlying cellular and molecular mechanisms of this disparity would be pivotal for further investigation in the area of animals and human mammary gland immunobiology and neoplasia.

The source of host and/or pathogen-derived cytokines in udder secretions and their impact on udder PMN function has been a subject of investigation. There is evidence of cytokines secretion by mammary macrophages and epithelial cells during both physiological and pathological conditions of the gland (Boudjellab et al., 1998; Mehrzad et al., 2001b; 2004; 2005a; 2005b; Rainard, 2002; Stevens et al., 2011a; 2011b; Pezeshki et al., 2011). These cytokines influence PMN function. For example, the IL-8 is involved in the recruitment of PMN and T lymphocytes into the gland (Barber et al., 1999). Proinflammatory cytokines, like TNF- α, IL-1β, and LPS suppress the gene expression of cytochrome P-450 1A1 (*cyp1a1*), by activating the transcription nuclear factor κB (NF-κB) (Notebaert et al., 2005). PMN also play a crucial role in the recruitment of other leukocytes such as CD4$^+$ T lymphocyte and CD8$^+$ T lymphocyte to the inflammation sites (Mehrzad et al., 2008a; 2008b). From bone marrow to the blood stream and the extravasation, the on time PMN influx to the site of inflammation is important in limiting injury and promoting recovery of severe inflammation (Carey et al., 1997; Mehrzad et al., 2001b; 2004; 2005a; 2005b).

4. Location of microbicidal weaponry in circulating and post-diapedetic neutrophils

Armed with an array of highly microbicidal weapons, such as enzymes that hydrolyze and destroy proteins, lipids and sugars of pathogens, the weaponry is mainly stored in, at least, three different kinds of granules in the cytoplasm as well as outside the cytoplasm. Additionally, neutrophils have powerful systems for generation of large amounts of free radicals or ROS. Microbial pathogens are taken up into an intracellular compartment, called phagolysosome, into which microbicidal agents are released. There are also many new forms of innate effector molecules like neutrophil extracellular traps (NETs), PRRs, opsonin receptors and plenty more that sense, bind and efficiently kill invading microbes, destroy virulence factors, or prevent them from spreading.

Following adherence of opsonized bacteria to surface receptors on the PMN, phagocytosis, respiratory burst and degranulation are triggered. The process of opsonization, though not essential for phagocytosis, certainly promotes the uptake of bacteria by PMN. The phagocytosis process is energy-dependent and requires the presence of a functional cytoskeleton. The cytoskeleton machinery, when sequentially activated following receptor stimulation, is thought to envelope the microorganism in a "zipper mechanism" (Griffin et al., 1975). Immunological recognition is mainly accomplished by specific antibodies (IgG_2 and IgM) which recognize the bacterium through Fab-regions and bind to PMN via Fc-receptors on the PMN plasma membrane (Paape et al., 1996). There is a synergy between the Fcγ and C3b receptors activity and neutrophils' ROS production (Newman & Johnston, 1979).

Neutrophils produce several proteolytic enzymes that degrade and destroy microbes in the phagolysosome. Two important proteases produced by neutrophils are the serine protease, elastase, and cathepsin G (Reeves et al., 2002; Mehrzad et al., 2005b). More importantly, neutrophils also destroy ingested microorganisms with ROS produced by the "phagocyte oxidase system (phox)," or "NADPH oxidase or NOX," which reduces molecular oxygen into ROS in the phagolysosome (Mehrzad et al., 2001a; 2001c; 2005a; Reeves et al., 2002). NOX pumps electrons from the oxidation of NADPH to NADP in the neutrophil cytosol, across the phagolysosome membrane via flavocytochrome b558 (the core component of phox) and onto molecular oxygen (O_2) in the phagolysosome reducing it to superoxide anion ($O_2^{\cdot -}$), and cascade reaction of respiratory burst starts. NOX activity and K^+ flux are important for provision of acidic pH in the phagolysosome for effective killing of engulfed microbes (Reeves et al., 2002). Normally, during intracellular killing pH of the phagolysosome (initially neutral) rapidly drops to ~4 within <10 min; this change in pH is very important for killing of engulfed microbes, because many enzymes and peptides necessary for microbicidal are activated at acidic pH.

After a complicated cascade of release of biological substances and activation of the endothelium, neutrophils migrate into the mammary gland and finally also appear in the fluid of the lactiferous sinus (Burvenich et al., 1994; 2003). Although several antimicrobial systems exist in the mammary gland (Burvenich et al., 1994; Paape et al., 1996; 2002), but, it is the massive influx of neutrophils that will resolve the infection through efficiently killing of the invading bacteria (Mehrzad et al., 2001b; 2005a; 2005b; Burvenich et al., 2003; Paape et al., 2002). Diapedesis will also affect binding of immunoglobulins to the PMN surface. An increased expression of Fc receptors and phagocytosis happens after *in vitro* migration of bovine PMN through membranes (Berning et al., 1993; and Worku et al., 1994). After *in vivo* migration of PMN into mammary quarters of nulliparous heifers, binding of IgG_1 and IgG_2 increased while binding of IgM decreased. Binding of IgA remained unchanged. The greatest change occurred with the binding of IgM. Seventy-six percent of the blood PMN bound IgM, whereas only 2% of the post-diapedetic PMN bound IgM. Interestingly, phagocytic activity of PMN increased after *in vitro* chemotaxis but not after *in vivo* chemotaxis of neutrophils. Activation of complement also promotes chemotaxis, extravasation, phagocytosis and killing capacities. The C3b and iC3b, generated on the surface of bacteria following antibody union, are recognized respectively by CR1 and CR3 receptors located on the PMN cell membrane. The type of bacteria also affects bovine PMN bactericidal capacity. For example, slime-producing *Staphylococcus aureus* hampers the killing capacity of PMN (Barrio et al., 2000; Mehrzad et al., 2009). The specific interactions between extracellular matrix proteins of *Staphylococcus aureus* and ICAM-1 inhibits further PMN recruitment, boosting anti-inflammatory reactions (Chavakis et al., 2002). This might be counterproductive for the killing activity of PMN. During migration of PMN into milk in response to infection increased binding of C3b was observed (DiCarlo et al., 1996). Thus, PMN are fully armed to confront invading bacteria, resulting in a more rapid ingestion and elimination of the pathogens. Once complement and immunoglobulins bind to receptors on the PMN surface, PMN become activated and generate ROS, such as $O_2^{\cdot-}$, H_2O_2 and halogen reactive species. This process associated with the respiratory burst is called the "oxygen-dependent" or "oxidative" killing, and that associated with neutrophil granules is also called "oxygen-dependent", but "non-oxidative" killing. Killing classified on the basis of these criteria has been explicitly addressed (e.g., Root & Cohen, 1981; Babior, 1984; Spitznagel & Shafer, 1985; Babior, 1994; Reeves et al., 2002; Mehrzad et al., 2001c; 2009; 2011). The pivotal role of ROS in all further events for killing of engulfed microbes by neutrophils is therefore indisputable.

ROS formed by neutrophils are critical microbicidal agents against infection as evidenced by individuals afflicted with Chronic Granulomatous Disease (CGD). Patients with CGD have mutations in key elements of NOX and are profoundly susceptible to bacterial and fungal infections (Heyworth et al., 2003), though this kind of mutation has not been observed in bovine. In addition, a number of proteolytic enzymes including elastase, cathepsin G, myeloperoxidase, gelatinase, and others contained in the azurophilic and specific granules fuse with the phagolysosome and also contribute to the intracellular killing of microbes and degradation of its contents.

Intracellular killing of phagocytosed microorganisms is accomplished by following adherence to the PMN surface, usually, but not necessarily, via specific receptors (Horwitz et al., 1982). Three different mechanisms are involved for intracellular bacterial destruction: 1) an oxygen-dependent mechanism (production of ROS), 2) a nitrogen dependent mechanism (RNS especially nitrogen oxide (NO) derived from L-arginine) and 3) an oxygen-and nitrogen-independent microbicidal mechanism e.g., lyzozyme, lactoferrin, proteases, pH changes and even neutrophil extracellular traps (NETs). Because of their essentiality for killing, here my prime focus is the oxygen-dependent microbicidal mechanisms and how these mechanisms are generated in neutrophils to efficiently destroy pathogens. Though not predominantly, pathogens are trapped and killed extracellularly, e.g., NETs, as well. Impaired neutrophil NETs formation would be considered as a novel innate immune deficiency of animals and human; the NETs are lattices of DNA, histones, granule enzymes, and antimicrobial proteins that are released by the PMNs in parallel with extrusion of nuclear material. It has been found that defect in NETs formation in neutrophils is substantially rescued by the ROS generation, confirming the broadly essential roles of ROS in NETs-related killing of pathogen. Similarly, NETs-related killing of pathogens and NETs formation occurs via pathways involving both ROS and RNS (Allport et al., 2002). Thus, ROS generation is always the most pivotal and prerequisite for all further events for efficient killing of invading microbes.

Baldridge and Gerard (1933) first reported that an increase in oxygen consumption by neutrophils takes place when phagocytosis is triggered. ROS generated by reduction-oxidation (redox) reactions, have been recognized as one of the major contributors to the killing of pathogens. This phenomenon is accompanied by an increase in oxygen consumption and the hexose monophosphate shunt (HMPS) activity by PMN and has been termed the "respiratory" burst. The oxygen molecule is central for PMN respiratory burst activity (Allen et al., 1972; Babior, 1984; 1994; Reeves et al., 2002); its importance in microbicidal activity of PMN was highlighted by the inefficient PMN bactericidal activity in anaerobic conditions (Mandell, 1974). One example: for each molecule of O_2 consumed 4 $O_2^{\cdot -}$ ions are generated; roughly 0.5 fmol of O_2 is consumed for each bacterium engulfed, resulting in an intravacuolar $O_2^{\cdot -}$ release of about 4 mol.l^{-1} (Reeves et al., 2002). Though still remains inconclusive, the application of ozone gass (O_3) would be further examined in domestic animals for treatment of infections such as mastitis, metritis, arthritis, cancer and increase many cell signaling pathways for tissue remodeling and repair; because it boosts milk PMN ROS production capacity (Ogata & Nagahata, 2000), cleaning pathogen/damage-associated molecular patterns PAMPs/DAMPs from inflamed site (Lai & Gallo., 2009; Alexandrova, 2009).

As shown in figure 5, the first step in the cascade of respiratory burst is the formation of O_2^-, requiring NOX, of which substrate (NADPH) is generated by HMPS to act as an electron donor (Rossi and Zatti, 1964; Babior, 1984; Rossi, 1986).

$$2\,O_2 + NADPH \rightarrow 2O_2^{\cdot -} + NADP^+ + H^+$$

Different stimuli (e.g., complement components, immunoglobulin, formyl-methionyl-leucyl-phenylalanine (fMLP), phorbol myristate acetate (PMA) and bacterial peptides) act via different specific receptors and thus have various signal transduction mechanisms to activate the NOX. Extensive research into activation by PMA has followed the identification of protein kinase-c (PK-C) as its cytosolic receptor (Nishizuka, 1984). PMA is a strong NADPH-oxidase and PK-C agonist (Tauber, 1987, Karlsson et al., 2000). Particulate stimuli may also act indirectly via PK-C (Cooke & Hallett, 1985) or via other intermediates such as arachidonic acid and its metabolites and phospholipase-A2 (Tauber, 1987). The next step is the formation of H_2O_2 by dismutation of $O_2^{\cdot -}$, which is mediated by superoxide dismutase (SOD):

$$2\,O_2^{\cdot -} + 2H^+ \rightarrow H_2O_2 + O_2$$

The O_2^- and H_2O_2, generated by NADPH-oxidase and SOD, are the precursors of variety of subsequent powerful ROS. Included among these ROS are a variety of oxidized halogens, including hypohalite ions or HOX (Thomas & Fishman, 1986; Weiss et al., 1986) and a variety of chloramines (Thomas et al., 1982) used by PMN as microbicidal agents. These are

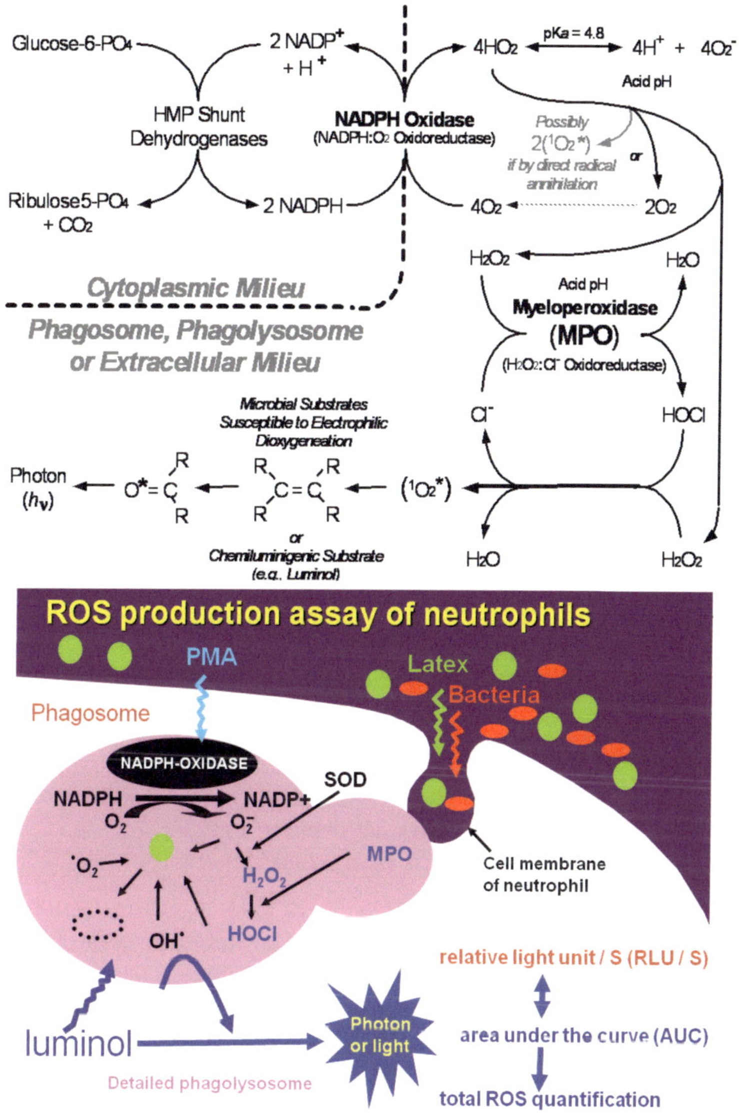

Fig. 5. Upper panel: Diagram depicting the major enzymatic systems responsible for microbicidal metabolism and oxygenation activities and the relationship of these activities to photon emission. In the scheme the activities of the cytoplasmic milieu are separated from those of the phagosome-phagolysosome-extracellular milieu. The superscripted number that precedes each molecular symbol (e.i., ^{1}for singlet, ^{2}for doublet, and ^{3}for triplet multiplicity) depicts the equation: $|2s| + 1$ = multiplicity (n). The diagram adapted from (Allen et al., 2000). Lower panel: Brief scheme of ROS production process by neutrophils during phagocytosis of bacteria. As shown the cell membrane of the neutrophils and bacteria (red). This is non-specefic phagocytosis of bacteria. The bacteria are engulfed by the neutrophils and form phagosome and fussion of phagosome to lysosome and then detialed phagolysosome is highlighted on the scheme. Activation of NADPH-oxidase (NOX) is the triger of neutrophil ROS production, the most fundametally powerful efferent arms of the

innate immune system .When bacteria are attached to the cell membrane ROS production starts and this continues when the pathogen are engulfed. Before engulfment most ROS are produced extracellularly, but afterwards it is produced intracellularly, both of which are pivotal for continuation of innate immune response against pathogens. This is a fundamental concept in the area of ROS-mediated phagocytosis and killing of microbes, in which NOX and MPO are central in this pathway; this is an interestingly big subjetc in innate immunophysiology. These ROS can be measured by chemiluminescence (CL) and this is the main technique that was highlighted in this chapter of the book. To conduct an assay on one of the pivotal efferent arms of neutrophils microbicidal capacity (light or photon produced by ROS), the pure neutrophils are activated artificially with phagocytosis-dependent (latex beads, bacteria etc.) or non-phagocytosis-dependent (PMA...) methods. Researchers routinly use photon enhancer like luminol, isoluminol, lucigenin and plenty more. The metabolites of, e.g., luminol (aminophtalate) is very unstable and can easily and immediately be oxidized by hydrogen peroxide-MPO-halide system and gain to the relaxation state and emit light. This light, which is unequivocal representative of PMN ROS production load, can be easily and precisely quatified by CL assay. The two units, which luminometer gives, are the ROS production in function of time.

generated by the H_2O_2-mediated oxidation of halide ions under catalysis by MPO or eosinophil peroxidase (EPO) and the subsequent oxidation of amines:

$$H_2O_2 + X^- \rightarrow HOX + OH^- \quad (X = Cl^-, Br^-, I^-)$$

$$HOX + R\text{-}NH\text{-}R' \rightarrow R\text{-}NX\text{-}R' + H_2O$$

Though not as crucial as PMN in infection and inflammation, the activity of compound I of EPO to react with H_2O_2 is similar to that of MPO but with substrates like Cl^-, however, it is far higher, yielding more HOX (Arnhold et al., 2001; Mehrzad et al., 2001a, 2005a; 2009; 20011).

Another group of ROS that are produced from $O_2^{\cdot -}$ are the hydroxyl radicals (OH°) generated in a transition metals (Fe or Cu) catalyzed reaction between $O_2^{\cdot -}$ and a hydroxyperoxide (a well-known Haber-Weiss reaction, if R = H):

$$O_2^{\cdot -} + ROOH \rightarrow RO + OH^- + H_2O_2 \qquad (R = H, \text{-}C, C(=O))$$

or in a reaction between previously generated oxidizing radical and another compound:

$$OH^\circ + RH \rightarrow R^\circ + H_2O$$

Eventually, singlet oxygen ($^1O_2$) has been found to be produced by neutrophils, and eosinophils (see e.g., Root & Cohen, 1981; Allen et al., 2000), possibly through a reaction between hypohalyte and H_2O_2:

$$HOX + H_2O_2 \rightarrow {}^1O_2 + X^- + H_2O$$

It is evident that the production of large quantities of ROS with a cascade of reactions will provide an environment that is destructive for any microorganims exposed to it, but it is also harmful to the nearby tissues. That is to say that ROS represent a "double-aged sword". Alternatively, ROS also enhance the activity of natural killer cell, T cell and dendritic cells

(DCs), neutralization of PAMPs and proinflammatory cytokines (Suthanthiran et al., 1984; Cemerski et al., 2002; Reth, 2002; Mehrzad et al., 2008a; 2008b; Lai & Gallo, 2009; Alexandrova, 2009), indicating that PMN ROS may not only damage cells and tissues but may also accelerate recovery of inflammation. The above reactions are tightly regulated so that the PMN releases its ROS under appropriate circumstances, depending on the physiological and pathological conditions of animals. What is not yet clear is whether there is a transient PMN ROS production change during physiopathological conditions, and if so, whether this change is or is not beneficial for animals and humans.

Neutrophils are capable of producing a range of ROS following activation of the membrane bound NOX. It is also generally agreed that ROS boost oxygen-independent microbicidal activity, like proteases (Reeves et al., 2002; Mehrzad et al., 2004; 2005a; 2009; 20011). Antimicrobial peptides especially proteases in the udder which is mainly released by neutrophils (Mehrzad et al., 2005b), will potentially promote angiogenesis, activation of macrophages, neutralization of PAMPs and pro-inflammatory cytokines, initiation of T-cell recruitment (Mehrzad et al., 2008a; 2008b) and immature (i)DCs and block of TLRs on iDCs (Lai & Gallo, 2009). Root and Cohen (1981) have suggested several possible direct sites of action for ROS, related to their microbicidal activity; these include: 1) unsaturated carbon bounds that may lead to toxic lipid peroxidation, 2) sulphydryl groups that lead to the destruction of sulphydryl containing enzymes, 3) amino group and possible peptide bound breakage and 4) nucleic acids. *In vitro* studies with $O_2^{\cdot-}$ generating systems in neutrophils such as xanthine oxidase (Rosen & Klebanoff, 1976) suggests that $O_2^{\cdot-}$ are far more toxic to bacteria if they operate in MPO H_2O_2-halide system (Reeves et al., 2002; Mehrzad et al., 2001a; 2001b; 2005a; 2009; 2011), which leads to the production of powerful chlorinated oxidising agents such as ClO^- which have a microbicidal effect by halogenating microbial proteins (see figure 5). Although the microbicidal mechanisms of neutrophils is very hugely broad and complex, but there are plenty mechanisms by which microbes evade and overcome the host's phagocytosis and killing mechanisms to succeed infections in the udder, like avoiding contact with phagocytes and inaccessible to phagocytes, inhibition of inflammatory responses and phagocyte chemotaxis and engulfment, even survival inside of phagocytes.

5. Techniques for neutrophils' ROS quantification versus their quality in the mammary gland

ROS production capacity of neutrophils is the most powerful efferent arms of the innate immune systems in blood stream and interstitial fluid for provision of further cascade of effective innate and adaptive immune responses. Several techniques of PMN ROS quantification are frequently applied. For example, the cytochrome c reduction test, flow cytometry method (Salgar et al., 1991), the scopoletine test (Root & Cohen, 1981) and chemiluminescence (CL) assay (Allen et al., 1972; Hoeben et al., 2000a; Mehrzad et al., 2000; 2001b; 2001c; 2002; 2004; 2005a; 2009; 20011). Also plenty laboratory kits available for precise neutrophils' functional tests both for genomics, proteomics and mechanomics related to the ROS production. The most widely used technique to quantify neutrophils' ROS production is CL (Mehrzad et al., 2000; 2001a; 2001b; 2002a; 2002b; 2004; 2005; 2009). As phagocytosis-induced and/or non-induced CL reflects intracellular and extracellular oxidation-reduction reactions (Mehrzad et al., 2001a; 2005a; 2009), changes might offer some evidence about the animals'/humans' susceptibility to infections.

Whereas many differential leukocyte count methods for blood leukocytes are available, study on the qualitative role of milk leukocytes in healthy and diseased animals and human is rare. The milk leukocytes differentiation also appears difficult. In addition, little attention has been paid to the standardization of particularly sample preparation procedures. To unequivocally evaluate PMN functional assays (from genomics to proteomics, mechanomics and metabolomics) appropriate isolation, differentiation and quantification of neutrophils in original or purified samples are essential. This is more special for neutrophils in non-inflammatory environment of milk/udder; not merely because a variety of cells e.g., PMN, macrophages, lymphocytes and epithelial cells, are existed but because their shapes, size and population could differ, compared to the blood. Milk sample processing varies from the use of centrifuged whole milk samples to dilution with a hypotonic buffer (Mehrzad et al., 2000; 2001a; 2001b; 2001c; 2002a; 2004; 2005a; 2009). Without microscopic confirmation, flow cytometric identification of milk cells based on forward and side scatter is inconclusive because phagocytosis of milk components may alter both size and intracellular granularity. Cellular debris may also interfere with the scatter pattern of normal milk cells. Even for blood leukocytes, their shapes and population changed significantly during mastitis. All of these changes could interfere with the assessment of PMN function. Therefore, developing an isolation, differentiation and enumeration of leukocytes in blood and milk in the laboratory to better assess PMN function is always critical. Nowadays, the problem of breast cancer in human is rising substantially, and particularly deep focus on the cellular and molecular aspects of interstitial fluid of mammary gland is urgently needed.

A functional udder immune system depends on the existence of high quality neutrophils in the interstitial fluid of mammary gland and/or milk, protecting the gland against invading pathogens (Burvenich et al., 1994; 2003; Mehrzad et al 2001a; 2001b; 2001c; 2002; 2005a; 2005b; 2009; 2011). Investigation on PMN viability can provide suitable information about PMN quality and tissue damage. This is more special for milk PMN, which migrate to the apparently unsuitable environment. PMN life span might be affected by many physiological and pathological factors in the gland. Many cellular and acellular signaling pathways are available in blood and mammary tissue for the modulation or inhibition of PMN survival. Till now, little attention has been paid on the neutrophils viability in the interstitial fluid of mammary gland/milk. Accordingly, the contribution of neutrophil enzymes (e.g., activity of NOX, MPO etc.) to the viability is critical (Mayer et al., 1989; Jankowski et al., 2002). This supports the assumption of the existence of a good correlation between PMN viability and CL. To obtain a better insight into the effects of (patho)physiology of mammary gland on non-specific defense mechanisms of the udder, assessment of viability of blood and milk PMN can be pivotal. Milk PMN viability assessment could also be an index for the detection of inflammation of the mammary gland.

To overcome any problem and to simplify PMN functional assay, researchers, who wants to work on this area in animals/human breast physioimmunology, should properly isolate targeted cells from blood and mammary gland for quantitative and qualitative assays (see figures 1-2 and 6); there are plenty references in these topics, and some appeared in the reference list. CL simplifies PMN ROS production measurement, and is a relatively recent technique. Application of CL technique to study PMN function helps to gain more insight into first line of immune defense mechanisms and the pathophysiology of physiological and environmental stresses-related infections and/or inflammations. For CL quantification, we need viable PMN, a PMN activator (e.g. PMA, fMLP, particles, etc.) and a CL substrate (e.g.,

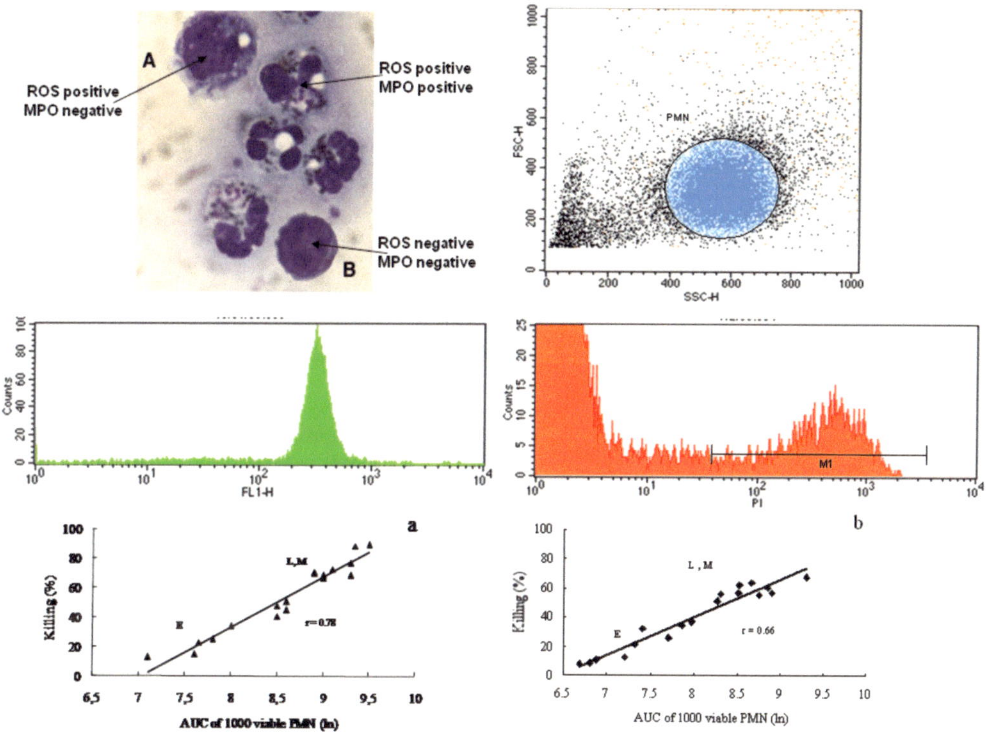

Fig. 6. Upper left: Light microscopic image of PMN (middle), a macrophage (A) and a lymphocyte (B) isolated from non-inflamed lactating udder stained with benzidine dihydrochloride plus H_2O_2 and counterstained with hematoxilin-eosin (× 1000). Because MPO is central to intracellular ROS-associated microbicidal and luminol dependent CL, the contribution of other cells especially macrophages on CL and MPO activity assays should also be considered. Bovine milk macrophages has no MPO activity in our assay, and in case of having mixed cells in the samples their contribution to the CL assay is little. Conversely, bovine post-diapedetic neutrophils has huge MPO activity, and they are main source of CL assay of milk cells. Flow cytometric analysis of isolated bovine milk neutrophils gated in the FS-SS dot plot (upper right). Green fluorescence of PMN labeled with a monoclonal antibody specific against bovine granulocytes and with a secondary FITC-labeled antibody (middle left). Red fluorescence of propidium iodide-incubated PMN selectively gated in the FS-SS dot plot; gate M1 is applied to determine the percentage of dead PMN (for the quantification of viability/quality of post-diapedetic neutrophils) (middle right). Lower panel shows correlation between PMA induced luminol-dependent CL (LDCL) of blood neutrophils (a) and post-diapedetic neutrophils in lactating udder (b) and their effectiveness towards killing of *S. aureus*. E: early lactogenesis period; L, M: late and mid lactogenesis periods, respectively. Partially adapted from (Mehrzad et al., 2001a; 2001c).

luminol, isoluminol, lucigenin etc). Luminol-dependent CL has been described as an appropriate probe for assessment of blood and milk PMN ROS production (Briheim et al., 1984). The PMN metabolic pathways responsible for O_2-dependent bactericidal activity and CL assays are depicted schematically in figure 5.

A flow cytometric technique has also been used to detect ROS production, necrosis, apoptosis and many immunological assays on bovine blood and interstitial fluid neutrophils (Mehrzad et al., 2001a; 2001b; 2001c; Dosogne et al., 2002; Vangroenweghe et al., 2001; Van Oostveldt et al., 2001; 2002a; 2002b Mehrzad et al., 2002; 2004; 2005a; 2009; 2011) applying propidium iodide (PI) exclusion method, Anexi V and JC-1 solution (5,5',6,6'-tetrachloro-1,1',3,3'-tetraethylbenzimidazolylcarbocyanine iodide) (Merhzad et al., 2001a; 2001b; 2001c; 2011; Van Oostveldt et al., 2002a; 2002b) (figures 6). Although many immunological assays can be done with flow cytometry, the assay of neutrophils' ROS production with flow cytometry has revealed some challenging results, compared to luminometry technique; also, with the flow cytometry it is hardly possible to measure the kinetics and the dynamics of the neutrophil-pathogen interaction 'during' neutrophil-pathogen interaction.

Methodological studies reveal a very well correlation between PMN viability and CL activity and killing capacities. Isolated blood and milk PMN can appropriately be identifiable on FS-SS dot plot (see figures 5, 6). Flow cytometry is an accurate and reproducible technique for the rapid quantification of PMN apoptosis and necrosis in physiological and pathological conditions of animals and human (figure 6). This can effectively facilitate further PMN functional assay, hence boosting insight into the first line defense mechanism of the host.

6. Lipopolysaccharide, TLR4, TNF-α and NO levels in inflammatory environment of the mammary gland

The compound of the bacterial outer membrane, peptidoglycan monomers and lipopolysaccharide (LPS) or endotoxins, are unique to all Gram-negative bacterial cell walls. In the case of Gram negative bacteria, the principal stimulator of the innate immune system is the LPS; this LPS evokes several functional responses in these short-lived, bone marrow myeloid-derived cells, neutrophils, to the site of inflammation or infection.

The PRRs are the main sensors of pathogens and danger signals in innate immunity. Though they are mainly highly expressed by macrophages and DCs of different organs, neutrophils also highly express these sensor molecules inside and outside their surface. Toll like receptors/proteins, homologues of the *Drosophila* protein Toll, are the most studied and best characterized PPRs, which are responsible for sensing PAMPs and also products of inflamed tissues, DAMPs. TLRs activation triggers signaling pathways that lead to activation of transcription factors such as NF-κB and the interferon regulatory factors. This, in turn, leads to induction of immune and inflammatory genes, including such important cytokines as TNF-α and type I interferons. The contribution of PRRs to inflammation induced by microbial infection, tissue damage and cancer are a hot topic in immunology, immunopathology and immunotherapy. Much evidence points to the role for PRRs and especially TLRs in immune and inflammatory diseases and increasingly in cancer detection and therapy (Bellocchio et al., 2004; Simons et al., 2008). For example, cancerous cell lines are one of the best models to study the biological roles of PRRs in cancer and tumor biology. Role of neutrophils on those points remained deeply unnoticed. Study also reports how, e.g., TLR2 expression by endothelia is locally upregulated by the action of activated neutrophils via an unprecedented mechanism involving cell-cell interaction and NOX, emphasizing yet another way in which the primordial innate immune system is remarkably complex.

The interaction of neutrophils in the sites of inflamed/infections with these key elements of the PAMPs, LPS, and bind to PRRs is pivotal to overcome pathogen and limit the severity of infection. The PRRs are present on a variety of defence cells of the body causing them to synthesise and release a variety of cytokines. Synergistically, the LPS interacts with LPS-binding protein and CD14, which in turn promotes the ability of particularily TLR4 on neutrophils and macrophages to respond to the LPS with the release of various pro-inflammatory cytokines and chemokines (Sohn et al., 2007a; 2007b; Rinaldi et al., 2010; Stevens et al., 2011a ; 2011b). These pro-inflammatory molecules bind on target cells via specific receptors and initiate inflammation. TLRs have been detected on the surface of mammalian cells (Beutler, 2002). They are important in the responses of phagocytes to bacterial, viral, and fungal antigens. TLR2 and TLR4 have candidate genes for resistance to several diseases as they recognise broad classes of PAMPs, such as peptidoglycans and LPS (Werling & Jungi, 2003; Bellocchio et al., 2004). Bovine and human neutrophils express substantial amounts of TLR4 and other TLRs, critical for response to PAMPs/DAMPs (Kurt-Jones et al., 2002 ; Hayashi et al., 2003; Werling. & Jungi, 2003; Rinaldi et al., 2010; Stevens et al., 2011a ; 2011b). TLR4 activates the inflammatory gene expression through NF-κB (Hayashi et al., 2003). GM-CSF and and G-CSF dramatically up-regulate TLR2 and CD14 expression (Kurt-Jones et al., 2002). Recent *in vitro* studies have shown that mammary epithelial cells actively participate in the immunoregulation during inflammation via mainly cytokine production (Sohn et al., 2007a; 2007b; Rinaldi et al., 2010; Stevens et al., 2011a; 2011b). A MAC-T cell line was utilised to investigate the expression of many innate immune mRNAs like IL-1 and its subsequent secretion after stimulation with PAMPs showed that these cells secrete IL-1 in response to LPS. IL-1 also appeared to be an important mediator for the release of the IL-8 and many other chemokines (Huynh et al., 1991; Boudjellab et al., 1998; 2000; Pezeshki et al., 2011).

During infection of mammary gland, IL-1, IL-6 and IL-8 (Shuster et al., 1997), platelet-activating factor (PAF), (Pezeshki et al., 2011), prostaglandins (Pezeshki et al., 2011; Shuster et al., 1997), activated complement C5 (C5a; Shuster et al., 1997; Rinaldi et al., 2010) NO (Blum et al., 2000), many ROS (Mehrzad et al., 2001; 2004; 2005a) and proteases (Mehrzad et al., 2005b) are released locally. In milk, an increase in TNF-α, a cytokine of particular interest in the pathogenesis of mastitis, is observed (Blum et al., 2000; Hoeben et al., 2000b; Shuster et al., 1997). The kinetics of cytokines in the inflammatory environment of udder shows that the increase in TNF-α and IL-1, the mother of proinflammatory cytokines, occurs faster during inflammation from endotoxins than from *E. coli* mastitis, though more pronounced in *E. coli* infection (Blum et al., 2000; Hoeben et al., 2000b). Absorption of this cytokine from the udder into the blood circulation is highest during *E. coli* mastitis. The level of these key cytokines in milk correlated well with the pyrexia and the severity of the udder infection (Shuster et al., 1997; Blum et al., 2000; Hoeben et al., 2000b; Pezeshki et al., 2011).

Many of the biological activities of LPS are mediated by TNF-α. LPS and cytokines stimulate the synthesis of NO, which is a vasodilator. Synthesised from L-arginine, this diatomic free radical, NO, is lipid soluble and easily diffuses through the cell membrane. It is short lived and usually reacts and degrades fast. The natural form is a gas that reacts with a variety of innate immune molecules and mediates a large spectrum of immunobiological effects in the body. An inducible NO synthase (E.C. 1.14.13.39, iNOS) is expressed by a variety of cells, especially phagocytes, as a result of triggering with substances of microbial origin such as LPS and TNF-α. In response to invading pathogens and PAMPs like LPS, bovine phagocytes produce NO (Adler et al., 1995; Stich et al., 1998), functioning as a strong anti-PAMP agent. When the NO is produced in excessive amounts, it can also induce cytotoxic and apoptosis in the cells (Moncada et al., 1991; Anggard, 1994)

Several studies on ruminants have shown a relationship between LPS, TNF-α and production of NO. The increase in TNF-α is followed by a delayed increase in NO_x (NO_2 + NO_3) (Blum et al., 2000; Bouchard et al., 1999). The NO_x production lasts longer in the udder. A causal relationship between TNF-α and NO_x production was observed in studies in which *E. coli* LPS was injected intravenously. It seems that severe forms of udder's inflamed environment are accompanied by the highest increase in blood stream's levels of both TNF-α and NO_x; the increase in NO_x and TNF-α during infection is not inhibited by antibiotics (Blum et al., 2000), supporting the notion that the release of NO_x is PAMP dependent rather than *E. coli*. Initially called endothelium derived factor (EDRF), NO causes many other vital physiological phenomena like vasodilation and subside of inflammation. It is released after the fever peak, and is involved in this delayed phase of hyperemia.

7. Neutrophil AOAH as a potent protector of mammary gland from pathogens

The contribution of circulating and postdiapedetic neutrophils' acyloxyacyl hydrolase (AOAH) to the outcome of infection in animals has recently been highlighted (Dosogne et al., 1998; Mehrzad et al., 2007). Apart from existence of many bactericidal mechanisms in the bovine neutrophils (Barrio et al., 2000; Burvenich et al., 2003; Mehrzad et al., 2001a; 2001b; 2001c; 2002; 2004; 2005a; 2005b; 2007; 2008a; 2009), there are many other soluble and insoluble proteins on the neutrophils in the mammary gland that protect the gland from invading pathogens. One of them is AOAH molecules. Endotoxins or LPS are released during bacterial growth and lysis of Gram-negative bacteria have been recognized as important mediators for the treatment and outcome of coliform mastitis (Pyörälä et al., 1994; Dosogne et al., 2002; Mehrzad et al., 2007). The role of the absorption of free LPS into the circulation is controversial (Dosogne et al., 2002; Mehrzad et al., 2004; 2005a; 2007). Conversely, it is accepted that the amount of released LPS into the mammary gland, its subsequent detoxification and TNF-α production significantly contribute to the outcome of coliform infection (Blum et al. 2000; Hoeben et al. 2000b; Mehrzad et al., 2007). Severity of *E. coli* infection seems to be related to the enhanced release of secondary induced inflammatory mediators such as TNF-α (Blum et al., 2000; Mehrzad et al., 2007), as a result of impaired LPS detoxification mechanisms in inflamed organ. It has been suggested (Burvenich et al., 1996; 2003; Paape et al., 1996; 2002) that local CD14 expression alleviates the toxic effects of LPS in the mammary gland. AOAH, an enzyme hugely produced by bovine neutrophils, hydrolyses LPS (McDermott et al., 1991; Mehrzad et al., 2007) and alleviate the inflammation. This neutrophils' arsenal, AOAH, hydrolyses two acyl chains of the lipid A of LPS, leading to substantial decreased toxicity of LPS while retaining much of the immunostimulatory potency of native toxicity of LPS (Munford and Hall, 1986).

Although there are some rare investigation of bovine blood PMN AOAH activity, but little has been done on post-diapedetic neutrophils' AOAH activity either during physiological or pathological conditions. Immediately after parturition, there is a decreased blood PMN AOAH activity (Dosogne et al., 1998) that coincides with the decreased PMN ROS production and number in circulation (Mehrzad et al., 2001b; 2002a; 2004; 2005a). This coincidence could be considered as a risk factor for Gram negative bacterial infections during especially physiological stress (Mehrzad et al., 2001b; 2004; 2005a). Indeed, intravenous LPS administration to rabbits resulted in a rapid (within 90 min) increase of plasma AOAH activity (Erwin and Munford, 1991). The finding that PMN AOAH activity is increased upon LPS stimulation may indicate the existence of a PMN-dependent self-regulatory protection mechanism against endotoxemia and sepsis. It is suggested that a decreased AOAH activity in post-diapedetic PMN can also contribute to the outcome of organ failure and even death, as we observed in bovine (Mehrzad et al., 2007).

Apart from AOAH, bovine neutrophils granules also contain different LPS binding cationic proteins such as lactoferrin, and a huge variety of cationic antimicrobial proteins (Levy et al., 1995; Mehrzad et al., 2005b). These proteins do not degrade the LPS molecule, but binding to LPS results in a decreased LPS bioavailibility and hence may attenuate its toxicity during Gram-negative bacterial infections. In a recent study, oral lactoferrin administration attenuated spontaneous TNF-α production by peripheral blood cells in human (Zimecki et al., 1999). Study on this topic would be very interesting for immunobiologists.

Several classes of phagocyte-derived antimicrobial peptides have been purified from mammalian phagocytes, and it is now clear that next to their production of ROS, bovine PMN also inactivate microorganisms by exposing them to these antimicrobial peptides and proteins within the phagolysosomal vacuoles. Bovine PMN granules contain a group of highly cationic proteins. Beta-defensins, a family represented by 13 cationic, tridisulfide-containing peptides with 38-42 residues, have potent antibacterial activities against both *S. aureus* and *E. coli in vitro*. Similar molecules have also been isolated from specialized epithelia. These polypeptides are structured through disulfide bonds of cysteine but can also be linear and unstructured; they remarkably contribute to host defense against pathogens. Because many bactericidal peptides like β-defensins etc. are stored in the dense granules of neutrophils, it is likely that they are discharged simultaneously during PMN activation. Although co-packaged in the dense granules, cathelicidins, but not β-defensins, are stored as inactive propeptides. Following PMN stimulation with PMA, the cathelicidins Bac5 and Bac7 are cleaved from their respective propeptides and released extracellularly. In contrast, β-defensins exist as fully processed peptides in bovine PMN.

The 46 kDa soluble CD14 (sCD14), which is shedding of membrane CD14 (mCD14) from phagocyte, is also available in interstitial fluid/milk (Wang et al., 2002; Sohn et al., 2007a; 2007b), and can bind LPS directly and prevent LPS from binding to mCD14, thus preventing over-secretion of TNF-α, thereby silencing the severity of inflammation and clinical symptoms. This potentially plays a role in neutralizing LPS and controlling the clinical symptoms associated with acute infection. *In vitro* incubation of recombinant bovine (rbo) sCD14 with PMN and LPS prevented LPS induced upregulation of CD18 adhesion receptors (Wang et al., 2002; Sohn et al., 2007a). Intramammary and systemic use of rbosCD14 may provide a means of eliminating the potential damaging effects of LPS during acute infection and sepsis; this approach would also be applicable in human inflammatory and infectious diseases.

Furthermore, iron-binding protein, lactoferrin, is small protein synergizes neutrophils' functions and LPS detoxification. Bovine lactoferrin does far beyond the binding of iron, and has considerable inhibitory effect on bacterial growth (Bishop et al., 1976). Lysozyme or muramidase can cleave the mucopeptide layer of most non-encapsulated Gram-positive bacterial cell walls resulting in cytoplasmic blebbing of the bacterial cell wall, leading to direct bacterial lysis, especially when the osmolarity of the infected microenvironment is sufficiently low. Lysozyme has also the capacity to neutralise and strongly interact with *E. coli* LPS; another non-oxidative antimicrobial agent in PMN, which directly/indirectly enhances LPS degradation, is PMN elastase. Elastase, cathepsin G and other granule-proteases degrade the outer membrane protein A of *E. coli*, which is located on the surface of the bacteria (Belaaouaj et al., 1998). PMN ROS production synergises activity of all above mentioned antimicrobial and anti-PAMP compounds. Overall, apart from the role of bovine PMN granules and enzymes, it is fully accepted that the PMN ROS production plays a major role in protection of udder from Gram negative bacterial infection (Burvenich et al., 2003; Mehrzad et al., 2004; 2005a) and detoxification of LPS.

8. Oscillatory events on neutrophils functions

Neutrophil dysfunction in animals and human has been associated with decreased immunocompetence, resulting in the suppression of host defense mechanisms and increased susceptibility to many infectious and non-infectious diseases. Nowadays, potential increasingly environmental stresses and worldwide-food scarcity issues have resulted in unstoppably intensive feed/food and dairy production. The intensive production system leads to unstoppable oscillatory events on innate immune systems, especially neutrophils in bone marrow, blood and udder of high yielding dairy cows, compromising innate defence system in udder, thereby making animals particularly sensitive to infections. Oscillatory events on neutrophils occurs in all stages of maturation and functions (see figures 7 and 8), not only in mature animals but also in neonate, e.g., in bovine (Mehrzad et al., 2001a; 2001c; 2002a; 2008a 2008b; 2008c). Relative magnitude of circulating and post-diapedetic PMN impairment differed from different physiopathological status of animals and humans. A dramatic reduction in random migration, iodination and ROS production of blood PMN were observed during the first week after parturition (Heyneman et al., 1990; Hoeben et al., 2000a; Mehrzad et al., 2001a; 2001b; 2001c). It was recently discovered that the adhesion molecule L-selectin is shed from the surface of bovine PMN at parturition (Diez-Frail et al., 2004). Surface expression of L-selectin remains low for several days following parturition and could contribute to the reported defect in bovine PMN chemotaxis during the period immediately following parturition (Berning et al., 1993; Diez-Frail et al., 2004). Regulation of bovine PMN adhesion molecules during mammary gland infection and possible use of immunomodulators has recently been studied (Diez-Frail et al., 2004).

Cumulative deficiencies in opsonin levels (IgG_1 and conglutinin) were observed in peak of physiological stress in animals, which closely coincided with impaired PMN oxidation-reduction reactions capacity (Detilleux et al., 1994; Burvenich et al., 2003). The proportion of all cases of infections especially mastitis, metritis, arthritis and laminitis that develop during period at which the animals encounter with maximal stress status; these period is coincided with maximal oscillatory events in circulating and post-diapedetic neutrophils (Burvenich et al., 1994; 2003; Mehrzad et al., 2001a; 2001c; 2002a; 2008b; 2008c).

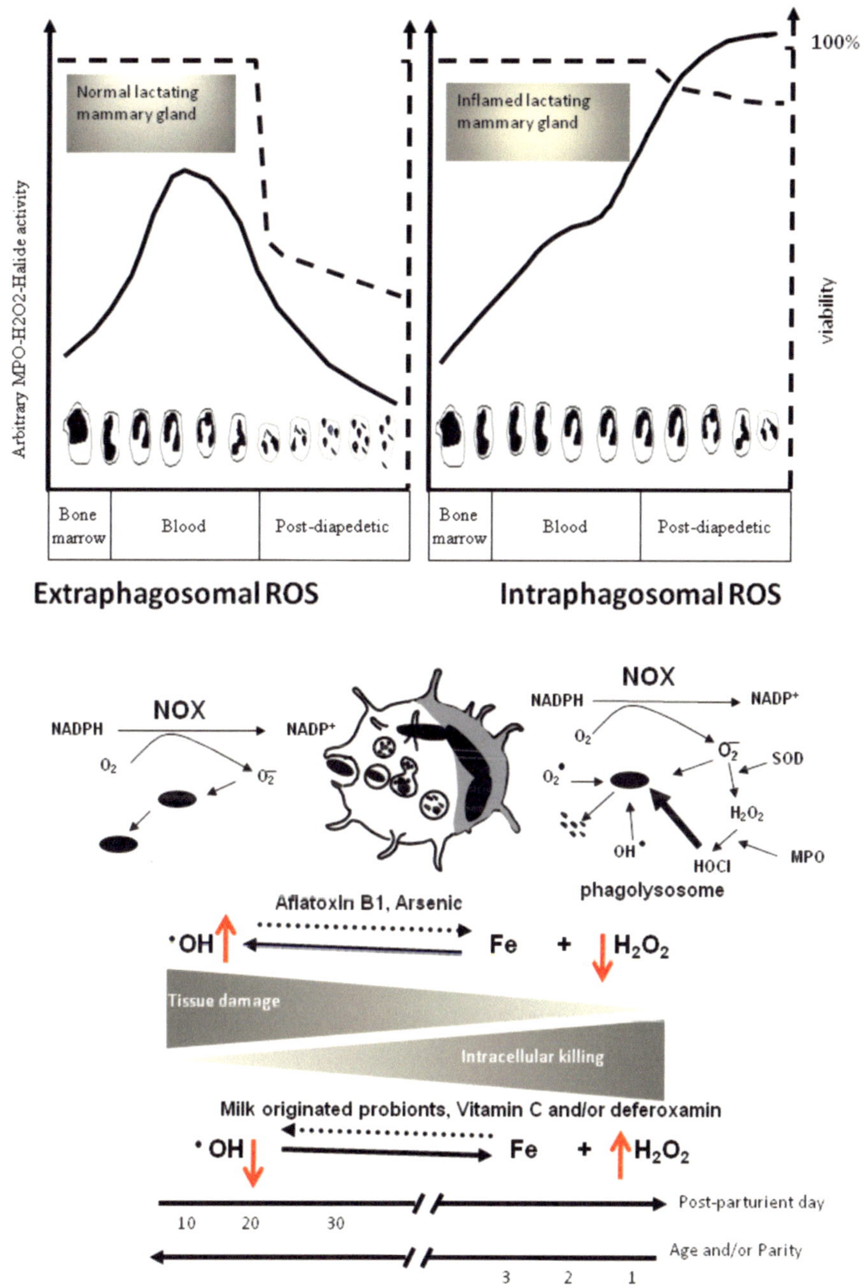

Fig. 7. Upper panel: An schematic overview on author's recent findings (together with literatures) about changes in neutrophils' MPO-H_2O_2-Halide system (solid lines), viability (dashed lines) and dynamics of neutrophils structure and maturity in healthy and mastitis dairy cows. Formed in bone marrow, blood neutrophils function and structure changed after normal extravasation. These changes differed in inflammatory environments. The most probable reason for these disparities would be the "rate of diapedesis", which is faster

during inflammation; pinpointing the aspects of molecular mechanisms of this classically mechanomical phenomenon of neutrophils in different physiological and pathological conditions in animals and humans is very interesting topics for further fundamental research in the area of innate immune system. Lower panel: Diagram illustrating the oscillatory events on neutrophils and some potential nutritional and environmental interventions (Ibeagha et al., 2009; Mehrzad et al., 2008c; 2011) in animals and human to modulate their neutrophils' ultimate functions. These provocative hypotheses address the points that during severe infection/inflammation of the udder extracellular production of ROS by neutrophils may be impaired and could lead to tissue damage in mammary gland. Normally, ROS for bactericidal activity is produced intracellularly for effective destruction of microbes with a minimal tissue damage. The hypothesis is based on the study of the kinetics of chemiluminescence: 1) there is a difference between extracellular and intracellular ROS production of both blood and post-diapedetic neutrophils during different stages of lactogenesis, and 2) in blood and milk, extracellular ROS production by neutrophils is more pronounced in old animals. This may lead to an impaired bactericidal capacity of resident udder neutrophils and boost tissue damage in aged animals (Mehrzad et al., 2001a; 2001b; 2002; 2004; 2005a; 2005b) and partially adapted from (Burvenich et al., 2003). Further, many environmental toxins cause oscillations on neutrophils' ultimate functions (Mehrzad et al., 2011); conversely potential nutritional intervention could reverse the oscillatory events in neutrophils (Ibeagha et al., 2009; Mehrzad et al., 2008c); what happens on the impacts of nanotubes, nanovectors, nanoneedles, nanoparticles and nanoadjuvants on this casecade of events can be very interesting to work. Promising photoredox and antioxidant properties of vitamin C, probionts and deferoxamin with huge quenching capacity mainly on $OH^{\bullet}$ with much less pronounced on H_2O_2 and $O_2^{\bullet -}$ (Mehrzad et al., unpublished data), and dietary supplementation with probiotics and peptides originated from bovine milk augments neutrophils' functions (Gill et al., 2000; 2001a; 2001b; Mehrzad et al., 2002b). Reverse results have been observed with aflatoxin B1 (Mehrzad et al., 2011), Arsenic, Lead (Mehrzad et al., unpublished data) and plenty more with marked oscillatory effects on neutrophils' ultimate functions. Both in animals and humans due to many environmental and physiological stresses influencing on the overall immune system of the body, switching the oxidant-antioxidant systems on the body from antioxidant status to prooxidant ones and excessive extracellular ROS will accumulate in the body. To remove excessive and unwanted ROS, especially $OH^{\bullet}$ in the body some antioxidants like vitamins C, E, A..., deferoxamin and probionts can be promisingly helpful and here immunobiologists are strongly encouraged to focus on those novel topics of nutritional and environmental immunology in animals and humans.

One of the most critically physiological associated stress periods would be periparturient period and early lactogenesis. Both in milk and blood PMN function is substantially decreased around parturition (Van Oostveldt et al., 2001; Mehrzad et al., 2001a; 2001c, 2002; 2009; Burvenich et al., 2003). Up till now the underlying mechanisms involved in periparturient immunosuppression remain unknown. However, metabolites (e.g. β-hydroxybutyrate) (Suriyasathaporn et al., 1999) and hormones (e.g. growth hormone, cortisol, pregnancy associated glycoprotein) (Gray et al., 1982; Burvenich et al.,1994; Suriyasathaporn et al., 1999) have been reported as attributable factors.

There are many reports demonstrating that at least some of hormones and metabolites contribute to the oscillatory events in PMN function, targeting both the afferent and efferent arms of PMN functions (Gray et al., 1982; Burvenich et al., 1994; Suriyasathaporn et al., 1999; Hoeben et al., 1999; 2000a). As these studies suggest, the link between periparturient immunosuppression and hormonal and metabolic changes is nevertheless apparent; most of which directly/indirectly affect PMN functions. Hormonal and metabolic changes such as glucocorticoids, ketone bodies and pregnancy associated glycoproteins play a causative role in oscillatory events on key efferent arms of PMN function, ROS production/microbicidal capacity (Dosogne et al., 1998; Hoeben et al. 2000a). These hormones and metabolites also inhibit the proliferation of bone marrow cells *in vitro* (Hoeben et al. 1999; Van Merris, et al., 2001a; 2001b 2002).

Our understanding of the precise ways in which the complex cascade of ROS production occurs in blood or milk PMN during physiological and pathological conditions is still in its infancy. This is especially true for the mechanism of in vivo effect of PMN functions by hormones and metabolites, especially the metabolomics aspects of neutrophils' dysfunction. Based on current understanding of impact of hormones on PMN function, the membrane, cytosolic and nuclear effects of hormones (e.g. growth hormone, sex hormones, cortisol, pregnancy associated glycoprotein) and metabolites (β-hydroxybutyrate, non-esterified fatty acid) on blood and post-diapedetic PMN functions are to be more fundamentally investigated.

Recombinant bovine somatotropin (bST) has been shown to boost cows' milk production and compositional performance following experimentally induced *E. coli* and *Streptococcus uberis* infection (Hoeben et al., 1999). Recombinant bST also prevented severe local and general clinical symptoms in cows suffering from *E. coli* mastitis, especially in severe responders. Prolactin, bST, and insulin-like growth factor-I (IGF-I) are thought to be involved in several immune functions (Elvinger et al., 1991; Hooghe et al., 1993; Kooijman et al., 1996). The function of bST on PMN can either be directly or indirectly mediated through IGF-I. Plasma and milk concentrations of IGF-I increase after bST administration (Zhao et al., 1992). Their concentration differs throughout lactation in milk (Campbell et al., 1991). An increased number of circulating leukocytes, band neutrophils, and an enhanced PMN functions in cows treated with bST after stress related to parturition. Also PMN ROS generation, chemotaxis, random migration, phagocytosis towards IgG-opsonised microorganisms is boosted by IGF-I and bST (Fu et al., 1991; Wiedermann et al., 1993; Warwick-Davies et al., 1995; Mehrzad et al., unpublished). The expression of complement receptors on neutrophils can be upregulated by bST and IGF-I. Increased chemotaxis and random migration (Wiedermann et al., 1993), increased numbers of circulating neutrophils (Clark et al., 1993), and increased proliferation of granulocyte and monocyte precursors (Merchav et al., 1993); *in vivo* bST administration leads to elevation in blood IGF-I lovel. Though *in vivo* might be different from *in vitro,* many recent studies revealed an increased PMN ROS production capacity after *in vivo* administration of bST in healthy animal model; similar results were observed *in vitro* (Mehrzad et al., 2002b). Thus, there is ample evidence that bST and IGF-I can boost neutrophils' functions. Concentration of some biomolecules like β-lactoglobulin in udder secreta is minimal during maximal stress condition of lactaogenssi (Caffin et al., 1984); this means that the β-lactoglobulin can be a potential immunomodulator in the mammary gland and good topic to further focus and apply in human breast and milk physioimmunobiology (Wong et al., 1998; Mehrzad et al., 2000). Hence the insight into PMN activators and/or inhibitors in milk during physiological and pathological conditions is crucial concern for udder's first line defense mechanism and neonatal passive immunity in animals and humans.

As explained before, blood and post-diapedetic neutrophils have the potential to produce substantial amounts of ROS to kill engulfed bacteria (Hoeben et al., 2000a; Mehrzad et al., 2001a; 2001c; 2002a; 2004; 2005a; 2005b; 2009). ROS production can be measured in resting (non-stimulated) neutrophils and after stimulation with e.g., PMA, zymosan, bacteria and latex beads.

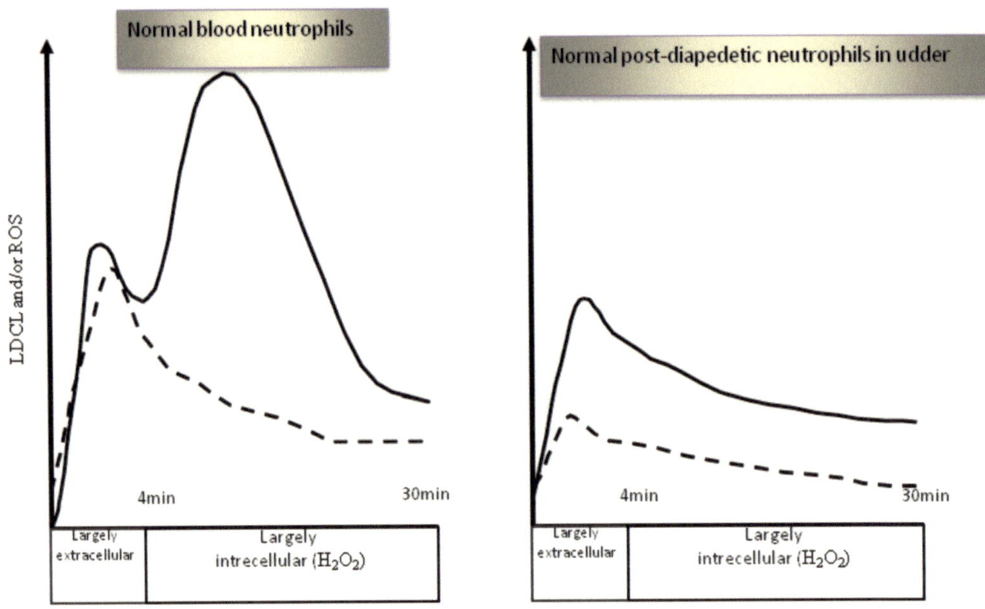

Fig. 8. A comparison between blood and post-diapedetic neutrophils chemiluminescence (CL) profiles of PMA-activated luminol-enhanced neutrophils during different physiological status of animals. The intra-and-extra-cellular ROS production of neutrophils and the concept of biphasic versus monophasic CL pattern of neutgrophils are overviewed. The first peak is the result of mainly initial extracellular reactions and the second peak is mainly a result of subsequent intracellular reactions of the MPO-H_2O_2 system. The Y-axes are the cumulative RLU / s in function of time, and the X-axes are the entire measurement period of CL. Based on the author's previous studies, curves are arbitrarily depicted to show how neutrophils microbicidal capacity changes after diapedesis through blood-milk barrier and during different physiological status. Oscillatory phenomenon observed in the postdiapedetic neutrophils specially the monophasic pattern with minimal ROS production peak. Throughout lactogenesis period of the lactating mammary gland, the kinetics of post-diapedetic PMN CL never exhibited double phase patterns. Further, blood PMN CL kinetics immediately after parturition gave neither double phase nor high intensity as in later phase of lactogenesis period. The plateau and shape of the blood and- post-diapedetic neutrophils' CL curves shows a biphasic pattern of the blood neutrophils CL during minimal stress condition (like later period of lactogenesis). The intensity of ROS production is lower in post-diapedetic neutrophils than in blood neutrophils, the plateau and shape of the milk- and blood CL curves were similar during maximal physiological and environmental

stresses. Thus, the oscillatory phenomenon of milk PMN ROS production/microbicidal capacity during parturition and lactation seems to be directly related to that of the blood PMN. This animal model of ineffectiveness of the oxygen-dependent intracellular killing mechanisms of neutrophils during inevitable physiological and environmental stresses is very interesting topic of efferent arms of neutrophils for further research in animals and human.

Production of ROS is effective in killing engulfed microbes (Burvenich et al., 1994; 2003; Reeves et al., 2002; Mehrzad et al;, 2001a; 2001c; 2002a; 2004; 2005a; 2005b; 2009). Also the most widely used technique to estimate oscillatory events in bovine and human PMN ROS production is the elegantly simple CL assay (Hoeben et al., 2000a; Mehrzad et al., 2001a; 2001b; 2001c; 2002a; 2004; 2005a; 2009; 2011).

Little comparison has been made between CL of circulating and post-diapedetic neutrophils. To interpret and assess the responsiveness of PMN to stimulating agents such as PMA, it is necessary to distinguish between stimulated and non-stimulated PMN. This offers information about the activity of protein kinase C and NADPH-oxidase, as PMA is a protein kinase C and NADPH-oxidase agonist (Karlsson et al., 2000; Mehrzad et al., 2001a; 2001b; 2001c; 2002; 2004; 2005a; 2009) in the lactating mammary gland. Ingestion of milk fat globules and casein micelles affects milk PMN quality (Mehrzad et al., 2001a; 2001b; 2004; Paape et al., 2002; Burvenich et al., 2003) and subsequent degranulation. No such a problem in blood stream is existed. Smits et al, (1999) have shown that *in vitro* transepithelial/endothelial diapedesis of PMN across mammary gland reduces ROS production of PMN. It has also been shown that the function of post-diapedetic neutrophils in udder differs from their blood counterparts (Smits et al., 2000; Mehrzad et al., 2001a; 2001b; 2001c; 2002a; 2009). Some physiological influencing factors such as lactogenesis (Mehrzad et al., 2001a; 2001c) and ageing (Mehrzad et al., 2002a; 2008b; 2009) are involved in overall PMN impairment. Some other contributing factors would be β-lactoglobulin (Mehrzad et al., 2000b), of which concentration in milk is minimal during maximal stress condition like early lactogenesis (Caffin et al., 1984). The PMN function impairment generally coincides with cow's susceptibility for environmental infection (van Werven et al., 1997; Burvenich et al., 1994; Burvenich et al., 2003; Mehrzad et al., 2004; 2005a). Dynamically, the topic is very important especially for human medicine and further research on this topic of mammary gland innate defence system is deeply needed.

Apart from the involvement of environmental and nutritional factors in hosts' PMN functions and resistance to infection, plenty of many other factors contribute to PMN oscillatory events and the outcome of infection/inflammation in humans and animals; one of the key and interestingly dynamic attributing factors would be the effect of genetics on the quantity and quality of circulating and and post-daipedetic neutrophils (Dietz et al., 1997; Riollet et al., 2000; Wall et al., 2005; Radwan et al., 2007; Rupp et al., 2007; Bannerman et al., 2008). Undoubtedly, all of above mentioned factors could become an important alternative for prophylactic measures of infectious and inflammatory diseases in animals and humans.

Another future increasingly challenging issue in the area of innate immunotoxicity is the environmental and artificial nanoparticles (Karathanasis et al., 2009; Sadikot & Rubinstein, 2009; Gonçalves et al., 2010; Paulsson et al., 2010; and plenty more), which can be both friend and foe for the innate immune system and cancer development. This can be more special for the oscillatory events on both afferent and efferent arms of blood and post-diapedetic neutrophils. Exposures to airborne nanosized particles have been frequently experienced by animals/humans throughout their evolutionary stages, affecting on, e.g., portals of body's entry (respiratory and gastrointestinal tracts and skin). To highlight potential mechanisms of nanotubes, nanovectors, nanoneedles, nanoparticles and nanoadjuvants and cancer nanomedicine, researchers should always focus on immune systems especially the issue of genomics, proteomics and mechanomics aspects of free radicals production of the phagocytes. Application of those potentially promising idea and hypotheses in relation to the neutrophils' oscillatory events versus neutrophils the medicines, eg, topical wound protectant and antiseptics for the treatment of human/animals blister wounds contaminated with microbes or to kill abnormal cells in the body would be very challengingly promising. The challenge is to integrate effectively all information from cellular to molecular events anthropogenically happening for animals/humans' health and performance may contribute to further oscillatory in neutrophils.

9. Conclusions and future perspectives

The issues on animals and humans' diseases are many; among them is neutrophil function that has been the researchers' past, current and future concern. It is clear that appropriate function of neutrophils in the body of animals and humans is very vital to enhance their health and performance. The concepts of neutrophil recruitment at the site of microbial invasion and the interesting phenomenon of nonspecifically engulfing and killing of microbes by neutrophils is still a complex cascade of many cellular and molecular events; molecularly, afferent (sensing) and efferent (effector and/or highly intracellular-and-extracellular microbicidal compounds) weapons of neutrophils are vital in protection of the hosts. Inevitable occurring of general and local immunocompromised conditions especially on the effector weaponry of neutrophils leads to countless infectious and non-infectious diseases. Most researchers see the immunocompromised condition of the organs like udder as a result of neutrophils' dysfunction in bone marrow, bloodstream and interstitial fluid. This chapter would make the complex oscillatory events happening in neutrophils a little bit more comprehensible.

Despite intense progress in molecular biology, medicine, nutrition, genetics and nanomedicine, animals and humans are still susceptible -more than before- to environmental bacteria; this susceptibility is maximal during stress, of which neutrophils dysfunction can be one of the most central attributable factors. Immunomodulation is still far from assured. The long-term and fundamental solution for the oscillatory event on neutrophils is to strengthen their functions by means of attainable physio-immunological approaches. This requires a comprehensive study on molecular and cellular aspects of physio-immunological alterations throughout gestation, lactation and diseases.

One of the focuses of the chapter was a comparative overview of blood and post-diapedetic neutrophils' functions. To uncover further evidence on neutrophils' oscillatory events during stress conditions the shape of blood and post-diapedetic PMN CL proven one more reason for high susceptibility of animals/humans to infections. On this topic, many more questions remain open for future research. Future research is also necessary to pinpoint the physiopathological influencing factors on post-diapedetic neutrophils' necrosis and apoptosis. The hypotheses of contribution of antioxidants like vitamins C, E, A, GHS and dynamic of phagolysosomal pH on post-diapedetic neutrophils' quality and first line defense during stress condition could be tested in the future research.

It is conclusive that blood PMN had stronger weaponry than that of post diapedetic PMN, when encountered with pathogens. It is also concluded that the relative magnitude of blood and post-diapedetic neutrohpils' oscillation/impairment differ from different physiopathological status of animals. For example, post-diapedetic PMN quality impairment is more pronounced in older animals/humans. This impairment coincided with the impairment of PMN microbicidal capacity in bloodstream; PMN ineffectiveness against invading pathogens not merely resulted from the quantity of PMN, but, more importantly, from the quality of PMN, which was identified via PMN CL kinetics and PMN viability. In healthy animals the lowest post-diapedetic PMN quality is found during stress conditions, which is more pronounced in older ones, proving one more reason for high susceptibility of aged animals and humans to infections during environmental and physiological stresses. The explanations in this chapter aimed to increase the insight into the first line defense mechanism of organs like mammary gland/breast, could further deepen our understanding at the complex physiopathology of mammary gland infections, cancers and other stress-related infectious and non-infectious diseases. It is conceivable, however, more novel findings and views on these topics remain for future research.

With the existed knowledge, it is clear that stressed animals and humans are relatively immunosuppressed. This could boost their susceptibility to environmental bacterial infections. Nowadays, the overstressed animals/humans are more susceptible to environmental pathogens than before. The main concern now is how to control and enhance these non-specific aspects of immune system. Clearly, the most appropriate treatment for infectious and non-infectious diseases is preventive treatment. The chapter clearly demonstrates that the severity of mammary gland infections is highly related to pre-infection neutrophils' functions, quick recruitment of neutrophils in the gland and their quality after diapedesis. All of these neutrophils' functions impaired during stress conditions. Therefore, preventive measures on animals around stress should be thoroughly performed. The preventive measures should be aimed at lowering stressful conditions and ensuring a high standard of nutrition and hygiene. Both in animals and humans zero stress status must be implemented for the future; this is hardly achievable. The long-term, environmentally friendly ways and fundamental solution for stress-related infectious diseases in animals/humans is "to strengthen their first line defense" by means of attainable physio-immunological approaches. This requires more insight into the first line defense mechanism, which is absolutely crucial. Perhaps one exciting and environmentally acceptable approach for infection/inflammation control would be application of "probionts". Protection of the organ from pathogens with less/non-pathogen bacteria, then further research on host-bacteria interactions would be promising.

As addressed, the protruding psuedopodes in blood differs from those of post-diapedetic neutrophils; it would be worth studying the impact of stress, age and infections on surface morphology of blood and post-diapedetic neutrophils. To further mimic the first line defense mechanism similar study should be conducted on "bone marrow-blood-barrier". Positive role of transient PMN impairments during parturition and early lactation in animals and humans should not be ignored as a good event, because this might be responsible for less damage on biomolecules, cells and tissue during periparturient period, potentially providing better passive immunity to neonates from invading pathogens. Study should also be focused on molecular mechanisms of higher blood and milk neutrophil's functions (both efferent and afferent arms) in younger animals and humans.

10. Acknowledgment

The author gratefully acknowledges the bureau (area) for Research & Technology of Ferdowsi University of Mashhad for granting the basic research studies in connection with neutrophil functions in animals and human. The author also gratefully thanks Prof. Dr. Christian Burvenich for his encouraging support.

11. References

Adler H., Frech B., Thony M., Peterhans E. & Jungi T.W. (1995). Inducible nitric oxide synthase in cattle. Differential cytokine regulation of nitric oxide synthase in bovine and murine macrophages, J. Immunol. 154: 4710-4718.

Alexandrova M. L. (2009). What happens with ageing: decline or remodeling of opsonin-independent phagocyte oxidative activity? Luminescence, 24: 340–347.

Allen R.C., Stjernholm R.L. & Steele R.H. (1972). Evidence for the generation of an electronic excitation state(s) in human polymorphonuclear leukocytes and its participation in bactericidal activity. Biochem. Biophys. Res. Commun. 47: 679-684.

Allen R.C., Dale D.C. & Taylor F.B. Jr. (2000). Blood phagocyte luminescence: gauging systemic immune activation. Method in Enzymol. 305: 591-629.

Allport J.R., Lim Y.C., Shipley J.M., Senior R.M., Shapiro S.D., Matsuyoshi N., Vestweber D. & Luscinskas F.W. (2002). Neutrophils from MMP-9- or neutrophil elastase-deficient mice show no defect in transendothelial migration under flow in vitro. J. Leukoc. Biol. 71: 821-828.

Anggard E. (1994). Nitric oxide: mediator, murderer, and medicine. The Lancet. 343 : 1199-1206.

Arnhold J., Furtmüller P.G., Regelsberger G. & Obinger C. (2001). Redox properties of the couple compound I/native enzyme of myeloperoxidase and eosinophil peroxidase. Eur. J. Biochem. 268: 5142-5148.

Babior B. (1984). The respiratory burst of phagocytes. J. Clin. Invest. 73: 599-601.

Babior B.M. (1994). Activation of the respiratory burst oxidase. Environmental Health Ptospectives. (suppl 10) 102: 53-56.

Baldridge C.W. & Gerard R.W. (1933). The extra respiration of phagocytosis. Am. J. Physiol. 103: 235-236.

Bannerman D.D., Springer H.R., Paape M.J., Kauf A.C. & Goff J.P. (2008). Evaluation of breed-dependent differences in the innate immune responses of Holstein and Jersey cows to Staphylococcus aureus intramammary infection. J. Dairy Res., 75:291-301.

Barber M.R., Pantschenko A.G., Hinckley L.S. & Yang T.J. (1999). Inducible and constitutive in vitro neutrophil chemokine expression by mammary epithelial and myoepithelial cells. Clin. Diagn. Lab. Immunol., 6: 791-798.

Barrio B., Vangroenweghe F., Dosogne H. & Burvenich C. (2000). Decreased neutrophil bactericidal activity during phagocytosis of slime-producing Staphylococcus aureus strain. Vet. Res., 31: 603-609.

Belaaouaj A., McCarthy R., Baumann M., Gao Z., Ley T.J., Abraham S.N. & Shapiro S.D. (1998). Mice lacking neutrophil elastase reveal impaired host defence against gram negative bacterial sepsis. Nature Med., 4: 615-619.

Bellocchio S, Moretti S, Perruccio K, Fallarino F, Bozza S, Montagnoli C, Mosci P, Lipford GB, Pitzurra L, & Romani L. (2004). TLRs govern neutrophil activity in aspergillosis. J Immunol. 173:7406-7415.

Berning L.M., Paape M.J. & Peters R.R. (1993). Functional variation in endogenous and exogenous immunoglobulin binding to bovine neutrophils relative to parturition. Am. J. Vet. Res., 54: 1145-1153

Beutler B., (2002). TLR4 as the mammalian endotoxin sensor, Curr.Top.Microbiol.Immunol. 270 108-120.

Bishop J., Schanbacher F., Ferguson L. & Smith K. (1976). In vitro growth inhibition of mastitis-causing coliform bacteria by bovine apo-lactoferrin and reversal of inhibition by citrate and high concentrations of apo-lactoferrin. Infect. Immun., 14 : 911-918.

Blum J.W., Dosogne H., Hoeben D., Vangroenweghe F., Hammon H.M., Bruckmaier R.M. & Burvenich C. (2000). Tumor necrosis factor-α and nitrite/nitrate responses during acute mastitis induced by Escherichia coli infection and endotoxin in dairy cows. Dom. Anim. Endocrinol., 19: 223-235.

Borregaard N., Sørensen O.E. & Theilgaard-Monch K. (2008). Neutrophil granules: a library of innate immunity proteins. TRENDS in Immunology, 28: 340-345.

Bouchard L., Blais S., Desrosiers C., Zhao X. & Lacasse P. (1999). Nitric oxide production during endotoxin-induced mastitis in the cow, J.Dairy Sci. 82: 2574-2581.

Boudjellab N., Chan-Tang H.S., Li X. & Zhao X. (1998). Bovine mammary epithelial cells secrete interleukin-8 in response to lipopolysaccharide stimulation. Am. J. Vet. Res., 59: 1563-156.

Boudjellab N., Chan-Tang H.S. & Zhao X. (2000). Bovine interleukin-1 expression by cultured mammary epithelial cells (MAC-T) and its involvement in the release of MAC-T derived interleukin-8, Comp. Biochem. Physiol. A. Mol. Integr. Physiol. 127: 191-199.

Bruhn O., Grötzinger J., Cascorbi I., & Jung S. (2011). Antimicrobial peptides and proteins of the horse - insights into a well-armed organism. Veterinary Research 2011, 42:98-120.

Burvenich C., Paape M.J., Hill A.W., Guidry A.J., Miller R.H., Heyneman R., Kremer W.D.J. & Brand A. (1994). Role of the neutrophil leukocyte in the local and systemic reactions during experimentally induced E. coli mastitis in cows immediately after calving. Vet. Q., 16: 45-50.

Burvenich C., Paape M.J., Hoeben D., Dosogne H., Massart-Leën A.M. & Blum J. (1999). Modulation of the inflammatory reaction and neutrophil defence of the bovine lactating mammary gland by growth hormone. Domest. Anim. Endocr., 17: 149-159.

Burvenich C., Van Merris V., Mehrzad J., Diez-Fraile A. & Duchateau L. (2003). Severity of E. coli mastitis is mainly determined by cow factors. Vet. Res., 34, 521-562.

Caffin J.P., Poutrel B. & Rainard P. (1984). Physiological and pathological factors influencing bovine α-lactalbumin and β-lactoglobulin concentrations in milk. J. Diary Sci., 68: 1086-1094.

Campbell P.G., Skaar T.C., Vega J.R. & Baumruker C.R. (1991). Secretion of insulin-like growth factor-I (IGF-I) and IGF-binding proteins from bovine mammary tissue in vitro. J. Endocr., 128: 219-228.

Carey L.A., Perkowski S.Z., Lipsky C.L., Cirelli R.A., Spath J.A. Jr. & Gee M.H. (1997). Neutrophil recruitment as a factor limiting injury or promoting recovery from acute lung injury. Am. J. physiol., 272: (Heart Circ. Physiol. 41) H179-H289.

Cemerski S., Cantagrel A., van Meerwijk J.P.M. & Romagnoli P. (2002). Reactive oxygen species differently affect T cell receptor signaling pathways. J. Biol. Chem. 277: 19585-19593.

Chavakis T., Hussain M., Kanse S.M., Peters G., Bretzel R.G., Flock J.I., Herrmann M. & Preissner K.T. (2002). Staphylococcus aureus extracellular adherence protein serves as anti-inflammatory factor by inhibiting the recruitment of host leukocytes. Nature Medicine. 8: 687-693.

Clark R., Strasser J., McCabe S., Robbins K. & Jardieu P. (1993). Insulin-like growth factor-1 stimulmation of lymphopoiesis. J. Clin. Invest., 92: 540-548.

Cooke E. & Hallett M.B. (1985). The role of C-kinase in the physiological activation of the neutrophil oxidase. Biochem. J. 232: 323-327.

Detilleux J.C., Koehler K.J., Freeman A.E.F., Kehrli M.E. & Kelley D.H. (1994). Immunological parameters of periparturient Holstein cattle: genetic variation. J. Dairy Sci., 77: 2640- 2645.

DiCarlo A.L., Paape M.J. & Miller R.H. (1996). Reactivity of purified complement component 3b with bovine neutrophils and modulation of complement receptor 1. Am. J. Vet. Res. 57: 151-156.

Dietz A.B., Cohen N.D., Timms L. & Kehrli M.E. Jr (1997). Bovine Lymphocyte Antigen Class II Alleles as Risk Factors for High Somatic Cell Counts in Milk of Lactating Dairy. J Dairy Sci., 80:406–412.

Diez-Fraille A., Mehrzad J., Meyer E., Duchateau L. & Burvenich C. (2004). Comparison of L-selectin and Mac-1 expression on blood and milk neutrophils during experimental Escherichia coli-induced mastitis in cows. Am. J. Vet. Res., 65:1164-1171.

Dosogne H., Capuco A.V., Paape M.J., Roets E., Burvenich C. & Fenwick B. (1998). Reduction of acyloxyacyl hydrolase activity in circulating neutrophils from cows after parturition. J. Dairy Sci., 81: 672-677.

Dosogne H., Meyer E., Sturk G., Van Loon J., Massart-Leën A.M. & Burvenich C. (2002). Effect of enrofloxacin treatment on plasma endotoxin during bovine Escherichiacoli mastitis. Inflammation Res., 51: 201-205.

Elvinger F., Hansen P.J., Head H.H. & Natzke R.P. (1991). Actions of bovine somatotropin on polymorphonuclear leukocytes and lymphocytes in cattle. J. Dairy Sci., 74: 2145-2152.

Erwin A.L. & Munford R.S. (1991). Plasma lipopolysaccharide-deacylating activity (acyloxyacyl hydrolase) increases after lipopolysaccharide administration to rabbits. Lab. Invest., 65: 138-144.

Fu Y. K., Arkins S., Wang B.S. & Kelley K.W. (1991). A novel role of growth hormone and insulin-like growth factor-I. Priming neutrophils for superoxide anion secretion. J. Immunol., 146: 1602-1608.

Gennaro R.B., Dewald B., Horisberger U., Gubler H.U. & Baggiolini M.A. (1983). A novel type of cytoplasmic granule in bovine neutrophils. J. Cell Biol., 96: 1651-1661.

Gill H.S., Doull F. & Rutherfurd K.J. (2000). Immunoregulatory peptides in bovine milk. Br. J. Nutr. 84 Suppl 1: S111-S117.

Gill H.S. &, Rutherfurd K.J. (2001a). Immune enhancement conferred by oral delivery of Lactobacillus rhamnosus HN001 in different milk-based substrates. J. Dairy Res. 68:611-616.

Gill H.S., Cross M.L., Rutherfurd K.J. & Gopal P.K. (2001b). Dietary probiotic supplementation to enhance cellular immunity in the elderly. Br. J. Biomed Sci. 58:94-96.

Gonçalves D.M, Chiasson S. & Girard D. (2010). Activation of human neutrophils by titanium dioxide (TiO2) nanoparticles. Toxicology in Vitro 24 (2010) 1002–1008.

Gray G.D., Knight K.A., Nelson R.D. & Herron M.J. (1982). Chemotactic requirements of bovine leukocytes. Am. J. Vet. Res., 43: 757-759.

Griffin F.M. Jr., Griffin J.A.., Leider J.E. & Silverstein S.C. (1975). Studies on the mechanism of phagocytosis. I. Requirements for circumferential attachment of particle-bound ligands to specific receptors on the macrophage plasma membrane. J. Exp. Med. 142: 1263-1282.

Hayashi F., Means T.K., & Luste A. D. (2003). Toll-like receptors stimulate human neutrophil function. Blood, 102: 2660-2669

Heyneman R., Burvenich C. & Vercauteren R. (1990). Interaction between the respiratory burst activity of neutrophil leukocytes and experimentally induced E. coli mastitis in cows. J. Dairy Sci., 73: 985-994.

Heyneman R. & Burvenich C. (1992). Kinetics and characteristics of bovine neutrophil alkaline phosphatase during acute Escherichia coli mastitis. J. Dairy Sci., 75: 1826-34.

Heyworth P.G., Cross A.R. & Curnutte J.T. (2003). Chronic granulomatous disease. Curr. Opin. Immunol. 15: 578-584.

Hoeben D., Burvenich C., Eppard P.J. & Hard D.L. (1999). Effect of recombinant bovine somatotropin on milk production and composition in bovine Streptococcus uberis mastitis. J. Dairy Sci., 82: 1671-1683.

Hoeben D., Monfardini E., Opsomer G., Dosogne H., De Kruif A., Beckers J.F. & Burvenich C. (2000a). Chemiluminescence of bovine polymorphonuclear leukocytes during the periparturient period and relation with metabolic parameters and bovine pregnancy-associated glycoprotein. J. Dairy Res., 67: 249-259.

Hoeben D., Burvenich C., Trevisi E., Bertoni G., Hamann J. & Blum J.W. (2000b). Role of endotoxin and TNF-α in the pathogenesis of experimentally induced mastitis in periparturient cows. J. Dairy Res., 67: 503-514.

Horwitz M.A. (1982). Phagocytosis of microorganisms. Rev. Infect. Dis. 4: 104-123.

Huynh H.T., Robitaille G. & Turner J.D. (1991). Establishment of bovine epithelial cells (MAC-T): an in vitro model for bovine lactation, Exp. Cell. Res. 197: 191-199.

Ibeagha A.E., Ibeagha-Awemu E.M., Mehrzad J., Baurhoo B., Kgwatalala P. & Zhao X. (2009). The effect of selenium sources and supplementation on neutrophil functions in dairy cows. Animal, 3: 1037-1043.

Jankowski A., Scott C.C. & Grinstein S. (2002). Determinants of phagosomal pH in neutrophils. J. Biol. Chem. 277: 6059-6066.

Karathanasis E., Geigerman C.M., Parkos C.A., Chan L., Bellamkonda R.V. & Jaye D.L. (2009). Selective Targeting of Nanocarriers to Neutrophils and Monocytes Annals of Biomedical Engineering, 37: 1984–1992

Karlsson A., Nixon J.B. & Mcphail L.C. (2000). Phorbol myristate acetate induces neutrophils NADPH-oxidase activity by two separate signal transduction pathways: dependent or independent of phosphatidylinositol 3-kinase. J. Leukocyte Biol. 67: 396-404.

Kurt-Jones E.A., Mandell L., Whitney C., Padgett A., Gosselin K., Newburger P.E., Finberg R.W., (2002). Role of toll-like receptor 2 (TLR2) in neutrophil activation: GM-CSF enhances TLR2 expression and TLR2-mediated interleukin 8 responses in neutrophils, Blood. 100: 1860-1868.

Lai Y., & Gallo R.L. (2009). AMPed up immunity: how antimicrobial peptides have multiple roles in immune defense. Trends in Immunology, 30: 131-141

Li Y., Karlin A., Loike J.D. & Silverstein S.C. (2002). A critical concentration of neutrophils is required fro effective bacterial killing in suspension. PNAS. 99: 8289-8294.

Liu Y, Walter S, Stagi M, Cherny D, Letiembre M, Schulz-Schaeffer W, Heine H, Penke B, Neumann H, & Fassbender K (2005). LPS receptor (CD14): a receptor for phagocytosis of Alzheimer's amyloid peptide. Brain. 128:1778-89.

Mandell G.L. (1974). Bactericidal activity of aerobic and anaerobic polymorphonuclear neutrophils. Infect. Immun. 9: 337-341.

Mayadas T. N. & Cullere X. (2005). Neutrophil β2 integrins: moderators of life or death decisions. Trends in Immunology. 26: 388-395.

Mayer S.J., Keen P.M., Craven N. & Bourn F.J. (1989). Regulation of phagolysosome pH in bovine and human neutrophils: the role of NADPH oxidase activity and an Na+/H+ antiporter. J. Leukocyte Biol. 45: 239-248.

Mehrzad J., Dosogne H., Meyer E., Hoeben D. & Burvenich C. (2000). Effect of α-lactalbumin and β-lactoglobulin on the supperoxide production of bovine milk neutrophils. Biotechnol. Argronomy Soc. Environ., 4: 22 (abstract).

Mehrzad J., Dosogne H., Meyer E., Heyneman R. & Burvenich C. (2001a). Respiratory burst activity of blood and milk neutrophils in dairy cows during different stages of lactation. J. Dairy Res., 68:399-415.

Mehrzad J., Dosogne H., Meyer E. & Burvenich C. (2001b). Local and systemic effects of endotoxin mastitis on the chemiluminescence of milk and blood neutrophils in dairy cows. Vet Res., 32:131-144.

Mehrzad J., Dosogne H., Vangroenweghe F. & Burvenich C. (2001c). A comparative study of bovine blood and milk neutrophil functions with luminol-dependent chemiluminescence. Luminescence., 16:343-356.

Mehrzad J., Duchateau L., Pyörälä S. & Burvenich C. (2002a). Blood and milk neutrophil chemiluminescence and viability in primiparous and pluriparous dairy cows during late Pregnancy, around parturition and early lactation. J. Dairy Sci., 85:3268-3276.

Mehrzad J., Dosogne H., Vangroenweghe F. & Burvenich C. (2002b). Effect of bovine somatotropin (bST) on bactericidal activity of bovine neutrophil. Biotechnol. Argronomy Soc. Environ. 6: 15 (abstract).

Mehrzad J., Duchateau L. & Burvenich C. (2004). Viability of milk neutrophils and severity of bovine coliform mastitis. J Dairy Sci., 87:4150-4162.

Mehrzad J., Duchateau L. & Burvenich C. (2005a). High milk neutrophil chemiluminescence limits the severity of bovine coliform mastitis. Vet. Res., 36:101-116.

Mehrzad J., Desrosiers C., Lauzon K., Robitaille G., Zhao X. & Lacasse P. (2005b). Proteases involved in mammary tissue damage during endotoxin-induced mastitis in dairy cows. J Dairy Sci., 88:211-222.

Mehrzad J., Dosogne H., De Spiegeleer B., Duchateau L. & Burvenich C. (2007). Bovine blood neutrophil acyloxyacyl hydrolase (AOAH) activity during endotoxin and coliform mastitis. Vet. Res., 38:655-668.

Mehrzad J., Janssen D., Duchateau L. & Burvenich C. (2008a). Increase in Escherichia coli inoculum dose accelerates CD8+ T-cell trafficking in the primiparous bovine mammary gland. J. Dairy Sci., 91:193-201.

Mehrzad J. & Zhao X. (2008b). T lymphocyte proliferative capacity and CD4+/CD8+ ratio in primiparous and pluriparous lactating cows. J. Dairy Res., 75:457-465.

Mehrzad J., Mohri M. & Burvenich C. (2008c). Excessive extracellular chemiluminescence and necrosis of neutrophils in bovine neonates and potentially supportive role of vitamin C. In: *Bioluminescence and Chemiluminescence, Light Emission: Biology and scientific applications*. Shen X., Yang, XL, Zhang XR, Cui ZJ, Kricka LJ and Stanley PE, (Ed.), (233-336), Published by World Scientific Publishing Co. Pte. Ltd, ISBN 978-912-8395-72, Shanghai, China

Mehrzad J., Duchateau L. & Burvenich C. (2009). Phagocytic and bactericidal activity of blood and milk-resident neutrophils against Staphylococcus aureus in primiparous and multiparous cows during early lactation. Vet. Microbiol., 134:106-112.

Mehrzad J., Klein G., J Kamphues., Wolf P., Grabowski N. & Schuberth H.J. (2011). In vitro effects of very low levels of aflatoxin B1 on free radicals production and bactericidal activity of bovine blood neutrophils. Vet. Immunol. Immunopathol. 141: 16–25.

Merchav S., Lake M. & Skottner A. (1993). Comparative studies of the granulopoietic enhancing effects of biosynthetic human insulin-like growth factors I and II. J. Cell Physiol., 157: 178-183.

Moncada S., Palmer R.M.J. & Higgs E.A. (1991). Nitric oxide: physiology, pathophysiology, and pharmacology, Pharmacol.Rev. 43: (1991) 109-142.

Nathan C. (2006). Neutrophils and immunity: challenges and opportunities. Nat. Rev. Immunol. 6: 173-182.

Newman S.L. & Johnston R.B. (1979). Role of binding through C3b and IgG in polymorphonuclear neutrophil function: studies with trypsin-generated C3b. J. Immunol. 123: 1839-1846.

Nishizuka Y. (1984). The role of protein kinase C in cell surface signal transduction and tumour promotion. Nature (London) 308: 693-698.

Ogata A. & Nagahata H. (2000). Intramammary application of ozone therapy to acute clinical mastitis in dairy cows. J. Vet. Med. Sci. 62: 681-686.

Paape M.J., Lillius E.M.P., Wiitanen A. & Kontio M.P. (1996). Intramammary defence against infections induced by Escherichia coli in cows. Am. J. Vet. Res., 57: 477-482.

Paape M.J., Mehrzad J., Zhao X., Detileux J. & Burvenich C. (2002). Defense of the bovine mammary gland by polymorphonuclear neutrophil leukocytes. J. Mammary Gland Biol. Neoplasia., 7: 109-121.

Paulsson J.M., Jacobson S.H. & Lundahl J. (2010). Neutrophil activation during transmigration in vivo and in vitro A translational study using the skin chamber model. J. Immunol. Methods. 361:82-88.

Pezeshki A., Stordeur P., Wallemacq H., Schynts F., Stevens M., Boutet P., Peelman L.J., De Spiegeleer B., Duchateau L., Bureau F. and Burvenich C. (2011). Variation of inflammatory dynamics and mediators in primiparous cows after intramammary challenge with Escherichia coli. Vet. Res. 42:15-25.

Pyörälä S., Kaartinen L., Käck H. & Rainio V. (1994). Efficacy of Two Therapy Regimes for Treatment of Experimentally Induced Escherichia coli Mastitis in the Bovine. J. Dairy Sci., 77: 453-461.

Rainard P. (2002). Bovine milk fat globules do not inhibit C5a chemotactic activity. Vet Res. 33(4):413-419.

Reth M. (2002). Hydrogen peroxide as second messenger in lymphocyte activation. Nature Immunol. 3: 1129-1134.

Rinaldi M., Li R.W., Bannerman D.D., Daniels K.M., Evock-Clover C., Silva M.V., Paape M.J., Van Ryssen B., Burvenich C. & Capuco A.V. (2010). A sentinel function for teat tissues in dairy cows: dominant innate immune response elements define early response to E. coli mastitis. Funct. Integr. Genomics. 10:21-38.

Root R.K. & Cohen M.S. (1981). The microbicidal mechanisms of human neutrophils and eosinophils. Rev. Infect. Dis. 3: 565-598.

Rosen H. & Klebanoff S.J. (1976). Chemiluminescence and superoxide production by myeloperoxidase deficient leukocytes. J. Clin. Invest. 58: 50-60.

Rossi F. and Zatti M. (1964). Changes in the metabolic pattern of polymorphonuclear leukocytes during phagocytosis. Br. J. Exp. Pathol. 45: 548-559.

Rossi F. (1986). The O_2^- forming NADPH oxidase of the phagocytes: nature, mechanisms of activation and function. Biochem. Biophys. Acta. 853: 65-89.

Sachs U.J., Andrei-Selmer C.L., Maniar A., Weiss T., Paddock C., Orlova V.V., Choi E.Y., Newman P.J., Preissner K.T., Chavakis T. & Santoso S. (2007). The neutrophil-specific antigen CD177 is a counter-receptor for platelet endothelial cell adhesion molecule-1 (CD31). J. Biol. Chem. 282: 23603-13612.

Sadikot R. T. & Rubinstein I. (2009). Long-Acting, Multi-Targeted Nanomedicine: Addressing Unmet Medical Need in Acute Lung Injury. Journal of Biomedical Nanotechnology. 5: 614-619.

Shuster D.E., Kehrli M.E.J., Rainard P. & Paape M. (1997). Complement fragment C5a and inflammatory cytokines in neutrophil recruitment during intramammary infection with Escherichia coli. Infect. Immun. 65: 3286-3292.

Simons, M. P., O'Donnell, M. A. & Griffith, T. S. (2008). Role of neutrophils in BCG immunotherapy for bladder cancer. Urol. Oncol. 26, 341–345

Smits E., Burvenich C., Guidry A.J., & Massart-Leen A. (2000). Adhesion receptor CD11b/CD18 contributes to neutrophil diapedesis across the bovine blood-milk barrier. Vet. Immunol. Immunopathol., 73: 255-265.

Smits E., Burvenich C., Guidry A.J., Heyneman R. & Massart-Leen A. (1999). Diapedesis across mammary epithelium reduces phagocytotic and oxidative burst of bovine neatrophils. Vet. Immunol. Immunopathol., 68: 169-176.

Spitznagel J.K. & Shafer W.M. (1985). Neutrophil killing of bacteria by oxygen-independent mechanisms: A historical summary. Rev. Infect. Dis. 7: 398-403.

Stevens MG, Peelman LJ, De Spiegeleer B, Pezeshki A, Van De Walle GR, Duchateau L & Burvenich C. (2011a). Differential gene expression of the toll-like receptor-4 cascade and neutrophil function in early- and mid-lactating dairy cows. J. Dairy Sci. 94:1277-1288.

Stevens MG, Van Poucke M, Peelman LJ, Rainard P, De Spiegeleer B, Rogiers C, Van de Walle GR, Duchateau L, & Burvenich C. (2011b). Anaphylatoxin C5a-induced toll-like receptor 4 signaling in bovine neutrophils. J. Dairy Sci. 94:152-164.

Stich R., Shoda L., Dreewes M., Adler B., Jungi T. & Brown W. (1998). Stimulation of nitric oxide production in macrophages by Babesia bovis, Infect. Immun. 66: 4130-4136.

Suriyasathaporn W., Daemen A.J.J.M., Noordhuizen-Stassen E.N., Nielen M., Dieleman S.J., & Schukken,YH (1999). ß-hydroxybutyrate levels in peripheral blood and ketone bodies supplemented in culture media affect the in vitro chemotaxis of bovine leukocytes. Vet. Immunol. Immunopathol., 68: 177-186.

Suthanthiran M., Solomon S.D., Williams P.S., Rabin A.L., Novogrodsky A. & Stenzel K.H. (1984). Hydroxyl radical scavengers inhibit human natural killer cell activity. Nature (Lond.). 307: 276-278.

Tauber A.I. (1987). proten kinase C and the activation of the human neutrophil NADPH-oxidase. Blood. 69: 484-488.

Thomas E.L., Jefferson M.M. & Grishman M. (1982). Myeloperoxidase-catalyzed incorporation of amino acids into proteins: role of hypochlorous acid, and chloramines. Biochemistry. 21: 6299-6308.

Thomas E.L. & Fishman M. (1986). Oxidation of choloride, and thiocyanate by isolated leukocytes. J. Biol. Chem. 261: 9694-9702.

Van Merris V., Lenjou M., Hoeben D., Nijs G., Van Bockstaele D. & Burvenich C. (2001a). Culture of bovine bone marrow cells in vitro. Vet. Q., 23: 170-175.

Van Merris V., Meyer E., Dosogne H. & Burvenich C. (2001b). Separation of bovine bone marrow into maturation related myeloid cell fractions. Vet. Immunol. Immunopathol., 83: 11-17.

Van Merris V., Meyer E. & Burvenich C. (2002). Functional maturation during bovine granulopoiesis. J. Dairy Sci., 85: 2859-68.

Van Oostveldt K., Vangroenweghe F., Dosogne H. & Burvenich C. (2001). Apoptosis and necrosis of blood and milk polymorphonuclear leukocytes in early and midlactating healthy cows. Vet. Res., 32: 617-22.

Van Oostveldt K., Paape M.J. & Burvenich C. (2002a). Apoptosis of bovine neutrophils following diapedesis through a monolayer of endothelial and mammary epithelial cells. J. Dairy Sci., 85: 39-147.

Van Oostveldt K., Tomita G.M., Paape M.J. & Burvenich C. (2002b). Apoptosis of neutrophils during Eschericha coli and endotoxin mastitis. Am. J. Vet. Res., 63: 448-453.

Van Werven T., Noordhuizen-Stassen E.N., Daemen A.J.J.M., Schukken Y.H., Brand A. & Burvenich C. (1997). Preinfection in vitro chemotaxis, phagocytosis, oxidative burst, and expression of CD11/CD18 receptors and their predictive capacity on the outcome of mastitis induced in dairy cows with Escherichia coli. J. Dairy Sci., 80: 67-74.

Vangroenweghe F., Dosogne H., Mehrzad J. & Burvenich C. (2001). Effect of milk sampling techniques on milk composition, bacterial contamination, viability and functions of resident cells in milk. Vet. Res., 32: 565-579.

Wall R.J., Powell A.M., Paape M.J., Kerr D.E., Bannerman D.D., Pursel V.G., Wells K.D., Talbot N. & Hawk H.W. (2005). Genetically enhanced cows resist intramammary Staphylococcus aureus infection. Nat. Biotechnol., 23:445-451.

Wang Y., Zarlenga D.S., Paape M.J. & Dahl G.E. (2002). Recombinant bovine soluble CD14 sensitizes the mammary gland to lipopolysaccharide. Vet. Immunol. Immunopathol., 86: 115-124.

Warwick-Davies J., Lowrie D.B. & Cole P.J. (1995). Growth hormone is a human macrophage activating factor. Priming of human monocytes for enhanced release of H_2O_2. J. Immunol., 154: 1909-1918.

Weiss S.J., Test S.T., Eckmann C.M., Roos D. & Regiani S. (1986). Brominating oxidants generated by human eosinophils. Science. 234: 200-202.

Werling D. & Jungi T.W. (2003). Toll-like receptors linking innate and adaptive immune response, Vet.Immunol.Immunopathol. 9 : 1-12.

Wiedermann C.J., Reinisch N. & Braunsteiner H. (1993). Stimulation of monocyte chemotaxis by human growth hormone and its deactivation by somatostatin. Blood., 82: 954-960.

Wong K.F., Middleton N., Montgomery M., Dey M. & Carr R.I. (1998). Immunostimulation of murine spleen cells by materials associated with bovine milk protein fraction. J. Dairy Sci., 81: 1825-1832.

Worku M., Paape M.J., Filep R. & Miller R., (1994). Effect of in vitro and in vivo migration of bovine neutrophils on binding and expression of Fc receptors for IgG2 and IgM, Am.J.Vet.Res. 55: 221-226.

Zarbock A & Ley K. (2008). Mechanisms and consequences of neutrophil interaction with the endothelium. Am. J. Pathol.172: 1-7.

Zhao X., McBride B.W., Trouten-Radford L.M. & Burton J.H. (1992). Specific insulin-like growth factor-1 receptors on circulating bovine mononuclear cells. J. Recept. Res., 12: 117-129.

Zimecki M., Spiegel K., Wlaszczyk A., Kubler A. & Kruzel M.L. (1999). Lactoferrin increases the output of neutrophil precursors and attenuates the spontaneous production of TNF-alpha and IL-6 by peripheral blood cells. Arch. Immunol. Ther. Exp. Warsz., 47: 113-118.

16

An Ag-Dependent Approach Based on Adaptive Mechanisms for Investigating the Regulation of the Memory B Cell Reservoir

Alexandre de Castro
Laboratory of Computational Mathematics, National Center of Technological Research on Informatics for Agriculture (Embrapa Agriculture Informatics), Brazilian Agricultural Research Corporation (Embrapa), Campinas, Brazil

1. Introduction

Twenty years ago, Farmer, Packard, and Perelson presented an elegant dynamical model [1] to study Idiotype Network theory [2-19], in which they showed that every molecular and cellular binding site (cell receptor) can be modeled by binary *bit-strings* of length ℓ. In such a model, an antibody molecule can always recognize an antigen when there is complementarity between their *bit-strings*. The coincidence of antigens and lymphocyte receptors (lock-and-key model) is determined by considering the number of complementary bits [8,20]. For instance, if a B lymphocyte is represented by a binary string 00010101 ($\ell = 8$) and an antigen is represented by the 11101010 binary string, the immune response is activated (Fig. 1). The match between bit-strings does not need to be perfect, however; some bit positions are allowed in which two strings differ. These differences between strings (mismatches) reflect the degree of affinity between the entities of the immune system in mammals and determine the quality of the response.

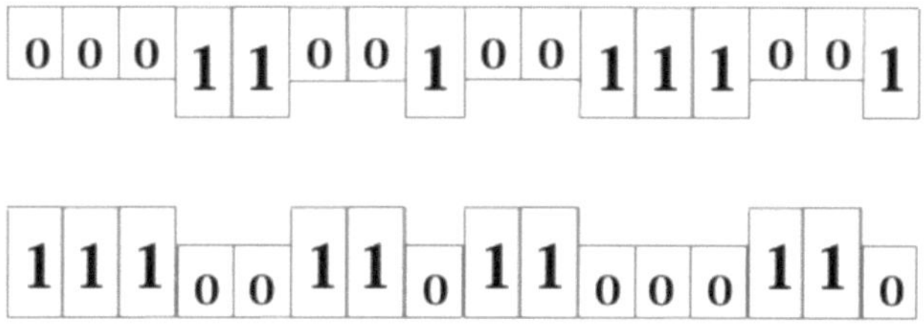

Fig. 1. Pictorial representation of the binding site (cell antigen) by means of a bit-string frame [6].

In another work, Lagreca *et al.* (2001) [21] also proposed a dynamic model that was based on the recognition of shapes or patterns using bit-strings, but used the iterative solution of a coupled map system that enabled the treatment of high dimensions. In the model created by

Lagreca *et al.* (2001), the B cell and the antibody populations are treated as a clone pools because their receptors are represented by the same bit-strings. Because a bit-string can be considered as the binary representation of an integer, the model indexes each clone to an entire σ, and the temporal evolution of the populations is described by the $N(\sigma, t)$ concentration. The model also considers a source term that simulates the role played by the bone marrow, where new bit-strings are presented. The death or depletion of clones occurs in two ways: 1) by means of natural death (apoptosis), described by the parameter d; and 2) by means of a general suppression mechanism, described by a Verhulst-like factor [22]. This factor is widely used in simulations of biological systems, because it limits the maximum population that can survive in a particular environment [22]. The Lagreca *et al.* model (2001) considers this maximum B cell population (N_{max}) to be the same for every clone, and the populations are normalized by the $y(\sigma,t) = N(\sigma,t) / N_{max}$ function.

Thus, considering a discrete temporal evolution, the following coupled map set proposed by Lagreca *et al.* [21] allows part of an adaptive immunological system to be simulated:

$$y(\sigma,t+1) = (1 - y(\sigma,t)).$$

$$.\left\{m + (1-d)y(\sigma,t) + b\frac{y(\sigma,t)}{y_{tot}(t)}\left[(1-a_h)(y(\bar{\sigma},t) + y_F(\bar{\sigma},t)) + a_h\sum_{i=1}^{B}(y(\bar{\sigma}_i,t) + y_F(\bar{\sigma}_i,t))\right]\right\}, \qquad (1)$$

where $(1 - y(\sigma,t))$ is the Verhulst-like factor; $y_F(\sigma,t)$ describes the antigen population, characterized by a σ bit-string which, in this case, represents distinct antigenic determinants; $\bar{\sigma}$ represents the perfect complementary shape of σ; and $\bar{\sigma}_i$ are the nearest neighbors of $\bar{\sigma}$ in a *B*-dimensional hypercube. The term m represents the population of cells produced by bone marrow; the (1-*d*) term represents the percentage of the lymphocyte population that survives a natural cell death (apoptosis); and the other terms describe the clonal proliferation $y(\sigma,t)$ that occurs because of interaction with complementary B cells and/or antigens.

The b parameter is a clonal proliferation constant (typically related to the mean number of new cells produced by the pre-existing cells), and $y_{Tot}(t)$ is the total population, given by equation 2:

$$y_{tot}(t) = \sum_{\sigma}\left[y(\sigma,t) + y_F(\sigma,t)\right] \qquad (2)$$

The parameter a_h is the connectivity factor between a specific *bit-string* and the specular image of its neighbors. When a_h = 0.0, only a perfect coincidence of complementary shapes is valid. When a_h = 0.5, a bit-string can recognize equally both its own specular image and the nearest neighbors of its specular image. The temporal evolution of the antigen pool is defined by equation 3.

$$y_F(\sigma,t+1) = y_F(\sigma,t) - k\frac{y_F(\sigma,t)}{y_{tot}(t)}\left\{(1-a_h)y(\bar{\sigma},t) + a_h\sum_{i=1}^{B} y(\bar{\sigma}_i,t)\right\}, \qquad (3)$$

where k is an antigen removal parameter that represents the interactions with the clonal populations.

In fact, it is well-known that the soluble antibody population is one of the essential mechanisms of immunological response regulation [23-25]. However, despite the pioneering work of Lagreca *et al.* (2001) in developing a coupled map for studying the behavior of the mammalian immune system, their model did not consider these populations [1-6], which makes the model incomplete with respect to the regulation of the immune response by adaptive mechanisms. This omission opens up the possibility of extending their work by taking the soluble antibody populations into account. We have performed that work and present our immunological modeling and simulation findings in this paper.

2. Materials and methods

In this section, we briefly describe the Verhulst approach and provide details of an extension to the Lagreca *et al. (2001)* model, which includes an antibody variable to address the regulation of the structural mechanisms that are mediated by the immunoglobulin population. This variable was not considered in the simplified model proposed by Lagreca *et al.* [21].

2.1 The Verhulst approach

Since the early nineteenth century, studies on population dynamics have been developed to identify possible nonlinear behaviors. One of the first efforts aimed at predicting biological population behavior was made by Pierre François Verhulst (1804-1849), a Belgian mathematician. He proposed a nonlinear model in which the death rate was proportional to the square of the number of individuals in the population. The model can be expressed by differential equations [26-30], as follows:

$$\frac{dN}{dt} = AN - BN^2$$

where N is the number of individuals, and A and B are constants related to the growth rate and the population growth limitation, respectively.

The Verhulst model was used again in 1976, by Robert May [27], to study insect population dynamics. In his experiments, he replaced the original differential method by what is now known as the *map* methodology, in which each value is obtained by its anterior value:

$$N_1 = AN_0 - B\,N_0^2$$

$$N_2 = AN_1 - BN_1^2$$

$$N_{n+1} = AN_n - BN_n^2$$

At the limit of saturation, $AN_{max} - BN_{max}^2 = 0$, then $N_{max} = 0$ or $N_{max} = A/B$.

Solving $\frac{N_{n+1}}{N_{máx}} = A\frac{N_n}{N_{máx}} - B\frac{N_n^2}{N_{máx}}\frac{N_{máx}}{N_{máx}}$ and inserting $x_n = \frac{N_n}{N_{máx}}$ results in the following:

$x_{n+1} = Ax_n - Bx_n^2.A/B$. Defining the parameter A (birth rate) = r (control parameter), we obtain:

$$x_{n+1}=rx_n(1-x_n)\,,\quad x_n \in [0,1] \tag{4}$$

In equation (4), known as a *logistic map*, the values for $x_n \in [0,1]$ and r are dimensionless and represent population fractions as a function of each of the n iterations, respectively, while r is a constant that represents the population growth rate in each new iteration. The term $(1-x_n)$ is known as the Verhulst factor [21,31,32].

The bifurcation diagram of the logistic map is built by the iterative resolution of the logistic equation, starting with an arbitrary x_0 initial value and choosing sequential values for the parameters r, $r \in [r_{min}, r_{max}]$. The bifurcation diagram of the logistic equation is shown in Fig. 2.

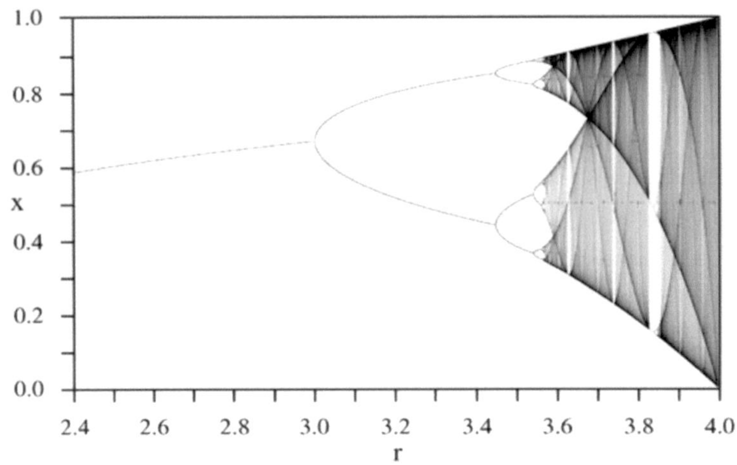

Fig. 2. Classical bifurcation diagram of a logistic map as a function of the parameter r [33].

In Fig. 2, the attractor is a fixed point up to the first bifurcation. For each bifurcation, there occurs a period of duplication before the system reaches the chaotic phase. However, to illustrate the dynamics of this simple model, it is important to show that, for r between 0 and 1, the population death rate is not dependent on the initial population. With r between 1 and 3, the population is prone to an attractor of a fixed point type. For r greater than 3.54, the population wiggles between values of 8, 16, 32, and so on. At approximately r=3.57, the end of the cascade duplication period occurs and chaos begins. From this value, small variations in the initial population produce very different results over time, which is the fundamental characteristic of chaos. For r greater than 4, the populations are outside the [0,1] interval.

It is possible to demonstrate that the Lagreca *et al.* (2001) model for clonal populations reduces to equation 4 when there is no further exposure of the system to the antigens. This reduction occurs because, under this one condition, the additive term (m) in equation 1, which represents the bone marrow contribution for the immune repertoire, is very small when compared with the clonal proliferation parameter (b) [34,35]. A detailed demonstration of this assertion is presented in subsection 3 of the section on the model parameters.

2.2 Simulation model

As in the Lagreca *et al.* (2001) model [21], our extended Ag-dependent model has molecular receptors of B cells that are represented by bit-strings with 2^B of diversity, where B is the number of bits in the string. The individual components of the immune system represented in the extended model are B cells, antibodies, and antigens located at the vertices of hypercubes of size B. B cells (clones) are characterized by their surface receptors and are modeled by a binary bit-strings. The epitopes [1,8,17-19], which are portions of an antigen that can be connected by the B cell receptor (BCR), are also represented by bit-strings. The antibodies have receptors (paratopes) [1,8,17-19] that are represented by the same bit-string models as the BCR B cell that produced them. Thus, the new dynamic equations that describe the behavior of the adaptive immune system, taking into account the inclusion of antibody populations, are the following:

$$y(\sigma,t+1)=(1-y(\sigma,t))\left\{m+(1-d)\,y(\sigma,t)+b\frac{y(\sigma,t)}{y_{tot}(t)}\zeta_{a_h}\left(\bar{\sigma},t\right)\right\}, \tag{5}$$

for a clonal population, with complementary shapes included in the term $\zeta_{a_h}(\bar{\sigma},t)$,

$$\zeta_{a_h}(\bar{\sigma},t)=(1-a_h)(y(\bar{\sigma},t)+y_F(\bar{\sigma},t)+y_A(\bar{\sigma},t))+a_h\sum_{i=1}^{B}(y(\bar{\sigma}_i,t)+y_F(\bar{\sigma}_i,t)+y_A(\bar{\sigma}_i,t)).$$

The clonal populations can range from the value generated by bone marrow (m) up to its maximum value (unity) because the Verhulst factor is a limiting factor [21,31,32].

In the model presented in this paper, the $y_{tot(t)}$ term represents the sum of the components that belong to an adaptive subset of the immune system, as described in the introduction to this work. Such elements, when added to antibody populations, are expressed as bit-string *concentrations.*

Therefore, the sum of every adaptive component considered by our model is given by equation (6).

$$y_{tot}(t)=\sum_{\sigma}\left[y(\sigma,t)+y_F(\sigma,t)+y_A(\sigma,t)\right] \tag{6}$$

The temporal evolution of the antigens can be defined by equation (7).

$$y_F(\sigma,t+1)=y_F(\sigma,t)-k\frac{y_F(\sigma,t)}{y_{tot}(t)}\left\{(1-a_h)\left[y(\bar{\sigma},t)+y_A(\bar{\sigma},t)\right]+a_h\sum_{i=1}^{B}\left[y(\bar{\sigma}_i,t)+y_A(\bar{\sigma}_i,t)\right]\right\}, \tag{7}$$

The antibody population is described by a group of 2^B variables, also defined by a B-dimensional hypercube, interacting with the antigen populations of equation (8).

$$y_A(\sigma,t+1)=y_A(\sigma,t)+b_A\frac{y(\sigma,t)}{y_{tot}(t)}\left[(1-a_h)\ y_F(\bar{\sigma},t)+a_h\sum_{i=1}^{B}y_F(\bar{\sigma}_i,t)\right]-k\frac{y_A(\sigma,t)}{y_{tot}(t)}\zeta_{a_h}(\bar{\sigma},t)\ ,(8)$$

where b_A is the antibody proliferation parameter; and k is the parameter related to the antibodies and antigens that will be removed.

In our model, equation 8, which considers the adaptive interactions that have been described in the specialized literature, is included. Thus, antibody proliferation is given by the recognition $y_A(\sigma,t)\Leftrightarrow y_F(\bar{\sigma},t)$ [1,8,17-19]. The antibody population is regulated by the intersection of $y_A(\sigma,t)\Leftrightarrow y(\bar{\sigma},t)$ [1,8,17-19], $y_A(\sigma,t)\Leftrightarrow y_F(\bar{\sigma},t)$ [1,8,17-19], and $y_A(\sigma,t)\Leftrightarrow y_A(\bar{\sigma},t)$ [19,36]. In all cases, the connectivity between the first two neighbors was considered. The factors $\frac{y_F(\sigma,t)}{y_{TOT}(t)}$ and $\frac{y_A(\sigma,t)}{y_{TOT}(t)}$ also help to regulate the antigen and antibody populations, while the term $\frac{y(\sigma,t)}{y_{TOT}(t)}$ is the corresponding clonal regulation factor involved in the formation of immunological memory.

The role performed by the clonal regulation factor, in addition to helping with the B cell response regulation, is fundamental to the regulation of the memorization ability and clonal homeostasis [37-39]. The importance of the effect of the clonal regulation factor over immune system memory evolution is shown in Fig. 3. Three distinct situations are possible:

1. antibody populations are included in the model (which corresponds to the model proposed in this work);
2. antibody populations are not included in the model (which corresponds to the Lagreca *et al.* [21] model);
3. memory expansion is not limited by the clonal regulation factor (which corresponds to the results obtained by P. G. Etchegoin [40]).

Fig. 3 illustrates the situation in which growth capacity increases indefinitely, which is when the clonal regulation factor is suppressed in the modeling phase. This shows that clonal regulation can be fundamental to the immune system reaching clonal homeostasis.

In the proposed Ag-dependent model, each bit-string is associated with an integer that is situated in an interval , $0\le M\le 2^B-1$, and each represents a clonal population, antigen, or antibody located in the B-dimensional hypercube vertex. The neighbors *i* of a specific σ or $\bar{\sigma}$ are expressed by the Boolean functions $\sigma_i=(2^i-1xor\sigma)$ or $\bar{\sigma}_i=(2^i-1xor\bar{\sigma})$, respectively. The complementary way of obtaining σ is obtained by $\bar{\sigma}=M-\sigma$ [21].

An example of the way in which the B cell, antibody, or antigen populations are localized in 3-dimensional space is shown in Fig. 4.

For the cubic configuration in Fig. 4, the following algorithm describes how to obtain the first neighbors and the complementary shape of the B cell population identified by the integer $\sigma=4$:

- For a cubic configuration (*B*=3), there exists a repertoire containing $2^B=8$ integer numbers arranged in the cube vertex. These integer numbers represent the 8 different B cell populations;

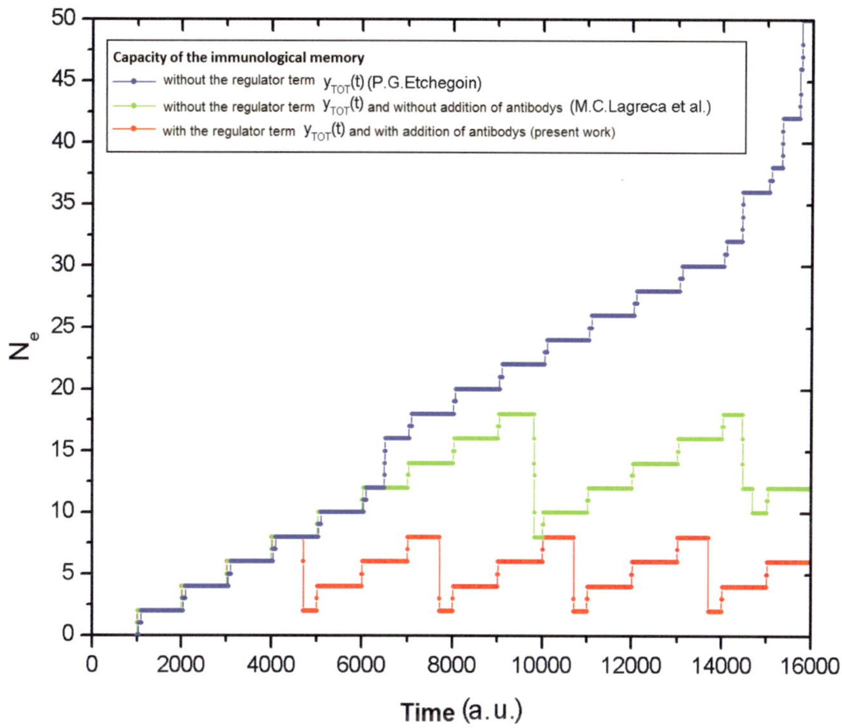

Fig. 3. Capacity of immune system memory in three distinct situations.

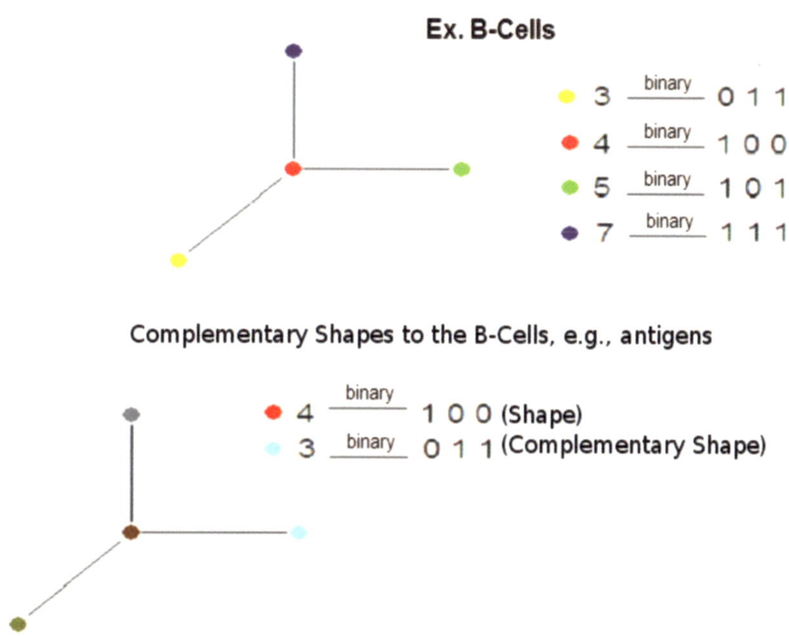

Fig. 4. Spatial arrangement of a B cell population that is identified by 4 integers. Antigens and antibodies also are spatially arranged in the same way, in various cubes.

- Each integer number M must be restrained in the interval $0 \le M \le 2^B - 1$; thus, each cube vertex is identified [16];
- With this condition, the smallest value of M is equal to 0 and the largest value is equal to 7. Consequently, the shape space S is equal to {0,1,2,3,4,5,6,7};
- To represent the reactions of the lock-and-key type described in the introduction, every cell population in a cubic configuration needs to be represented by 8 bit-strings;

$$\sigma = 4 = \sum_{i=0}^{2} 2^i a_i = 2^0 a_0 + 2^1 a_1 + 2^2 a_2 = 4$$

If, for example, $a_2 = 1$, $a_1 = 0$ and $a_0 = 0$, then in this case 4 in the decimal base corresponds to (1 0 0) in the binary base;

- For the other 7 vertices of the cube:

$$\sigma = 0 = (000),$$

$$\sigma = 1 = (001),$$

$$\sigma = 2 = (010),$$

$$\sigma = 3 = (011),$$

$$\sigma = 4 = (100),$$

$$\vdots$$

$$\sigma = 7 = (111);$$

- For a lock-and-key reaction to occur, there must be another shape $\overline{\sigma}$ that is complementary to $\sigma = 4$, i.e., $\overline{\sigma} = M - \sigma$ [16,21]. Then, $M = 2^B - 1 = 7$ and $\sigma = 4 \rightarrow \overline{\sigma} = M - \sigma = 7 - 4 = 3$, or (0 1 1), in a binary base. This complementary shape is, in principle, an antigen population. However, based on Immune Network Theory, B cells also recognize antibodies and other complementary lymphocytes [1,8,17-19,36];
- Last, search for the first neighbors of the complementary shape $\overline{\sigma} = 3$. If $\sigma_i = (2^i - 1 xor \sigma)$ [16,21], then, for B = 3 (i = 1,2,3), we get the following:

$$\sigma_1 = (2^1 - 1 xor 3) = 2(010),$$

$$\sigma_2 = (2^2 - 1 xor 3) = 0(000),$$

$$\sigma_3 = (2^3 - 1 xor 3) = 4(100).$$

In this example, a B cell population identified by $\sigma = 4$ or (1 0 0) would have recognized an antigen population that is perfectly complementary and is identified by $\overline{\sigma} = 3$ (0 1 1). The antigen populations identified as the first neighbors for $\overline{\sigma} = 3$ are 0, 2, and 4 and can be recognized by the $\sigma = 4$ B cell population, depending on the value of the connectivity parameter a_h, which is included both in our proposed model and in the Lagreca *et al.* model [21].

Also, for better visualization, we used a 3-dimensional spatial configuration. Similar constructions for this work were made for *B*-dimensional spaces. Therefore, equations (5) to (8) constitute a set of maps that describes the main interactions of the immune system between the entities that interact through the lock-and-key type of connection, in other words, adaptive immune system entities that self-recognize. Such an equation set is iteratively resolved, considering various initial conditions.

2.3 Simulation dynamics

In this section, we present the dynamics of the simulations that were used to reproduce the proposed experiments *in silico*, and we evaluate the behavior of the proposed model.

To simulate the behavior of the immune system by means of the proposed mathematical model, we developed computational applications in the Fortran programming language (IBM's Mathematical FORmula TRANslation System). The source code was compiled with GFortran (GNU Fortran Compiler) on a Linux Operating System platform. Simulations were performed by a 2 GHz processor, with 4 GB of random-access memory (RAM).

To establish the relationship between antigen mutation and the memory of the lymphocyte population, we performed 3 *in silico* experiments with 30 samples $E_{j,k} = E(j=1,\beta)(k=1,\gamma)$.

The same parameters were used in every $E_j = E(j=1,\beta)$ experiment to represent identical individuals. The antigens were identified by the following expression: $V_i E_{j,k} = V(i=1,\alpha)E(j=1,\beta)(k=1,\gamma)$, where the *i, j, and k* indexes describe the inoculation order, the experiment, and the sample, respectively. The number α is the number of inoculations in each experiment, β is the number of experiments, and γ is the number of samples in each experiment.

The antigen injection simulations were performed every 1,000 temporal steps (in arbitrary units - a.u.), representing the administration of a new antigen dose in a hypothetical mammal. In the first experiment, we injected 110 different antigen populations in the sample, in the second, 250, and, in the third, 350. To represent the mutation within a population of the same antigen, we used 10 different seeds for the pseudo-random number generator. In the first experiment, a seed was associated with each sample, and the same set of seeds was used to perform the other experiments. In this way, to represent the mutation, we considered that inoculated antigens in the same position belonged to the same species and underwent a mutation for each different sample. The difference between the samples is in the bit-string variation of the inoculated antigens, and the difference between the experiments is in the duration of the time steps. The design of the experiments and the antigen identification used in this work are shown in Fig. 5.

In the schematic diagram shown in Fig. 5, the antigen (i.e., a virus strain) is identified as V1E12, which is the mutation of the antigen V1E11 (belonging to an antigen population of the same species), and the antigen V2E11 is different from the V1E11 antigen (which belongs to various antigen populations).

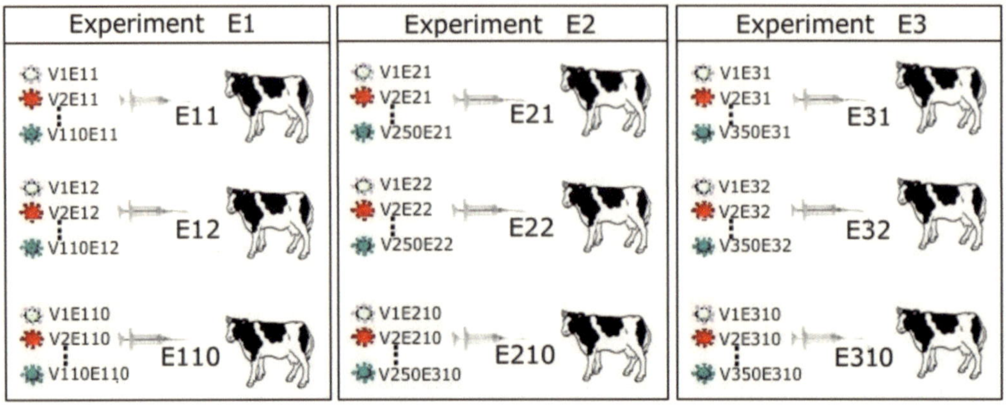

Fig. 5. In each experiment, different lifetimes were considered for individual hypothetical mammals. The lifetime ("lifespan") for E1, E2, and E3 is 110000, 250000, and 350000 respectively.

2.4 Model parameters

The following table shows the ranges for the parameters used in our simulations, based on the literature.

Symbol	Function	Value used in the model	Information obtained from the literature
d	Apoptosis	0.99	De Boer *et al.* [41] (2001): 0.95 Bueno *et al.*[42] (1999): 0.95 Lima *et al.* [43] (2007): $d > 0.95$
m	Source term	$10^{-7} if\ p < 0.1 \quad 0.0 if\ p \geq 0.1$	Lagreca *et al.*[21] (2001): 0.0005 von Laera *et al.* [34] (2005): 0.01 Monvel et *al.*[38] (1993): $m \approx 0.0$
b	Clonal proliferation	2.0	De Boer *et al.* [41] (2001): 2.5-3.0 Utzny *et al.* [44] (2001): 2.0 von Laera *et al.* [34] (2005): 1.2
k	Removal of antibodies and antigens	0.1	von Laera *et al.* [34] (2005): 0.01-0.1

Table 1. Parameters used in the proposed model.

2.4.1 The apoptosis clonal parameter (*d*)

In the extended model presented in this paper, d represents the fraction of cells that is subjected to natural death (apoptosis) or programmed death; thus, $s + d = 1$, where $s = 1 - d$

is the fraction of cells that avoids apoptosis. In the literature, the apoptosis of lymphocytes is typically assumed to occur in percentages not less than 95% [41.43]. For the simulations developed in this study, the natural death parameter was fixed at 0.99 (99%). To give an idea of the effect of varying this parameter, the performances of the model for two different apoptotic events and for the first inoculation antigen were compared (See Fig. 6).

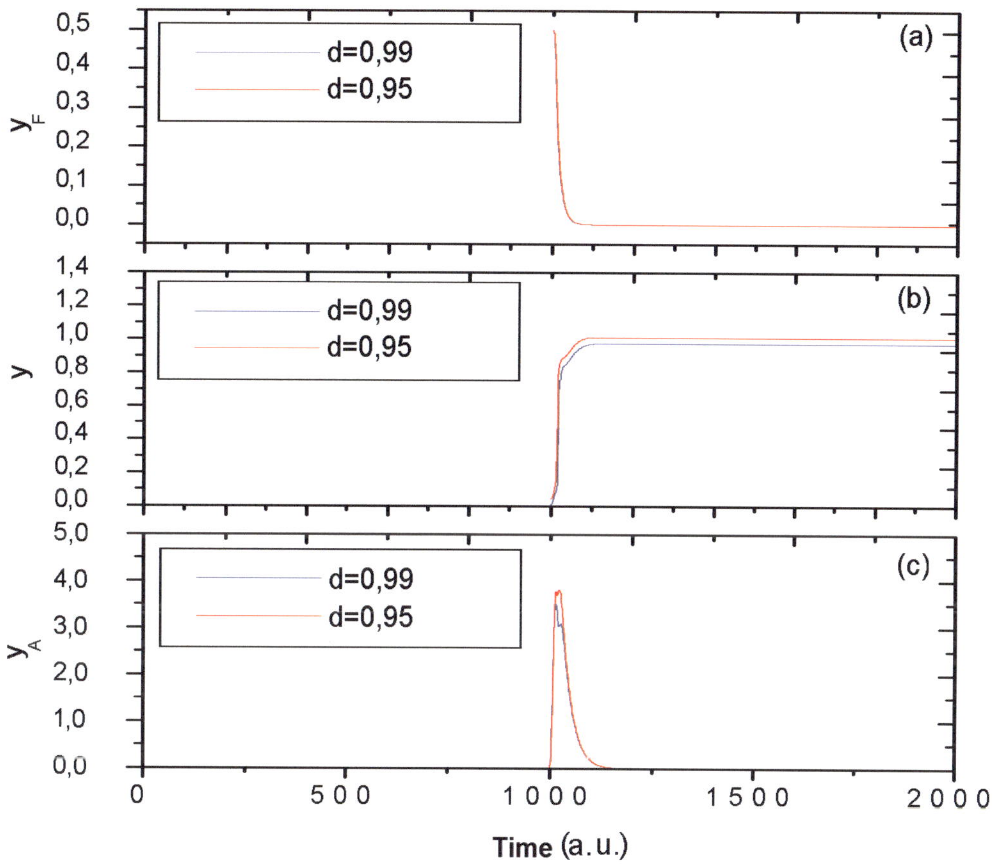

Fig. 6. Evolution of populations of antigens, B lymphocytes, and antibodies with respect to natural death parameter d = 0.99 and d = 0.95. The parameter $b_A = 100$ and initial antigen dosing $Ag_{inicial} = 0.5$. The virgin state of the system is the range of 0 to 1000.

2.4.2 The source term (*m*)

The source term m simulates the stochastic behavior of the bone marrow in the production of new lymphocytes [21.38].

In the model described in this work, if the pseudo-random number generator returns a value less than o r equal to $p = 0.1$, the source term takes the value $m = 10^{-7}$, because m is experimentally small compared with the levels of lymphocytes produced in the immune response [34,35,38]. If the generator returns values greater than $p = 0.1$, the source term takes the value $m = 0.0$ [21].

2.4.3 The clonal proliferation parameter (*b*)

Both the pioneering work and the recent work in the literature on theoretical immunology present results on the dynamics of the immune system and the search for attractors of the fixed point type to determine *in machine* clonal homeostasis (equilibrium) in the virgin state (antigen without inoculation) and in the excited state (when an antigen is recognized by some clonal population) [37,38,40].

The condition $y_F = y_A = 0$ is satisfied when the virgin state of the immune system is considered, i.e., without the presentation of antigens, no antibodies are produced. Also, considering that the system only allows high-affinity connections (connections between perfectly complementary shapes), the connectivity factor $a_h = 0$.

In the virgin state, the sum total of the immune populations is restricted to B lymphocytes:

$$y_{Tot}(t) = \sum_{\sigma}[y(\sigma,t) + y_F(\sigma,t) + y_A(\sigma,t)] = \sum_{\sigma} y(\sigma,t)$$

Hence, equation 5 reduces to the following:

$$y(\sigma,t+1) = [1 - y(\sigma,)]\{m + (1-d)y(\sigma,t) + b\frac{y(\sigma,t)}{\sum_{\sigma} y(\sigma,t)}y(\bar{\sigma},t)\}. \cdot$$

As in the dynamic simulation used in this work, the virgin state occurs in the interval of 0 to 1000 time steps, and only a pseudo-random number is drawn. Then,

$$\sum_{\sigma} y(\sigma,t) = y(\sigma,t) = y(\sigma^*,t) = y(t) = y_t \text{ and } y_t = y(\bar{\sigma},t),$$

because, according to Immune Network Theory, for each lymphocyte population, there is another complementary population [17,18,19]. A more detailed explanation can be found in the results section.

Because the bone marrow term in the absence of infection (virgin state of the immune system) is much smaller than the clonal proliferation parameter (m<<b) [34,35], we have the following:

$$y_{t+1} = [(1-d)y_t + by_t](1-y_t) \text{ or } [1-d+b]y_t(1-y_t). .$$

Defining $r \equiv 1-d+b$, the equality results in the following: ($y_{t+1} = ry_t(1-y_t)$, a logistic map-type equation). Moreover, for the system under study to evolve to a fixed point, the condition $1 < 1-d+b < 3$ must be satisfied.

Consequently, taking into account an apoptosis parameter equal to $d = 0.99$, the clonal proliferation parameter b must be located within the following range: $1 < 1+b-0.99 < 3 \rightarrow 0.99 < b < 2.99$. In the simulations presented in this paper, the clonal proliferation parameter b was set to 2.0.

2.4.4 The antibody and antigen removal parameter (*k*)

The parameter for the removal of antigens and antibodies k was set to 0.1, to ensure that the populations of antigens and antibodies decay to zero before the antigen is presented.

This procedure, which is adopted for a new antigen, is applied only after the previous antigen has been completely removed [21.45].

2.4.5 Connectivity (a_h)

The connectivity parameter used was 7, so that 99% of the populations are coupled to their perfect complement, and only 1% of the populations are coupled to the first neighbors of their complement. The quality of the immune response is directly related to the degree of affinity among the elements of the adaptive system [8].

2.4.6 Bit-string length (*B*)

Considering the available hypercube immune populations represented by the model, the length of the bit-string B was set at 12. This value corresponds to $2^{12} = 4{,}096$ different antigens.

2.4.7 Antibody proliferation parameter (b_A)

In the model presented in this work, the initial antigenic dose $(Ag_{initial})$ was set to study the influence of parameter b_A on the immune memory in some simulations.

In other simulations, this parameter was set to study the consequences to the memory of varying the antigen dosage. To clarify, the limit value of $b_A = 0.0$ corresponds to the model previously proposed by Lagreca et al. [21], and the limit value of $Ag_{initial} = y_F = 0.0$ corresponds to the virgin state of the immune system.

3. Results

The clonal populations that were excited after selection by an antigen (or an antigen population) are shown in Fig. 7, as follows: (a) for the first antigen inoculation; and (b) for the second antigen inoculation, with a dosage of 0.1. In this evolution, two populations were excited with the first antigen inoculation at step 1000: the clonal population that recognized the specific antigen (B1 - Burnet idiotypic cells [18.19]) and the clonal population (J1 - Jerne anti-idiotypic cells [18.19]) complementary to B1. At step 2000, the second antigen was inoculated, and four populations survived: the clonal population that was selected by the second antigen (B2), the clonal population (J2) that is complementary to B2, the clonal population that was selected by the first antigen (B1), and the clonal population (J1) that is complementary to B1.

At step 1000, clonal populations B1 and J1 are excited when they are selected by the first antigen, as shown in Fig. 7 (a). However, in step 2000, when populations B2 and J2 are excited, the clonal populations B1 and J1 are already memories of the first antigen. To maintain the homeostasis of the system, there is a decrease in the concentrations of the four remaining populations, as shown in Fig. 7 (b).

3.1 Antigen persistence

The temporal evolution (kinetics) of the Burnet cells is shown in Fig. 8 for each antigen i. Fig. 8 shows that the population selected by the first antigen begins to decrease after the second inoculation.

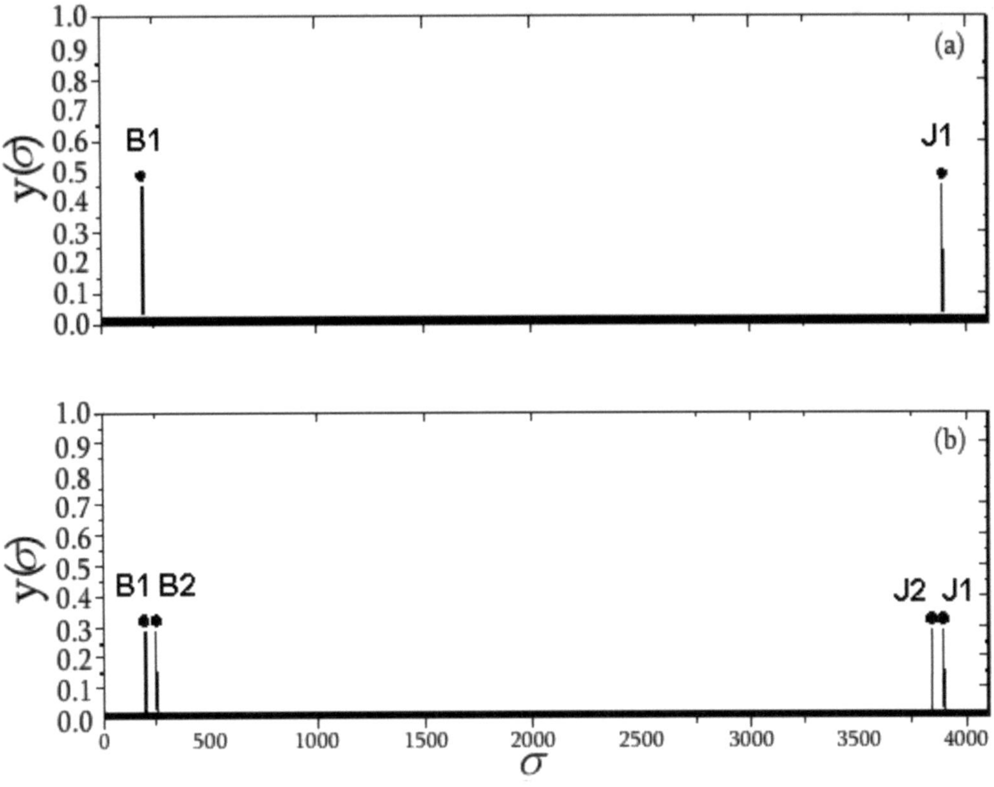

Fig. 7. Surviving clonal populations: (a) for the first antigen inoculated, and (b) for the first and second antigens inoculated.

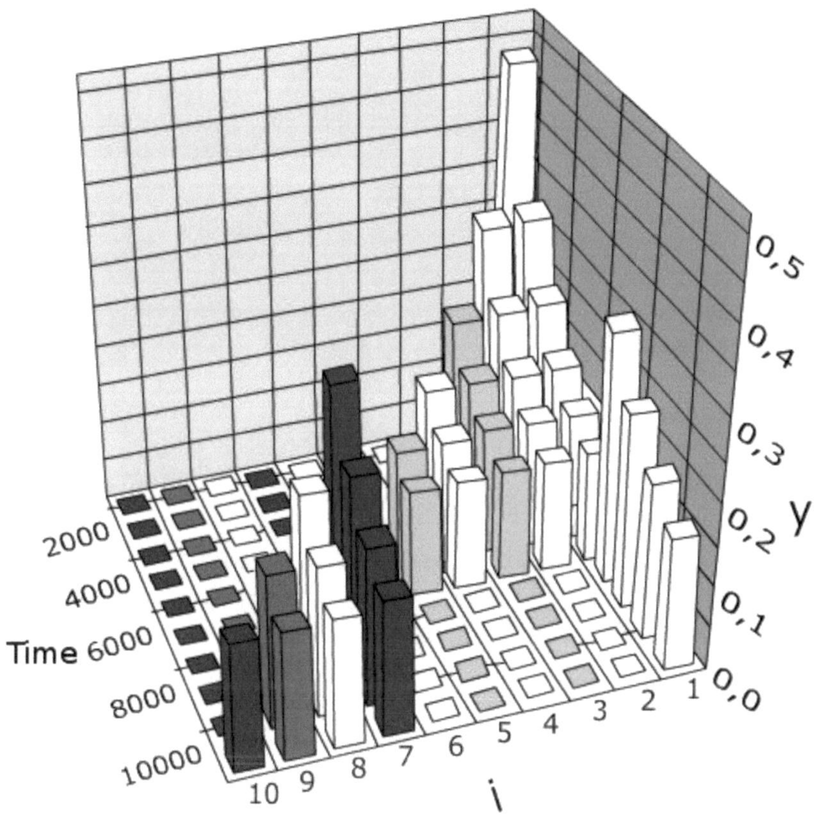

Fig. 8. Evolution of populations in memory, up to 11,000 time steps (concentration of antigens equal to 0.10 a.u.). The first and seventh clonal populations remain excited, while the others disappear - except for the last populations, which were excited near the end of the range.

This behavior occurs because the immune system has a maximum number of cells that it can support; in other words, when new antigens are memorized, others need to be forgotten (immune homeostasis turnover). At time step 7,000, when the seventh inoculation is performed, the first population begins to increase, indicating that it can be stored for a long period. In our Ag-dependent approach, this behavior indicates that an increase in the lifetime (lifespan) of memory can be generated by antigen survival (antigenic dependence).

3.2 Antigen mutation

To study the influence of antigenic mutation on memory (B cell antigen-dependent memory), simulations of inoculations of the 30 samples were also performed, with an antigenic dosage of

$Ag_{initial} = 0.1 a.u.$ The durations of memory populations in each experiment (E1, E2, and E3) are shown in Fig.9.

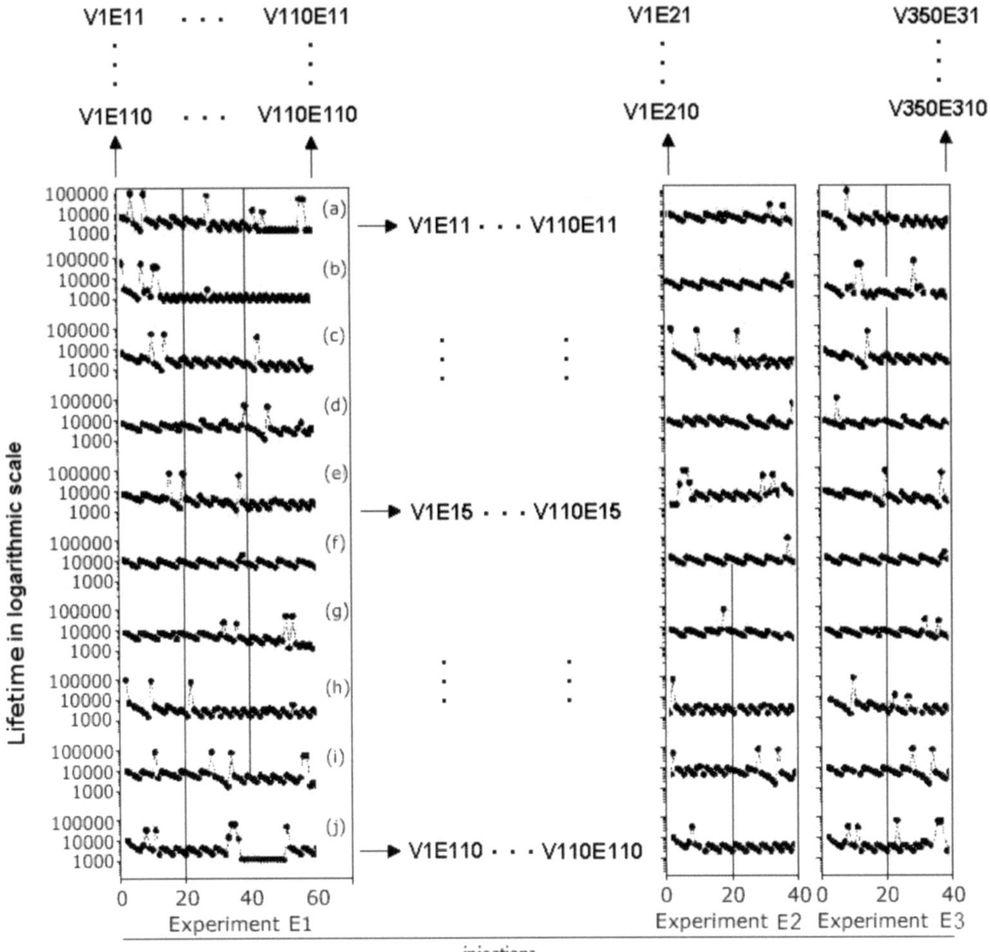

Fig. 9. Lifetime on a logarithmic scale for the clonal populations in each sample and in three experiments. For best viewing results, the graphs were truncated at 60 time steps (experiment E1) and 40 time steps (experiments E2 and E3). The arrows indicate the antigen populations that led to the production of immune memory.

In Fig. 9 (a), for example, all of the lifetimes (lasting memories) are related to antigens of different species (V1E11...V110E11). In contrast, the first lifetime in Fig. 9 (a)-(j) refers to an antigen that has already undergone mutation (V1E11...V1E110). Similar memory developments for experiments E2 and E3 are also shown in Fig. 9. The behavior of the average durability of the memories is shown in Fig. 10 (a) - (c).

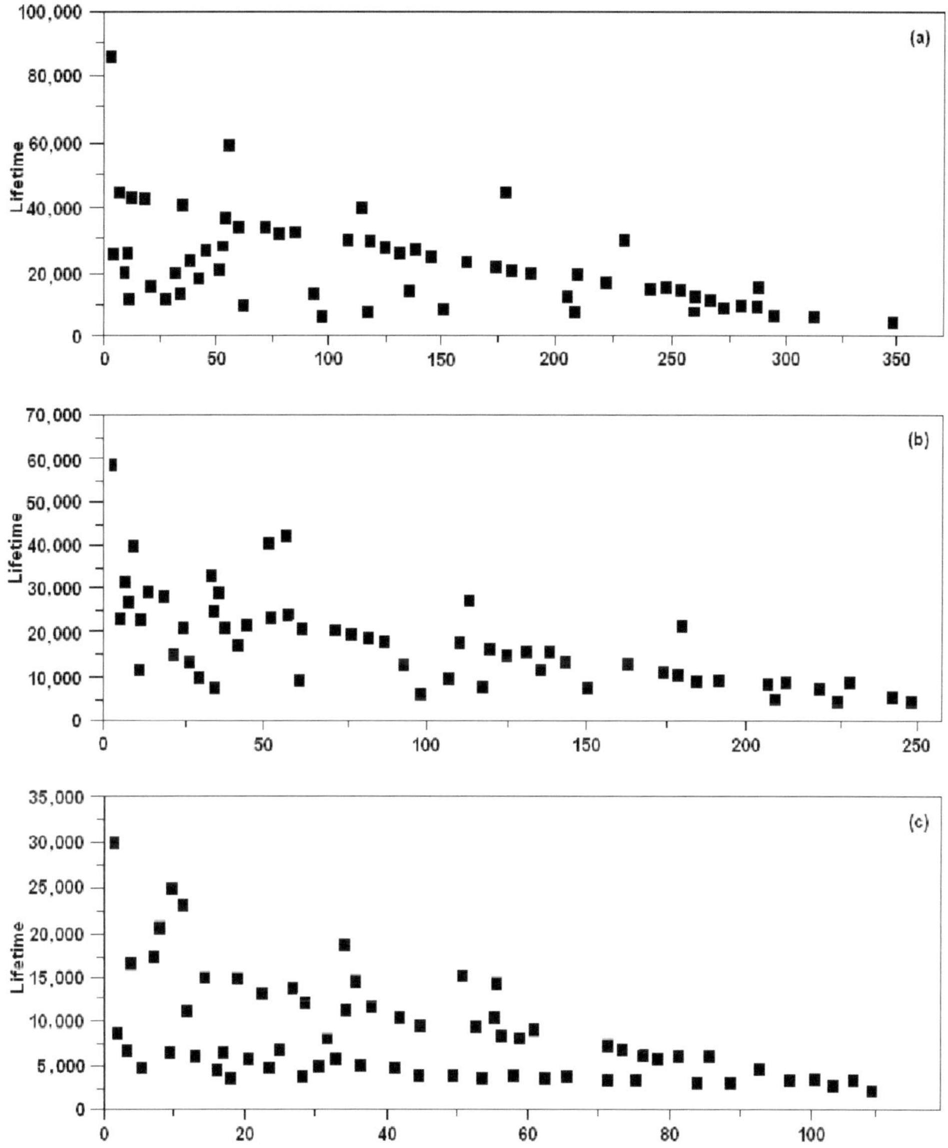

Fig. 10. Temporal averages of memory lifespans. In (a), to 350 antigen inoculations; in (b), to 250 antigen inoculations; and in (c), to 110 antigen inoculations.

The average lifespans are calculated from the memory lifespans generated by each mutated antigen, as follows:

- For experiment E1 (Fig. 10 (c)), the first average lifetime is obtained by $\frac{1}{10}\sum_{k=1}^{10} V_1 E_{1,k}$ and the last average lifetime is obtained by $\frac{1}{10}\sum_{k=1}^{10} V_{110} E_{1,k}$;

- For experiment E2 (Fig. 10 (b)), the first average lifetime is obtained by $\frac{1}{10}\sum_{k=1}^{10} V_1 E_{2,k}$ and the last average lifetime is obtained by $\frac{1}{10}\sum_{k=1}^{10} V_{250} E_{2,k}$;
- For experiment E3 (Fig. 10 (a)), the first average lifetime is obtained by $\frac{1}{10}\sum_{k=1}^{10} V_1 E_{3,k}$ and the last average lifetime is obtained by $\frac{1}{10}\sum_{k=1}^{10} V_{350} E_{3,k}$.

From Figs 9 and 10, the resulting set for this dynamics suggests that different antigens, and mutated antigens, generate different lifespans for immunological memory.

4. Discussion and conclusion

In this paper, an Ag-dependent mathematical model was used to explore how the key elements of the adaptive immune system function. The same model was also used to investigate the factors that are potentially responsible for maximum immunization capacity [40-55].

Inspired by the following statement of Elgueta et al.: "After 20 years, the role for persisting antigens, immune complexes, and FDCs is still not satisfactorily resolved [...] It is completely unknown how the memory B cell compartment is sustained [...] The role of antigens, FDCs, and immune complexes is still open to further investigation" [56], we have paid special attention to the phenomenon of immune memory and its relationship to antigen mutation and antigenic persistence.

Our results suggest that not only antigen type but also antigen mutation can influence the durability of immunizations, indicating that the role of antigen persistence is important for prolonging immune memory. These results were discussed with respect to recent work, and we refer to the adoption of parameter values chosen among data gathered from the literature. The model used in this study took into consideration that the immune system is a network of molecules and cells that can recognize itself [1-6,17]. The cells that recognize antigens select a complementary set of clones (anti-idiotypic antibodies) that can react with the idiotypes of other cells. Thus, the clonal expansion of complementary cells can also occur when these two types of cells interact through lock-and-key connections [8]. In the results presented here, such behavior was observed when an antigen was inoculated into the system and two B cell populations were excited: the population of cells that recognized the antigen and the population of cells that recognized its complementary shape, as shown in Fig. 7.

The results also show that an important factor in the durability of immunological memory is the mutation of antigen populations. In 2009, Tarlinton *et al.* [49] published a review paper, suggesting that the homeostasis of immune memory can only occur if new memory populations arise over others, i.e., to create dynamic equilibrium among memory cells, some need to disappear for others to arise, because the immune system has a maximum memory capacity [40-55]. Choo *et al.*, in a recent paper published in *The Journal of Immunology* [57], reported the same finding, based on the Ag-independent premise. Choo *et al.* (2010) have determined, by means of a quantitative analysis, that the homeostatic turnover of Ag-specific CD8 memory T cells is stochastic rather than deterministic.

Then, the results we show in Fig. 8 indicate, in part, an alignment with the work of Choo *et al.*(2010) and with that of Tarlinton et al., because some populations were "forgotten" so that others could be "memorized", thereby complying with the principle of homeostatic turnover. However, Tarlinton *et al.*(2008) [49] and Choo *et al.* (2010) [57] suggest that the mechanism for achieving homeostasis is stochastic, contrary to earlier work of Matzinger (1995)[50] and Nayak *et al.* (2001)[19], who indicated that the durability of memory depends on the antigen type.

The results presented in Figs. 9 and 10 suggest that the homeostatic turnover of a memory B cell depends on the antigen type and also on their mutation(s). Thus, our model aligns best with the earlier work of Nayak *et al.*(2001) and Matzinger *et al.* (1995), and it also aligns to some extent with the work of Tarlinton *et al.*, specifically with respect to storage capacity (homeostatic turnover). However, our results do not line up with a hypothesis of randomness (stochastically) for the kinetics of immune memory, as inferred by Choo *et al.*

The results presented here considered a pool of B cells, but similar conclusions can be drawn from a pool of CD4 T cells. In our simulations, memory lifespan is dependent on the antigen, and the dynamic behavior of memory is strongly deterministic. These results are especially interesting, because they may suggest a deterministic chaotic behavior for the immune memory. In chaotic behavior, there is a mix of stochasticity and determinism, i.e., there exists a well-defined mathematical function for the problem, but small changes in initial conditions can lead to unpredictable results. In conclusion, our results have shown that Choo *et al.*(2010) may have inferred an "apparent" stochastic behavior for homeostatic turnover in their work; however, this behavior may be linked to a deterministic-chaotic dynamic equilibrium. Nevertheless, this finding also indicates that, although the memory behavior is deterministic, just is possible to predict the durability of immunization inferred by a vaccine within a limited interval of antigenic concentration, i.e., outside chaotic region.

5. References

[1] Farmer, J. D., Packard, N. H., Perelson, A. S. *The Immune System, Adaptation, and Machine Learning*. Physica D, Amsterdam, v. 22, pp. 187-204, July 1986.

[2] Roitt, I., Brostoff, J., Male, D. *Immunology*. 4th Ed. New York: Mosby, 1998.

[3] Hofmeyr, S. A. *An Interpretative Introduction to the Immune System Design. In: Principles for the Immune System and Other Distributed Autonomous Systems*. Cohen, I., Segel, L. A. (eds.). Oxford: Oxford University Press, pp. 302-340, 2000.

[4] Klein, J. *Immunology*. Oxford: Blackwell Scientific Publications, 1990.

[5] Lederberg, J. *Ontogeny of the Clonal Selection Theory of Antibody Formation*. Annals of the New York Ac. of Sc., v. 546, pp. 175-182, 1988.

[6] Perelson, A. S., Weisbuch, G. *Immunology for Physicists*. Rev. of Modern Physics, Seattle, v. 69, n. 4, pp. 1219-1267, Oct. 1997.

[7] Celada, F., Seiden, P. *A computer model of cellular interaction in the immune system.* Immunology Today, Amsterdam, pp. 1356-1362, February 1992.

[8] Perelson, A. S., Mirmirani, M., Oster, G. F. *Optimal Strategies in Immunology II. B Memory Cell Production*. J. Math. Biol., Oxford, v. 5, pp. 213-256, October 1978.

[9] Kaufman, M., Urbain, J., Thomas, R. *Towards a logical analysis of the immune response.* J. Theor. Biol., Amsterdam, v. 11, pp. 527-561, January 1985.

[10] Kaufman, M., Weinberg, E. D. *The NK Model of Rugged Fitness Landscapes and Its Application to Maturation of the Immune Response*, J. Theor. Biol., Amsterdam, v. 141, pp. 211-245, December 1989.

[11] Celada, F., Seiden, P. *Affinity maturation and hypermutation in a simulation of the humoral immune response.* Eur. J. Immunol., Weinheim, v. 26, pp. 1350-1358, June 1996.

[12] Menchón, S. A., Ramos, R. A., Condat, C. A. *Modeling subspecies and the tumor-immune system interaction: Steps toward understanding therapy.* Physica A: Statistical Mechanics and its Applications, v. 386, pp. 713-719.

[13] MO, H. *Review of Modeling and Stimulating Human Immune Sysytem. Artificial Intelligence Applications and Innovations.* IFIP International Federation for Information Processing, 2005, v. 187/2005, pp. 845-854.

[14] Rapin, N., Lund, O., Bernaschi, M., Castiglione, F. *Computational Immunology Meets Bioinformatics: The Use of Prediction Tools for Molecular Binding in the Simulation of the Immune System* . PLoS One. v. 5(4), p. e9862, 2010.

[15] Lundegaard, C., Lund, O., Kesmir, C., Brunak, S., Nielsen, M. *Modeling the adaptive immune system: predictions and simulations.* Bioinformatics. v. 23, pp. 3265-3275, 2007.

[16] Boer, R. J., Oprea, M., Rustom. A., Murali-Krishna, K., Ahmed, R., Perelson, A. *Recruitment Times, Proliferation, and Apoptosis Rates during the CD8+ T-Cell Response to Lymphocytic Choriomeningitis Virus.* JOURNAL OF VIROLOGY, v. 75, pp. 10663-10669, 2001.

[17] Jerne, N. K. *Towards a Network Theory of the Immune System.* Ann. Immunol. v. 125C, pp. 373-389, October 1974.

[18] Shibani Mitra-Kaushik, S., Shaila, M. S., Anjali K. Karande, A. K., Nayak, R. *Idiotype and Antigen-Specific T Cell Responses in Mice on Immunization with Antigen, Antibody, and Anti-idiotypic Antibody.* Cellular Immunology v. 209, pp. 109-119, 2001.

[19] Nayak, R., Mitra-Kaushik, S., M. S. Shaila. *Perpetuation of immunological memory: a relay hypothesis.* Immunology v. 102, pp. 387-395, 2001.

[20] Castro, L. N. *Fundamentals of Natural Computing: Basic Concepts, Algorithms, and Applications.* Chapman & Hall/CRC Computer & Information Science Series, 2006.

[21] Lagreca, M. C., Almeida, R. M. C., Santos, R. M. Z. A Dynamical Model for the Immune Repertoire, Physica A, v. 289, pp. 191-207, 2001.

[22] Ausloos, M., Dirickx, M. *The Logistic Map and the Route to Chaos.* 413 p. Springer, 2006.

[23] Heyman, B. *Feedback regulation by IgG antibodies.* Immunology Letters, v. 88, pp. 157-161, 2003.

[24] Hjelm, F., Carlsson, F., Getahun, A., Heyman, B. *Antibody-Mediated Regulation of the Immune Response.* Scandinavian Journal of Immunology, v. 64, 177-184, 2006.

[25] Nimmerjahn, F., Ravetch, J. V. *Antibody-mediated modulation of immune responses,* v. 236, pp. 265-275, 2010.

[26] Ferrari, P. C., Angotti, J. A. P., Tragtenberg, M. H. R. *Introdução ao Caos em Sistemas Dinâmicos.* Mini-curso. Instituto de Física - UFG, 2006.

[27] May, R. M. *Simple Mathematical Models with Very Complicated Dynamics.* Nature, V. 261, p. 459, 1976.

[28] Aubin, D., Dalmedico, A. D. *Writing the History of Dynamical Systems and Chaos: Longue Dureé and Revolution, Disciplines and Cultures.* Historia Mathematica, v. 29, pp. 273-339, 2002.

[29] Erneux, T. *Applied delay differential equations.* In: Surveys and Tutorials in the Applied Mathematical Sciences. Springer, p. 210, 2009.

[30] Moreira, I. C. *Os primórdios do Caos Determinístico.* Ciência Hoje, v. 14, pp. 10-16, 1992.

[31] Dudek, M. R. *Lotka-Volterra PopulationModel of Genetic Evolution.* Communications in Computational Physics, v. 2, pp. 1174-1183, 2007.

[32] Bagnoli, F., Bezzi, M. Eigen's Error Threshold and Mutational Meltdown in a Quasi-species Model, International Journal of Modern Physics C, v. 9, pp. 1-7, 1998.

[33] Gould, H., Tobochnik, J. *An Introduction to Computer Simulation Methods: Applications to Physical Systems.* Addison-Weley Publishing Company. 1996.

[34] von Laer, D., Hasselmannb, S., Hasselmannb, K. *Impact of gene-modified T cells on HIV infection dynamics.* Journal of Theoretical Biology, v. 238, pp. 60-77, 2008.

[35] Walker, R. E., Carter, C. S., Muul, L., Natarajan, V., Herpin, B. R., Leitman, S. F., Klein, H. G., Mullen, C. A., Metcalf, J. A., Baseler, M., Falloon, J., Davey, R. T., Kovacs, J. A., Polis, M. A., Masur, H., Blaese, R. M., Lane, H. C. *Peripheral expansion of pre-existing mature T cells is an important means of CD4þ T-cell regeneration HIV-infected adults.* Nat. Med. v. 4, pp. 852-856, 1998.

[36] Heyman, B. *Regulation of Antibody Responses via Antibodies, Complements, and FC Receptors.* Annu. Rev. Immunol. v. 18, pp. 709-737, 2000.

[37] Rustom Antia, r., Pilyugin, s. s., Ahmed, r. *Models of immune memory: On the role of cross-reactive stimulation, competition, and homeostasis in maintaining immune memory.* Immunology, v. 95, pp. 14926-14931, 1998.

[38] Monvel, J. H. B., Martin, O. M. *Memory capacity in large idiotypic networks.* Bulletin of Mathematical Biology. v. 57, pp. 109-136, 1995.

[39. Vani, J., Elluru, S., Negi, V., Lacroix-Desmazes, S.. Michel D. *Role of natural antibodies in immune homeostasis: IVIg perspective.* Autoimmunity Reviews, *v. 7, pp. 440-444, 2008.*

[40] Etchegoin, P. G. *Vaccination pattern affects immunological response.* Physica A: Statistical Mechanics and its Applications, v. 354, pp. 393-403, 2005.

[41] Boer, R. J., Oprea, M., Rustom. A., Murali-Krishna, K., Ahmed, R., Perelson, A. *Recruitment Times, Proliferation, and Apoptosis Rates during the CD8+ T-Cell Response to Lymphocytic Choriomeningitis Virus.* Journal of Virology, v. 75, pp. 10663-10669, 2001.

[42] Bueno, V., Pacheco-Silva, A. *Tolerância oral: uma nova perspectiva no tratamento de doenças autoimunes.* Revista da Associação Médica Brasileira, v. 45, pp. 79-85, 1999.

[43] Lima, F. A., Carneiro-Sampaio, M. *The role of the thymus in the development of the immune system.* Reviews and Essays, v. 29, pp. 33-42, 2007.

[44] Utzny, C., Burroughs, N. J. *Long-term Stability of Diverse Immunological Memory.* J. Theor. Biol., v. 211, pp. 393-402, 2001.

[45] Yao, W., Hertel, L., Wahl, L. M. *Dynamics of recurrent viral infection.* Proc. R. Soc. B, v. 273, pp. 2193-2199, 2006.

[46] Dimitrijevic, L., Zvancevic-Simonovic, S., Istojanovic, M., Inic-Kanada, A., Ivkovic, I. *The Possible Role of Natural* Idiotopes *in Immune Memory.* Clinical & Developmental Immunology, v. 11, pp. 281-285, 2004.

[47] Obukhanych, T. V., Nussenzweig, M. C. *T-independent type II immune responses generate memory B cells.* Journal of Experimental Medicine, v. 203, pp. 305-310, 2006.

[48] Lanzavecchia, A., Sallusto, F. *Human B cell memory.* Current Opinion in Immunology, v. 21, pp. 298-304, 2009.

[49] Tarlinton, D., Radbruch, A., Hiepe, F., Thomas Dorner, T. *Plasma cell differentiation and survival.* Current Opinion in Immunology, v. 20, pp. 162-169, 2008.

[50] Matzinger, P. *Immunology: memories are made of this?* Nature, pp. 369-605, 1995.

[51] Hendrikxa, L. H., Berbersa, G. A. M., Veenhovenb, R. H., Sandersc, E.A.M., Buismana, A. M. *IgG responses after booster vaccination with different pertussis vaccines in Dutch children 4 years of age: Effect of vaccine antigen content.* Vaccine, v. 27, pp. 6530-6536, 2009.

[52] Tizard, I. R. *Immunology: An Introduction.* 4th ed. Philadelphia: Saunders College Publishing, 1995.

[53] Abbas, A. K., Lichtman, A. H., Pober, J. S. *Cellular and Molecular Immunology.*

[54] Kamradt, T., Avrion, M. N. *Advances in immunology: Tolerance and Autoimmunity.* N Engl J Med, v. 344, pp. 655-64, 2001.

[55] Peter, D., Roitt, I. M. *Advances in immunology: The Immune System.* New Engl. J. Med., v. 343, pp. 37-49, 2000.

[56] Elgueta, R., Vries, V. C., Noelle, R. J. The immortality of humoral immunity. Immunological Reviews, v. 236, pp. 139-150, 2010.

[57] Choo, D. K., Murali-Krishna, K., Anita, R., Ahmed, R. Homeostatic Turnover of Virus-Specific Memory CD8 T Cells Occurs Stochastically and Is Independent of CD4 T Cell Help. Journal of Immunolody, v.185, pp. 3436-44, 2010. Esta precisa ser a referência número 1.

17

Toll Like Receptors in Dual Role: Good Cop and Bad Cop

Saba Tufail[*], Ravikant Rajpoot[*] and Mohammad Owais
Aligarh Muslim University
India

1. Introduction

Every living organism tends to protect itself from harmful effects of pathogens or molecules of pathogenic origin that can disturb its well-being state. The first line of defence that comes into action upon encounter with the pathogen is referred to as innate immune defence mechanism. It had been a matter of great inquisitiveness how innate immune defence mechanism is able to render the body protected against such a diverse variety of pathogens. But with the discovery of germ line encoded pattern recognition receptors (PRRs) that can sense the pathogen associated molecular patterns (PAMPs), it is to an extent possible to answer the query, how innate immune system copes to recognise such a wide variety of micro-organisms and harmful microbial elements. PAMPs are usually of pathogenic origin and absent from the cells of host origin. PRRs can be transmembrane receptors like Toll like receptors (TLRs) (Beutler & Rietschel, 2003; Janeway & Medzhitov, 2002), C-type lectin receptors (CLRs) or these can be cytosolic receptors like Nod like receptors (NLRs) and Rig like helicases (RLRs). Every PRR is capable of recognising specific conserved molecular patterns on the micro-organism and later can start a downstream signalling process upon proper interaction of PAMP and PRR that leads to synthesis of effector molecules like antimicrobial peptides and pro-inflammatory cytokines that prevent the body from otherwise harmful microbes.

In the late 90's a protein was discovered in *Drosophila* named as Toll. Toll is a transmembrane receptor that is required for the establishment of proper dorso-ventral polarity during embryo formation in *Drosophila* (Hashimoto et al., 1988). Mutation in Toll gene results in a weird phenotype of the fruitflies. Later it was found that signalling pathways of *Drosophila* Toll and mammalian IL-1 receptor showed marked resemblance leading to the assumption that Toll may be involved in the regulation of immune responses. Now, it is well established that Toll signalling is required for the defence against Gram-positive, Gram-negative bacterial and fungal infections. Toll is responsible for the production of Drosomycin, antifungal peptide (Lemaitre et al., 1996). Mutants lacking in components of Toll mediated signalling pathway (Toll, Spatzle, Tube, Pelle) are highly susceptible to fungal infections. A year succeeding the discovery of Toll in *Drosophila*, through database searches, Toll homologues in mammals as well were revealed known as

---

[*] Saba Tufail and Ravikant Rajpoot contributed equally to this work

Toll like receptors (TLRs). TLRs recognise PAMPs of diverse origin from bacteria, virus, fungi, protozoa and others. TLRs can also sense the molecules that are generated within the host cells alarming a sort of danger signal like heat shock proteins (Hsp60, Hsp70, Hsp90), fibrinogen, surfactant protein A, heparin sulphate and others. Thirteen TLRs are reported so far, out of which TLR1 to TLR9 are conserved between human and mice. TLR10 is only functional in human while TLR11 is found to be functional only in mice. Upon interaction with their cognate ligands, TLRs either homodimerise or heterodimerise to further proceed the downstream signalling.

2. Structure of TLRs

Toll like receptors are type-I transmembrane receptors having an extracellular domain containing multiple leucine rich repeats (LRRs). There are about 19-25 tandem repeats of LRR motif each having 20-29 residue sequence motif LXXLXLXXNXLXXLXXXXXXXLXX where X is any amino acid (Bell et al., 2003). LRR motifs are responsible for interacting and recognising specific ligands and thereby initiating downstream signal transduction. LRRs are varied among different TLRs enabling them to sense a wide variety of PAMPs. Interaction of the pathogen with the LRR motif is supposed to take place at the concave side of the horse shoe shaped LRR motif. Mammalian TLRs are found to have homology with IL-1 receptor in cytoplasmic domain known as Toll/IL-1R or TIR domain while extracellular regions are devoid of any homology having three immunoglobulin domains in IL-1R and LRR motifs in TLRs. TIR domain consists of about 200 amino acids (Slack et al., 2000) and is composed of five β strands (βA, βB, βC, βD and βE) alternated with five α helices (αA, αB, αC, αD and αE) (Xu et al., 2000) connected via 8 loops. Box1, Box2 and Box3 are three highly conserved regions found to be present in TIR domain. BB loop is formed when Box2 forms a loop connecting the second β strand and α helix. This BB loop is of primary importance in further downstream signalling because any single amino acid residue substitution in this loop can lead to the complete impairment of its function. In C3H/HeJ mice, a point mutation in BB loop replacing conserved proline leads to hypo-responsiveness to the LPS resulting in loss of function of BB loop (Poltorak et al., 1998).

3. Distribution of TLRs

TLRs are generally expressed on the cells of innate immune system like dendritic cells, monocytes and macrophages (Beutler & Rehli, 2002) that are likely to have interacted with the pathogen earlier. TLR expression is found to be highest on the phagocytic cells like tissue macrophages, neutrophils and dendritic cells. Macrophages express all TLRs except TLR3. However, not all TLRs are expressed by all cell types i.e. TLR expression is tissue specific eg. TLR5 is shown to be exclusively expressed on the intestinal epithelial cells' basolateral surface. Also TLR expression may vary with the maturation stage of the cell, eg. TLR1, 2, 4 and 5 are shown to be expressed on the immature dendritic cells but there expression decreases as the cells undergo maturation. TLR3 is shown to be expressed only on mature dendritic cells. Yet tissue specific demarcation of TLR expression is not clear, it is observed that most of the tissues express atleast one type of TLR. Also TLR expression is found to be different in the two subsets of blood dendritic cells i.e. Myeloid dendritic cells express TLR1, 2, 4, 5 and 8 while plasmacytoid dendritic cell express TLR7 and TLR9 exclusively. TLR2 and 4 are highly expressed on the surface of macrophages but are also reported to be expressed on the endothelial cells, smooth muscle cells, intestinal cells and

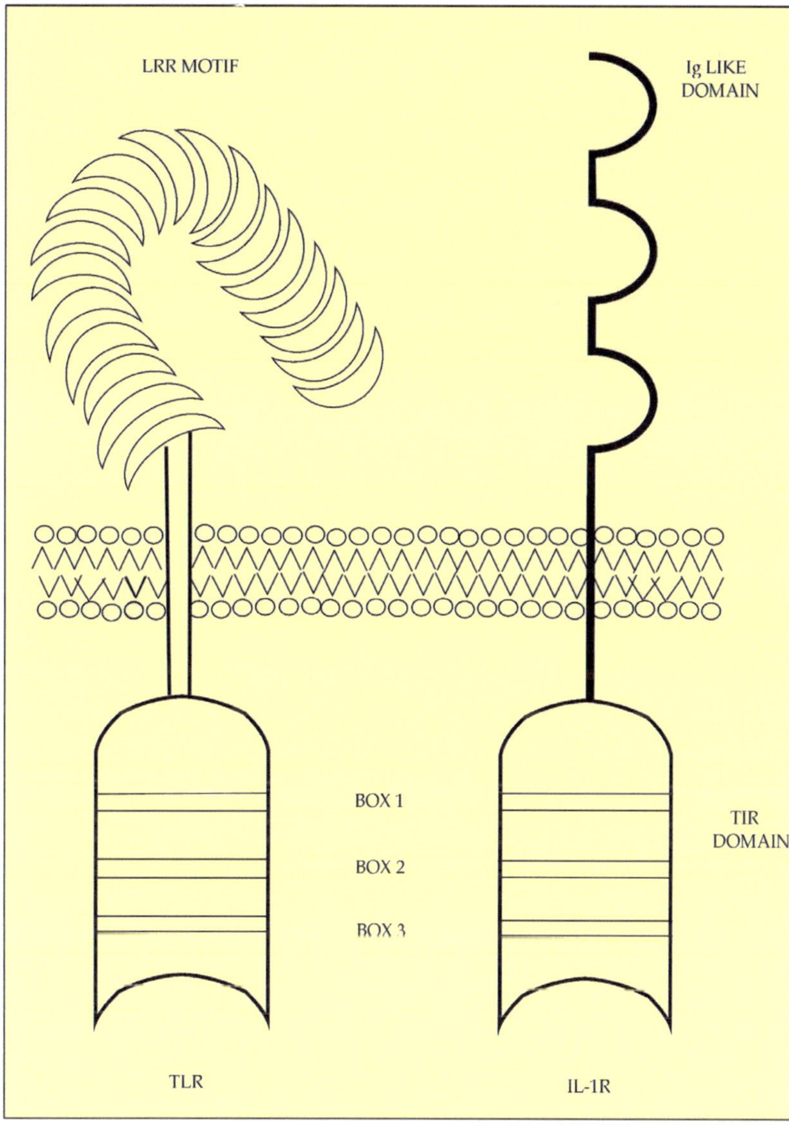

Fig. 1. Toll like receptors and IL-1R are transmembrane receptors both having a conserved region of about 200 amino acids in their cytoplasmic domain known as TIR domain. Three highly conserved regions in TIR domain are referred to as Box1, Box2 and Box3. TLRs and IL-1R though similar in their cytoplasmic domains are markedly different in their extracellular components; TLRs have LRR motif and IL-1R has Ig like domain extracellularly.

others. Studies also indicate subcellular location of TLRs. TLR1, TLR2, TLR4, TLR5 and TLR6 have been found to be expressed on the cell surface, as demonstrated by positive staining of the cell surface by specific antibodies and these recognize bacterial products while TLR3, TLR7, TLR8 and TLR9 have been shown to be expressed in intracellular compartments such as endosomes and recognize microbial nucleic acids (Takeda & Akira, 2005).

4. Phylogenetic relationship among TLRs

A sequence similarity search of different human TLRs revealed that TLRs can be subdivided into five subfamilies i.e. TLR2, TLR3, TLR4, TLR5 and TLR9 subfamilies. While the TLR3, TLR4 and TLR5 are the only respective members of their subfamily, TLR2 subfamily comprises of four members viz. TLR1, TLR2, TLR6 and TLR10; TLR9 family has three members TLR7, TLR8 and TLR9. Members within a subfamily exhibit high ratio of similar sequences than members of other subfamily eg. TLR1 and TLR6 show about 70% similarity in their amino acid sequence, identity approaches about 90% in their TIR domains.

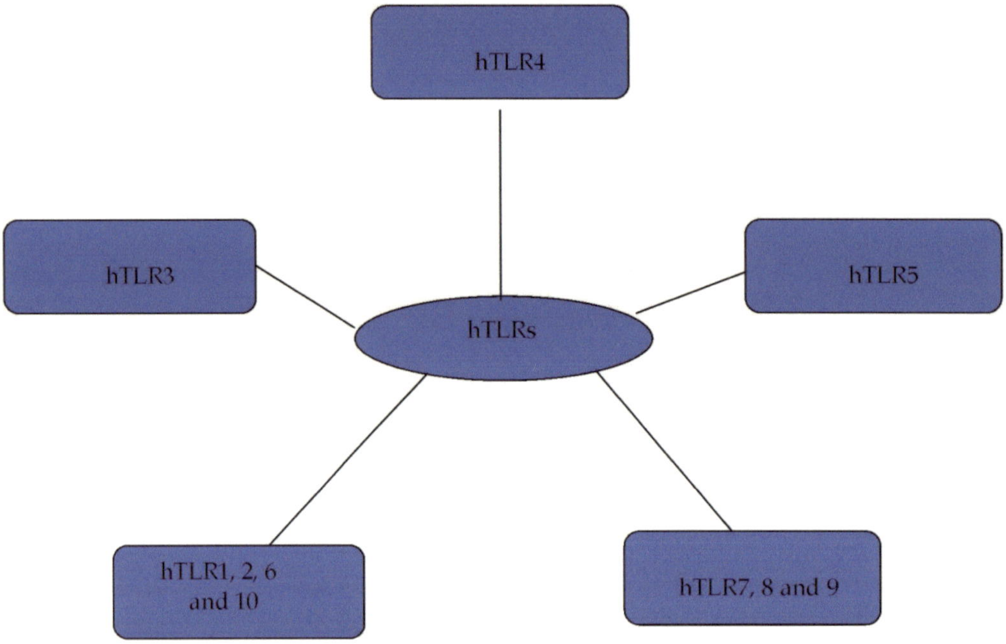

Fig. 2. Human TLRs can be divided into five subfamilies- TLR2, TLR3, TLR4, TLR5 and TLR9. Division is based on the amino acid sequence similarity.

5. Ligands of TLRs

TLRs are able to recognise a wide variety of pathogens and thereafter signal transduction commences that leads to mounting of desirable immune response against the pathogen like expression of inflammatory cytokines, chemokines, antibacterial peptides, enhanced expression of co-stimulatory molecules etc. Generally every TLR recognises more than one type of PAMP e.g. TLR4 (first TLR to be discovered in mammals) has the ability to recognise a variety of PAMPs diverse in nature, for instance it can recognise LPS from bacteria, taxol from plant, different proteins of viral origin, Hsp 60 and 70 from the host cell itself etc. Like TLR4 other TLRs are also able to recognise a wide variety of pathogens which is briefly summarised in Table 1.

TLR	LIGANDS
TLR1	Tri-acyl lipopeptides (bacteria, mycobacteria)
	Soluble factors (Neisseria meningitides)
TLR2	Lipoprotein/lipopeptides (a variety of pathogens)
	Peptidoglycan (Gram-positive bacteria)
	Lipoteichoic acid (Gram-positive bacteria)
	Lipoarabinomannan (mycobacteria)
	A phenol-soluble modulin (Staphylococcus epidermidis)
	Glycoinositolphospholipids (Trypanosoma Cruzi)
	Glycolipids (Treponema maltophilum)
	Porins (Neisseria)
	Zymosan (fungi)
	Atypical LPS (Leptospira interrogans)
	Atypical LPS (Porphyromonas gingivalis)
	HSP70 (host)
TLR3	Double-stranded RNA (virus)
TLR4	LPS (Gram-negative bacteria)
	Taxol (plant)
	Fusion protein (RSV)
	Envelope proteins (MMTV)
	HSP60 (Chlamydia pneumoniae)
	HSP60 (host)
	HSP70 (host)
	Type III repeat extra domain A of fibronectin (host)
	Oligosaccharides of hyaluronic acid (host)
	Polysaccharide fragments of heparan sulfate (host)
	Fibrinogen (host)
TLR5	Flagellin (bacteria)
TLR6	Di-acyl lipopeptides (mycoplasma)
TLR7/8	Imidazoquinoline (synthetic compounds)
	Loxoribine (synthetic compounds)
	Bropirimine (synthetic compounds)
TLR9	CpG DNA (bacteria)
	Hemozoin (protozoa)
TLR10	?
TLR11	Component of uropathogenic bacteria (bacteria)
	Profilin like molecule (protozoa *Toxoplasma gondii*)

Table 1. TLRs and their corresponding ligands.

6. TLRs bridge innate and adaptive immunity

TLRs serve as a link between innate and adaptive immunity by induction of dendritic cell (DC) maturation and directing T helper responses (Parker et al., 2006). It has been reported that stimulation of specific TLRs leads to induction of either IL-10 or IL-12 that results in a response biased towards either Th1 or Th2 cytokines. TLR2 mediated response preferentially leads to release of Th2 cytokines while TLR4 induces Th1 cytokine release. DCs have been reported to express TLRs on their surfaces which respond to different microbial antigens differently. Immature DCs have high phagocytic activity but low T cell activation potential and these are capable of detecting, capturing and phagocytosing pathogens that ultimately leads to activation of TLRs and cytokine release. A signalling cascade commences after TLR activation (as described later) which serves as a complex differentiation programme for DCs, collectively termed DC maturation. This DC maturation is characterised by up-regulation of co-stimulatory molecules such as CD40, CD80, and CD86. CD80 and CD86 are the two requisite signals for naïve T cell activation (Banchereau & Steiman, 1998; Parker et al., 2006).

Also, when TLRs on many cell types are stimulated by TLR agonists, bacteria and viruses, it leads to the production of type I interferon (IFN-α/β) (Parker et al., 2006). This response is popularly attributed to be part of first line of defence against infection and a central modulator of adaptive immunity. Proliferation of memory T cells, inhibition of T cell apoptosis, enhanced IFN-γ secretion, B-cell isotype switching and differentiation into plasma cells and NK cell activation are some of the attributes of IFNs owing to their diverse functions in the development of adaptive immunity.

In addition to up-regulation of CD80/CD86 molecules on DCs and production of type I interferon (IFN-α/β) to control T cell activation, another mechanism of T cell activation exists in which T cell responses are regulated by $CD4^+$ $CD25^+$ suppressor or regulatory T cells (Treg cells). The Treg cells function to induce tolerance in peripheral T cells (both self-reactive and non-self-reactive T cells), a malfunctioning of these cells leads to autoimmune diseases. It has been reported that DCs produce IL-6 in response to TLR activation that is critical for T cell activation as it relieves suppression of effector T cells (non-self-reactive T cells) by Treg cells (Pasare & Metzitov, 2003). Pasare & Metzitov also report that T cell activation occurs even in the absence of IL-6 when Treg cells are removed. This suggests that induction of co-stimulatory molecules on DCs is enough for T cell activation in the absence of Treg cells.

7. TLR signalling

Toll like receptors after recognising PAMPs initiate intracellular signalling that leads to the activation of NF-κB (Nuclear factor kappa B) or IRF3 (Interferon regulating factor 3) and subsequently expression of genes under their control takes place. To induce intracellular signal transduction, TLRs either homodimerise or heterodimerise upon interaction with PAMPs. Probably there are two pathways regarding TLR signal transduction, MyD88 (Myeloid Differentiation Factor 88) dependent and MyD88 independent.

MyD88 dependent signalling pathway is found to be central to all TLRs except TLR3. TIRAP (TIR domain containing adaptor protein) is essential for MyD88 dependent signalling through TLR2 and 4 as revealed by the studies with TIRAP deficient mice.

MyD88 dependent signalling involves a number of molecules which are briefly described below.

MyD88

It is encoded by MyD88 gene (Muzio et al., 1997; Wesche et al., 1997; Burns et al., 1998). This protein is utilised by all TLRs except TLR3 as an adaptor to transmit the signal inside the cell resulting in activation of transcription factor NF-κB. Data indicates that another protein TIRAP also known as MAL (MyD88 adaptor like protein) is required by MyD88 to be recruited to TLR2 and TLR4. MyD88 protein has two domains- N terminal death domain (DD domain) and C terminal TIR domain. It interacts with the TIR domain of TLR via its C terminal TIR domain. MyD88 is also reported to interact with IL-1R, IRAK1, IRAK2, RAC1 (Ras mediated C3 botulinum toxin1) and many other proteins.

IRAK

IRAKs (IL-1R associated protein kinases) are protein kinases that act downstream of MyD88. Four IRAKs are identified in mammals- IRAK1, 2, 4 and M (Janssens & Beyaert, 2003). While IRAK1 and 4 are expressed in all cell types, IRAK2 shows narrower distribution and IRAK M is reported to be only expressed in cells of myeloid origin. IRAKs have an N terminal death domain but lack a TIR domain. But a central serine threonine kinase domain is present. IRAK1 and 4 have intrinsic kinase activity while IRAK2 and M are with no kinase activity.

TRAF

TRAFs (TNF receptor associated factors) are proteins having an N terminal coiled coil domain known as TRAF-N and a conserved C terminal domain known as TRAF- C (Bradley & Pober, 2001). There are six members in the mammalian TRAF family (TRAF1, TRAF2, TRAF3, TRAF4, TRAF5 and TRAF6). Binding of TRAF to its interacting proteins require that proteins should contain TRAF binding motif of which consensus sequence is identified and found to be as Pro-X-Glu-X-X-(aromatic/acidic residue) (Ye et al., 2002). This motif is found to present in CD40, IRAK1, IRAK2, IRAK4, TRANCER (TNF related activation induced cytokine receptor).

TAK1 and TABs

Activation of IKK complex (Inhibitor of NF-KB kinase complex) by TRAF6 requires two factors TRIKA1 (TRAF6 regulated IKK activator1) and TRIKA2 (TRAF6 regulated IKK activator2). Further studies revealed that TRIKA1 is composed of Ubc13 (Ubiquitin conjugating enzyme 13) and Uev1A (Ubiquitin conjugating enzyme variant1) which act as ubiquitin conjugating enzyme complex. Polyubiquitination of TRAF6 is done by TRIKA1 complex with lysine 63 (K63) of ubiquitin. This polyubiquitination directly activates the TAK1 in a proteasome independent manner. TRIKA2 is composed of TAK1, TAB1 and TAB2. TAK1 (TGF-β activated kinase) belongs to a MAPKKK family of protein kinases (Yamaguchi et al., 1995). TABs are TAK1 binding proteins (Shibuya et al., 1996; Takaesu et al., 2000). TAB1 acts as co-activator of TAK1 enhancing its kinase activity while TAB2 has an adaptor function linking TAK1 to TRAF6.

NF-κB

NF-κB (Nuclear factor kappa B) is a transcription factor that controls the expression of genes involved in inflammation, immunity and apoptosis. It was discovered as a transcription factor for the K chains in immunoglobulins. About 100 genes are under the transcriptional control of NF-κB. It belongs to rel family of proteins. NF-κB is an evolutionary conserved protein having five members in mammals- p50, p52, RelA/p65, RelB and RelC. All these function either as homodimer or heterodimer for e.g. p50 homodimer and p50/p65 heterodimer. Their ability to regulate and control transcription also differs markedly, for instance p65 and Rel-C are most potent transcriptional activators while p50 homodimers seem to repress transcription. NF-κB is composed of two subunits p50 and p65. It is bound to an inhibitory protein IκB via non-covalent interaction which hampers its activity. Studies indicate that p50 and p65 dimerise around a 10 base pair region referred to as κB sites. Sequence of this site is 5'GGGRNNYYCC3' where R, Y and N refer to purine, pyrimidine and any base respectively.

7.1 MyD88 dependent signalling pathway

MyD88 is an adaptor protein that is recruited to the TIR domain of TLR upon its activation via C terminal TIR domain. MyD88 also has a death domain at its N terminal end spaced with a short linker sequence from its C terminal. MyD88 then recruits IRAK4 (IL-1R associated protein kinase 4) at its death domain via its N terminal. IRAK4 has N terminal death domain and a central serine/threonine kinase domain that is essentially required for its kinase activity and downstream signalling. This recruitment of IRAK4 to MyD88 induces conformational changes in IRAK4 that allows the interaction of IRAK1 with it and then IRAK4 acts on IRAK1 to phosphorylate it. Also upon activation, IRAK1 starts auto-phosphorylating itself (Takeda & Akira, 2005). To this assembly, TRAF6 (TNF receptor associated factor 6) further associates via phosphorylated IRAK1. TRAF6 acts as a signalling mediator for both IL-1R/TLR superfamily and TNF receptor superfamily. Association of TRAF6 with phosphorylated IRAK1 leads to the dissociation of both these mediators from the assembly and binding to TAK1 (Transforming growth factor β activated kinase), TAB1(TAK1 binding protein 1) and TAB2 (TAK1 binding protein 2). TAK1 belongs to MAPKKK (Mitogen activated protein kinase kinase kinase) family. TAB1 acts as an activator of TAK1 while TAB2 functions as an adaptor molecule linking TAK1 to TRAF6. Recently, another TAK1 binding protein, TAB3 came into being and might function similar to TAB2. This causes phosphorylation of TAB2 & TAK1 and degradation of IRAK1. This remaining complex i.e. TAK1, TAB1, TAB2 and TRAF6 now gets associated with ubiquitin ligase UBC13 (Ubiquitin conjugating enzyme 13) and UEV 1A (Ubiquitin conjugating enzyme E2 variant 1). This leads to activation of TRAF6 which in turn activates TAK1. TAK1 activation takes place through linkage of a lysine63 linked polyubiquitin chain via TRAF6-UBC13 complex where TRAF6 acts as an E3 Ubiquitin ligase (Wang et al., 2001). Activated TAK1 is responsible for the phosphorylation of MAPK and IKK complex (Inhibitor of NF-κB (IκB) kinase complex). IKK has three subunits, IKK1 or IKKα, IKK2 or IKKβ and IKKϒ or NEMO (NF-κB essential modulator) (Karin & Ben-Neriah, 2000). This kinase complex phosphorylates IκB at conserved serine residues in N terminal which mark it for ubiquitination and its subsequent degradation via proteasome. Removal of inhibitor from NF-κB leads to its activation and translocation from cytosol to nucleus where it binds to NF-κB binding regions (present in the genes under the control of NF-κB transcriptional activation) and induce the transcription of genes responsible for synthesis of effector molecules that act against the invading pathogen or PAMPs and lead to their destruction.

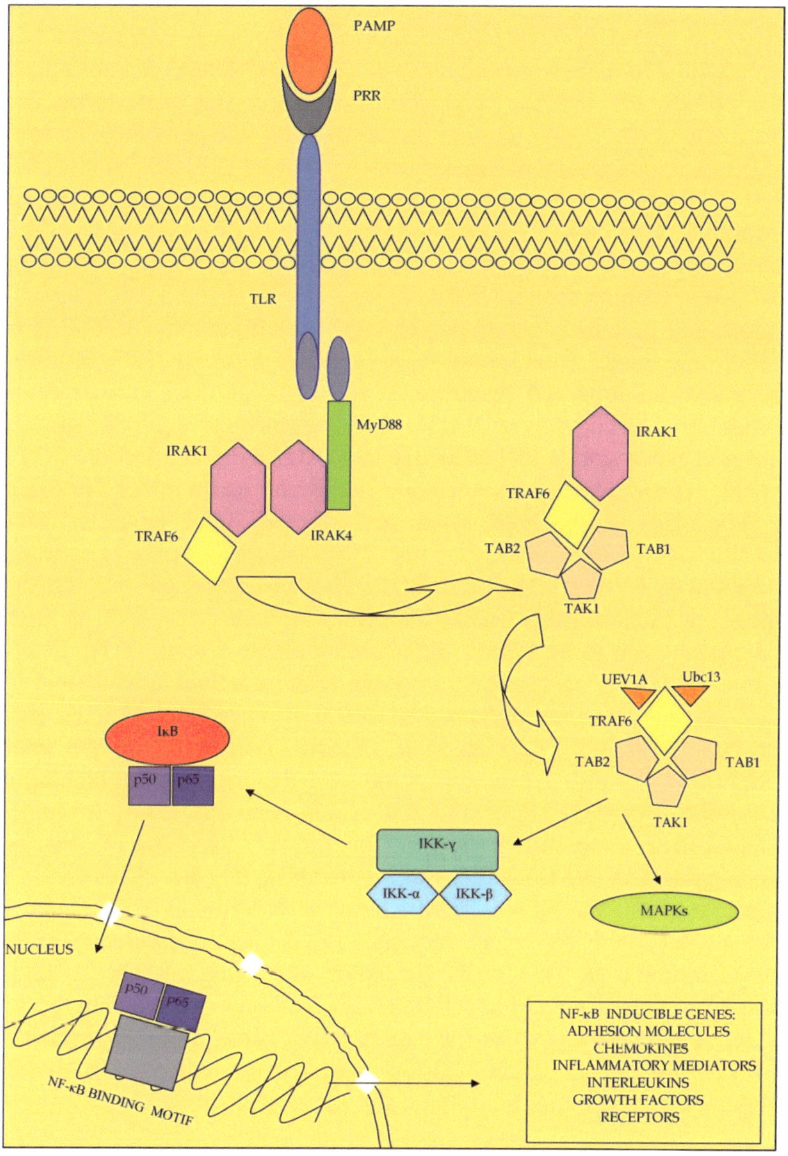

Fig. 3. Upon stimulation of TLR with suitable PAMP, MyD88 is recruited to TIR domain of TLR. IRAK4 then associates with MyD88. This causes IRAK1 to attach with IRAK4 which causes its phosphorylation. TRAF6 then joins this complex and thereafter causes IRAK1 to dissociate from IRAK4 along with it. Later TRAF6 and IRAK1 bind to TAK1, TAB1 and TAB2. Later IRAK1 is degraded and remaining complex joins Ubc13 and Uev1A which causes polyubiquitination of TRAF6 and activates TAK1 in a proteasome independent manner. Activated TAK1 phosphorylates both MAPK and IKK complex. IKK complex phosphorylates IκB that leads to its ubiquitination and then degradation in proteasome. Release of IκB from NF-κB activates it which then translocates into the nucleus and causes the expression of genes which are under its transcriptional control including genes involved in apoptosis, inflammation and immunity.

7.2 MyD88 independent signalling pathway

Studies have revealed that upon stimulation with LPS in MyD88 deficient cells, there is still production of NF-κB, although the production is delayed. This leads to the fact that TLR signalling can also occur in the absence of MyD88 i.e. independently of MyD88. TLR3 utilizes MyD88 independent signalling pathway to activate IRF3 that is responsible for the up-regulation of interferon (IFN) inducible genes and the production of IFN-β. This MyD88 independent signalling pathway utilizes another adaptor molecule known as TRIF/TICAM1 (TIR domain containing adaptor protein inducing IFN-β/ TIR domain containing molecule 1). TRIF has TRAF6 binding motifs (T6BM) in its N terminal and a TIR domain and RHIM (Receptor interacting protein 1 homotypic interaction motif) domain at its C terminal. TRIF is the only molecule meant to be involved in signalling through TLR3. Studies with TRIF deficient mice showed impaired response in activation of IRF3 and expression of IFN inducible genes only with ligands of TLR3 and TLR4 (Hoebe et al.,2003). IRF3, 5 and 7 play important roles in expression of IFN inducible genes during viral infection. IRF3 is typically required for the expression of genes encoding IFN-β and genes under the control of other interferons (Yoneyema et al., 1998). Upon activation of TLR3 with its ligand, TRIF is recruited to the TIR domain of TLR3. Then TRIF associates at its N terminus via two molecules- TRAF6 and TBK1 (TRAF family member associated NF- κB activator (TANK) binding kinase 1). TBK1 is responsible for phosphorylating the IRF3 at its C terminal regulatory domain which leads to their dimerization (Sharma et al., 2003). Dimers are then able to translocate into the nucleus and associate with co-activators p300 and CBP(cAMP responsive element binding protein).This then causes the expression of genes encoding IFN-β and other TypeI interferons (Taniguchi & Takaoka, 2002). These TypeI interferons via JAK-STAT signalling pathway are capable of inducing the expression of IFN inducible genes like GARG16 (Glucocorticoid attenuated responsive gene 16), IPG1(Immunoresponsive gene1) and CXCL10 etc. Also, IRF7 is produced later in viral infections via interferons whose expression is regulated by IRF3. TRAF6, another molecule that associates with TRIF at its N terminal is meant to activate NF-κB. TRAF6 binds to N terminal of TRIF via its TRAF-C. TRIF has three T6BM with consensus sequence Pro-X-Glu-X-X-(aromatic/acidic residue). Also, to the C terminal of TRIF, RIP1 (Receptor interacting protein 1) binds which is discovered recently and also found to activate NF- κB (Meylan et al., 2004). Activated NF-κB then is able to translocate and causes the expression of genes under its control. It has been found that transcriptional activation of IFN-β encoding gene needs both NF-κB and IRF3. However, inflammatory cytokine production still remains impaired.

Search for adaptors containing TIR domain led to the discovery of a new adaptor molecule known as TRAM/TICAM2 (TRIF related adaptor molecule/TIR domain containing molecule2) (Bin et al., 2003). Studies with TRAM deficient mice revealed that TRAM is involved in signalling through TLR4 in a MyD88 independent/TRIF dependent manner (Yamamoto et al., 2003). TRAM has a TIR domain in the C terminal and it acts upstream of TRIF while mediating TLR4 signalling exclusively. Studies showed that siRNA mediated inhibition of TRAM expression causes impairment of IRF3 activation and expression of IFN inducible genes only in response to TLR4 ligand, eg. LPS. However, TRAM knockout mice shows normal activation of IRF3 and expression of IFN inducible genes in response to TLR3 activation. Hence, TRAM is only involved in signalling through TLR4 but not TLR3. MyD88 deficient macrophages when stimulated with LPS show activation of IRF3 and also production of NF-κB, although production is delayed. Also, the production of inflammatory cytokines is impaired in these cells. Studies with TRIF and TRAM deficient mice showed that for the production of inflammatory cytokines via TLR4, activation of both the signalling pathways is required i.e. MyD88 dependent and independent, although the mechanism is not clear. However, the production is not affected via MyD88 dependent pathway in response to ligands of TLR2, 7 and 9. Another adaptor that is involved in signalling via TLR4 is TIRAP/MAL (TIR domain containing adaptor protein/MyD88 adaptor like protein) (Horngs et al., 2001). TIRAP deficient mice show impaired production of inflammatory cytokines in response to TLR2 and 4 ligands but not to TLR3, 5, 7 and 9 ligands. This confirms its role in signalling through TLR2 and 4. TIRAP deficient mice also show IRF3 activation and production of late phase NF-κB as seen in the studies with MyD88 deficient mice. TIRAP has a C terminal TIR domain but it lacks a death domain that is present in MyD88. It acts upstream of MyD88.

LPS signalling through TLR4 is mediated with the help of several other proteins eg. MD-2 is a novel protein that mediates the TLR4 signalling in response to LPS. MD2 functions to bind LPS and then presents this LPS to TLR4 via physically interacting with it. MD2 is found to attach with TLR4 extracellular domain. Also, another protein CD14 is found to facilitate LPS signalling via TLR4. CD14 along with LBP (LPS binding protein) binds to LPS (Wright et al., 1990) and can initiate signalling via transmembrane receptors like TLR4.

7.2.1 Genes under transcriptional control of NF-κB

NF-κB is crucial for the expression of genes which are involved in immune responses (both innate and adaptive), inflammation, viral infection, stress, cytokine signalling, acute phase responses etc. Genes under the regulation of NF-κB have NF-κB binding sites in their promoter region. Adhesion molecules like ICAM-1, VCAM-1, E-selectins are expressed as a result of NF-κB transcriptional activation. ICAM-1/CD54 (Intercellular adhesion molecule -1) is expressed on endothelial and immune system cells. ICAM-1 expression upon required stimulus is enhanced via NF-κB activity. ICAM-1 binds to LFA1 (Lymphocyte function-associated antigen1), a receptor on leukocytes. Leukocytes adhere and then migrate into the tissues via ICAM-1 and LFA-1 interaction and carry out the required actions. VCAM-1(Vascular cell adhesion protein-1) is present in the endothelial cells and function to adhere lymphocytes, basophils, monocytes etc. to vascular endothelium. E-selectin/CD62E/ELAM-1(Endothelial leukocyte adhesion molecule-1) is expressed on vascular endothelium in response to TNF-α and IL-1β. It binds to carbohydrate moieties on some leukocytes. Genes expressing growth factors are also up-regulated by NF-κB like genes for GM-CSF (Granulocyte macrophage colony stimulating factor), M-CSF/CSF1 (Macrophage colony stimulating factor/ Colony stimulating factor3) and G-CSF(Granulocyte colony stimulating factor/ Colony stimulating factor 3). GM-CSF is a cytokine that stimulates stem cells to differentiate into neutrophils, eosinophils, basophils, granulocytes and monocytes. M-CSF is also a cytokine that stimulates stem cells to differentiate into macrophages and related cell types. G-CSF acts on bone marrow to form more of granulocytes and stem cells. Various chemokine genes also show enhanced expression in response to NF-κB like genes for Eotaxin, RANTES (Regulated upon activation, normal T cell expressed and secreted), MIP 1α (Macrophage inflammatory protein 1 α) etc. Eotaxin is a chemokine that recruits eosinophils while RANTES is a chemoattractor for T cells, K cells, eosinophils, dendritic cells and is also responsible for recruiting leukocytes at inflammatory sites. Several cell surface receptor genes are up-regulated eg. CCR5 (C-C chemokine receptor

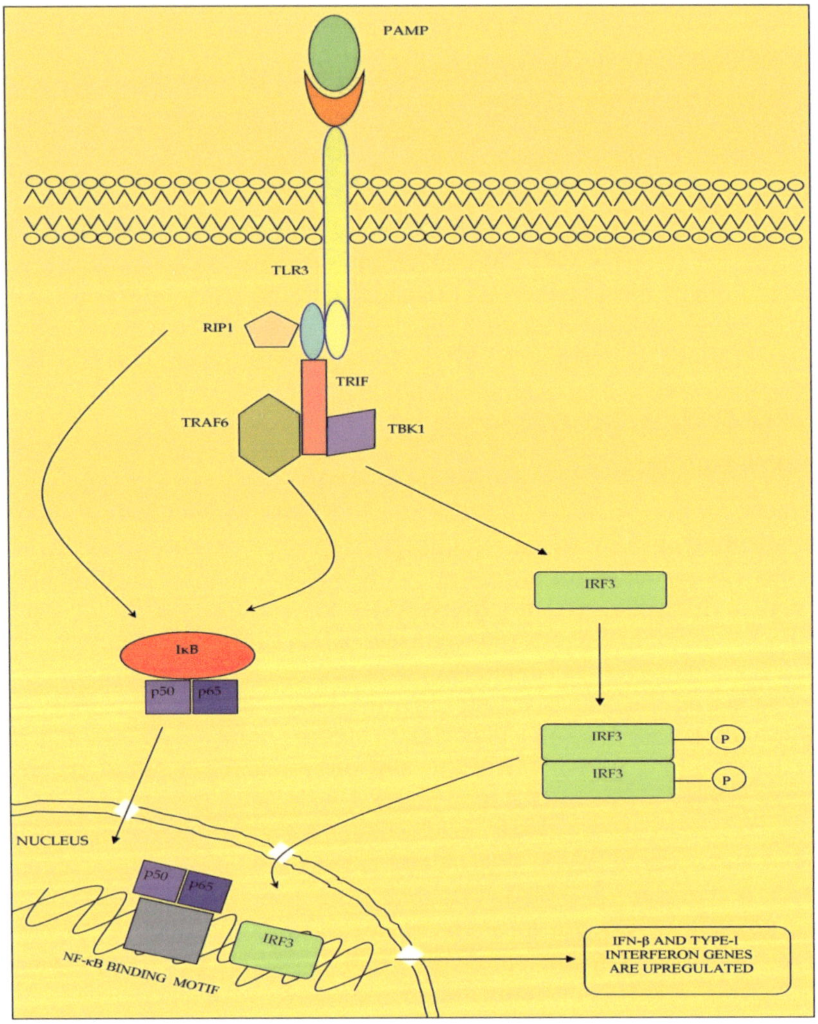

Fig. 4. TLR3 recruits TRIF upon stimulation with its ligand. To N terminal of TRIF, TBK1 associates which carries out later phosphorylation of IRF3. Upon phosphorylation, IRF3 forms dimer and translocates into nucleus and causes the expression of genes of IFN-β and Type I interferons. Also, to the N terminal of TRIF, TRAF6 binds which activates NF-κB which is then able to translocate and causes the transcription of genes under its control. Genes encoding IFN-β require activation of both NF-κB and IRF3.

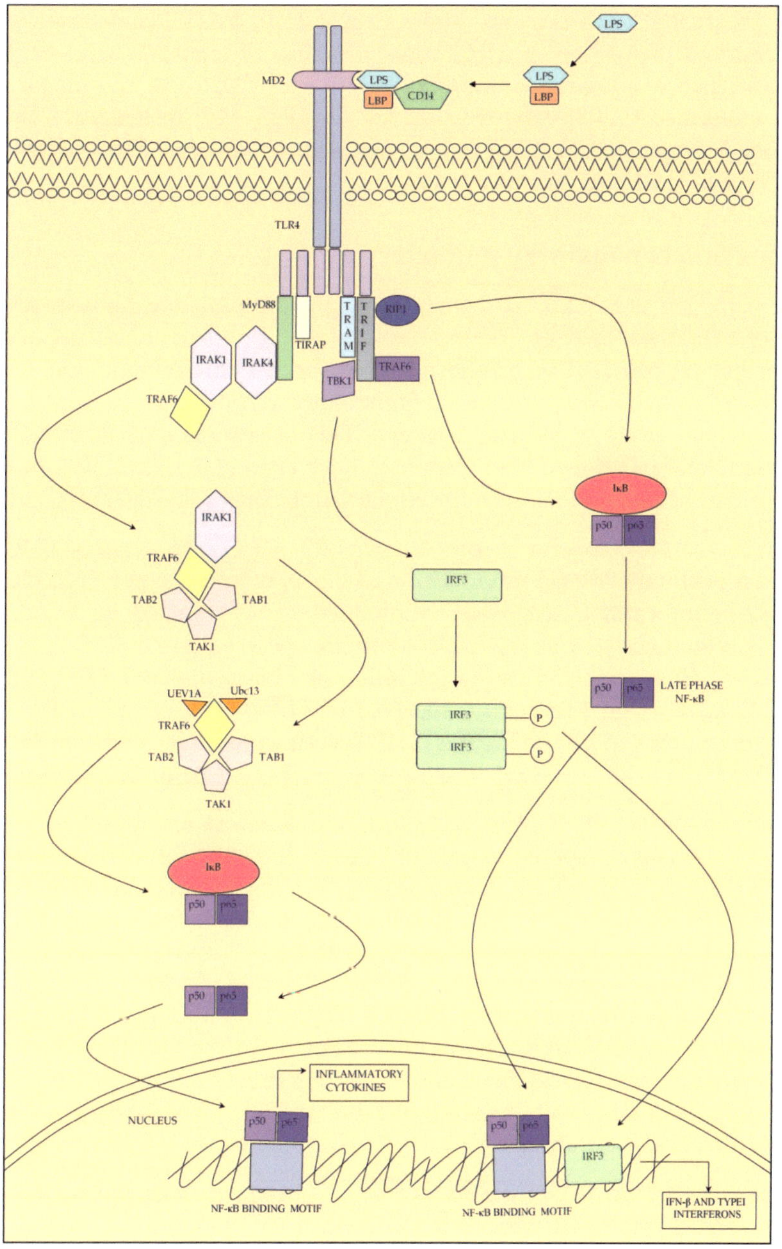

Fig. 5. Response to LPS is mediated through TLR4; LPS binds to LBP, and then forms a complex with CD14. This complex interacts with MD-2 which is able to interact physically with TLR4. Signalling downstream afterwards proceeds either via MyD88 dependant or MyD88 independent pathway. In MyD88 dependant pathway, NFκB is activated which induces transcription of several genes including genes of inflammatory cytokines. On the other hand, in TIRAP and MyD88 knockout mice, activation of IRF3 and late phase NFκB takes place both of which are able to initiate transcription of the genes under their respective control.

type 5), CD86, TCR(T cell receptor), MHC class I & II, PAF(Platelet activating factor) receptor. Enhanced expression of MHC molecules and TCR means to up-regulate T cell activation and hence adaptive immunity. CD80 and CD86 are the major T cell co-stimulatory molecules. CCR5 is the receptor for RANTES, MIP 1α and 1β. Cytokine IL-1β, IL-2, IL-6 and TNFα show enhanced expression after NF-κB activation. NF-κB dependent stimulation of iNOS promoters also takes place.

8. TLR signalling is negatively regulated

Docking of pathogen onto TLRs and their subsequent stimulation induces production of inflammatory cytokines such as TNF-a, IL-6 and IL-12. An uncontrolled and excessive cytokine production can lead to manifestation of serious autoimmune and inflammatory diseases. Hence, to avoid an excessive inflammatory response, organisms have evolved mechanisms which make a balance between TLR activation and inactivation. Several molecules modulating TLR-mediated responses have been unravelled. Negative regulators of TLRs can either be extracellular or intracellular (Arancibia et al., 2007).

Extracellular regulators comprise of soluble form of TLRs. Soluble form of TLR2, sTLR2, is produced by a post-translational modification of the membrane bound TLR2. It is reported that if sTLR2 splice variant expression is inhibited, an augmented response to bacterial lipopeptide is seen (Lebouder et al., 2003). Alternate splice variant of TLR4 (soluble TLR4), sTLR4, is shown to be involved in the inhibition of LPS-mediated TNFα production and NFκB activation, blocking MD-2 (a co-receptor of TLR4) recruitment to the TLR4-CD14 complex. Also, soluble product of TLR5, sTLR5, is seen to be implicated in cellular response of flagellin that induces an increased NF-κB activation by an unknown cellular mechanism.

A variety of intracellular molecules (adaptors and kinases) are found to regulate TLR signalling. An alternatively spliced variant of MyD88 that lacks the intermediary domain of MyD88 (MyD88s) is induced in monocytes upon LPS stimulation. Overexpression of MyD88s results in impaired LPS-induced NF-κB activation through inhibition of IRAK-4-mediated IRAK-1 phosphorylation. IRAK-M is another negative regulator of TLR signalling cascade and it lacks catalytic kinase activity. IRAK-M inhibits expression of pro-inflammatory cytokines by preventing IRAK-1/IRAK-4 dissociation from MyD88, hence causing inhibition of IRAK-1-TRAF6 complex formation. The fact that IRAK-M plays a crucial role in regulating MyD-88 dependant signalling pathway can be established from the information that IRAK-M-/- mice overproduce inflammatory cytokines in response to LPS and CpG DNA (Arancibia et al., 2007).

A protein associated with Toll-Like Receptor 4 (PRAT4A) regulates cell surface expression of TLR4. PRAT4A is associated with the immature form of TLR4 but not with MD-2 (a TLR4 co-receptor) or TLR2. PRAT4A knockdown led to the profound defect in LPS responsiveness in a cell line expressing TLR4/MD-2, probably due to impaired maturation of TLR4, leading to the lack of mature TLR4/MD-2 on the cell surface. PRAT4A is likely to be a component of the machinery facilitating TLR4/MD-2 trafficking to the cell surface. Hence, PRAT4A is another negative regulator of TLR4.

SOCS1 and SOCS3 belong to SOCS (Suppressor of cytokine signaling) family of proteins. These proteins themselves induced by cytokines, negatively regulate TLR4/NFκB signalling pathways (Gingras et al. 2004). In SOCS 1-/- mice defective induction of LPS tolerance was observed as they were found to be hypersensitive to LPS-endotoxin. In the same manner, LPS induced TNF-α production was found to be suppressed in macrophages exposed to IL-10 and IL-6 isolated from SOCS3-/-(Arancibia et al., 2007).

PI3K, implicated in TLR signalling, has been found to suppress both MAPKs and NFκB induced by LPS, thereby decreasing TNF-α production (Arancibia et al., 2007). Tollip (Toll interacting protein) has also been found to play an inhibitory role in TLR signalling. Tollip when in association with TIR domain decreases IRAK-1 phosphorylation upon LPS activation. A plausible role of PI3K in regulating inhibitory effects of Tollip has been proposed. PI3K does that by interacting with 3′ phosphorylated phosphatidylinositides (Arancibia et al., 2007).

SIGIRR (single immunoglobulin IL-1 receptor-related molecule) and T1/ST2, membrane bound proteins adhered to the TIR domain, have also been found to be negative regulators of TLR signalling (Takeda & Akira, 2005). Nucleotide oligomerization domain receptor (NOD2), a mammalian PRR, too seems to be a negative regulator as NOD2-/- macrophages when stimulated by TLR agonists produce significantly higher amount of cytokines but on restoration of NOD phenotype, cytokine expression is lowered (Arancibia et al., 2007).

Activating Transcription Factor-3 (ATF-3) has also been found to negatively regulate TLR-signalling pathways (Whitmore et al., 2007). It has been observed that different TLR ligands (i.e., zymosan for TLR2/3, pIC for TLR3, LPS for TLR4, and CpG-ODN for TLR9) stimulate rapid induction of ATF3 in cultured mouse macrophages. It is reported that primary macrophages of mice lacking *atf3* gene (ATF3-knockout (KO)) show enhanced expression of TLR-induced IL-12 and IL-6 when compared to wild type macrophages. In a reporter assay, ectopic expression of ATF3 was found to antagonize TLR-stimulated IL-12p40 activation. Further, CpG oligodeoxynucleotide, a TLR9 agonist when introduced in ATF3-KO mice resulted in enhanced cytokine production from splenocytes. Hence, it can be concluded that *atf3* deficiency leads to altered pattern of immunological response and ATF-3 is a negative regulator of TLR pathways.

In addition to these, degradation of TLRs (either ubiquitination mediated or lysosomal) is also proposed as a mechanism for negatively regulating TLR signaling (Takeda & Akira, 2005; Wang et. al., 2007). A RING finger protein, Triad3A, has been found to act as an E3 ubiquitin ligase, ligating ubiquitin molecules onto the TLR4 and TLR9 and enhancing their proteolytic degradation. A recent study by Wang et. al. (Wang et. al., 2007) reveals another mechanism of negative regulation of TLR4 signalling, by lysosomal degradation of TLRs. They propose that Rab7b, a lysosome associated small GTPase negatively regulates NF-κB and IRF3 signalling pathways in macrophages by promoting lysosomal degradation of TLR4 and decreasing the cell surface expression of TLR4. These complex mechanisms of negative regulation of TLRs emphasize that it is important for prevention of uncontrolled immune activation in the host.

9. TLRs in various diseases

9.1 TLRs in nervous system diseases

TLRs have been considered earlier as receptors expressed solely on antigen presenting cells of the immune system i.e. B cells, dendritic cells, monocytes, macrophages etc. and mediate innate immunity. However, with advancement in techniques, it is clear that nearly all cells within the body express TLRs, including different brain cell types such as microglial cells, astrocytes, oligodendrocytes and neurons within the CNS (Central Nervous System). The present section will focus the role of TLRs in these brain cells.

Microglia

Microglial cells are bone marrow-derived macrophage-like cells constituting about 10% of the adult CNS and mediate neuronal immune interactions under both physiological and pathological conditions (Pessac et al., 2001). Microglial cells are the key defence against invading pathogens within the CNS, and it is not surprising, therefore, that activation of these cells either by a single type of ligand or a combination of ligands, leads to secretion of a milieu of cytokines and chemokines. It is now well known that microglial cells express wide receptors of TLRs in addition to their adapter proteins, required for functional downstream TLR signalling. Recent studies showed that TLR1-9 are expressed in microglia (Jack et al., 2005). Upon activation, TLR mRNA and protein expression is increased in microglia. As a result of TLR activation, these cells secrete higher amounts of pro-inflammatory cytokines and hence show pathogen specific responses. TLR signalling in microglia may also have a role in cell death and survival following inflammatory activation which suggests a paradigm in which auto-regulation of the innate immune system exists in the CNS which helps to prevent excessive inflammation during pathogen infection (Jack et al., 2007; Tanaka et al., 2008; Okun et al., 2009).

Astrocytes

Astrocytes are characteristic star-shaped glial cells in the brain and spinal cord and perform many functions, including biochemical support to endothelial cells that form the blood–brain barrier provision of nutrients to the nervous tissue, maintenance of extracellular ion balance, and a role in the repair and scarring process of the brain and spinal cord following traumatic injuries. Similar to microglial cells, astrocytes exhibit a wide expression of TLRs. Astrocytes express robust TLR 3 with low expression of TLR 1, TLR4, TLR5 and TLR9, and with rare expression of TLR2, TLR6, TLR7, TLR8 and TLR10. Several cytokines and chemokines are reportedly produced following TLR activation in astrocytes. TLR 3 signalling induces strongest pro-inflammation polarizing response by secreting increased levels of IL-12, TNF-alpha, IL-6, CXCL-10, IFN-beta and IL-10 (Jack et al., 2005). Both cytokines and TLR agonists induce expression of chemokine ligands i.e. CCL2, CCL3, CCL5, ICAM-1 and vascular cell adhesion molecule-1 (VCAM-1) (Carpentier et al., 2005 ; Okun et al., 2009).

Oligodendrocytes

Oligodendrocytes are a type of neuroglia and function as an insulation of axons in the CNS. As compared to other CNS cell types, very little is known regarding the expression and function of TLRs in oligodendrocytes. The first report on TLRs in these cells has shown the predominant expression of TLR2 and 3 as evidenced by promotion of survival, differentiation, and myelin-like membrane formation and induction of apoptosis by TLR2 agonist, zymosan and TLR3 agonist, poly-I:C respectively (Bsibsi et al., 2002). While the exact role of TLR2 in oligodendrocytes is unknown, *in vivo* evidences suggest that activation of this receptor is involved in CNS repair by enhancing myelination of neurons in the CNS and damage repair after spinal cord injury (Okun et al., 2009).

Neurons

Neurons are the core components of the CNS which processes and transmits information by electrical and chemical signalling. During the past few years, evidence for the neuronal expression of TLRs has increased, suggesting a role for this receptor family in neurons during physiological as well as pathological conditions. The expression of the mRNA for TLRs1-9 as well as protein levels of TLR 2, 3 and 4 has been shown *in vivo* following infection in a parasitic model of neurocysticercosis (Tang et al., 2007). Studies provide evidence that neurons from both the central and peripheral nervous systems express TLR3 and that it is concentrated at the growth cones of neurons. In addition to TLR expression in brain diseases, it is known that neuronal TLR activation plays a role in development. It has been reported recently that treatment of cultured embryonic cortical neurospheres with a TLR3 ligand significantly reduced proliferating (BrdU-labeled) cells and neurosphere formation, whereas neural progenitor cells (NPC) from TLR3-deficient embryos formed greater numbers of neurospheres compared to neurospheres from wild-type embryos (Okun et al., 2009). A distinct difference is apparent between the effects of TLR activation in differentiated neurons and neuronal progenitor cells. Apart from the classical TLR ligands such as LPS (TLR4) or Pam3CSK4 (TLR2), it is considered that neuronal TLRs respond to endogenous ligands but not to pathogen-derived ligands (Okun et al., 2009).

9.1.1 TLRs in neurodegeneration

TLRs generally respond against invading pathogens, however, they can also be activated in the absence of microbial infection and regulate neurogenesis. Studies examining inflammatory markers in normal brain aging have also suggested a dynamic regulation of TLRs and hence, showed its participation in aging and age-related disease. Despite the emerging role of TLRs in stokes, AD (Alzheimer's disease) and MS (Multiple sclerosis), very little is known regarding the function of these receptors in other neurodegenerative disorders. In this context, the role of TLRs in brain diseases such as, Alzheimer's disease, multiple sclerosis and other neurodegenerative conditions is discussed herewith.

9.1.2 TLRs in Alzheimer's disease

Alzheimer's disease (AD) is a progressive neurodegenerative disease characterized by gradual onset and advancement of memory loss and other cognitive deficits. Definitive diagnosis of AD is based on the presence of extracellular amyloid plaques comprised of neurotoxic amyloid β-peptide (Aβ) which is generated by proteolysis of the β-amyloid precursor protein (APP), and intracellular neurofibrillary tangles composed of hyper-phosphorylated insoluble forms of *tau* protein. TLR expression is up-regulated and increased in the AD brain. A screening of TLRs in murine models of AD revealed an up-regulation of TLR2 and TLR7 transcription levels compared to wild-type controls. Further, multiple TLR genes (1-8) are expressed in microglia in post-mortem tissue from AD patients, with varying levels of expression. The increased expression of TLRs in AD positions them as potential players in neurodegenerative mechanisms and disease progression. The TLR4 gene has emerged as a candidate susceptibility gene for AD. A common missense polymorphism occurs at the TLR4 gene locus resulting from an adenine to guanine substitution 896 nucleotides downstream of the transcription start site. This substitution causes the replacement of glycine for aspartic acid at amino acid 299 (Asp299Gly), and alters the structure of the extracellular domain of TLR4. This mutation attenuates TLR4 signalling in response to LPS and diminishes the ability to induce inflammation (Arbour et al, 2000). In AD brain, activated glia expressing high levels of TLR4 and TLR2 surround Aβ plaques. The close association between Aβ plaques and reactive astrocytes and microglia has led to the assertion that these cells contribute to plaque formation (Walter et al., 2007). TLR4 expression increases during exposure to Aβ and the lipid peroxidation product 4-hydroxy-nonenal (HNE). Further, c-Jun N-terminal kinases (JNK) and caspase-3 activity levels are augmented in neurons exposed to Aβ and HNE. Selective elimination of TLR4 function significantly suppresses the abilities of Aβ and HNE to induce activation of JNK and caspase-3 (Tang et al., 2007) suggesting that TLR4 expression increases neuronal vulnerability to Aβ-induced damage (Okun et al., 2009). Neurons expressing TLR4 have increased sensitivity to Aβ and are vulnerable to degeneration in AD. In addition to epidemiological studies that suggest mutations in TLR4 lead to decreased susceptibility to neurodegeneration, several data indicate that activation of TLR4 is required for clearance of Aβ in AD. In addition to TLR4, activation of other TLRs may also contribute to Aβ clearance. Whereas TLRs are activated by exogenous pathogens, mounting evidence indicates that Aβ itself activates TLRs and mediates microglial activation. At present, it still remains to be determined if the activation of TLRs by Aβ contributes to and/or inhibits AD progression. Contrasting data exist on the precise role of TLRs in Aβ deposition. Therefore, there may be a balance of TLR activation in which mild activation is beneficial, promoting Aβ uptake and breakdown. However, excessive activation of TLRs on microglia may lead to the accumulation of cytotoxic compounds such as reactive oxygen species, cytokines, complements and proteases causing damage and eventual neuronal loss. TLR signalling pathways are a potential therapeutic target in AD; however more work remains to delineate the complex interaction of TLRs in Aβ deposition and clearance and its precise role in AD development (Okun et al., 2009; Akiyama et al., 2000).

9.1.3 TLRs in Multiple Sclerosis

Multiple Sclerosis (MS) is a chronic inflammatory and demyelinating disease of the CNS and characterized by recurrent neurological dysfunction. It is believed to be an immune-mediated disease in which auto-reactive T cells enter the CNS and drive a pro-inflammatory reaction resulting in tissue injury after infection. There is a marked increase in TLR expression in multiple sclerosis lesions. Microglial cells from MS patients express TLRs 1-8, while, healthy white matter from patients does not contain TLRs. Examination of TLR3 and TLR4 localization revealed that early active MS lesions are associated with vesicular localization of TLR3 and TLR4 within microglia, located near blood vessels at the outer edges of lesions. In contrast, late active lesions also contain astrocytes bearing surface TLR3 and TLR4. This suggests that early lesions are characterized by microglia infiltration, while astrocytes are also active in later MS lesions. Researchers showed that TLR expression is up-regulated in the brain and spinal cord in animal models of MS. The exact role and mechanism of TLRs and its activation in these lesions is still unclear. One hypothesis asserts that in response to pro-inflammatory cytokines, microglial cells are capable of serving as antigen-presenting cells which can activate CD4+ T cells and facilitate neuroinflammation. Therefore, TLR activation may be an essential step in converting microglia to antigen presenting cells and facilitate T cell infiltration of MS lesions. Alternatively, TLRs may induce production of pro-inflammatory cytokines and thereby inflict damage. It can also happen that endogenous ligands like ganglioside and sialic acid containing glycosphingolipids released from apoptotic neurons may bind to TLR4 present on microglia and activate it resulting in either neurodegeneration by releasing pro-inflammatory molecules or provide neuroprotection by attracting oligodendrocyte progenitor cells to lesion sites in MS to promote remyelination. Although TLRs often recognize pathogen-associated molecular patterns and protect the body from invasion of microbial pathogens, the expression of TLRs within multiple sclerosis suggests novel roles for these receptors in mediating neurological disease and hence can be used as a biomarker of the neurodegenerative disorders (Okun et al., 2009). Moreover, it is important to determine the precise role of distinct TLRs in Aβ recognition and clearance, and the activation of glial cells. This may open a window of hope (Arroyo et al, 2011).

9.1.4 Therapeutic approaches

TLRs are not only activated in response to microbial infection, but are critically involved in mediating neurological dysfunction. The extensive involvement of TLRs in neurodegenerative disorders provides wide opportunity for promoting and inhibiting their signalling to intervene the progression of the disease. However, it may be difficult to achieve the correct balance and appropriate timing of such interventions. There is huge variation in the TLR expression and hence the modifications will be varied across different disorders and there may exist variability within patients of the same disease. Proper TLR targeting will require extensive understanding of the pathways, mechanism activated, cell-specific responses and the course of disease progression. Both human and animal studies implicating TLRs in neural degeneration suggest direct modulation of TLR signalling as an ideal therapy. Specific strategies are necessary to circumvent this barrier and allow administration of TLR treatments to the CNS. Targeting TLRs in neurological disease will not be without difficulties. One potential obstacle to targeting TLR signalling in disease is that virtually all cells in the body express TLRs. If chronic administration of TLR agonists is necessary, it may result in overstimulation of the immune system, which limits dosage capability as well as frequency of application. CNS- specific isoforms of TLR agonists which possess high selectivity could prevent such overstimulation of peripheral immune responses. In addition, partial agonists may be useful in preventing overstimulation of TLRs in the same tissues. Another potential hurdle to TLR- directed therapeutics is cross-talk between receptor subtypes. Alternatively, specific TLR activation can induce tolerance to stimulation for other TLRs sharing same cascade. Therefore, the consequences of targeted TLR stimulation on similar signalling pathways must be carefully considered while adapting the therapeutic approaches (Okun et al., 2009).

9.2 TLRs in cancer and anti-cancer immunotherapy

Tumour cells in order to survive try to modulate their microenvironment by providing signals for uncontrolled growth, anti-apoptosis, angiogenesis and metastasis. Despite all these efforts tumour cells get noticed by the immune system which treat cancer cells as foreign. The studies have shown that tumour cells have devised sets of strategies to escape the surveillance by immune system. TLRs were earlier thought associated only with immune cells but recent findings have suggested that tumour cells too have TLRs on their surface and may play important role in tumour growth and immune surveillance escape.

The tumour cells are able to escape the immune surveillance probably by inhibitory cytokines, inflammatory factors, proteinases, and other small molecules such as nitric oxide, IL-6 and IL-12. These molecules in conjugation with TLRs may play role in development of cancer by providing resistance to tumour cells to apoptosis and immune surveillance. It has been seen that upon activation of TLR4, level of X-linked inhibitor of apoptosis and phosphorylated Akt (Protein Kinase B, PKB) are increased. Apoptosis inhibition has been seen as the case also in lymphoma and lung cancer cells. Previous studies have given evidence in support of LPS as tumour growth promoter through the NF-κB resulting in up-regulation of iNOS and MMP2 and the β1 integrin subunit (Harmey et al, 2002; Wang et al, 2003). Apart from microbial origin ligands for TLRs, the source of endogenous ligands which may promote tumour growth is not clear. The answer to the endogenous source of ligands may not only provide some insight to tumour growth but may also help to understand autoimmune diseases. It has been proposed that the TLR-4-MyD88 signalling pathway may be a risk factor for developing cancer and may represent a novel target for the development of bio-modulators. Heat shock proteins such as Hsp60, Hsp70 and Hsp90 may induce the production of pro-inflammatory cytokines such as TNF-α, IL-1, IL-6 and IL-12, release of NO and chemokines by monocytes, macrophages and dendritic cells (Neill., 2008; Asea et al., 2000; Kol et al., 2000; Singh-Jasuja et al., 2000) . There are strong possibilities of Hsp60, Hsp70 and Hsp90 being putative endogenous ligands for TLR4. Ulcerative colitis, a chronic inflammatory disease of the colon may put an individual at risk of colorectal carcinoma. Chronic hepatitis and cirrhosis, pose a risk for the development of hepatocellular carcinoma. Research in the past few years have given strong evidence that an inflammatory profile of cytokines and chemokines persisting at a particular site would lead to the development of a chronic disease. The innate immune system may give in to the promotion of tumour growth through inflammation-dependent mechanisms. Recognition of molecules either of viral or bacterial origin bearing molecular signature or pattern by TLRs on immune cells may induce an inflammatory response associated with tumour promotion. It has been observed that bacterial infection post-surgery may promote metastasis of previously dormant tumour, and LPS have implicated in leading to this situation (Hsu et al, 2011). The MyD88-independent TLR signalling involves the activation of the late phase of NF-κB in addition to the activation of IFN regulatory factor 3, which ultimately leads to the production of type I IFN (IFN a/h), IFN-inducible gene products, and an immune regulatory response. Activated TLRs on the surface of tumour cells not only promote their own proliferation but also help to build resistance to apoptosis. Further, rouge TLRs may enhance tumour cell invasion and metastasis by regulating metalloproteinases and integrins. Moreover, the control of TLRs may also lie beyond the traditional boundaries of protein molecules into world of miRNA, and their role is still being uncovered. In fact, the discovery of miRNAs has indeed brought a paradigm shift in our understanding towards the eukaryotic gene regulation. Their uniqueness lies in the fact that these molecules show cell or tissue specific expression. In principle, the miRNAs fine tune the gene expression, and similar to the classical oncogenes and tumour suppressor genes, miRNA may play part in promotion or suppression of malignancies. They act mainly by inhibiting the translation or by promoting the degradation of mRNA. For example, miRNAs like miR-146, which targets two proteins involved in TLR signalling, TRAF6 and IRAK1, negatively regulates mRNAs of both TRAF6 and IRAK1 proteins whereas its own level gets up-regulated in response to LPS. Another miRNA, miR-155 targets Src domain containing inositol 5-phophate 1(SHIP-1) and negatively regulates NF-κB signalling. Owing to their role of fine tuner of gene expression pattern, the administration of single miRNA may affect the expression pattern of the target gene. Despite some apprehensions over the safety and efficacy of miRNA based therapies, a judicial extrapolation to TLR regulated miRNAs may provide some therapeutic solution. Also the role of innate immune system in cancer development is being looked into more seriously.

TLRs, tumour cells and Treg cells have been linked. TLR agonists can induce differentiation, proliferation or activation of Treg cells. Several TLR agonists such as Streptococcal agent OK-432, double stranded RNA and CpG DNA have anti-tumour activity (Chen & Oppenheim, 2009). TLR agonists overcome tolerance to self-antigens or tumour-antigens by directly or indirectly relieving suppression of effector T cells by Treg cells. A TLR2 agonist has been reported to transiently suppress FoxP3 (a member of forkhead/winged helix family of transcription factors and a master regulator of Treg development) expression and render resistance to suppression by Treg cells of $CD4^{+}CD25^{+}$ effector T cells. Treg cells express TLR4, 5, 7 and 8 in mice. It has been reported that transfer of Treg cells enhanced tumour growth in mice but it was reversed upon stimulation of Treg cells with a TLR8 ligand. Administration of LPS also abrogates Treg activity reveals latent anti-tumour immunity ((Chen & Oppenheim, 2009). The biggest problem in using TLRs as anti-cancer targets lies in the fact that many cancer patients have very low immunity because of anti-cancer therapy side effect, thus it becomes very difficult to get innate immune response. The quest to arrive at a point where innate immune system's stimulatory compounds are used along with anticancer agents may bear some fruit. The TLR3 has been shown to be receptor for viral dsRNA, and also seems to be potentially promising in anti-cancer therapy. Reports have shown that cancer cells themselves express TLR3 *in vivo* and agonist ploy (I:C) is activating the signalling pathway leading to the anticancer effects (Elizabeth et al., 2010; O'Neill et al., 2011). Hence, this complex relationship of tumour cells and TLRs seems to be crucial to determine the balance between beneficial and pathological roles of TLRs.

9.3 TLRs in asthma and allergy

Lungs are continuously exposed to microbial pathogens because of their constant relationship with the surrounding environment. Therefore, innate immune response in lungs to eliminate the pathogen requires expression of TLRs which would be activated upon pathogen exposure and subsequently commencing in signalling cascade. This signalling culminates in the elevated expression of IL-1-β, TNF-α, IL-12, and IFN-γ. The nature and intensity of response is regulated by the display of polarized cytokine profiles, either Th1 or Th2. Th2 cytokines are reported to play a crucial role in initiation and perpetuation of allergy and asthma (Bauer et al., 2007). Exposure to low doses of LPS results in Th2 biased response leading to onset of allergic response. On the contrary, high doses of LPS show protective effect. This is confirmed by the studies revealing an inverse relationship between allergy and asthma and early childhood exposure to rural farm environment. Although the exact mechanistic pathway is yet to be explored, but it becomes quite evident that LPS-TLR4 complex can either protect or aggravate the severity of asthma, depending on the timing of the LPS exposure. This is supported by "hygiene hypothesis" that favours that development of asthma and allergies is executed by the reduction in microbial exposure in early childhood and decrease in naturally occurring infections. Asthma and allergies are found to be less prevalent among individuals brought up in rural farm areas in their childhood (Gehring et al., 2002). Such early exposure to farms and barns or early exposure to microbes and microbial components is attributed to the protection rendered in development of allergies in later life. This might be because of the induction of regulatory T cells that down-regulate the adaptive immune responses.

Apart from the role of TLR4 in allergies, recently it has been reported that TLR2 too modulates the development of allergic disease (Bauer et al., 2007). Studies conducted on children of farmers of Germany who have decreased risk of developing allergies were found to have augmented expression of TLR2 mRNA. The presence of asthma and allergies in the children of farmers was co-related with the genetic variation in TLR2. It was found that asthma and atopy were less prevalent in the children carrying T allele in TLR2/-16934 (Chen et al., 2007).

9.3.1 TLRs, regulatory T cells and allergy

A few studies recently have sparked widespread interest in the regulation of allergy as they claim that control of allergy is not only restricted to Th1/Th2 bias but other mechanisms as well are responsible for controlling inflammatory response and regulatory T cells (Treg cells) play a pivotal role in this regulation (Akbari et al., 2002). TLRs are expressed on Treg cells (Bauer et al., 2007). A study shows that in adults allergic to pollen, a significant reduction in the number of Treg cells and their capacity to restrain allergic response occurs when compared to healthy controls. Another finding supports that Treg cells can block allergic responses by demonstrating that activation of TLR4 expressed on the $CD4^+CD25^+$ subset of Treg cells in response to high doses of LPS may prevent activation of pathogenic T effector cells and airway inflammation and hyper-reactivity can be overcome by $CD4^+CD25^+$ Treg cell function in IL-10 dependant manner (Chen et al., 2007). Recently, a report elaborates a link between TLR2 and Treg cells as well because in TLR2 mice, $CD4^+CD25^+$ Treg cell subset was found to be significantly reduced when compared to wild type mice (Sutmuller et al., 2006).

9.3.2 Therapeutic potential of TLR ligands in allergy

The discovery that TLR signalling culminates in the activation of DCs leading to increased Th1 bias can also be applied in the treatment of allergic diseases. Particularly, TLR9 stimulation by un-methylated CpG-motif that promotes a Th1 response has been explored as potential treatment for atopic diseases like asthma and allergic rhinitis (Horner et al., 2001). In mice sensitized with allergen, CpG administration has been shown to inhibit the development of airway hyper-responsiveness and eosinophilia. It has also been demonstrated that CpG-DNA when conjugated to allergen offer a new anti-allergic strategy in which the complexes so formed show a more promising result by augmenting the immunotherapeutic effect when compared CpG-DNA given alone or CpG-DNA given mixed to allergen (Tighe et al., 2000; Horner et al., 2001). These studies encourage usage of selectively targeted allergen TLR-fusion proteins for manipulating and eliciting specific immune responses and studies are also suggestive that CpG-DNA might be a valuable and potent agent for treatment of allergies. Interestingly, imidazoquinoline resiquimod (R-848), a ligand for TLR8 has the potential to revert Th2 allergic response to Th1 because of its exceptional capability to induce Th1 response

(Hemmi et al., 2002). Hence, ligands like imidazoquinoline resiquimod too can be therapeutic targets for allergic reactions.

9.4 TLRs in autoimmune and inflammatory diseases

9.4.1 Systemic Lupus Erythematosus (SLE)

SLE is an autoimmune disorder in which antibodies are directed against a range of self-antigens. Out of these, autoantibodies to nuclear antigens are of keen importance to the clinical diagnosis of SLE. Nuclear antigens include dsDNA, ssDNA, nucleolar RNA, histone proteins and others. Emerging researches have revealed the involvement of TLRs in the progression of autoimmune diseases like SLE, rheumatoid arthritis, diabetes mellitus etc. TLR7 and TLR9 are of particular interest in the studies of SLE which are located in the endosomal compartments (Anders, 2005; Christensen et al., 2005). It has been seen that unregulated or misregulated activation of TLRs can lead to an autoimmune phenotypic appearance. Nucleic acids which are usually not immunogenic are not able to induce an immune response, but these can become immunogenic via several chemical modifications like hypo-methylation, increased oxidation and high CpG content. Immune complexes having DNA or RNA which are formed as a consequence of necrosis thus are capable of activating TLRs. It has been reported that DNA found in immune complexes has 5-6 times more of CpG content and is hypo-methylated in SLE patients. Release of autoantibodies and inflammatory cytokines which are responsible for chronic inflammation (Christensen et al., 2007; Savarese et al., 2008) can be traced to the improper activation of TLR7. In SLE patients, levels of IFNα and TypeI interferons are excessively high and it is found that higher levels of IFNα are beneficiary to the disease progression. Nowadays, TLR signalling pathways are directed for therapeutic intervention. Various key molecules of TLR7 and TLR9 signalling pathways are targeted to block downstream signalling and hence the effector responses. Molecules targeted are MyD88, TRAF6, IRAK1 & 4. Other approaches are monoclonal antibodies directed against IFNα. Also immunoregulatory DNA sequences (IRS) bind to TLRs and block their activation. Hence, these can be used as effective strategies in reduction of SLE progression molecules. Research for absolute treatment is still in its early stages.

9.4.2 Rheumatoid Arthiritis (RA)

RA is an autoimmune disorder which affects the joints most severely. RA is caused due to generation of autoantibodies against the Fc region of IgG. Usually these autoantibodies are of IgM type and referred to as rheumatoid factors. Recent studies have revealed that TLRs play a significant role in the development of RA. TLR2 & 4 seems to play a crucial role in RA. TLR2 & 4 over expression is found in the blood monocytes, synovial fluid macrophages and fibroblasts in RA (Iwahashi et al., 2004). Patients with RA are found to have presence of TLR ligands in the joints synovial fluid. These ligands can be endogenous (Heat shock proteins, HMGB1, hyaluronan etc) (Huang et al., 2009) or can be exogenous like peptidoglycan. It has been seen that MyD88 and TLR2/4 deficient mice show reduced severity of RA. Currently various approaches are investigated to treat RA effectively. TLR antagonists and various TLR signalling molecules are targeted as a promising agent for treating RA.

9.4.3 Inflammatory Bowel Disease (IBD)

TLR2, TLR4 and TLR5 have been found to play a role in the pathogenesis of IBD. IBD comprises of Crohn's disease (CD) and ulcerative colitis (UC). Elevated expression of TLR4 is seen in the colonic tissue of UC and CD patients (Cairo & Podolsky, 2000), but TLR2 is found to be highly expressed in mouse manifested with colitis (Singh et al., 2005). This shows that IBD may be a consequential result of mutations and dysregulation in TLRs. Another family of PRRs, nucleotide binding oligomerization domain proteins (Nod) have been reported to contribute to IBD pathogenesis in conjunction with TLRs (Chen et al., 2007). Polymorphism in Nod2 is attributed to the development of CD.

9.4.4 Psoriasis

Psoriasis is a dermatological disorder of chronic autoimmune inflammatory nature. Expression of TLR2, TLR5 and TLR1 is altered in psoriatic individuals when compared to normal individuals (Chen et al., 2007). TLR2 is found to be highly expressed in the upper epidermis in contrast to normal skin where TLR2 is expressed in basal keratinocytes. Basal keratinocytes of the lesions also show reduced expression of TLR5 (Baker et al., 2003) and an enhanced and diffused expression of TLR1 when compared to normal skin (Curry et al., 2003). One of the mechanistic explanations of inflammatory response to psoriasis can be that the DNA released from keratinocytes in psoriatic skin binds to antimicrobial peptide cathelicidin LL37 thus mimicking bacterial DNA and triggers TLR expression on surface of immune cell/dendrocytes to activate NF-kB which controls the inflammation.

9.5 TLRs in infectious diseases

Apart from inflammatory and immune diseases associated with TLRs, TLRs are vital players in infectious diseases as well. One of these is *Mycobacterium tuberculosis* infection in which TLR2, TLR4 and TLR9 have been found to play some role. At an early stage of infection TLR2- and TLR4-knockout mice showed an increased susceptibility to the bacteria but it subsided at the later stage of infection (Tjarnlund, 2006). It has also been reported that absence of TLR2 in mice leads to aggravated inflammatory response (Drennan et al., 2004). A study reports that mice double deficient in TLR9 and TLR2 are highly susceptible to mycobacterial infection, however, single knockouts in either TLR2 or TLR9 did not show this phenomenon (Bafica et al., 2005). Another mycobacterial species, *Mycobacterium leprae,* results in various clinical manifestations associated with host immune response (Chen et al., 2007). TLR1 and TLR2 have been found to be highly expressed in patients with tuberculoid lesions whereas lepromatous lesions lack these TLRs indicating their role in the progression of tuberculoid form of the disease (Krutzik et al., 2003).

Altered expression of TLR4, TLR5 and TLR9 has been observed in *Helicobacter pylori* infection (Chen et al., 2007). TLR4 and MD-2 have been found to be expressed at significantly higher levels in gastric mucosa. This indicates the possible role of TLR4/MD-2 complex in host response to *H. pylori* derived LPS (Ishihara et al., 2004). Interestingly, TLR5 and TLR9 are located on both apical surface and basolateral surface but during *H. pylori* infection, these TLRs are not found to be expressed at the apical surface (Schmausser et al., 2005). TLR adaptor protein, MyD88, is found to be crucial in eliciting a protective host innate response against *Cryptococcus neoformans* and *Legionella pneumophila* infections (Archer et al., 2006; Yauch et al., 2004). The response is generated via activation of TLR2. Also *Chlamydia pneumonia* infection is prevented by TLR2 and TLR4 expression (Rodriguez et al., 2006).

Lyme disease, caused by infection by spirochete *Borrelia* is also associated with TLRs. Outer surface protein A lipoprotein (OspA) is an antigen belonging to *Borrelia burgdorferi* that when docks onto TLR2 and TLR6 culminates in the induction of NFκB in human dermal endothelial cells (HMEC) (Bulut et al., 2001). TLR2/1heterodimerization is essential for the macrophages to recognize OspA and initiate desirable immune response against *B. Burgdorferi* (Chen et al., 2007). Absence of chemokine receptor XCR2 results in decreased inflammation which is considered as a novel therapeutic target for lyme disease.

Role of TLRs in viral disease progression is not yet completely elucidated, however, TLR3, TLR7, TLR8 and TLR9 have been associated with viral sensing (Kanwar et al., 2011). TLR3 and TLR9 have been conferred the foremost place in generating viral immunity. TLR3 and TLR9 recognize viral double stranded RNA and non-methylated CpG di-nucleotides (both of viral and bacterial origin) respectively. TLR7 and TLR8 too leave their signature in viral immunity by initiating IFN-α and IFN-β production in DCs and monocytes through IRAK-4 TLR adaptor (Kanwar et al., 2011). Role of TLR3 has been of prime importance in the immune response of lung epithelial cells to Influenza A virus (IAV). Influenza infection causes enhanced pulmonary expression of TLR3 in mice. However, IAV-infected TLR3-/- mice exhibited significantly reduced levels of inflammatory mediators and lower number of $CD8^+$ T lymphocytes in broncho-alveolar space (Le Goffic et al., 2006). Therefore, it can be concluded that TLR3-IAV interaction renders the body protected against debilitating host inflammatory response.

10. TLRs as adjuvant vaccines and their role in immune stimulation

Adjuvant is an agent that may stimulate the immune system and increase the response to an antigen or a vaccine without showing any antigenic property of its own. Adjuvants are used to augment the effect of a particular vaccine by putting in action the innate and then adaptive immune system in action so that the response to a vaccine is more vigorous. Adjuvants mimic molecules of bacterial or viral origin which are conserved and bear molecular signatures called PAMPs or pattern in terms of conservation. These pattern bearing molecules act as a ligand for toll like receptors (TLRs). When TLRs come in contact with their appropriate ligands, the receptor-ligand complex gives rise to innate immune response which in turn activates adaptive immune system. Since the distribution of TLRs is not limited to the innate cells such as DCs, macrophages, natural killer cells, but are also found on B cells, T cells, and other non-immune cells such as epithelial, endothelial and fibroblast, the importance of giving adjuvant based vaccines can be gauged from the fact that ligands will be able to elicit strong immune response from innate to adaptive immunity. The adjuvant simply mimics natural infection, which in turn first puts the innate then adaptive immune system on, subsequently the purpose of generation of memory cells against the desired target is achieved (Kaisho & Akira, 2002).

The role of TLRs as adjuvant receptors may be exploited to control the TLR signalling using immunity modulating reagents which may be used against the pathogens, autoimmune diseases, inflammation and cancers. Since TLRs are crucial in recognition of viral and bacterial pathogens, current treatment aims at activating these receptors, generation of pro-inflammatory response and finally destruction of these pathogens. Ribavarin in combination with IFNα and resiquimod are currently being used as antiviral drugs. But these molecules have their own sets of limitations in terms of side effects. Agonist molecules like ANA773 and IMO-2125 have shown promising results with their respective receptors TLR7 and TLR9. TLR agonists have also been supplemented to boost immune responses to cancer vaccines. TLR7 imidazoquinoline ligand 3M-019 has been found to be a potent adjuvant for pure protein prototype vaccines (Johnston et al., 2007). TLR2 agonist SMP-105 has been approved for the bladder cancer treatment. The compound has shown strong adjuvant and antitumor activities. In experimental model, SM-105 has shown anti-tumour property. Thus TLRs as adjuvant receptors may open up new avenues of medical treatments. MPL has been approved in Europe as adjuvant vaccine. This molecule is a component of the hepatitis B vaccine and papillomavirus virus vaccine. It act as a ligand to TLR4 and activates the TRAM/TRIF pathway leading to the induction of IFNβ and regulation of CD80/86. MGN-1703 and MGN-1706 are double stem loop, non-coding DNA based adjuvants which ligate with TLR9 are being developed as anticancer agents. Another vaccine adjuvant, VAX-102, which acts as TLR5 agonist is also under trial to treat the viral infections (Elizabeth., 2010). This adjuvant vaccine if successful will provide protection from all strains of seasonal and pandemic influenza. Synthetic TLR agonists poorly reproduce the essential 'pattern' component of the larger natural ligands. To overcome this, an agonist PolyMAP, has been generated in which individual ligand is presented in a more natural linear pattern along the length of a biocompatible polymer. PolyMAP agonists can boost the immune response up to 200 times higher on a per molecule basis. PolyMAP has three key properties that contribute to the enhanced adjuvant activity and safety: (1) increased receptor avidity through cooperative, multi-valent interactions, (2) clustering of receptors through cross-linking and (3) improved solubility of TLR ligands that are otherwise difficult to use in their free form. Recently, Kasturi et al. (Kasturi et al., 2011) have reported synthetic nanoparticle adjuvant that stimulates TLR4 and TLR7, ensuing in enhanced generation of antigen-specific antibodies by synergistic action. Hence, conferring protection to lethal viral challenges in mice and inducing robust immunity against the pandemic H1N1 influenza strain in *Rhesus macaques*. Researchers developed poly(d,l-lactic-co-glycolic acid) (PGLA), a biodegradable polymer based nanoparticle to administer the TLR4 and TLR7 ligands, it was found that in comparison to the stimulation of either TLR4 or TLR7 alone, the double TLR stimulation significantly enhanced antibody response and was found to be evident even after secondary immunization.

Overall it can be concluded that adjuvants mimicking the natural molecules of viral or bacterial origin may be used to modulate the immune system resulting in the treatment of autoimmune diseases, cancers, other diseases, and when combined with vaccines, they may help in the generation of memory cells against a particular invader. The potential of adjuvant alone or as an adjuvant vaccine is yet to be fully exploited.

11. TLRs in transplantation

Transplantation is a surgical procedure by which cells, tissues or organs can be moved from one part of body to another or from one individual to another. Despite the advancement in surgical and medical sciences, the immune system remains the biggest barrier to transplantation. Till recently, the rejection of a transplant was taken as an adaptive immune response mediated by killer T cells capable of inducing apoptosis as well as antibody secreting B cells with only small and finishing role of innate immune system like phagocytosis and complement activation. However, the emerging results have shown the importance of innate immune system in the transplant rejection via TLRs. Although direct role of TLRs are yet to be found but the activation of adaptive immune system because of TLRs may be the reason. As we know that TLRs need specific ligands to activate the signalling pathway and it is quite possible that during transplantation there is release of putative endogenous ligands such as heat shock proteins (Hsp), uric acid, hyaluronan, fibrinogen and chromatin (Goldstein, 2006). Some of these putative ligands have been seen to work with the TLRs. At the same time the role of exogenous ligands cannot be ruled out completely, which may be because of infection contracted while surgery. LPS from gram negative bacteria has been shown to activate the TLR mediated signalling pathway and create complications in graft or transplant acceptance. The recognition of alloantigen by adaptive immune system, in principle, made active because of TLRs may show increased level of complications on the development of cross reactivity with alloantigen and viral molecules. Previous studies have shown that lung, intestine and skin are more prone than kidney, heart and pancreas to acute rejection after transplantation (Wang et al., 2010). This observation may be explained that these organs which are less likely to be accepted as graft have commensals or pathogens, which in turn may activate innate immune system through TLRs leading finally to the activation of adaptive immunity. The identification of endogenous and control of exogenous TLR ligands may pave way for longer period of acceptance of transplants.

12. TLRs in trophoblast

During pregnancy the placenta is not only exposed to the maternal immune system, but also to microorganisms. It has been shown recently that in first trimester trophoblastic cells have TLR2 and TLR4 on their surface by which they can recognize and respond to invading pathogens. Interestingly, both of these TLRs show divergent response. TLR4 activation results in a more classical response, characterized by the induction of cytokine production whereas activation of TLR2 results in the induction of apoptosis. This induction of apoptosis by TLR2 may provide a mechanism by which pathogens may give rise to complicated pregnancies in the first trimester, although a clear picture remains elusive. It has been seen that in several complicated pregnancies the case of intrauterine infection was found to be the leading cause. It has been seen that during first trimester TLR2 assisted trophoblastic cell apoptosis level rises. In turn this may give rise to several medical conditions like preterm labour, IUGR, and preeclampsia. Usually, the uterine infection takes place before the implantation of trophoblast. The pathogen gets the recognition only when it is able to penetrate the placental wall and is able to reach the layer where trophoblastic cells are expressing TLRs. The TLR expression is not limited to the cell surface but has been seen also in cytoplasm may be to facilitate emergency call on infection or to face the intracellular infections, if any. The TLR4 when comes in contact with its ligand, LPS, triggers classical response whereas TLR2 induces apoptosis by coming in contact with Gram positive bacterial peptidoglycan or lipoteichoic acid, but at the same time it has been reported that recognition of these bacterial products by TLR2 requires recruitment of TLR6 or TLR1. Further studies have shown that TLR6 may show increased effect but is not essential for TLR2 mediated response and response may be executed through

TLR2 homodimer or TLR1/TLR2 heterodimer. The TLR2 induces apoptotic effect through the activation of caspases. The TLR4 interaction with LPS does not give rise to pro-apoptotic signals during first trimester because the anti-apoptotic signals generated may outweigh the pro-apoptotic signals leading to the survival of trophoblastic cells. There is also a possibility of indirect induction of apoptosis due to the high level of cytokine production such as TNF and IFN to which placenta cells are sensitive (Vikki et al., 2006).

13. Conclusion

Earlier confusion of innate immunity being nonspecific as compared to adaptive immunity got cleared with the discovery of Toll like Receptors (TLRs) which ligate with the molecules having either exogenous origin like viral or bacterial or endogenous origin like Hsp. These ligands bear molecular patterns or signatures which make them unique for their receptors. The induction by these molecules may have either positive or negative effect on the body depending on the type of ligand and TLR. It has been seen that though ligands get recognised because of molecular pattern by a specific receptor, occasionally the same receptor may ligate with two to three different molecules with each having its own signature or pattern. This may be possibly due to assistance by some co-receptors. Further study is needed to arrive at some conclusion about this enigma. The protein-ligand complex crystal structures may provide insight into the still unclear picture of TLR signalling. The TLRs have been implicated in the development of cancers, autoimmune diseases, nervous system disorders and other inflammatory diseases. TLRs agonist or antagonist may help to get the desired result. Also their role as receptor for adjuvant alone or adjuvant vaccine is being explored much vigorously than before. Role of TLRs from premature birth, complicated pregnancies to transplant rejection cannot be ignored. Moreover, their roles along with miRNA need to be probed further. Also the sources of endogenous ligands need to be discovered. Apart from receptors, the other molecules of signalling pathway too need attention to understand the process much better. The need of the time is to push the TLR research into next level where better animal models (knockout) are ready to rule out artefacts. Lastly, to design drugs, vaccines and fine tune them for lesser or ideally no side effects. Therefore, in the light of emerging information about the complexity of TLRs in immune system regulation, it can be concluded that TLRs are in fact a necessary evil. Sometimes, from their usual behaviour as a good cop by being a part of an innate immune system, a first line of defence, may turn rouge due to several compelling reasons and play bad cop. Hence, activation of TLRs is a double edged sword in therapeutics, it has the potential to mount immunity against various autoimmune, inflammatory and cancerous diseases etc. but can also promote their development and dampen immune response against them.

14. References

Akbari, O., Freeman, G.J., Meyer, E.H., Greenfield, E.A., Chang, T.T., Sharpe, A.H., Berry, G., DeKruyff, R.H. & Umetsu, D.T. (2002). Antigen-specific regulatory T cells develop via the ICOS-ICOS-ligand pathway and inhibit allergen-induced airway hyperreactivity. *Nat. Med.*, Vol. 8, pp. 1024–1032.

Akiyama, H. et al. (2000) Inflammation and Alzheimer's disease. *Neurobiol Aging*, Vol.21, pp. 383-421.

Anders, H.J. (2005). A toll for lupus. *Lupus*. Vol. 14, pp. 417–422.

Arancibia, S.A., Beltran, C.J., Aguirre, I.M., Silva, P., Peralta, A.L., Malinarich, F. & Hermoso, M.A. (2007). Toll-like receptors are key participants in innate immune responses. *Biol Res.* Vol.40, pp. 97-112.

Arbour, N.C. (2000). TLR4 mutations are associated with endotoxin hyporesponsiveness in humans. *Nat Genet*, Vol.25, pp. 187–191.

Archer, K.A. & Roy, C.R. (2006) MyD88-dependent responses involving toll-like receptor 2 are important for protection and clearance of *Legionella pneumophila* in a mouse model of Legionnaires' disease. *Infect Immun*, Vol.74, pp. 3325–33.

Arroyo, S.D., Soria, A.J., Gaviglio, A.E., Rodriguez-Galan, C.M., Iribarren,P. (2011) Toll-like receptors are key players in neurodegeneration. *Inter. Immunopharmacology*, Vol.11, pp. 1415–1421.

Asea, A., Kraeft, S.K., Kurt-Jones, E.A., Stevenson, M.A., Chen, L.B. & Finberg RW et al. (2000). Hsp70 stimulates cytokine production through a CD-14-dependent pathway, demonstrating its dual role as a chaperone and cytokine. *Nat Med*, Vol.6, pp. 435–442.

Bafica, A., Scanga, C.A., Feng, C.G., Leifer, C., Cheever, A. & Sher, A. (2005). TLR9 regulates Th1 responses and cooperates with TLR2 in mediating optimal resistance to Mycobacterium tuberculosis. *J Exp Med*, Vol.202, pp. 1715–24.

Baker, B.S., Ovigne, J.M., Powles, A.V., Corcoran, S. & Fry L. (2003) Normal keratinocytes express Toll-like receptors (TLRs) 1, 2 and 5: modulation of TLR expression in chronic plaque psoriasis. *Br J Dermatol*, Vol.148, pp. 670–9.

Banchereau, J. & Steiman, R.M. (1998). Dendritic cells and the control of immunity. *Nature*, Vol.392, pp. 245-52.

Bauer, S., Hangel, D. & Yu, P. (2007). Immunobiology of toll-like receptors in allergic disease. *Immunobiology*, Vol.212, pp. 521-533.

Bell, J. K., Botos, I., Hall, P.R., Askins, J., Shiloach, J., Segal, D.M.,et al (2003).Leucine-rich repeats and pathogen recognition in Toll-like receptors. *Trends Immunol*. Vol.24, pp. 528–533.

Beutler, B. & Rietschel, E. T. (2003). Innate immune sensing and its roots: the story of endotoxin. *Nature Rev. Immunol.*, Vol.3, pp. 169–176.

Beutler, B., Rehli, M. (2002). Evolution of the TIR, tolls and TLRs: functional inferences from computational biology. *Curr. Top Microbial. Immunol.* Vol.270, pp. 1-21.

Bin, L. H., Xu, L. G. & Shu, H. B. (2003).TIRP, a novel Toll/interleukin-1 receptor (TIR) domain-containing adapter protein involved in TIR signaling. *J. Biol. Chem.*, Vol.278, pp. 24526–24532.

Bradley, J. R. & Pober, J. S. (2001).Tumor necrosis factor receptor associated factors (TRAFs). *Oncogene*, Vol.20, pp. 6482–6491.

Bsibsi, M.(2002) Broad expression of Toll-like receptors in the human central nervous system. *J Neuropathol Exp Neurol*, Vol.61, pp. 1013–1021.

Bulut ,Y., Faure, E., Thomas, L., Equils, O. & Arditi M. (2001). Cooperation of Toll-like receptor 2 and 6 for cellular activation by soluble tuberculosis factor and Borrelia burgdorferi outer surface protein A lipoprotein: role of Toll-interacting protein and IL-1 receptor signaling molecules in Toll-like receptor 2 signaling. *J Immunol*, Vol.167, pp. 987–94.

Burns, K., Martinon F., Esslinger C., Pahl H., Schneider P., Bodmer J.L., Marco F.D., French L. & Tschopp J. (1998). MyD88, an adapter protein involved in interleukin-1 signaling. *J. Biol. Chem.*, Vol.273, pp. 12203–12209.

Cario, E. & Podolsky, D.K. (2000). Differential alteration in intestinal epithelial cell expression of toll-like receptor 3 (TLR3) and TLR4 in inflammatory bowel disease. *Infect Immun*, Vol.68, pp. 7010–7.

Carpentier PA, et al. (2005) Differential activation of astrocytes by innate and adaptive immune stimuli. *Glia*, Vol.49, pp. 360-374.

Chen, K., Huang, J., Gong, W., Iribarren P., Dunlop, N.M. & Wang, J.M. (2007). Toll like receptors in inflammation, infection and cancer. *International Immunopharmacology*, Vol.7, pp. 1271-1285.

Chen, X. & Oppenheim, J.J. (2009). Regulatory T cells, Th17 cells, and TLRs: Crucial role in Inflammation, Autoimmunity, and Cancer. *Pathways*, 888.503.3187, Issue 10.

Christensen, S.R. & Shlomchik, M.J. (2007). Regulation of lupus-related autoantibody production and clinical disease by Toll-like receptors. *Seminars in Immunology*. Vol.19, pp. 11–23.

Christensen, S.R., Kashgarian, M., Alexopoulou, L., Flavell, R.A., Akira, S. & Shlomchik, M.J. (2005) Toll-like receptor 9 controls anti-DNA autoantibody production in murine lupus. *Journal of Experimental Medicine*. Vol.202, pp. 321–331.

Curry, J.L., Qin, J.Z., Bonish, B., Carrick, R., Bacon, P. & Panella, J. et al. (2003) Innate immune-related receptors in normal and psoriatic skin. *Arch Pathol Lab Med* ,Vol.127, pp. 178–86.

Drennan, M.B., Nicolle, D., Quesniaux, V.J., Jacobs, M., Allie, N. & Mpagi, J. et al.(2004). Toll-like receptor 2-deficient mice succumb to Mycobacterium tuberculosis infection. *Am J Pathol*. Vol.164, pp. 49–57.

Elizabeth, J., Hennessy, Andrew, E., Parker, Luke A.J.O., Neill. (2010) Targeting Toll-like receptors: emerging therapeutics, *Nature Rev. Drug Discovery*, Vol. 9, pp. 293-307.

Gehring, U., Bischof, W. & Fahlbusch, B., et al. (2002). House dust endotoxin and allergic sensitization in children. *Am J Respir Crit Care Med.*, Vol.166, pp. 939-944.

Gingras, S., Parganas, E., Pauw, A.D., Ihle, J.N. & Murray, P.J. (2004). Re- examination of the role of suppressor of cytokine signaling 1 (SOCS1) in the regulation of toll-like receptor signaling. *J Biol Chem*, Vol.279, pp. 54702-7.

Goldstein, D.R. (2006) Toll like receptors and acute allograft rejection, *Transplant Immuno.* Vol. 17, pp. 211–215.

Harmey, J.H., Bucana, C.D., Lu, W., Byrne, A.M., McDonnell, S. & Lynch, C. et al. (2002). Lipopolysaccharide-induced metastatic growth is associated with increased angiogenesis, vascular permeability and tumor cell invasion. *Int J Cancer* . Vol.101, pp. 415–422.

Hashimoto, C.; Hudson, K. L. & Anderson, K. V. (1988). The *Toll* gene of *Drosophila*, required for dorsal–ventral embryonic polarity, appears to encode a transmembrane protein. *Cell*, Vol.52, pp. 269–279.

Hemmi, H., Kaisho, T., Takeuchi, O., Sato, S., Sanjo, H., Hoshino, K., Horiuchi, T., Tomizawa, H., Takeda, K., Akira, S. (2002). Small anti-viral compounds activate immune cells via the TLR7 MyD88-dependent signaling pathway. *Nat. Immunol.* Vol.3, pp. 196–200.

Hoebe, K., Du, X., Georgel, P., Janssen, E.M., Tabeta, K., Kim, S.O., Goode, J., Lin, P., Mann, N., Mudd, S., Crozat, K., Sovath, S., Han, J. & Beutler, B. (2003). Identification of

Lps2 as a key transducer of MyD88-independent TIR signalling. *Nature,* Vol.424, pp. 743–748.

Horner, A.A., Van Uden, J.H., Zubeldia, J.M., Broide, D. & Raz, E. (2001). DNA-based immunotherapeutics for the treatment of allergic disease. *Immunol. Rev.* Vol.179, pp. 102–118.

Horng, T., Barton, G. M. & Medzhitov, R. (2001). TIRAP: an adapter molecule in the Toll signaling pathway. *Nature Immunol.,* Vol.2, pp. 835–841.

Hsu, Y. C. Rich., Chan, H. F. Carlos, Spicer, D. J., Rousseau, C. M., Giannias, B., Rousseau, S., Ferri, E. L., (2011) *Cancer Res,* Vol. 71(5), pp. 1989-98.

Huang, Q.Q., Sobkoviak, R., Jocheck-Clark, A.R., Shi, B., Mandelin, A.M. & Tak, P.P.et al. (2009). Heat shock protein 96 is elevated in rheumatoid arthritis and activates macrophages primarily via TLR2 signaling. *J Immunol.* Vol.182, pp. 4965-73.

Ishihara, S., Rumi, M.A., Kadowaki, Y., Ortega-Cava, C.F., Yuki, T. & Yoshino N, et al. (2004). Essential role of MD-2 in TLR4-dependent signaling during Helicobacter pylori-associated gastritis. *J Immunol* ,Vol.173, pp. 1406–16.

Iwahashi, M., Yamamura, M., Aita ,T., Okamoto, A., Ueno, A. & Ogawa, N., et al. (2004). Expression of Toll-like receptor 2 on CD16+ blood monocytes and synovial tissue macrophages in rheumatoid arthritis.*Arthritis Rheum.* Vol.50, pp. 1457–67.

Jack, C.S., Arbour, N., Manusow, J., Montgrain, V., Blain, M., McCrea, E., Shapiro, A., Antel JP. (2005) TLR signaling tailors innate immune responses in human microglia and astrocytes. *JImmunol,* Vol.175, pp. 4320-4330.

Jack, C.S. et al. (2007) Th1 polarization of CD4+ T cells by Toll-like receptor 3-activated human microglia.*J Neuropathol Exp Neurol,* Vol.66, pp. 848-859.

Janeway, C. A. & Medzhitov, R. (2002). Innate immune recognition. *Annu. Rev. Immunol.,* Vol.20, pp. 197–216.

Janssens, S. & Beyaert, R. (2003). Functional diversity and regulation of different interleukin-1 receptor-associated kinase (IRAK) family members. *Mol. Cell,* Vol.11, pp. 293–302.

Johnston, D., Zaidi, B., Bystryn, J.C. (2007). TLR7 imidazoquinoline ligand 3M-019 is a potent adjuvant for pure protein prototype vaccines. *Cancer Immunol Immunother,* Vol.58, Issue 8, pp.1133-41.

Kaisho, T., Akira, S., (2002) Toll-like receptors as adjuvants receptors, *Biochimica et Biophysica Acta,* Vol.1589, pp. 1-13.

Kanwar, J.R., Zhou, S.F., Gurudevan, S., Barrow, C.J., Kanwar, R.K. (2011). Toll Like Receptors Play a Role in General Immunity, Eye Infection and Inflammation: TLRs for Nanodelivery. *J Clin Cell Immunol,* Vol.2, Issue 4.

Kasturi, S.P., Skountzou, I., Albrecht, R.A., Koutsonanos, D., Hua, T., Nakaya, H.I. et. al.(2011). Programming the magnitude and persistence of antibody responses with innate immunity. *Nature,* Vol.470, pp.543-547.

Kol, A., Lichtman , A.H., Finberg, R.W., Libby, P. & Kurt-Jones EA. (2000). Cutting edge:heat shock protein (HSP) 60 activates the innate immune response:CD14 is an essential receptor for HSP60 activation of mononuclear cells. *J Immunol,* Vol.164, pp. 13–17.

Krutzik, S.R., Ochoa, M.T., Sieling, P.A., Uematsu, S., Ng, Y.W. & Legaspi A, et al.(2003) Activation and regulation of Toll-like receptors 2 and 1 in human leprosy. *Nat Med,* Vol.9, pp. 525–32.

Le Goffic, R., Balloy, V., Lagranderie, M., Alexopoulou, L., Escriou, N. & Flavell, R. et al. (2006) Detrimental contribution of the Toll-like receptor (TLR)3 to influenza Avirus-induced acute pneumonia. PLoS *Pathog* Vol.2, pp. e53.

Lebouder, E., Rey-Nores, J.E., Rushmere, N.K., Grigorov, M., Lawn, S.D., Affolter, M., Griffin ge, Ferrara, P., Schiffrin, E.J., Morgan, B.P. & Labeta , M.O. (2003) Soluble forms of Toll-like receptor (TLR)2 capable of modulating TLR2 signaling are present in human plasma and breast milk. *J Immunol*, Vol.171, pp. 6680- 9.

Lemaitre, B.; Nicolas, E., Michaut, L., Reichhart, J.M. & Hoffmann, J. A. (1996).The dorsoventral regulatory gene cassette *spatzle/Toll/cactus* controls the potent antifungal response in *Drosophila* adults. *Cell*, Vol.86, pp. 973–983.

Meylan, E., Burns, K., Hofmann, K., Blancheteau, V., Martinon, F., Kelliher, M., et al. (2004).RIP1 is an essential mediator of Toll-like receptor 3-induced NF-κB activation. *Nature Immunol.*, Vol.5, pp. 503–507.

Muzio, M.; Ni, J.; Feng, P. & Dixit, V. M. (1997). IRAK (Pelle) family member IRAK-2 and MyD88 as proximal mediators of IL-1 signaling. *Science*, Vol.278, pp. 1612–1615.

Neill, L.O., (2008) Toll-like receptors in cancer, *Nature Oncogene*, Vol. 27, pp. 158–160s.

Okun, E., Griffioen, J.K., Lathia, D.J., Tang, S., Mattson, P.M., Arumugam, V.T. (2009). Toll like receptors in Neurodegenration, *Brain Res. Rev*. Vol. 59, pp. 278–292.

O'Neill, L. A., Sheedy, F. J., & Claire E. McCoy, C. E. (2011). MicroRNAs: the fine-tuners of Toll-like receptor signalling.*Nature Rev. Immunol.* Vol.11, pp. 163-175.

Parker, L.C., Prince, L.R. & Sabroe, I. (2006). Translational mini-review series on toll like receptors: networks regulated by toll like receptors mediate innate and adaptive immunity. *Clinical and Experimental Immunology.* Vol.147, pp. 199-207.

Pasare, C., Medzhitov, R. (2003). Toll pathway-dependent blockade of $CD4^+$ $CD25^+$ T cell-mediated suppression by dendritic cells. *Science*, Vol.299, pp.1033–1036.

Pessac, B. (2001) Microglia origin and development. *Bull Acad Natl Med*, Vol.185, pp. 346-33.

Poltorak, A., He, X., Smirnova, I., Liu M., Huffel C.V., Du X., Birdwell D., Alejos E., Silva M, Galanos C., Freudenberg M., Castagnoli P.R., Layton B. & Beutler B. (1998). Defective LPS signaling in C3H/HeJ and C57BL/10ScCr mice: mutations in *Tlr4* gene. *Science*, Vol.282, pp. 2085–2088.

Rodriguez, N., Wantia, N., Fend, F., Durr, S., Wagner, H. & Miethke T. (2006) Differential involvement of TLR2 and TLR4 in host survival during pulmonary infection with Chlamydia pneumoniae. *Eur J Immunol*, Vol.236, pp. 1145–55.

Savarese, E., Steinberg, C. & Pawar, R.D., et al. (2008). Requirement of Toll-like receptor 7 for pristane-induced production of autoantibodies and development of murine lupus nephritis. *Arthritis and Rheumatism*. Vol.58, pp. 1107–1115.

Schmausser, B., Andrulis, M., Endrich, S., Muller-Hermelink, H.K. & Eck M. (2005). Toll-like receptors TLR4, TLR5 and TLR9 on gastric carcinoma cells: an implication for interaction with Helicobacter pylori. *Int J Med Microbiol*, Vol.295, pp. 179–85.

Sharma, S., R. tenOever , B., Grandvaux, N., Zhou, G.P., Lin, R. & Hiscott , J. (2003). Triggering the interferon antiviral response through an IKK-related pathway. *Science*,Vol. 300, pp. 1148–1151.

Shibuya, H., Yamaguchi, K., Shirakabe, K., Tonegawa, A., Gotoh, Y., Ueno, N., Irie, K., Nishida, E. & Matsumoto, K.(1996).TAB1: an activator of the TAK1 MAPKKK in TGF-β signal transduction. *Science*, Vol.272, pp. 1179–1182.

Singh, J.C., Cruickshank, S.M., Newton, D.J., Wakenshaw, L., Graham, A. & Lan, J., et al. (2005). Toll-like receptor-mediated responses of primary intestinal epithelial cells during the development of colitis. *Am J Physiol Gastrointest Liver Physiol*, Vol.288, pp. G514–24.

Singh-Jasuja, H., Scherer, H.U., Hilf, N., Arnold-Schild, D., Rammensee, H.G. & Toes, R.E. et al. (2000). The heat shock protein gp96 induces maturation of dendritic cells and down-regulation of its receptor. *Eur J Immunol*; Vol.30, pp. 22 11–221.

Slack, J. L., Schooley, K., Timothy, P. B., Jennifer, L. M., Eva, E. Q., John E. S. & Steven K. D. (2000). Identification of two major sites in the type I interleukin-1 receptor cytoplasmic region responsible for coupling to pro-inflammatory signaling pathways. *J. Biol. Chem.*, Vol. 275, pp. 4670–4678.

Sutmuller, R.P., den Brok, M.H., Kramer, M., Bennink, E.J., Toonen, L.W., Kullberg, B.J., Joosten, L.A., Akira, S., Netea, M.G. & Adema, G.J. (2006). Toll-like receptor 2 controls expansion and function of regulatory T cells. *J. Clin. Invest.* Vol.116, pp. 485–494.

Takaesu, G., Kishida, S., Hiyama, A., Yamaguchi, K., Shibuya, H., Irie, K., Tsuji, J.N. & Matsumot, K. (2000). TAB2, a novel adaptor protein, mediates activation of TAK1 MAPKKK by linking TAK1 to TRAF6 in the IL-1 signal transduction pathway. *Mol. Cell*, Vol. 5, pp. 649–658.

Takeda, K. & Akira, S. (2005). Toll like receptors in innate immunity. *The Japanese Society for Immunology*. Vol.17, pp. 1-14.

Tanaka T, et al. (2008). NF-kappaB independent signaling pathway is responsible for LPS-induced GDNF gene expression in primary rat glial cultures. *Neurosci Lett*; vol.431, pp. 262-267.

Tang SC, et al. (2007). Pivotal role for neuronal Toll-like receptors in ischemic brain injury and functional deficits. *Proc Natl Acad Sci U S A*, Vol. 104, pp. 13798-13803.

Taniguchi, T. & Takaoka, A. (2002).The interferon-α/β system in antiviral responses: a multimodal machinery of gene regulation by the IRF family of transcription factors. *Curr. Opin. Immunol.*, Vol.14, pp. 111–116.

Tjarnlund, A., Guirado, E., Julian, E., Cardona, P.J. & Fernandez C. (2006). Determinant role for Toll like receptor signalling in acute mycobacterial infection in the respiratory tract. *Microbes Infect*, Vol.8, pp. 1790–800.

Vikki, M., Abrahams, Paulomi B.A., Kim, Y.M., Shawn, L., Chavez, S., Chaiworapongsa, T., Romero, R., Mor G. (2006) *The J. Immunology*, Vol.173, pp. 4286 - 4296.

Walter ,S., et al. (2007) Role of the toll-like receptor 4 in neuroinflammation sin Alzheimer's disease. *Cell Physiol Biochem*, Vol.20, pp. 947-956.

Wang, C., Deng, L., Hong, M., Akkaraju, G.R., Inoue, J. & Chen Z.J. (Jul 2001). TAK1 is a ubiquitin-dependent kinase of MKK and IKK. *Nature*, Vol.412, pp. 346-51.

Wang, J.H., Manning, B.J., Wu, Q.D., Blankson, S., Bouchier-Hayes, D. & Redmond, H.P. (2003). Endotoxin/lipopolysaccharide activates NF-kappaB and enhances tumor cell adhesion and invasion through a beta 1 integrin-dependent mechanism. *J Immunol*. Vol.170, pp. 795–804.

Wang, S., Schmaderer, C., Kiss, E., Schmidt, C., Bonrouhi, M., Porubsky, S., Gretz, N., chaefer, L., Carsten, J., Kirschning, Zoran V., Popovic, Gröne, H.J. (2010) Recipient Toll-like receptors contribute to chronic graft dysfunction by both MyD88- and TRIF-dependent signaling, *Disease Models & Mechanisms*, Vol. 3, pp. 92-103.

Wang, Y., Chen, T., Han, C., He, D., Liu, H., An, H., Cai, Z. et. al. (2007) Lysosome-associated small Rab GTPase Rab7b negatively regulates TLR4 signaling in macrophages by promoting lysosomal degradation of TLR4. *Blood,* Vol. 110, pp. 962-971.

Wesche, H.; Henzel, W. J.; Shillinglaw, W.; Li, S. & Cao, Z. (1997). MyD88: an adapter that recruits IRAK to the IL-1 receptor complex. *Immunity,* Vol.7, pp. 837–847.

Whitmore, M.M., Iparraguirre, A., Kubelka, L., Weninger, W., Hai, T. & Williams, B.R.G. (2007). Negative Regulation of TLR-Signaling Pathways by Activating Transcription Factor-3. *J Immunol* , Vol.179, pp.3622-3630.

Wright, S.D., Ramos, R.A., Tobias, P.S., Ulevitch, R.J. & Mathison, J.C. (1990). CD14, a receptor for complexes of lipopolysaccharide (LPS) and LPS binding protein. *Science,* Vol.249, pp. 1431–1433.

Xu, Y., Tao, X., Shen, B., Horng, T., Medzhitov, R., Manley, J.L. & Tong, L. (2000). Structural basis for signal transduction by the Toll/interleukin-1 receptor domains. *Nature,* Vol.408, pp. 111–115.

Yamaguchi, K. , Shirakabe, K., Shibuya, H., Irie, K., Oishi, I., Ueno, N., Taniguchi, T., Nishida, E. & Matsumoto K. (1995). Identification of a member of the MAPKKK family as a potential mediator of TGF-β signal transduction. *Science,* Vol. 270, pp. 2008–2011.

Yamamoto, M., Sato, S., Hemmi, H., Hoshino, K., Kaisho, T., Sanjo, H., Takeuchi, O., Sugiyama, M., Okabe, M., Takeda, K. & Akira, S. (2003). Role of adaptor TRIF in the MyD88-independent Toll-like receptor signaling pathway. *Science,* Vol.301, pp. 640–643.

Yauch, L.E., Mansour, M.K., Shoham, S., Rottman, J.B. & Levitz ,S.M. (2004).Involvement of CD14, toll-like receptors 2 and 4, and MyD88 in the host response to the fungal pathogen Cryptococcus neoformans in vivo. *Infect Immun* , Vol.72, pp. 5373–82.

Ye, H., Arron, J.R., Lamothe, B., Cirilli, M., Kobayashi, T., Shevde, N.K., Segal, D., Dzivenu, O.K., Vologodskaia, M.,Yim, M., Du, K., Singh, S., Pike, J.W., Darnay, B.G., Choi ,Y. & Wu, H. (2002). Distinct molecular mechanism for initiating TRAF6 signalling. *Nature,*Vol. 418, pp. 443–447.

Yoneyama, M., Suhara, W., Fukuhara, Y., Fukuda, M., Nishida, E. & Fujita, T. (1998). Direct triggering of the type I interferon system by virus infection: activation of a transcription factor complex containing IRF-3 and CBP/p300. *EMBO J.,* Vol.17, pp. 1087–1095.

18

Immunology of Leishmaniasis and Future Prospective of Vaccines

Rakesh Sehgal[1], Kapil Goyal[1], Rupinder Kanwar[2], Alka Sehgal[3] and Jagat R. Kanwar[2]
[1]*Department of Parasitology, Postgraduate Institute of Medical Education & Research, Chandigarh,*
[2]*Nanomedicine-Laboratory of Immunology and Molecular Biomedical Research (LIMBR), Centre for Biotechnology and Interdisciplinary Biosciences (BioDeakin), Institute for Technology & Research Innovation (ITRI), Deakin University, Geelong, Technology Precinct (GTP), Waurn Ponds, Geelong, Victoria,*
[3] *Government Medical College & Hospital, Sector 32, Chandigarh,*
[1,3]*India*
[2]*Australia*

1. Introduction

Leishmaniasis causes human suffering on a global scale and there are more than 12 million current cases with 2 million additional cases annually. There is a serious threat to get infected cases of 350 million in endemic areas specifically in South East Asia. The epidemiological studies revealed that there are 20 protozoan parasite species of the genus *Leishmania* known to cause leishmaniasis in humans (Table 1)(WHO 2004). Leishmaniasis is prevalent in tropical and subtropical regions and endemic in more than 88 countries where annually 2 million new cases are reported. The geographic distribution of each *Leishmania* species affects the type of disease that occurs in each region of the world. Visceral leishmaniasis (VL; commonly known as kala-azar) is caused by *Leishmania donovani* in South Asia and Africa, while *Leishmania infantum* causes VL in the Mediterranean, the Middle East, Latin America and parts of Asia too (Table 2)(WHO 2010). Other mammals can also be infected with *Leishmania* spp., dogs develop canine visceral leishmaniasis (CaVL) and they serve as an important parasitic reservoir in these regions. Cutaneous leishmaniasis (CL) is caused by *L. major* in Africa, the Middle East and parts of Asia, by *Leishmania tropica* in the Middle East, the Mediterranean and parts of Asia, and by *Leishmania aethiopica* in parts of Africa. Many different species may be involved in the Americas, where CL can be found throughout South America and as far as Mexico in the north (Table 1 and 2). Infection have also been reported in Canada and the US. Australia is free of *Leishmania* spp. but infection among local animals like captive kangaroos, wallabies and other marsupials have been reported recently and there are chances of transmission of this disease to human through infected meat and also due to close proximity with these native animals (Gelanew, Kuhls et al. 2010).

***Old world, subgenus* Leishmania**	
Visceral leishmaniasis	*Leishmania donovani, L. infantum*
Cutaneous leishmaniasis	*L. major, L. tropica, L. aethiopica*
***New world, subgenus* Leishmania**	
Visceral leishmaniasis	*L. infantum*
Cutaneous leishmaniasis	*L. infantum, L. mexicana, L. pifanol, L. amazonensis*
Diffuse cutaneous leishmaniasis	*L. mexicana, L. amazonensis*
***New world, subgenus* Viannia**	
Cutaneous leishmaniasis	*L. braziliensis, L. guyanensis, L. panamensis, L. peruviana*
Mucocutaneous leishmaniasis	*L. braziliensis, L. panamensis*

Table 1. Main species of *Leishmania* that affect humans.

2. Immunology of leishmaniasis

Leihmaniasis is caused by one of several species of *Leishmania.* The clinical spectrum depends upon both the parasite species and the host's immune response. Some *Leishmania* spp. cause cutaneous, mucocutaneous or diffuse cutaneous leishmaniasis whereas others may disseminate to internal organs such as the liver, spleen and bone marrow to cause visceral leishmaniasis. The main species of *Leishmania* that affect humans are given Table 1&2.

Leishmania parasite exists in two different morphological forms i.e. promastigotes (flagellate form) and amastigote (aflagellated form). Promastigotes develops inside the midgut of sandfly and become infective, non-dividing metacyclic promastigotes which are located near stomodeal valve (an invagination of the foregut into midgut). During blood feeding metacylic promastigotes are regurgitated along with immunomodulatory parasite-derived proteophosphoglycans and various salivary components. The metacyclic promastigotes are rapidly phagocytosed by one of several possible cell types that are found in the local environment. The various cell types may include neutrophils, tissue-resident macrophages or dendritic cell (DC) or monocyte derived DCs (moDCs). After establishing an intracellular niche, metacyclic promastigotes are transformed to non motile amastigote form. These amastigotes replicate within the host cells, which rupture to release too many amastigotes, allowing reinfection of phagocytes. The transmission is complete when infected phagocytes are taken up by another sandfly with the blood meal and amastigotes then convert into promastigotes in the sandfly midgut. (Fig 1: Life cycle of *Leishmania* parasite)

Disease	*Leishmania sp.(CFSPH 2009)*	Geographical burden
Cutaneous Leishmaniasis (CL)	*L. mexicana* complex (ZCL)	Argentina, Belize, Bolivia, Brazil. Colombia, Costa Rica, Ecuador, French Guiana, Guatemala, Mexico, Peru, Suriname, USA, and Venezuela
	L. tropica complex (ACL)	Afghanistan, Azerbaijan, India, Iran, Iraq, Israel, Morocco, Pakistan, Syria, Turkey, and Uzbekistan
	L. major complex (ZCL)	Afghanistan, Algeria, Azerbaijan, Burkina Faso, Cameroon, Chad, Egypt, Ethiopia, Gambia, Georgia, Ghana, Guinea Bissau, India, Iran, Iraq, Israel, Jordan, Kazakhstan, Kenya, Kuwait, Libya, Mali, Mauritania, Mongolia, Morocco, Niger, Nigeria, Oman, Pakistan, Saudi Arabia, Senegal, the Sudan, Syria, Tunisia, Turkey, Turkmenistan, Uzbekistan, and Yemen
	L. aethiopica complex (ZCL)	Ethiopia, Kenya, and Uganda
	L. brazilensis complex (ZCL)	Argentina, Belize, Bolivia, Brazil. Colombia, Costa Rica, Ecuador, French Guiana, Guatemala, Honduras, Mexico, Nicaragua, Panama, Paraguay, Peru, and Venezuela
	L. guyanensis complex (ZCL)	Argentina, Belize, Bolivia, Brazil. Colombia, Costa Rica, Ecuador, French Guiana, Guatemala, Guyana, Honduras, Nicaragua, Panama, Peru, Suriname, and Venezuela
Mucosal/mucocutaneous Leishmaniasis (ML)	*L. braziliensis* complex	Argentina, Belize, Bolivia, Brazil. Colombia, Costa Rica, Ecuador, French Guiana, Guatemala, Honduras, Mexico, Nicaragua, Panama, Paraguay, Peru, and Venezuela
	L. guyanensis complex	Colombia, Costa Rica, Ecuador, Guatemala, Honduras, Nicaragua, and Panama
Visceral Leishmaniasis (VL; Kala-azar)	*L. donovani* complex (AVL, ZVL)	Afghanistan, Albania, Algeria, Argentina, Armenia, Azerbaijan, Bangladesh, Bhutan, Bolivia, Bosnia & Herzegovina, Brazil, Bulgaria, Chad, Central African Republic, China, Colombia, Croatia, Cyprus, Djibouti, Egypt, El Salvador, Eritrea, Ethiopia, France, Gambia, Georgia, Greece, Guatemala, Honduras, India, Iran, Iraq, Israel. Italy, Jordan, Kazakhstan, Kenya, Kyrgyzstan, Lebanon, Libya, Macedonia, Malta, Mauritania, Mexico, Monaco, Montenegro, Morocco, Nepal, Nicaragua, Oman, Pakistan, Paraguay, Portugal, Romania, Saudi Arabia, Senegal. Slovenia, Somalia, Spain, Sri Lanka, the Sudan, Syria, and Yemen
Post-Kala-azar Dermal Leishmaniasis (PKDL)	*L. donovani* complex	Bangladesh, China, Nepal, India, Iran, Iraq, Kenya, Pakistan, the Sudan

Table 2. Disease phenotype and geographical burden attributed to various *Leishmania* species (WHO 2010).

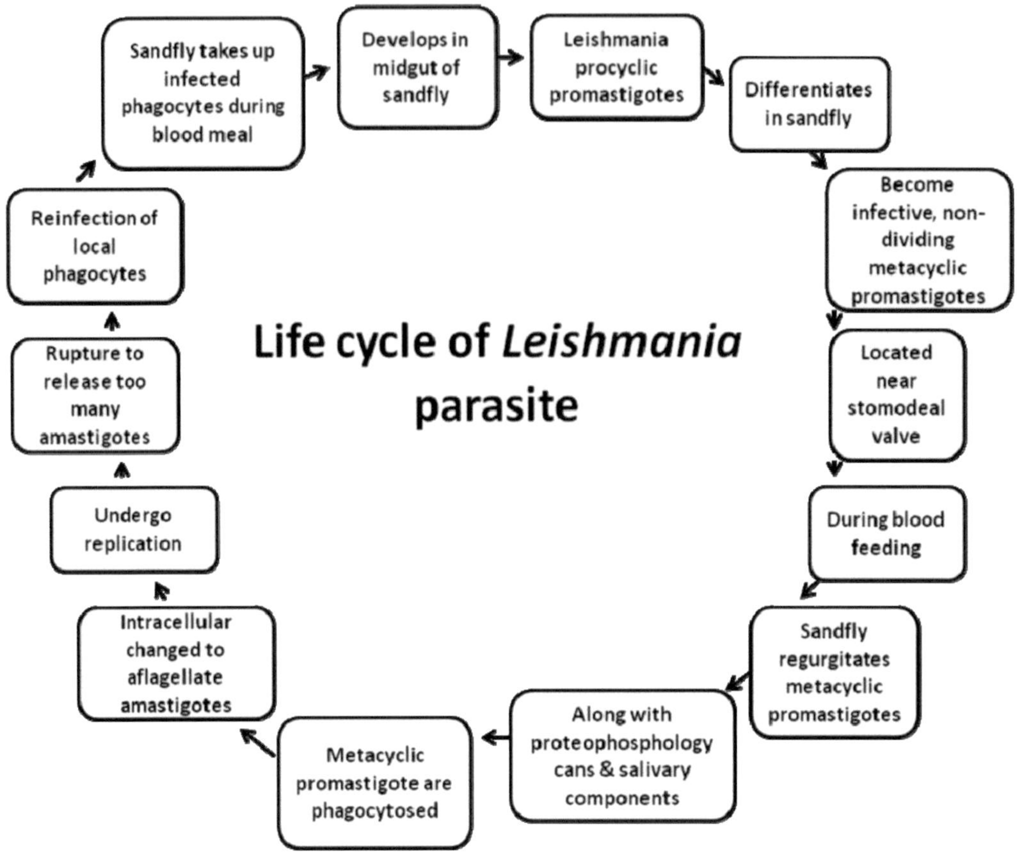

Fig. 1. Life cycle of Leishmania parasite.

3. Host cells for *Leishmania* parasites

Leishmania spp. is an obligate intracellular pathogen which mainly infects macrophages. Recent studies have shown that it can infect multiple cell types. Neutrophils have been regarded as Trojan Horses which help promastigotes to establish intracellular niche in macrophages without triggering their antimicrobial defences. The promastigotes are phagocytosed by neutrophils and they reside in their phagosomes. They become phagocytic meal for the macrophages when undergo apoptosis. Since these apoptotic bodies are phagocytosed through receptor mediated pathways that fail to trigger antimicrobial defences.(Ravichandran and Lorenz 2007) The neutrophils are attracted at local site of sandfly bite due to alarmins(IL-33,IL1β,high mobility group protein B1-HMGB1), which are endogenous molecules that provide signal of tissue damage.(Haraldsen, Balogh et al. 2009) Mononuclear phagocytes which are infected with Leishmania parasites also produce various chemokines which help in recruitment of neutrophils.(Lopez Kostka, Dinges et al. 2009; Xin, Vargas-Inchaustegui et al. 2010)

Leishmania promastigotes have a dense covering of glycocalyx which is attached to the plasma membrane with the help of GPI (glycophosphoinositol). Lipophosphoglycan (LPG) is an important molecule which promotes the infectivity of the parasite in mammalian host.

It is a long phosphoglycan molecule having repeated sugar residues, glycan side chains and a capping oligosaccharide. It shows a great variability in its structure which helps in immune evasion. Another important surface glycoprotein is zinc metalloproteinase(GP-63) which acts as a virulence factor (Gomez, Contreras et al. 2009). *Leishmania donovani* promastigotes stimulate neutrophil extracellular traps (NETs) by a LPG independent pathway (Gabriel, McMaster et al. 2010). These NETs are filamentous DNA which are decorated with antimicrobial peptides.

Though the neutrophils play an important role but mononuclear phagocytes are equally essential for the replication and long term survival of parasites. Dermal DCs uptake the parasite within first few hours of infection by pseudopodium formation (Ng, Hsu et al. 2008). As the number of resident macrophages and dendritic cells is limited in the skin, the parasitic multiplication is accompanied by the recruitment of monocytes (precursor of DCs) (Charmoy, Brunner-Agten et al. 2010). Infected inflammatory moDCs may facilitate parasite to reach the draining lymph node. *Leishmania* parasite can hide itself in skin and lymph node fibroblasts.

In human neutrophils, phagosomes containing promastigotes fuse with myeloperoxidase(mpo) containing primary granules. It is an additional fusion of phagosome with tertiary and specific granules which lead to parasite degradation. These tertiary and specific granules are responsible for acidification and superoxide generation (Fig 2).

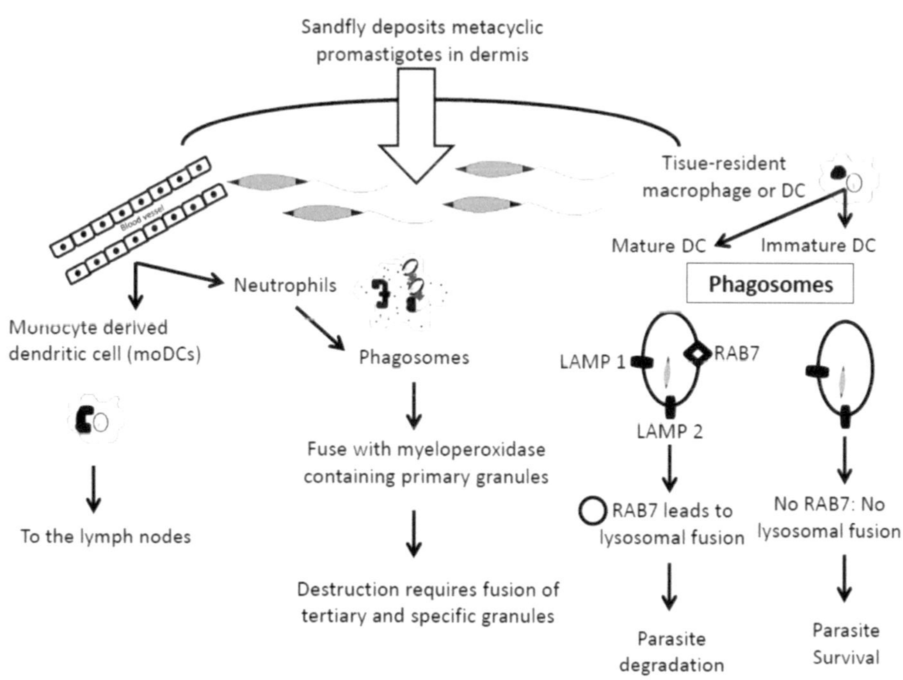

Fig. 2. Different cell types involved in Leishmaniasis and fate of phagosome. Metacyclic promastigotes are deposited in the dermis and taken up by various cells like neutrophils, monocyte derived dendritic cells, macrophages. Small GTPase RAB 7 helps in lysosomal fusion and its degradation. This fusion is inhibited in immature dendritic cells. This could be a mechanism to ensure the transport of live parasites to lymphnodes. Adapted from (Kaye and Scott 2011).

Inside macrophages parasite containing phagosomes mature to form phagolysosome but promastigotes inhibit this process. Lysosomal-associated membrane protein 1 (LAMP 1) and LAMP 2 are found in phagosomes containing *Leishmania* promastigotes in both immature DCs and mature DCs. Maturation of parasite containing phagosomes is arrested at late endosomal stage. Fusion of lysosome occurs with the help of GTPase RAB7 which is observed in mature DCs only. Thus, inhibition of RAB7 recruitment could be a mechanism used by *Leishmania* to transport the live parasites safely to lymph nodes (Lippuner, Paape et al. 2009).

LPG also provides an opportunity for the parasite to survive inside phagosomes by altering acidification (Vinet, Fukuda et al. 2009). Integration of LPG into phagosome membrane leads to extrusion of synaptotagmin V, which helps in acidification of pagosome by recruiting vesicular portion of ATPase. Thus, LPG-deficient parasites die rapidly before they fully adapted to an intracellular lifestyle.

Size of the parasite containing phagosomes also helps in parasite survival. Larger the size more is the dilutional effect on lesihmanicidal factors like nitric oxide. Lysosomal size is regulated by a Beige protein; also known as lysosomal trafficking regulator (LYST). Mutations in LYST gene (Chediak-Higashi syndrome) leads to increase in size of lysosomes whereas induction of this gene (Leishmaniasis) leads to decrease in size of lysosomes. Thus, LYST behaves as an inducible innate response gene during Leishmaniasis, leading to increased susceptible to killing by nitric oxide (Wilson, Huynh et al. 2008).

Iron has an important role in survival of *Leishmania* parasite as it is used by amastigotes (Huynh and Andrews 2008). There is an efflux pump present in phagosomal membrane which translocates Fe^{2+} and Mn^{2+} ions into the cytosol and thus limits iron availability to the parasite (Blackwell, Goswami et al. 2001). To overcome this decrease in iron availability, there occurs an upregulation of iron transporters, after its entry into macrophages. Thus intra-phagosomal competition for iron leads to activation of cytosolic iron sensors which helps in increased production of iron-binding protein transferrin and transferrin-mediated iron uptake (Das, Biswas et al. 2009).

Lipid microdomains present on macrophage surface helps the promastigotes of *Leishmania* to enter into macrophages (Fig 3). It also directs the entry of various virulence factors such as major surface protein also known as GP63 (Joshi, Rodriguez et al. 2009). These virulence factors can also be transferred to the macrophages by parasite-produced exosomes (Silverman and Reiner 2010). When promastigote enters into the phagosome, LPG inserts itself into lipid rafts and inhibits phagosome-lysosome fusion (Winberg, Holm et al. 2009). The inhibition of fusion is accompanied by accumulation of periphagosomal filamentous actin (F-actin) near lipid microdomains. Various virulence factors also use lipid microdomains to channel themselves into cytoplasm of macrophages. Altered lipid rafts may also be responsible for defective antigen presentation and CD40 signalling, MHC class II, major histocompatibility complex class II.

Leishmania is known to activate various inhibitor molecules that inhibit intracellular signaling spathways such as a negative regulatory molecule is the PTP SHP-1 (Src homology 2 domain containing tyrosine phosphatase)(Yi, Cleveland et al. 1992). SHP-1 is responsible for the negative regulation of many signaling pathways (Gregory and Olivier 2005). The majority of documented SHP-1effects are the result of the inhibition by

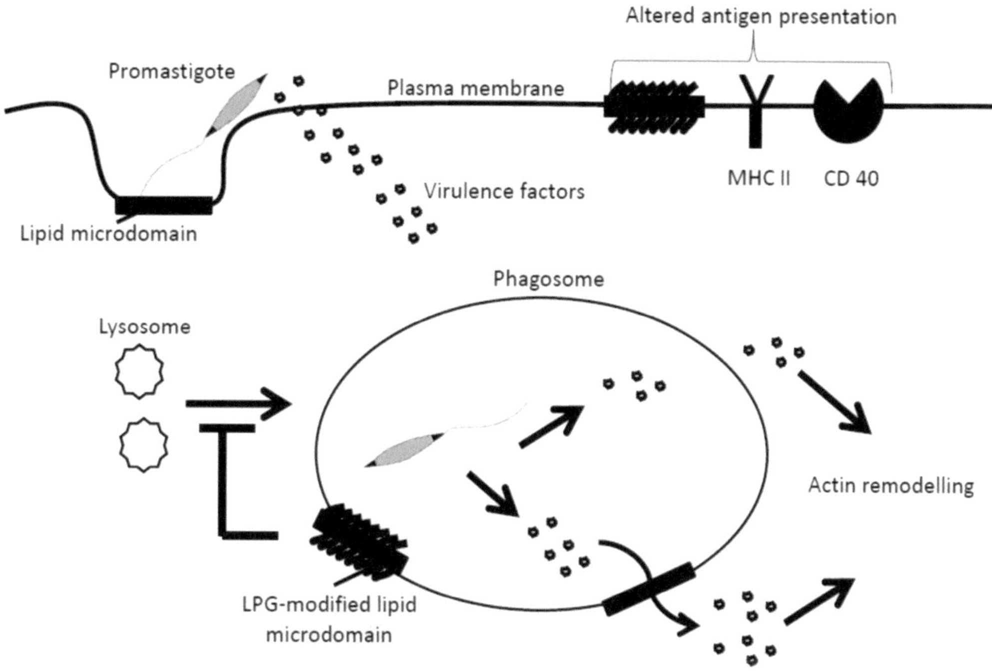

Fig. 3. Lipid microdomains, Leishmania parasite and macrophages. Role of lipid microdomains in transporting parasite and its virulence factors inside macrophages. Altered lipid domains by lipophosphoglycan (LPG) inhibits phagosome-lysosome fusion and also responsible for defective antigen presentation and CD40 signalling, MHC class II. Adapted from (Kaye and Scott 2011).

dephosphorylation of various kinases and their signaling pathways (Frearson and Alexander 1997). SHP-1 plays a vital role in limiting the activation of the JAK/STAT pathways following cytokine receptor stimulation. SHP-1 is known to be activated by MSP (major surface protein, GP63). *Leishmania spp.* contains multiple MSPs and can be found on the promastigote surface as well as in the parasite cytoplasm. Surface MSP is involved in parasite development within sandfly and the cytoplasmic MSP which is in preformed form is ready to use by the mammalian host (Yao, Donelson et al. 2007). This action is analogous to various effectors that are used by type III secretion system in bacteria which behaves like syringe and needle to inject various factors into cells (Winnen, Schlumberger et al. 2008). SHP-2 also known as PTPN 11 also shares many downstream targets with SHP-1 and provides anti-leishmanial immunity. The first line anti-leishmanial drug (sodium stibogluconate) also targets SHP-1 at concentrations that are used for chemotherapy in humans (Pathak and Yi 2001).

Another mechanism used by *Leishmania* parasite when inside the macrophages is by interference with host cell signalling at the level of macrophage protein C (PKC)(Olivier, Baimbridge et al. 1992). After initial contact with the target cells *Leishmania* parasite leads to leads to transient activation of MAPK and NF-kB. These signalling pathways lead to stimulation of cytokines and chemokines required for the efficient control of invading pathogen. Thus, amplitude and duration of this immune response must be maintained under strict control to avoid harmful effects on host itself. Important mechanism by which cells protect themselves is by developing refractoriness state to repeated stimulation. It is well known that prolonged stimulation of toll like receptors and macropahges by microbial components such as LPS (lipopolysaccharide), lead these cells to hyporesponsiveness to the same stimulus (Ben-Othman, Guizani-Tabbane et al. 2008). This phenomenon is termed as LPS tolerance similar phenomenon of and similar hyporesponsiveness is seen in macrophages infected by *L. major* promastigotes. *Leishmania* parasite is able to induce a state of tolerance which correlates with a blockade of intracellular MAPK and/or NF-kB signalling pathway (Ben-Othman, Guizani-Tabbane et al. 2008).

Type 1 interferon response is usually associated with viral infections but their role in leishmaniasis is increasingly becoming important. Such response has been seen in infection with *Leishmaniasis*, which induces the expression in macrophages of PKR, a protein kinase that is activated by double stranded RNA. PKR appears to promote parasite survival through induction of the macrophage-deactivating cytokine IL-10 (Pereira, Teixeira et al. 2010).

$CD4^{+}T_{H}1$ cells are important for the control of *Leishmania* infections, owing their ability to make IFNγ, which activates macrophages and DCs, leading to parasite death (Fig 4). $CD8^{+}$ T cells are known to provide immunity in visceral leishmaniasis and play an important role in resistance to reinfection (Muller, Kropf et al. 1993). $CD8^{+}$ T cells are not always associated with disease resolution as seen in patients infected with *L. braziliensis*. These cells are correlated with disease progression when they express the granule-associated serine protease granzyme B. The factors that determine when $CD8^{+}$ T cells are protective and when they promote disease remain puzzle to the investigators. Chronicity of infection with *L. donovani* appears to be caused by depletion of $CD8^{+}$ T cells (Joshi, Rodriguez et al. 2009). Activation of $CD8^{+}$ T cells depend upon dermal DCs and $CD8^{+}$ T cells activated during Leishmaniasis infections can provide increased resistance to previously encountered pathogens.

Inspite of robust immune response, small number of parasites persist following disease resolution. The production of IL-10 dampens the immune response and allows the some parasites to escape destruction. The IL-10 is produced by a variety of cells following Leishmanial infection, such as regulatory T cells, T helper 1 cells, CD 8^{+} T cells, B cells, natural killer cells, DCs, macrophages and neutrophils. $CD8^{+}CD40^{+}$ T cells may act against regulatory T cells, limiting the production of IL-10 during the early phase of infection, but themselves become susceptible to IL-10 as the infection progresses (Belkaid, Piccirillo et al. 2002; Charmoy, Megnekou et al. 2007; Maroof, Beattie et al. 2008). Exactly how these immune mechanisms operate still remains unanswered and is an active area of research.

Dramatic remodelling occurs when leishmaniasis involve infection of lymphoid tissues like spleen and lymph nodes. Immune suppression occurs due to loss of architectural integrity. Interventions which can restore tissue microarchitecture can have important immune restorative functions.

A concept of concomitant immunity has been proposed in Leishmaniasis. It is a situation in which immunological resistance to reinfection co-exists at the same time as persistence of the original infection. The T cells which contribute to such immunity include CD4+T cells

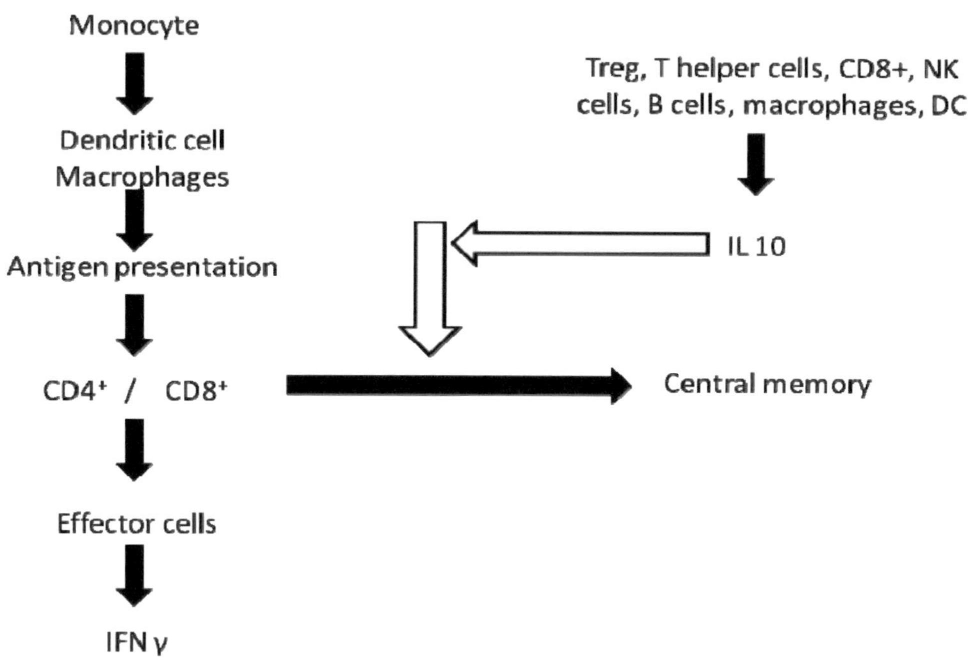

Fig. 4. Cellular components of immune response. Control of response is produced by IL 10, produced by different cell types. Effector cells produce interferon-γ which mediate parasite killing.

with a phenotype of central memory T cells, effector T helper type 1 cells, and resting effector T helper type 1 cells. CD8+ T cells are important in providing resistance to reinfection. Till date no successful vaccine has been developed but recent studies have shown that most protective CD4+ T cells are those which are multifunctional, capable of producing IFNγ, IL-2 and TNF. IL-10 appears to limit the generation of these protective T cells during vaccination (Kedzierski 2010). In future, the application of genomic approaches and study of host factors will lead to a better understanding of pathogenesis and immunology related to leishmaniasis. Further studies are required to investigate unanswered questions related to innate and T cell response in leishmaniasis.

4. *Leishmania* vaccines

WHO has classified Leishmaniasis is an emerging disease. The available treatment options are various chemotherapeutic drugs which are not only costly but also have many adverse side effects. Safe and cost effective vaccine is a need of an hour. Various vaccine strategies have been tried but these are of a little hope. The classical vaccinology or first generation vaccines have been tried in the past which includes infectious material for inoculation, live attenuated parasites and killed parasites for vaccination. Leishmanization, was based on the fact that individual is refractory to reinfection after the lesions of primary illness heals. Initially, infectious lesion material was used but later it was replaced by culture of parasites to inoculate uninfected individuals. This method was abandoned due to poor quality control, parasite persistence, emergence of HIV and ethical issues. Killed parasites replaced leishmanization, but they showed poor efficacy in clinical trials (Noazin, Modabber et al. 2008). Second generation vaccines (modern vaccinology) using subunit vaccines, DNA vaccines and recombinant vaccines are being tried but their efficacy in field trials have not been reported. The major hurdle in vaccine designing is the translation of data from animal models to human disease, and the transition of laboratory experiments to field trials. Table 3 summarizes the important vaccine candidates tested for the cure of leishmaniasis.

Killed vaccines

Vaccination trials in Brazil and Ecuador with killed *Leishmania* stocks have shown to provide immunity from natural infection. Killed vaccination induced Th1 type of immune response and delayed type of hypersensitivity skin test conversion can be used as a surrogate marker for protective immune response (Olivier, Baimbridge et al. 1992; Mendonca, De Luca et al.1995).

Convit and colleagues used a combination of killed *L. mexicana* or *L. braziliensis* promastigotes and *M. bovis* BCG to induce the immunity against South American leishmaniasis. High cure rate have been documented with the induction of Th1 type of immune response (Castes, Moros et al. 1989; Convit and Ulrich 1993). Recombinant IL-12 has been tried as an adjuvant in monkeys to provide the immunity against cutaneous leishmaniasis using killed *L. amazonensis* (Kenney, Sacks et al. 1999)

Live attenuated

Live attenuated vaccines are well known for their better immunogenicity but there are chances of reverting back to virulent forms. However, recent advances in genomics have provided an opportunity to manipulate the *Leishmania* genome by eliminating the virulent genes to produce the attenuated forms. Genes required for long term survival have been manipulated to produce the short lived forms in humans. In a mouse model, *L. major* parasites lacking the gene encoding for enzyme dihydrofolate reductase-thymidylate synthetase DHFR-TS have been produced to induce the protection against infection with either *L. major* or *L. amazonensis.* Mutant lacking genes encoding for cysteine proteases cpa and cpb have also been studied. Thus, the use of attenuated organisms is very useful as it closely mimics to natural infection and can lead to similar immune responses (Titus, Gueiros-Filho et al. 1995).

Synthetic recombinant vaccines:

These newer vaccines include recombinant DNA-derived antigens and peptides. The targets used as antigens may be species or life cycle stage specific. Recombinant antigens can be delivered as purified proteins, as the naked DNA encoding them, or as bacteria manufacturing the proteins of interest. These can be used as a potential vaccine candidate. Bioinformatics can be used to predict the immunogenic peptides which can be synthetically constructed. Though this approach sounds better but it suffers from many disadvantages such as the magnitude of the T-cell memory induced, the inability of all individuals in the population to respond to the peptide, and the high cost of production on large scale. Despite these limitations gp63 peptides have been successfully tested in animals (Campbell et.al 201; Carrión J. 2011).

Immunogens expressing Bacteria and Viruses as vaccines

Leishmaniolysin or gp63 is the first recombinant antigen to be used against as a vaccine candidate against leishmaniasis (Chang, Chaudhuri et al. 1990). The surface expressed glycoprotein leishmaniolysin (gp63) is one of the parasite receptors for host macrophages and mutants lacking this protein are avirulent. However, the T-cell responses to gp63 have been variable in animals and human studies (Olobo, Anjili et al. 1995). Parasite surface antigen have also been tested as a vaccine candidate. gp46/M2 or parasite surface antigen 2 (PSA-2) is expressed in all *Leishmania* species except *L. braziliensis.* Thus, providing an opportunity for developing pan-*Leishmania* vaccine (Handman, Symons et al. 1995). The leishmanial eukaryotic ribosomal protein (LeIF), a homologue of the ribosomal protein cIF4A, is an another important vaccine candidate as it can induce Th1-type cytokines in humans (Skeiky, Coler et al. 2002). This protein is highly conserved in evolution, but parasite specific epitopes can be used for vaccination, so that autoimmune responses can be avoided. Other vaccine candidates are amastigote specific proteins, such as A2, P4, and P8 of *L. mexicana pifanoi* (Soong, Duboise et al. 1995). Another vaccine candidate is a flagellar antigen, lcr1, from *L. donovani chagasi* (Streit, Recker et al. 2000) but its role in humans is debatable as asmastigote forms have a rudimentary flagellum.

Candidate vaccine	Advantages	Disadvantages
Whole killed	Cost effective Good safety profile in South America and Sudan	Quality control, difficult to standardize, variable potency
Surface expressed glycoprotein leishmaniolysin (gp63)	Good results in animals	Poor T cell response in humans
GPI-anchored membrane protein gp46 or Parasite Surface Antigen 2 (PSA-2)	Native polypeptides derived from promastigotes provide protection in mice	Recombinant protein derived from either promastigotes or amastigotes protein showed poor efficacy
Leishmania homologue for receptors of activated C kinase (LACK)	Promote IL-4 secreting T cells (Th2 responses)	Fails to provide protection against visceral leishmaniasis.
Leish-111f: Single molecule constructed by fusion of three molecules: *L. major* homologue of eukaryotic thiol-specific antioxidant (TSA *L. major* stress-inducible protein-1 (LmSTI1) *L. braziliensis* elongation and initiation factor (LeIF) Leish-110f: improved version of Leish-111f	Provides protection in mice against *L. major* and *L. amazonensis* infection Provides partial protection against visceral leishmaniasis in animal models Phase I and II clinical trials done	Failed to protect dogs against infection
Sandfly saliva components: maxadilan, 15 kDa protein, SP15, LJM19	LJM 19: protection in hamsters Dogs: IgG2 and IFN-γ	Experimental stage

Table 3. Summary of important vaccine candidates for leishmaniasis.

DNA vaccine

Vaccinations with DNA encoding gp63and PSA-2 have been tried. It has shown a good protection in animal models which is accompanied by Th1 immune responses (Gurunathan, Sacks et al. 1997; Walker, Scharton-Kersten et al. 1998). The genes encoding the vaccine candidate is cloned into mammalian expression vector, and the DNA is injected directly into muscle or skin. The plasmid DNA is taken up by cells and translocated to the nucleus, where it is transcribed into RNA and then translated in the cytoplasm. It has shown to induce both $CD4^+$ and $CD8^+$ T cell responses and they also ensure proper folding of proteins. Another advantage is that production on large scale is cheap and DNA is highly stable, so does not require cold chain. Research is still going on for developing a vaccine which can provide life long immunity without any side effects. Newer adjuvants are also being tried. Till date no successful vaccine has been developed but recent studies have shown that most protective CD4+ T cells are those which are multifunctional, capable of producing IFNγ, IL-2 and TNF. IL-10 appears to limit the generation of these protective T cells during vaccination (Kedzierski 2010). In future, the application of genomic approaches and study of host factors will lead to a better understanding of pathogenesis and immunology related to leishmaniasis. Further studies are required to investigate unanswered questions related to innate and T cell response in leishmaniasis.

5. Conclusions

Recent studies have provided new and important information on the biology of *Leishmania*. The *Leishmania* genome sequence is now available as well as new methods for its manipulation. We have learned that *Leishmania* can exchange genetic material during its journey in the sand fly, and we understand better the molecular mechanisms that allow *Leishmania* promastigotes and amastigotes to survive in their respective environments. Recent investigation have provided new insight into the role of cells of the innate immunity, such as neutrophils, monocytes, NK, and DCs, as well as 'non-immune' cells such as keratinocytes. Now we have better understand how *Leishmania* evade the mammalian immune response and avoid the development of sterilizing immunity, therefore increasing its chances to secure transmission to a new host. The identification of a greater range of antigen candidates with broad species coverage, and a greater understanding of the immunology of protective immunity, these arguments should be balanced by the need to develop a stronger base in clinical vaccinology. This end is only likely to be accomplished by an accelerated programme of well-defined clinical trials, and in this context the use of therapeutic vaccine trials as a first step has much to offer. New generation vaccines hold promises to control leishmaniasis and data suggest that prophylactic vaccination in humans and dogs could generate protection and may able to interrupt transmission, ultimately reducing disease incidence. These new generation vaccines in a therapeutic setting as an adjunct with various chemotherapies have demonstrated safety and efficacy against various manifestations of *Leishmania* infection. New generation's refined antigens and adjuvants for vaccines may provide the best range of vaccines aimed at controlling disease incidence and severity to *Leishmania* infection.

6. References

Belkaid, Y., C. A. Piccirillo, et al. (2002). "CD4+CD25+ regulatory T cells control Leishmania major persistence and immunity." Nature 420(6915): 502-507.

Ben-Othman, R., L. Guizani-Tabbane, et al. (2008). "Leishmania initially activates but subsequently down-regulates intracellular mitogen-activated protein kinases and nuclear factor-kappaB signaling in macrophages." Mol Immunol 45(11): 3222-3229.

Blackwell, J. M., T. Goswami, et al. (2001). "SLC11A1 (formerly NRAMP1) and disease resistance." Cell Microbiol 3(12): 773-784.

Castes, M., Z. Moros, et al. (1989). "Cell-mediated immunity in localized cutaneous leishmaniasis patients before and after treatment with immunotherapy or chemotherapy." Parasite Immunol 11(3): 211-222.

CFSPH (2009). "The Center for Food Security and Public Health, I.S.U., Leishmaniasis (cutaneous & visceral). Animal Disease Resource Index. Fact Sheet."

Chang, K. P., G. Chaudhuri, et al. (1990). "Molecular determinants of Leishmania virulence." Annu Rev Microbiol 44: 499-529.

Charmoy, M., S. Brunner-Agten, et al. (2010). "Neutrophil-derived CCL3 is essential for the rapid recruitment of dendritic cells to the site of Leishmania major inoculation in resistant mice." PLoS Pathog 6(2): e1000755.

Charmoy, M., R. Megnekou, et al. (2007). "Leishmania major induces distinct neutrophil phenotypes in mice that are resistant or susceptible to infection." J Leukoc Biol 82(2): 288-299.

Convit, J. and M. Ulrich (1993). "Antigen-specific immunodeficiency and its relation to the spectrum of American cutaneous leishmaniasis." Biol Res 26(1-2): 159-166.

Das, N. K., S. Biswas, et al. (2009). "Leishmania donovani depletes labile iron pool to exploit iron uptake capacity of macrophage for its intracellular growth." Cell Microbiol 11(1): 83-94.

Frearson, J. A. and D. R. Alexander (1997). "The role of phosphotyrosine phosphatases in haematopoietic cell signal transduction." Bioessays 19(5): 417-427.

Gabriel, C., W. R. McMaster, et al. (2010). "Leishmania donovani promastigotes evade the antimicrobial activity of neutrophil extracellular traps." J Immunol 185(7): 4319-4327.

Gelanew, T., K. Kuhls, et al. (2010). "Inference of population structure of Leishmania donovani strains isolated from different Ethiopian visceral leishmaniasis endemic areas." PLoS Negl Trop Dis 4(11): e889.

Gomez, M. A., I. Contreras, et al. (2009). "Leishmania GP63 alters host signaling through cleavage-activated protein tyrosine phosphatases." Sci Signal 2(90): ra58.

Gregory, D. J. and M. Olivier (2005). "Subversion of host cell signalling by the protozoan parasite Leishmania." Parasitology 130 Suppl: S27-35.

Gurunathan, S., D. L. Sacks, et al. (1997). "Vaccination with DNA encoding the immunodominant LACK parasite antigen confers protective immunity to mice infected with Leishmania major." J Exp Med 186(7): 1137-1147.

Handman, E., F. M. Symons, et al. (1995). "Protective vaccination with promastigote surface antigen 2 from Leishmania major is mediated by a TH1 type of immune response." Infect Immun 63(11): 4261-4267.

Haraldsen, G., J. Balogh, et al. (2009). "Interleukin-33 - cytokine of dual function or novel alarmin?" Trends Immunol 30(5): 227-233.

Huynh, C. and N. W. Andrews (2008). "Iron acquisition within host cells and the pathogenicity of Leishmania." Cell Microbiol 10(2): 293-300.

Joshi, T., S. Rodriguez, et al. (2009). "B7-H1 blockade increases survival of dysfunctional CD8(+) T cells and confers protection against Leishmania donovani infections." PLoS Pathog 5(5): e1000431.

Kaye, P. and P. Scott (2011). "Leishmaniasis: complexity at the host-pathogen interface." Nat Rev Microbiol 9(8): 604-615.

Kedzierski, L. (2010). "Leishmaniasis Vaccine: Where are We Today?" J Glob Infect Dis 2(2): 177-185.

Kenney, R. T., D. L. Sacks, et al. (1999). "Protective immunity using recombinant human IL-12 and alum as adjuvants in a primate model of cutaneous leishmaniasis." J Immunol 163(8): 4481-4488.

Lippuner, C., D. Paape, et al. (2009). "Real-time imaging of Leishmania mexicana-infected early phagosomes: a study using primary macrophages generated from green fluorescent protein-Rab5 transgenic mice." Faseb J 23(2): 483-491.

Lopez Kostka, S., S. Dinges, et al. (2009). "IL-17 promotes progression of cutaneous leishmaniasis in susceptible mice." J Immunol 182(5): 3039-3046.

Maroof, A., L. Beattie, et al. (2008). "Posttranscriptional regulation of Il10 gene expression allows natural killer cells to express immunoregulatory function." Immunity 29(2): 295-305.

Mendonca, S. C., P. M. De Luca, et al. (1995). "Characterization of human T lymphocyte-mediated immune responses induced by a vaccine against American tegumentary leishmaniasis." Am J Trop Med Hyg 53(2): 195-201.

Muller, I., P. Kropf, et al. (1993). "Gamma interferon response in secondary Leishmania major infection: role of CD8+ T cells." Infect Immun 61(9): 3730-3738.

Ng, L. G., A. Hsu, et al. (2008). "Migratory dermal dendritic cells act as rapid sensors of protozoan parasites." PLoS Pathog 4(11): e1000222.

Noazin, S., F. Modabber, et al. (2008). "First generation leishmaniasis vaccines: a review of field efficacy trials." Vaccine 26(52): 6759-6767.

Olivier, M., K. G. Baimbridge, et al. (1992). "Stimulus-response coupling in monocytes infected with Leishmania. Attenuation of calcium transients is related to defective agonist-induced accumulation of inositol phosphates." J Immunol 148(4): 1188-1196.

Olobo, J. O., C. O. Anjili, et al. (1995). "Vaccination of vervet monkeys against cutaneous leishmaniosis using recombinant Leishmania 'major surface glycoprotein' (gp63)." Vet Parasitol 60(3-4): 199-212.

Pathak, M. K. and T. Yi (2001). "Sodium stibogluconate is a potent inhibitor of protein tyrosine phosphatases and augments cytokine responses in hemopoietic cell lines." J Immunol 167(6): 3391-3397.

Pereira, R. M., K. L. Teixeira, et al. (2010). "Novel role for the double-stranded RNA-activated protein kinase PKR: modulation of macrophage infection by the protozoan parasite Leishmania." Faseb J 24(2): 617-626.

Ravichandran, K. S. and U. Lorenz (2007). "Engulfment of apoptotic cells: signals for a good meal." Nat Rev Immunol 7(12): 964-974.

Silverman, J. M. and N. E. Reiner (2010). "Exosomes and other microvesicles in infection biology: organelles with unanticipated phenotypes." Cell Microbiol 13(1): 1-9.

Skeiky, Y. A., R. N. Coler, et al. (2002). "Protective efficacy of a tandemly linked, multi-subunit recombinant leishmanial vaccine (Leish-111f) formulated in MPL adjuvant." Vaccine 20(27-28): 3292-3303.

Soong, L., S. M. Duboise, et al. (1995). "Leishmania pifanoi amastigote antigens protect mice against cutaneous leishmaniasis." Infect Immun 63(9): 3559-3566.

Streit, J. A., T. J. Recker, et al. (2000). "BCG expressing LCR1 of Leishmania chagasi induces protective immunity in susceptible mice." Exp Parasitol 94(1): 33-41.

Titus, R. G., F. J. Gueiros-Filho, et al. (1995). "Development of a safe live Leishmania vaccine line by gene replacement." Proc Natl Acad Sci U S A 92(22): 10267-10271.

Vinet, A. F., M. Fukuda, et al. (2009). "The Leishmania donovani lipophosphoglycan excludes the vesicular proton-ATPase from phagosomes by impairing the recruitment of synaptotagmin V." PLoS Pathog 5(10): e1000628.

Walker, P. S., T. Scharton-Kersten, et al. (1998). "Genetic immunization with glycoprotein 63 cDNA results in a helper T cell type 1 immune response and protection in a murine model of leishmaniasis." Hum Gene Ther 9(13): 1899-1907.

WHO (2004). "Scientific working group on Leishmaniasis. Meeting report. 2–4 February 2004, Geneva, Switzerland. http://apps.who.int/tdr/publications/tdr-research-publications/swg-report-leishmaniasis/pdf/swg_leish.pdf.".

WHO (2010). "WHO, Control of the Leishmanises, in WHO Technical Report Series 2010, World Health Organization: Geneva. ."

Wilson, J., C. Huynh, et al. (2008). "Control of parasitophorous vacuole expansion by LYST/Beige restricts the intracellular growth of Leishmania amazonensis." PLoS Pathog 4(10): e1000179.

Winberg, M. E., A. Holm, et al. (2009). "Leishmania donovani lipophosphoglycan inhibits phagosomal maturation via action on membrane rafts." Microbes Infect 11(2): 215-222.

Winnen, B., M. C. Schlumberger, et al. (2008). "Hierarchical effector protein transport by the Salmonella Typhimurium SPI-1 type III secretion system." PLoS One 3(5): e2178.

Xin, L., D. A. Vargas-Inchaustegui, et al. (2010). "Type I IFN receptor regulates neutrophil functions and innate immunity to Leishmania parasites." J Immunol 184(12): 7047-7056.

Yao, C., J. E. Donelson, et al. (2007). "Internal and surface-localized major surface proteases of Leishmania spp. and their differential release from promastigotes." Eukaryot Cell 6(10): 1905-1912.

Yi, T. L., J. L. Cleveland, et al. (1992). "Protein tyrosine phosphatase containing SH2 domains: characterization, preferential expression in hematopoietic cells, and localization to human chromosome 12p12-p13." Mol Cell Biol 12(2): 836-846.

19

Adaptive Immunity from Prokaryotes to Eukaryotes: Broader Inclusions Due to Less Exclusivity?

Edwin L. Cooper
Laboratory of Comparative Neuroimmunology
Department of Neurobiology, David Geffen School of Medicine at UCLA
University of California, Los Angeles
USA

1. Introduction

1.1 The prevailing view: blurring, innate and adaptive

The currently held view of the immune system proposes generally acceptable descriptions supported by strong evidence. There are two primary systems: innate and adaptive but distributed "unequally" among the two major animal groups (ignoring mostly all plants). Animal groups include the multitudinous invertebrates and vertebrates with vertebrates being the greatest beneficiaries of a fully functional complex immune apparatus that combines the two systems. Despite this super armamentarium, the overwhelming problems of possessing this dual system, as the vertebrates i.e. the innate and adaptive does not seem to guard or even prevent the development of one internal threat to survival. This is the scourge: development of cancer. By contrast invertebrates whose immune system is primarily of the innate type manage to eat, reproduce and survive without developing cancer. Briefly the immune system consists of: Innate: natural, nonspecific, no memory, non-anticipatory, non-clonal, germ line; Adaptive: acquired, specific, memory, anticipatory, clonal, somatic. In general, both systems and in the simplest reductionist terms, each must possess a cell that recognizes an antigen and digests it. The second cell if appropriately stimulated must react to destroy a potentially detrimental antigen. During evolution more cells were added to this armamentarium giving rise to increasing functions associated with effector activity. Emerging information supports the view that overlap or blurring exists between these two sometimes rigidly defined systems. Clearly evidence suggests that lines of demarcation within and between innate and adaptive may not be so strictly delineated—there is immunologic flexibility designated as blurring, not "black and white".

1.2 Evolution of the immune systems

1.2.1 The agnathans (jawless fish)

We have been alerted to numerous analyses of the vertebrate and more specifically the mammalian immune system that reveal profound interrelationships and fundamental differences between the adaptive and innate systems of immune recognition (Fig.) [Du

Pasquier and Litman, 2000]. There is increasing experimental accessibility of non-mammalian jawed vertebrates (*gnathosomes; cartilaginous* and bony fish), jawless vertebrates (*agnathans*) (hagfish, lampreys), protochordates and invertebrates and an enthusiasm by comparative immunologists to explore. Thus we have intriguing new information that suggests likely patterns that reveal emergence of immune-related molecules during metazoan phylogeny. Moreover there is the promise that we may find evolution of alternative mechanisms that ensure receptor diversification. These such findings have already blurred traditional distinctions between adaptive and innate immunity. The adaptive must rely on the innate throughout evolution, the immune system has benefited by using a remarkably extensive variety of well-equipped mechanistic solutions to meet fundamentally similar requirements for host protection.

The range of such molecules, which includes the fibrinogen-related proteins (FREPs) in a mollusk, variable regioncontaining chitin-binding proteins (VCBPs) in a cephalochordate, variable lymphocyte receptors (VLRs) in jawless vertebrates, and novel immune-type receptors (NITRs) in bony fish, encompasses both the immunoglobulin gene superfamily (IgSF) and leucine-rich repeat (LRR) proteins. Although these molecules vary markedly in form and likely in function, growing evidence suggests that they participate in various types of host immune responses. These results represent significant alternatives to prevailing paradigms of innate and adaptive immune receptors. Thus unusual genetic mechanisms may support mechanisms for diversifying recognition proteins and it may be a ubiquitous characteristic of animal immunity (Fig. 2) (Theodor, 1970; Hildemann et al, 1977; Franc et al, 1996; Pancer, 2000; Watson et al, 2005; Sun et al, 1990; Flajnik and Pasquier, 2004; Zhang et al, 2004), not restricted rigidly to innate and adaptive.

Our immune system rarely acts alone but functions in association with the other two linked regulating systems (the nervous and endocrine systems; not to be examined in this review). Second, when we examine the immune systems close up, there are several generalizations that emerge. The immune system is ubiquitous, found in all creatures including plants and is therefore not restricted to humans. If carefully traced stepwise during evolution treating extremely limited fossil forms, reveals progressively more complex development after we critically examine various levels of plant and animal evolution. There is evidence for innate immunity in plants. According to Luke and O'Neill (2011), "Every organism has to contend with the risk of infection. To cope, organisms have evolved two types of immune responses: the more recent "adaptive" system, found only in vertebrates; and the more ancient "innate" system, which is present in both plants and animals. Researchers have uncovered remarkable evolutionary conservation of innate immune mechanisms between plants and animals. (Figure 3) They use similar receptor molecules to sense pathogens and for immune system signaling (Luke and O'Neill 2011).

This review will: 1) for the first time present an emerging view that "adaptive immunity" mechanisms need not be restricted to complex eukaryotic organisms. Although this may be revolutionary, we might ask: why not since microbes survive? In fact, there is compelling information that prokaryotes may possess adaptive immune mechanisms; 2) deemphasize the over reliance on embryologically defining the animal kingdom and forcing the immune system's evolution into two separate categories, i.e. the protostomes and deuterostomes; 3) support concepts that propelled the immune system into prominent discourse in the life sciences; 4) indicate that the concern for immunologic memory, development of cancer, autoimmunity, and clonal selection may not be essential for effective immunity to evolve; 5) consider analogous mechanisms in prokaryotes that concern CRISPR that are direct repeats found in the DNA of many bacteria and archaea; 6) to understand the mechanism of action of CRISPR systems reveals a prokaryotic analog of eukaryotic RNA supporting the view that bacteria possess a form of acquired immunity; 7) suggest a molecular mechanism by which the nervous system may sense inflammatory responses and respond by controlling stress response pathways at the organismal level; This supports the interconnectedness of two of the three monitoring systems: immune<>nervous<> endocrine to maintain a balanced internal milieu.

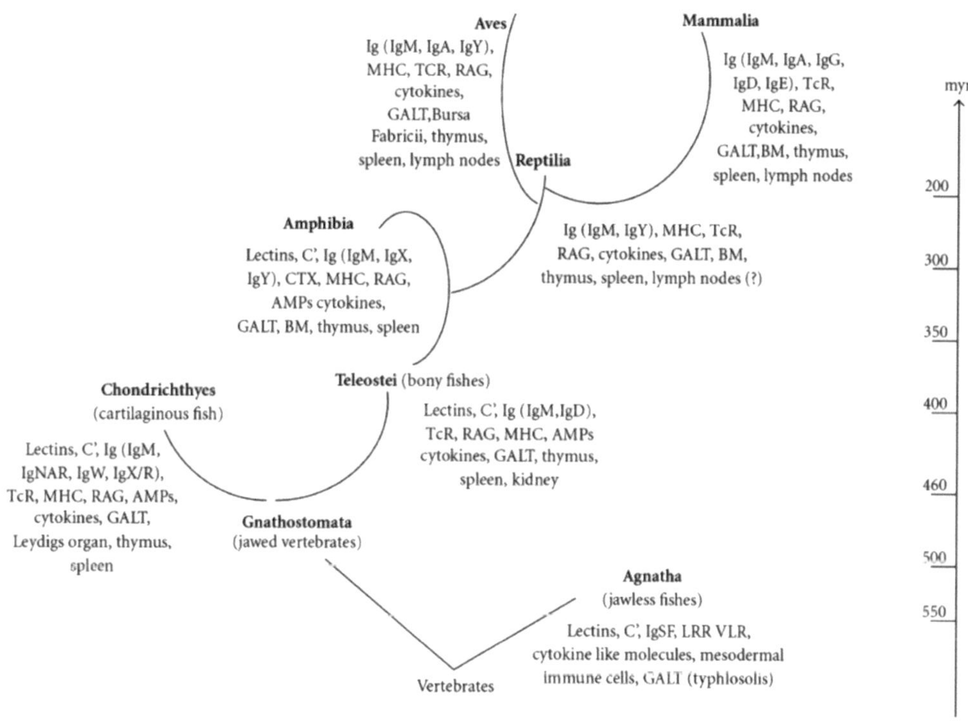

AMP: antimicrobial peptides
C': complement pathway elements
Ig: immunoglobulin
CTX: cortical thymocyte marker in *Xenopus*
LRR VLR: variable lymphocyte receptors with leucine rich repeats
MHC: major histocompatibility complex
GALT: gut associated limphoid tissue
BM: bone marrow
NAR: new ("nurse shark") antigen receptor
RAG: recombination activating genes
TCR: T cell receptor

Fig. 1. Evolution of molecular and histological structures of the vertebrate immune system. Regarding lymphatic tissues, the thymus, and spleen appeared early in fishes, while lymph filtering lymph nodes are observed only in birds and mammals. Among the development of various immunoglobulin isotypes, IgD is expressed in bony fishes, later only mammals are using this B-cell receptor. Reproduced by permission from (Kvell K, Cooper EL, Engelmann P, Bovari J, Nemeth P. Blurring borders: Innate immunity with adaptive features. Clin Dev Immunol (2007):836–71).

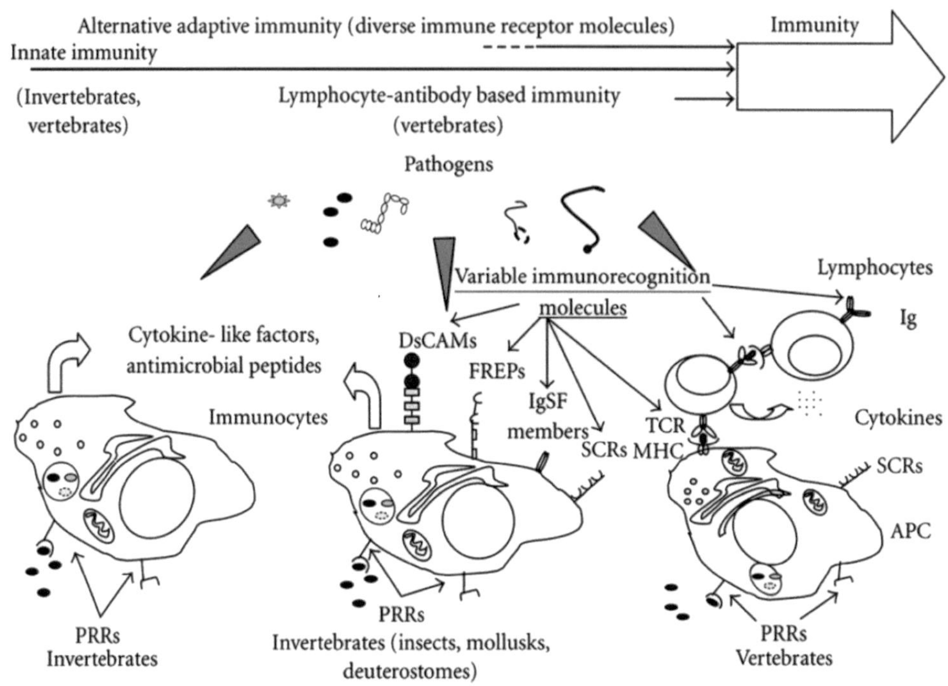

Fig. 2. Schematic representation of innate and adaptive immune feature development in animals. All immune cells express nonspecific receptors, for example, pattern recognition receptors that recognize pathogen associated molecular patterns (PAMPs). Several clusters of innate receptors are conserved from plants to humans and are essential components in the defense of self-integrity. Immune cells of invertebrates also express various scavenger receptor-like proteins (Croquemort, SCRs), immunoglobulin superfamily members (hemolin, DsCAM), and fibrinogen-related peptides (FREPs); all involved in immune functions (eliminating apoptotic cells, parasites, etc.). Invertebrate immune systems also exhibit receptors with high diversity involved in immune functions: FREPs, SCRs, and DsCAMs have extreme individual variability-like vertebrate adaptive immune recognition molecules (Ig, TcR). Reproduced by permission from (Kvell K, Cooper EL, Engelmann P, Bovari J, Nemeth P. Blurring borders: Innate immunity with adaptive features. Clin Dev Immunol (2007):836–71).

1.3 Self/ not-self

Now *Self/not self, adaptive immunity* and a fresh and renewed vision of a vigorous *innate immunity* are acceptable first for invertebrates and now essential for mammals. However, self/not self is now challenged by the controversial, alternative *danger hypothesis*. (Cooper, 2010; Cooper et al, 2002; Engelmann and Nemeth, 2010; Cossarizza, 2010; Parrinello 2010 Pradeu and Carosella 2004; 2006). Since Metchnikoff discovered phagocytosis, controversy persisted concerning two points. First, innate immunity was accorded minor significance to most of immunology while adaptive immunity emerged as predominant, perhaps due to anthropocentricity of 19th and early 20th century immunologists. Later adaptive immunity acquired a significant hypothetical base. Second, clonal selection and specific memory cast a shadow over Metchnikoff's leukocytes, perhaps bolstered by discovering them in invertebrates and not in mammals (Cooper, 2008; Cooper 2010)

Pradeu and Carosella criticize origins and legitimacy of self/non-self. They advocate a critical analysis both conceptually and experimentally to redefine self/non-self that reveals certain shortcomings; they even advocate possibly rejecting that model in favor of an alternative theoretical view for immunology: *continuity*. The *'continuity hypothesis'* attempts to support immunogenicity that avoids criticism of the self-model. Pradeu and Carosella assert that the main objective of immunology is to establish why (teleological?) and when an immune response occurs: to support immunogenicity. Is there an experimental model?

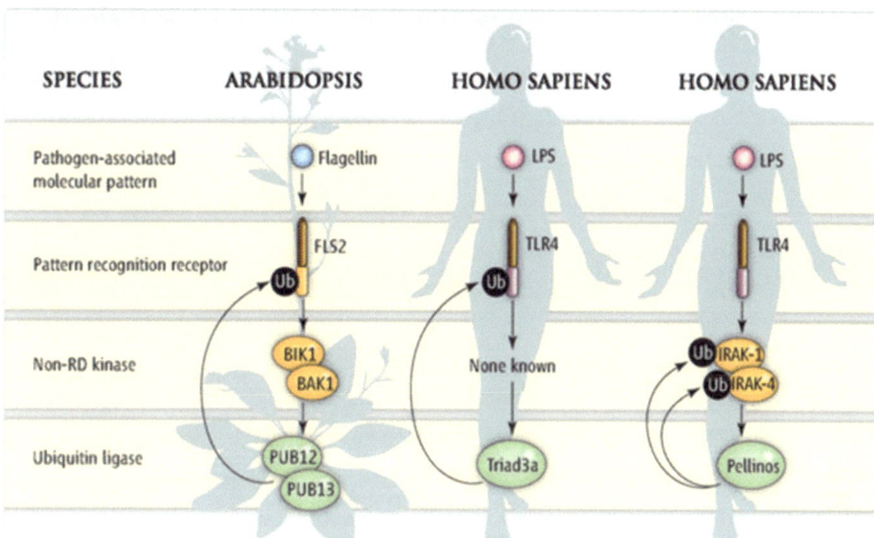

Fig. 3. Innate immunity, conserved.

Arabidopsis and humans have evolutionarily conserved innate immune signaling processes that involve a posttranslational modification process called ubiquitination. In Arabidopsis, bacterial flagellin is sensed by FLS2, which recruits the non-arginine/aspartate (Non-RD) kinases BAK1 and BIK1. BAK1 phosphorylates and activates PUB12/13, which ubiquitinates (Ub) FLS2 and leads to degradation. In humans, TLR4 senses lipopolysaccharide (LPS). This can activate Triad3a (third column), which ubiquitinates TLR4 and leads to its degradation. TLR4 can also activate IRAK-1 and IRAK-4 (fourth column), which activates nuclear factor kappa B (not shown), and also Pellino proteins (Pellinos), which ubiquitinate the IRAKs and lead to their degradation.

1.4 Clonal selection

Another view pertinent to prevailing immunologic concepts includes clonal selection which is a Darwinian corollary. In other words lymphocytes with appropriate receptors could be stimulated to divide leaving progenitor offspring lymphocytes. Now we may be able to deconstruct clonal selection since it may be not applicable to invertebrate mechanisms; all evidence indicates that clonal selection is purely a vertebrate strategy. Some views may insist that anthropocentric mammalian immunologists utilized a tool to propel: the universal innate immune system of ubiquitous and plentiful invertebrates as an essential system for vertebrates. Immunology benefited and innate immunity acquired an extended *raison d'être*. Innate immunity should help if there is a failure of the adaptive immune system. As an internal threat cancer would be subject to the immune system's efficiency. Still to be answered are questions concerning immunologic surveillance that includes clonal selection. According to the question does immunologic surveillance play a role in the survival of invertebrates that seem to not develop cancer as we identify metastasizing transplantable vertebrate type? As a possible explanation, perhaps invertebrate efficient innate immune systems and short life spans evolved certain "canceling devices" that maintain survival, thus precluding their demise by metastasis. (Cooper et al, 2002; Burnet, 1959; Burnet 1962)

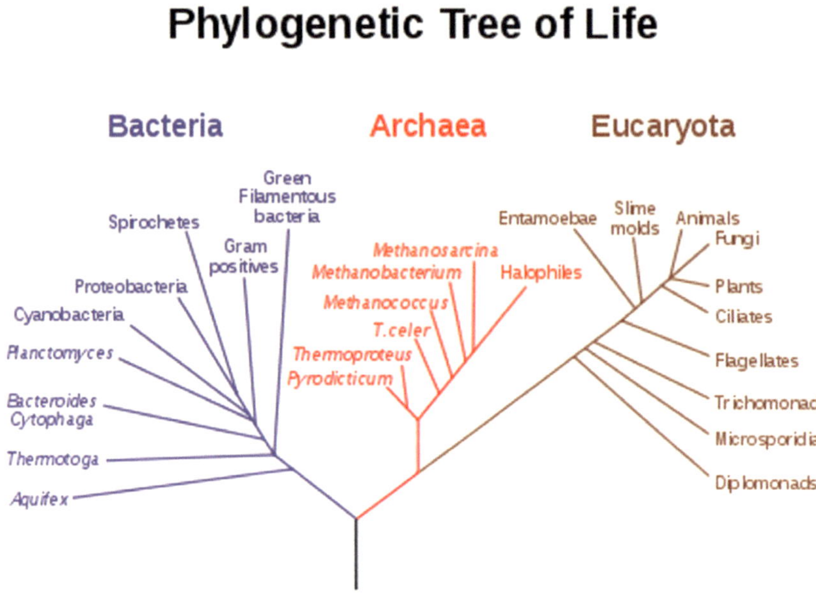

Fig. 4. A phylogenetic tree of living things, based on RNA data and proposed by Carl Woese, showing the separation of bacteria, archaea, and eukaryotes. Trees constructed with other genes are generally similar, although they may place some early-branching groups very differently, thanks to long branch attraction. The exact relationships of the three domains are still being debated, as is the position of the root of the tree. It has also been suggested that due to lateral gene transfer, a tree may not be the best representation of the genetic relationships of all organisms. For instance some genetic evidence suggests that eukaryotes evolved from the union of some bacteria and archaea (one becoming an organelle and the other the main cell). Author : Eric Gaba. Published : Sep. 2006. Nasa Astrobiology Institute. http://en.wikipedia.org/wiki/File:Phylogenetic_tree.svg

2. What are prokaryotes?

It is essential to define prokaryotes. The prokaryotes are a group of organisms that lack a cell nucleus (= karyon), or any other membrane-bound organelles. The organisms that have a cell nucleus are called eukaryotes. (Figure 4) Most prokaryotes are unicellular, but a few such as myxobacteria have multicellular stages in their life cycles. The word *prokaryote* comes from the Greek *πρό- (pro-)* "before" + *καρυόν (karyon)* "nut or kernel". Prokaryotes do not have a nucleus, mitochondria, or any other membrane-bound organelles. In other words, neither their DNA nor any of their other sites of metabolic activity are collected together in a discrete membrane-enclosed area. Instead, everything is openly accessible within the cell, some of which is free-floating. Prokaryotes belong to two taxonomic domains: the bacteria and the archaea. Archaea were recognized as a domain of life in 1990. These organisms were originally thought to live only in inhospitable conditions such as extremes of temperature, pH, and radiation but have since been found in all types of habitats."

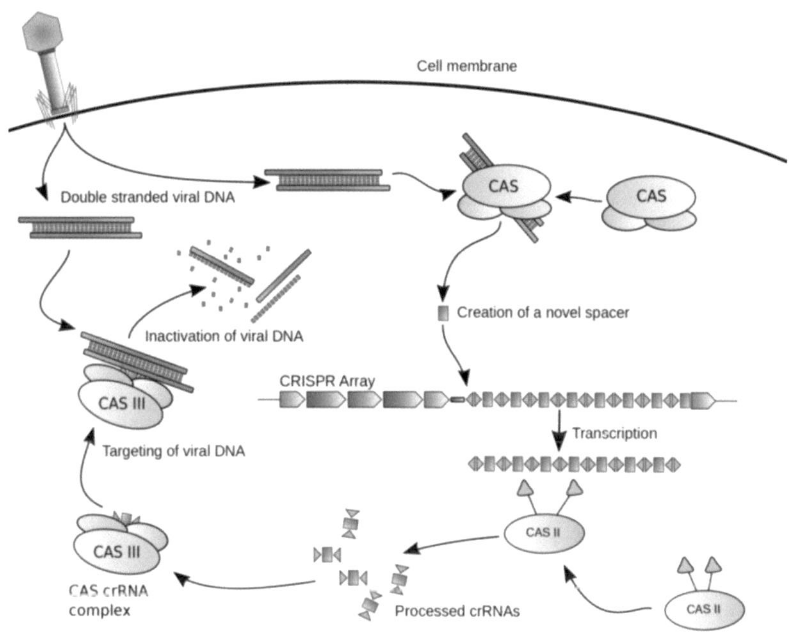

Fig. 5. Diagram of the possible mechanism for CRISPR. http://en.wikipedia.org/wiki/File:Crispr.png Author: James Atmos 15 September 2009.

3. CRIPSR: Clustered, Regularly Interspaced Short Palindromic Repeat

3.1 CRIPSR (Clustered Regularly Interspaced Short Palindromic Repeats)

CRISPRs are loci containing multiple short direct repeats that are found in the genomes of approximately 40% of bacteria and 90% of archaea. CRISPR functions as a prokaryotic immune system, in that it confers resistance to exogenous genetic elements such as plasmids and phages. The CRISPR system provides a form of acquired immunity. Short segments of foreign DNA, called spacers, are incorporated into the genome between CRISPR repeats, and serve as a 'memory' of past exposures. CRISPR spacers are used to recognize and silence exogenous genetic elements in a way analogous to RNAi in eukaryotic organisms (Fig 5) (2, Grissa et al 2007; Barrangou et al 2007; Marraffini and Sontheimer 2010; Marraddini and Sontheimer 2010).

3.2 Self versus non-self discrimination during CRISPS RNA-directed immunity

All immune systems must distinguish self from non-self to repel invaders without inducing autoimmunity. Clustered, regularly interspaced, short palindromic repeat (CRISPR) loci protect bacteria and archaea from invasion by phage and plasmid DNA through a genetic interference pathway. CRISPR loci are present in ~ 40% and ~90% of sequenced bacterial and archaeal genomes respectively and evolve rapidly, acquiring new spacer sequences to adapt to highly dynamic viral populations. Immunity requires a sequence match between the invasive DNA and the spacers that lie between CRISPR repeats[1]. Each cluster is genetically linked to a subset of the *cas* (CRISPR-associated) genes that collectively encode >40 families of proteins involved in adaptation and interference. CRISPR loci encode small CRISPR RNAs (crRNAs) that contain a full spacer flanked by partial repeat sequences. CrRNA spacers are thought to identify targets by direct Watson-Crick pairing with invasive "protospacer" DNA, but how they avoid targeting the spacer DNA within the encoding CRISPR locus itself is unknown. Here we have defined the mechanism of CRISPR self/non-self discrimination. In *Staphylococcus epidermidis*, target/crRNA mismatches at specific positions outside of the spacer sequence license foreign DNA for interference, whereas extended pairing between crRNA and CRISPR DNA repeats prevents autoimmunity. Hence, this CRISPR system uses the base-pairing potential of crRNAs not only to specify a target but also to spare the bacterial chromosome from interference. Differential complementarity outside of the spacer sequence is a built-in feature of all CRISPR systems, suggesting that this mechanism is a broadly applicable solution to the self/non-self dilemma that confronts all immune pathways" (Marrafini & Sontheimer 2010).

3.3 CRISPR based adaptive and heritable immunity in prokaryotes

The recently discovered CRISPR (clustered regularly interspaced short palindromic repeat) defense system protects bacteria and archaea against mobile genetic elements. This immunity system has potential to continuously adjust its reach at the genomic level, implying that both gain and loss of information is inheritable. The CRISPR system consists of typical stretches of interspaced repetitive DNA (CRISPRs) and associated cas genes (van der Oost et al. 2009).

3.4 Hallmark of ingenious antiviral defense mechanisms

According to Al-Attar et al, many prokaryotes contain the recently discovered defense system against mobile genetic elements. (i) CRISPR-Adaptation, the invader DNA is encountered by the CRISPR/Cas machinery and an invader-derived short DNA fragment is incorporated in the CRISPR array. (ii) CRISPR-Expression, the CRISPR array is transcribed and the transcript is processed by Cas proteins. (iii) CRISPR-Interference, the invaders' nucleic acid is recognized by complementarity to the crRNA and neutralized (2011). An application of the CRISPR/Cas system is the immunization of industry-relevant prokaryotes (or eukaryotes) against mobile-genetic invasion. In addition, the high variability of the CRISPR spacer content can be exploited for phylogenetic and evolutionary studies. Despite impressive progress during the last couple of years, the elucidation of several fundamental details will be a major challenge in future research. (Fig 5)

3.5 Structural basis for CRIPSR RNA-guided DNA recognition by cascade and biology seahorse vs. pathogen

Here is the composition and low-resolution structure of casecade and how it recognizes double-stranded DNA (dsDNA) targets in a sequence-specific manner. Cascade is a 405-kDa complex comprising five functionally essential CRISPR-associated (Cas) proteins (CasA(1)B(2)C(6)D(1)E(1)) and a 61-nucleotide CRISPR RNA (crRNA) with 5'-hydroxyl and 2',3'-cyclic phosphate termini. Cascade recognizes target DNA without consuming ATP, which suggests that continuous invader DNA surveillance takes place without energy investment. The structure of Cascade shows an unusual seahorse shape that undergoes conformational changes when it binds target DNA (Jore et al. 2011). Jore et al. have analyzed the composition and low-resolution structure of the Cascade complex, which lies at the heart of the CRISPR Immune response. The snippets of invader sequence are transcribed and converted into CRISPR RNA (crRNA), which is bound by the Cascade complex. The overall structure of the Cascade complex surprisingly resembled the shape of the seahorse, with the spine and head consisting of a tight curved polymer of six CasC protein subunits, which might binf the crRNA- GR (Riddihough 2011).

3.6 Structures of the RNA-guided surveillance complex from a bacterial immune system

According to Wiedenheft et al (2011), bacteria and archaea acquire resistance to viruses and plasmids by integrating short fragments of foreign DNA into clustered regularly interspaced short palindromic repeats (CRISPRs). In *Escherichia coli*, crRNAs are incorporated into a multisubunit surveillance complex called Cascade (CRISPR-associated complex for antiviral defence), which is required for protection against bacteriophages. They used cryo-electron microscopy to determine the subnanometre structures of Cascade before and after binding to a target sequence. Cascade engages invading nucleic acids through high-affinity base-pairing interactions near the 5′ end of the crRNA. Base pairing extends along the crRNA, resulting in a series of short helical segments that trigger a concerted conformational change. This conformational rearrangement may serve as a signal that recruits a trans acting nuclease (Cas3) for destruction of invading nucleic-acid sequences.

4. What are eukaryotes?

A eukaryote is an organism whose cells contain complex structures enclosed within membranes (Figure 4). Eukaryotes may more formally be referred to as the taxon Eukarya or Eukaryota. The defining membrane-bound structure that sets eukaryotic cells apart from prokaryotic cells is the nucleus, or nuclear envelope, within which the genetic material is carried. The presence of a nucleus gives eukaryotes their name, which comes from the Greek ευ (eu, "good") and κάρυον (karyon, "nut" or "kernel"). Most eukaryotic cells also contain other membrane-bound organelles such as mitochondria, chloroplasts and the Golgi apparatus. All species of large complex organisms are eukaryotes, including animals, plants and fungi, although most species of eukaryote are protist microorganisms.[Cell division in eukaryotes is different from that in organisms without a nucleus (prokaryotes). It involves separating the duplicated chromosomes, through movements directed by microtubules. There are two types of division processes. In mitosis, one cell divides to produce two genetically identical cells. In meiosis, which is required in sexual reproduction, one diploid

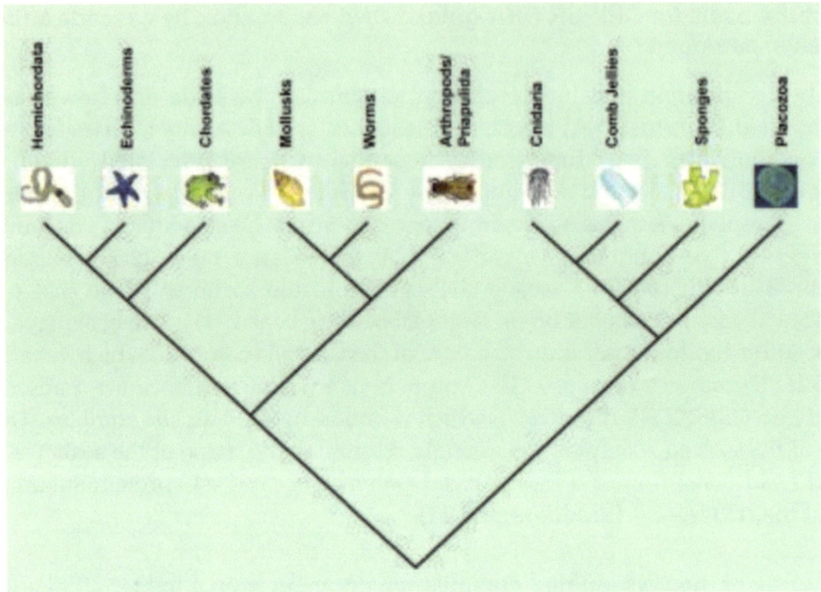

Fig. 6 New metazoan tree of life presented in Schierwater, et al. 2009
http://www.amnh.org/science/papers/metazoan.php Credit: AMNH

cell (having two instances of each chromosome, one from each parent) undergoes recombination of each pair of parental chromosomes, and then two stages of cell division, resulting in four haploid cells (gametes). Each gamete has just one complement of chromosomes, each a unique mix of the corresponding pair of parental chromosomes Eukaryotes appear to be monophyletic, and so make up one of the three domains of life. The two other domains, Bacteria and Archaea, are prokaryotes and have none of the above features. Eukaryotes represent a tiny minority of all living things; even in a human body there are 10 times more microbes than human cells.However, due to their much larger size their collective worldwide biomass is estimated at about equal to that of prokaryotes

5. Why was the 19th century crucial to the birth of immunology?

This provides an appropriate background for the analysis of eukaryotes. Darwin and Metchnikoff were laying the foundation for the "big bang" in immunology. It is not crystal clear when that occurred but surely whether directly or indirectly this revelation was the product of a coalescence of all the ferment that the 19th century inspired. In a sense, both were field biologists highly observant and meticulous - willing to take chances on the unexplored and to express their ideas. The inquisitiveness of Darwin and the consequence of Metchnikoff's single prescient observation by the sea both represent a *tour de force* in the annals of biology (Cooper et al 2002) The origin of species by natural selection underwent metamorphosis in its application to immunology and became the clonal selection theory with its inherent application to and explanation of adaptive immunity (Ribatti 2009] By contrast, Metchnikoff's phagocytosis in starfish larvae became the ancestor of innate immunity, even with the much later advent of T-cells (Silverstein 1989;, Tauber and Chernyak 1991, Besredka 1979). Darwin's well-known epic *The Origin of Species* was first published in 1859 when he was 50 years old and when Metchnikoff was only 14 years old.

The crossings and crisscrossing do continue. At 14 years Metchnikoff was already the budding zoologist imbued with an interest in animals, their lives and habitats quite the central thesis of Darwin's work as well that resulted from his now famous expeditions. Metcnikoff's observation split the monolithic field of immunology into two main camps, cellular and humoral giving cause to celebrate both investigations in 2008-2009.

6. From Darwin and Metchnikoff to Burnet and beyond

Phagocytosis in unicellular animals represents the most ancient and ubiquitous form of defense against foreign material. Unicellular invertebrates can phagocytose for food and defense. Multicellular invertebrates and vertebrates possess phagocytic cells and have evolved more complex functions attributed to immunodefense cells that specialized into sources of cellular and humoral immune responses. Thus all animals possess: innate, natural, nonspecific (no memory) nonanticipatory, nonclonal, germline (hard wired) host defense functions. In addition, all vertebrates possess: adaptive, induced, specific (memory), anticipatory, clonal, somatic (flexible) immune responses. A similar situation exists with respect to components of the signaling system, immunity and development. With multicellularity, clearly numerous immune response characteristics are not possible in unicellular forms or even those that straddle the divide between unicellularity and multicellularity, beginning with colonial/social protozoans. Still, it is instructive to elucidate a hierarchy of animals based upon immunologic characteristics and how they parallel other physiological traits. Evidence is presented that the most primitive of invertebrates prior to the evolution of multicellular organisms possess varying degrees of complexity at the molecular level of those hallmarks that now characterize the immune system.

According to Cooper (2008) we can now explore easily how potential external threats to life by continuously mutating microbes are first perceived, recognized, and the resulting signals interpreted and presumably survival from infection insured - or the blocking of cancer development an internal threat averted. This chapter will focus primarily on unicellular (Protozoa) and examples of multicellular animals (Sponges, Cnidarians); more complex invertebrates are excluded. Three reasons are presented. First, these two animal groups are situated at the nexus between single cell life and the emergence of multicellularity. Second, the unjustified thinking of immunologists would discredit these two groups with having evolved any semblance of an immune response other than phagocytosis. Third, the information that is included, i.e. the recent discovery of Toll-like receptors (TLRs) justified their inclusion. Finally, TLRs correlate with earlier information that substantiated the immunodefense capabilities as we knew them long ago and credit them today (Tables 1 and 2, Cooper 2008)

6.1 Emergence of modern immunology may be indebted to invertebrates?

This discovery of invertebrate phagocytosis dramatically changed the monolithic world of immunology. His careful and detailed observations of white cell motility toward and engulfment of foreign bodies in transparent larvae of starfish and in the water flea *Daphnia* provoked a major re-evaluation of the nature of immune systems, admittedly restricted to the human good. Before his prescient observations, immune systems were believed to be wholly humoral and there was little emphasis on the role of leukocytes or white cells. Metchnikoff's discovery, however, added cellular immunity to the known armory of

Genus & Species	Assessment of self and non- self activity	Results	Adhesion protein families and/or recognition system
Amoeba (*Amoeba preteus*) Amoeba discordes	Transplantation Allogeneic nuclei Xenogeneic nuclei	90% clones 0% clones 0% clones	-
Social amoebae (*Dictyostelium discoideum*) Slime molds	S cells Phagocytosis of bacteria	-	TIR domain proteins
Choanoflagellates (Unicellular colonial)	-	-	C-type lectins Tyrosine kinase signaling components
Ciliata Stentor Stenor coeruleus *Stentor polymorphus*	Lack of Chimera formation	Ejection of symbiotic *Chlorella*	-

Table 1. Recent evidence of signaling systems supported by early evidence of self and nonself recognition in unicellular species.

Genus & Species	Assessment of self and non- self activity	Results	Adhesion protein families and/or recognition system
Porifera Sponges *Microciona prolifera* *Cliona celata*	Mixing of red and yellow sponges	Disaggregated sponges to not reaggregate together	-
Demosponges *Suberites Domuncula*	Response to bacterial lipopeptides	-	TLR, IRAK-41, effector caspase sequence (SDCA, SL) Homologies in family-specific domains
Cnidaria Hydrozoa *Hydra* *Chlorphydra* *Pelmatohydra*	Allografts and xenografts	Incompatible transplant reactions	-
Anthozoa *Aborescent Cnidarians*	Autografts Allografts	Compatible Incompatible	-
Staghorn corals Acropora	Autografts Isografts Allografts	Compatible Incompatible Incompatible	-
Hydra magnipapillata *Nematostella vectensis*	- -		- -
Coral (*Acropora millepora*)			Canonical Toll/TLR Receptor C3, MAC/PF

Table 2. Evidence of signaling systems and early evidence of self and non-self recognition in multicellular animals (Porifera and Cnidaria).

humoral immunodefense mechanisms. Serendipity surely intervened and there was probably the impulse to shout Archimedes' *eureka* when the interpretation of why cells were moving toward a foreign body was easily visualized. Thus, the foundation for invoking the concept of self non-self recognition was laid (Cooper 1993).

Moreover, there is a much greater willingness to accept that invertebrate model systems have much more to contribute than was thought, even in the early 1960s when modern immunology was beginning to develop. Broadly interpreted, Darwin led us into the field and Metchnikoff into the laboratory at least with respect to comparative immunology (Cooper 1974; Cooper et al 1992). Evolutionary immunology reaped the benefits of Metchnikoff and modern immunology advanced conceptually when the clonal selection theory of Burnet was advanced - in essence a Darwinian corollary (Cooper 1974, Perlovsky 2010). According to Burnet (1962), 'The clonal-selection theory is a generalization about a wide range of biological phenomena but may suffer from the inherent weakness of all biological generalizations. The essence of the clonal-selection theory is that immunity and antibody production are functions of clones of mesenchymal cells. Each clone is characterized by the ability of its component cells to react immunologically with a very small number of antigenic determinants (Ribatti 2009).

Contact with the right antigenic configuration acts as a trigger to action and it is the essence of a clonal theory that such stimulation plays a major part in determining the observed changes in type and numbers of the mesenchymal cells of the body. The trigger of immunological contact is believed to provoke actions which, depending on many associated factors, may take one or other several forms. The cells may be killed or damaged, with release of cell-damaging or stimulating products; they may be stimulated to proliferate, with or without change of morphological type; or they may be converted to the plasma-cell form, with its capacity for active synthesis and liberation of antibody. Which particular reaction ensures will depend essentially on the physiological state of the cell and the nature of the internal environment to which it is exposed after stimulation.' (Burnet 1970) .

6.2 Origins of immunc system components

6.2.1 Unicellular colonial protozoans

One approach to origin of animals is to determine which developmental proteins predated them and were subsequently co-opted for their development. Another strategy involves comparative genomics that can identify the minimal set of intact genes from the beginning of animal evolution that reveals those shared by all animals and their nearest relatives. Resolving the mystery of origins, these workers have sampled gene diversity expressed by choanoflagellates, unicellular and colonial protozoa that are closely related to metazoa, crucial for providing a possible clue into early animal evolution. Results revealed that choanoflagellates express representatives of a surprising number of cell-signaling and adhesion protein families not previously isolated from nonmetazoans; these include cadherins, C-type lectins, several tyrosine kinases and tyrosine kinase signaling pathway components. Choanoflagellates have a complex and dynamic tyrosine phosphoprotein profile, and tyrosine kinase inhibitors selectively affect cell proliferation. The expression in choanoflagellates of proteins involved in cell interaction in metazoa demonstrates that these proteins evolved before the origin of animals and were later co-opted for development. A similar situation exists with respect to components of the signaling system with respect to immunity and development. (Fig 6)

6.2.2 Emergence of multicellularity: social amoeba

Social amoebae feed on bacteria in the soil but aggregate when starved to form a migrating slug. Chen et al (2007) discovered an unknown cell type in social amoeba that is apparently involved in detoxification and immune-like functions; they call it the sentinel (S) cells. S cells engulf bacteria and sequester toxins while circulating within the slug, eventually being sloughed off. A Toll/interleukin-1 receptor (TIR) domain protein, TirA, is also required for certain S cell functions and for vegetative amoebae to feed on live bacteria. This apparent innate immune function in social amoebae, and the use of TirA for bacterial feeding, suggests an ancient cellular foraging mechanism that may have been adapted to defense functions well before the diversification of animals. Multicellularity likely increased the selective pressure on an organism's ability to avoid exploitation by pathogens. The role of TirA in *Dictyostelium's* response to bacteria provides t he first glimpse of an immune-related signaling system in amoeba and suggests that the use of TIR domain based signaling for defense represents an ancient function present in the progenitor of all crown group eukaryotes. If true, it would suggest that this system of pathogen recognition was advantageous to organisms before the evolution of multicellularity.

6.2.3 Sponges

Sponges (phylum Porifera) are filter feeders, therefore they are extremely exposed to microorganisms that represent a potential threat. Examining sponges, therefore moving to a higher taxonomic level, Wiens et al. 2007 have identified, cloned and deduced the protein sequence from 3 major elements of the poriferan innate response (to bacterial lipopeptides according to these definitions): the TLR, the interleukin-1 (IL-1) receptor-associated kinase-4-like protein (IRAK-4l), and a novel effector caspase from the demosponge *Suberites domuncula*. Each molecule shares significant sequence similarity with its homologues in higher metazoa. There are sequence homologies within the family-specific domains Toll/IL-1 receptor/resistance (TLR family), Ser/Thr/Tyr kinase domain (IRAK family), and CASc (caspase family).

6.2.4 Hydra and corals

Recently, whole genome sequences became available for two cnidarians, *Hydra magnipapillata* and *Nematostella vectensis*, and large expressed sequence tag datasets are available for them and for the coral *Acropora millepora*. (Powell 2007) A canonical Toll/TLR pathway in representatives of cnidarians of the class Anthozoa was observed. Neither a classic Toll/TLR receptor nor a conventional nuclear factor-β was identified in *Hydra* - an anthozoan. The detection of complement C3 and several membrane attack complex/perforin domain (MAC/PF) proteins suggests that a prototypic complement effector pathway may exist in anthozoans, but not in hydrozoans. Together with information for several other gene families, they suggest that *Hydra* may have undergone substantial secondary gene loss during evolution. Such patterns of gene distribution may underscore possible significance of gene loss during animal evolution but indicate ancient origins for components of vertebrate innate immune systems. (Miller et al 2007)

6.3 Toll-like receptors: innate sensing

Chen et al. (2007) review the earliest work in relation to current views. Phagocytes that engulf bacteria form part of the innate immune system of animals in the defense against pathogens. According to Beutler et al (2003), in humans innate immune sensing usually proceeds through the activation of 10TLRs, and these in turn lead to the production of cytokine mediators that create the inflammatory milieu and collaborate in developing an adaptive immune response. Each TLR senses a different molecular component of microbes that have invaded the host.

TLR4 senses bacterial endotoxins (lipopolysaccharide), TLR9 unmethylated DNA, and TLR3 double-stranded RNA. Each receptor has a conserved signaling element called the TIR (Toll/IL-1 receptor/resistance) motif that transduces a signal through five cytoplasmic adapter proteins, each of which has a homologous motif. (Hoffman 2004). With respect to TLRs, the integration of signals that receptors emit is a crucial mechanism that requires resolution. (Ferrandon et al 2004) By creating random germline mutations in mice and screening for individuals with differences in signaling potential, the complex biochemical circuitry of the innate immune response can be unraveled. Up to now, more than 35,000 germline mutants have been produced, and approximately 20,000 have been screened to predict innate immunodeficiency states (Medzhitov 2000).

6.3.1 Toll-like receptors in invertebrates and vertebrates: application to human diseases seems real

6.3.1.1 Annelids

Toll-like receptors (TLRs) are an important component of the innate immunity system and are found throughout the animal kingdom, but have not yet been fully analyzed in annelids. We searched shotgun reads of the genomes of the leech *Helobdella* and polychaete *Capitella* for TLR homologs. We found 10^5 TLR homologs in *Capitella* and 16 in *Helobdella* (Davidson et al 2011). The deduced phylogeny of these sequences, together with TLRs from other animal phyla, reveals three major clades (A clade is a group consisting of a species [extinct or extant] and all its descendants.). One clade consists of a mixture of both vertebrates and invertebrates, including sequences from *Capitella* and *Helobdella*, while the other two clades contain only invertebrate TLRs. Now these represent a beginning in need of further analysis especially with respect to p53 (TLR) and existence of cancer. This is needed since earthworm immune responses are well defined (Cooper et al 2002). Moreover early attempts to induce cancer were not successful (Cooper 1969); new trials are proposed combined with analyses of p53.

6.3.1.2 Molluscs

Toll-like receptor (TLR) signaling pathway is an important and evolutionarily conserved innate immune pathway. Phylogenetic lineage of this pathway in the Lophotrochozoans is still less understood. (The Lophotrochozoa comprise one of the major groups herein annelids and molluscs within the animal kingdom, In turn, the Lophotrochozoa belongs to a larger group within the Animalia called the Bilateria, because they are bilaterally symmetrical with a left and a right side to their bodies) is still less understood. Zhang and Zhang (2011) have cloned a novel TLR, a key component of TLR pathway, from the oyster, and named it CgToll-1. Real-time reverse transcription polymerase chain reaction analysis revealed that the highest CgToll-1 expression level was in hemolymph, and this pattern increased dramatically in the presence of bacteria *Vibrio anguillarum*. TLR pathway core genes of molluscs were searched and compared with model invertebrates revealing that their genes were closer to the fruit fly *Drosophila melanogaster* than to the purple sea urchin *Strongylocentrotus purpuratus*, while three upstream genes (MyD88, IRAK, TRAF6) were not closer. They also found that these two downstream genes were significantly more conserved than the three upstream genes based on amino acid sequence alignment. Results suggests that CgToll-1 is a constitutive and inducible protein that could play a role in immune responses against bacterial infection.

6.3.1.3 Ascidians

It is appropriate to present information on the ascidian since they are the nearest invertebrate relative of vertebrates (see Figs 1 and 2). According to Sasake et al (2009), key transmembrane proteins in the innate immune system, Toll-like receptors (TLRs), probably occur in the genome of non-mammalian organisms including invertebrates. However, authentic invertebrate TLRs have only been recently investigated structurally and functionally. Inflammatory cytokine production of the ascidian *Ciona intestinalis*, designated as Ci-TLR1 and Ci-TLR2 have been analyzed. The amino acid sequence of Ci-TLR1 and Ci-TLR2 possessed unique structural organization with moderate sequence similarity to functionally characterized vertebrate TLRs. *ci-tlr1* and *ci-tlr2* genes were mostly expressed in the stomach, and in hemocytes. Both Ci-TLR1 and Ci-TLR2 stimulate NF-κB induction in response to multiple pathogenic ligands such as double-stranded RNA, and bacterial cell wall components that are differentially recognized by respective vertebrate TLRs.This revealed that Ci-TLRs recognize broader pathogen-associated molecular patterns than vertebrate TLRs. The Ci-TLR-stimulating pathogenic ligands also induced expression of Ci-TNFα in intestine and stomach where Ci-TLRs are expressed. These results provide evidence that TLR-triggered innate immune systems are essentially conserved in ascidians, and that Ci-TLRs possess "hybrid" biological and immunological functions, compared with vertebrate TLRs. This is significant since ascidians are the nearest ancestor to vertebrates.

6.3.1.4 Birds

The Toll-Like receptor (TLR) pathway plays is crucial in innate immunity and is maintained with amazing consistency in all vertebrates. Considering this background of substantial conservation, any subtle differences in this pathway's composition may have important implications for species-specific defense against key pathogens. Cormican et al (2009) used a homology-based comparative method to characterize the TLR pathway the employed the recently sequenced chicken and zebra finch genomes from two distantly related bird species. Primary features of the TLR pathway are conserved in birds and mammals, despite some clear differences. TLR receptors show a pattern of gene duplication and gene loss in both birds when compared to mammals. They found avian specific duplication of both TLR1 and TLR2 and a duplication of the TLR7 gene in zebra finch. Both positive selection and gene conversion may shape evolution of avian specific TLR2 genes. Results contribute to characterization of differing immune responses that have evolved in individual vertebrates in response to their microbiological environment. Birds have been considered since they usually receive less coverage than mammals. Moreover without them we would have been slow to recognize the T and B system.

6.3.1.5 Disease and TLR

Now we consider an example of another disease related to the immune system, having presented cancer as the first example. It is well to remember however that cancer can now be considered to occur in invertebrates. This is a major resolution after many years of speculation concerning its absence. Ngoi et al (2001) have raised awareness of the incidence of allergic disorders and increased autoimmune diseases especially in developed nations. The hygiene hypothesis suggests that as a living environment becomes more sanitized, children are not exposed to microbial and parasitic stimulations that were once commonly acquired since early in life; this caused a lack of immune sensitization tending towards T helper 2 (Th2) dominance. Thus we can conclude that the immune system perhaps like the nervous system requires early learning experiences in order to respond to antigen stimulation. This view may explain allergic disorders, which mostly result from hyper Th2 responses, but inadequate in explaining Th1 or Th17-based autoimmunity increases.

With respect to signaling, recent advances in experimental mouse models revealed that stimulation of Toll-like receptors (TLRs) by pathogen-associated molecular patterns could reduce symptoms of allergic airway disease and prevent the onset of autoimmunity. For one explanation, the underlying mechanism for protective effects of TLR ligands is currently under investigation and there are indications that IL-10-producing B cells, regulatory T cells, and innate immune cells play an important role during this process. That early exposure to microbial byproducts probably contributes to modulation of immunological disorders may once again modify our interpretation of the hygiene hypothesis.

7. Cancer development in invertebrates may be linked to the presence of tumor suppressor genes independent of the innate immune system?

According to immunosurveillance, the adaptive immune system evolved to protect multicellular organisms against harmful invaders (bacteria, viruses, fungi—any disturbance of *non-self* material not acceptable to *self*) earlier thought of exclusively as threats from the external environment; however, internal threats may now include cancer cells growing out of control. These characteristics were restricted to vertebrates with adaptive immune responses. And invertebrates were not considered since it was assumed based mostly upon field observations that invertebrates with an innate system did not develop cancer. Some even assumed that the short life span of countless invertebrates precluded the development of any visible tumors. Thus the generalization: innate immunity either protects against cancer or it is so fast acting and efficient, more than the seemingly more complex vertebrate system that they do not develop cancer. Now it is becoming increasingly clear that invertebrates may also develop cancer. It seems safe to conclude that the influence may rest partially on **p53** or its family members: **p63, 73.**

p53 (also known as **protein 53** or **tumor protein 53**), is a tumor suppressor protein that in humans is encoded by the *TP53* gene. **p53** is crucial in multicellular organisms, where it regulates the cell cycle and, thus, functions as a tumor suppressor that is involved in preventing cancer. As such, **p53** has been described as "the guardian of the genome", the "guardian angel gene", and the "master watchman", referring to its role in conserving stability by preventing genome mutation. *p53* continues to be one of the most intensively studied genes in cancer biology. **p53** was initially identified >20 years ago as a binding partner for the SV40 T oncoprotein. Further studies revealed that **p53** is a tumor suppressor gene that is mutated or inactivated in >50% of human cancers. Furthermore, germ-line **p53** mutations cause hereditary cancer in both mice and humans. Molecular and biochemical assays revealed that the **p53** protein is a sequence-specific DNA-binding transcription factor. **p53** plays a central role in cellular responses to aberrant growth signals and certain cytotoxic stresses, such as DNA damage, by enhancing the transcription of genes that regulate a variety of cellular processes including cell cycle progression, apoptosis, genetic stability, and angiogenesis.

According to Walker et. al., (2011) the human **p53** tumor suppressor protein is inactivated in many cancers; it is also crucial in apoptotic responses to cellular stress. **p53** protein and the two other members (**p63, p73**) are encoded by distinct genes, whose functions have been extensively documented for humans and other vertebrates. The structure and relative expression levels for members of the **p53** superfamily have also been reported for most invertebrates. Using classical model organisms (nematodes, anemones and flies) reveal that the gene family originally evolved to mediate apoptosis of damaged germ cells or to protect germ cells from genotoxic stress. Analyses of **p53** signaling pathways in marine bivalve cancer and stress biology studies suggest that **p53** and **p63/73**-like proteins in soft shell clams (*Mya arenaria*), blue mussels (*Mytilus edulis*) and Northern European squid (*Loligo forbesi*) have identical core sequences. Still we know little about the molecular biology of marine invertebrates to address molecular mechanisms that characterize particular diseases. Understanding the molecular basis of naturally occurring diseases in marine bivalves is a virtually unexplored aspect of toxicoproteomics and genomics and related drug discovery. Marine bivalves could provide the most relevant and best understood models for experimental analyses by biomedical and marine environmental researchers.

The *Drosophila* tumor-suppressor gene lethal malignant brain tumor [l(3)mbt] (Bonasio et al., 2010) was first identified as a temperature-sensitive mutation that caused malignant growth in the larval brain (Gateff, et al 1993). These long awaited observations provided ample background for further analysis after discovery of tumor suppressors. According to Janic et al (2010), model organisms such as the fruit fly *Drosophila melanogaster* can help to elucidate the molecular basis of complex diseases such as cancer. Mutations in the *Drosophila* gene lethal malignant brain tumor (mbt) cause malignant growth in the larval brain. It has been shown that l(3)mbt tumors exhibited a soma-to-germline transformation through the ectopic expression of genes normally required for germline stemness, fitness, or longevity. Orthologs of these genes are also known to be expressed in human somatic tumors. Moreover, inactivation of any of the germline genes *nanos, vasa, piwi,* or *aubergine* suppressed l(3)mbt malignant growth. There was a consensus: results demonstrated that germline traits are necessary for tumor growth in this *Drosophila* model. Moreover inactivation of germline genes might have tumor-suppressing effects in other species which could inspire further investigations especially in those other invertebrates such as earthworms in which innate immune systems are well defined (Cooper et al 2002).

Receiving support for the work of Janic et al, Wu and Ruykun (2010) suggest that cancer cells and germ cells share several characteristics. For instance, both have the ability to rapidly proliferate, typically do not lose the ability to divide as they age (lack senescence), and exist in undifferentiated states. Although some genes involved in cancer may initiate disease simply by activating cell division, others may promote tumors by activating early developmental pathways associated with programming for multipotency (the ability to differentiate into different cell types). Janic et al. (2010) have revealed that in fruit flies several genes typically involved in early programming of germline cells also play a role in the formation of malignant brain tumor. Moreover by inactivating these germ cell genes—some of which have related genes abnormally expressed in certain human cancers—can suppress tumor growth, suggesting new and future avenues for developing therapy.

If the expression of germline characteristics is common in tumors, for instance, it should be observable in gene expression analyses of human tumors. Indeed, the Piwil2 protein, a human Piwi family member, is widely expressed in several solid tumors. It should be feasible to examine more carefully the expression of germ cell genes, including *vasa* and *nanos*, in human tumors by microarray or deep RNA sequencing. The retinoblastoma tumor that stimulated analysis of this pathway provides a suitable candidate for studying germline gene activity in tumorigenesis. In addition, mutations in the human homologs of L(3)MBT, Rb, and its chromatin cofactors may be common in cancer genomes as they are sequenced. A query of the human homologs of these genes at the Cosmic web site (www.sanger.ac.uk/genetics/CGP/cosmic), for instance, revealed somatic mutations in L(3)MBT, Rb, and CHD3 (an Mi2 homolog) in a small fraction of tumors. Because there are so many mutations in these tumors, however, a more sophisticated statistical analysis is needed. The up-regulation of germline pathways in the l(3)mbt brain tumors and the required role for some of these genes in tumor growth also suggest new possibilities for tumor therapy. These genes are also conserved in mammals and could be potential targets for drugs that treat tumors similar to those analyzed by Janic et al. (2010)

Let us focus on new information that correlates with an animal model and cancer development. According to Read, (2011) glioblastomas (GBM), the most common primary brain tumors, infiltrate the brain, grow rapidly, and are refractory to current therapies. To analyze the genetic and cellular origins of this disease, a novel *Drosophila* GBM model is now available; Glial progenitor cells give rise to proliferative and invasive neoplastic cells that create transplantable tumors in response to constitutive co-activation of the EGFR-Ras and PI3K pathways. Since there is relevance of *Drosophila* to human cancer, neurological disease, and neurodevelopment, this fly model represents a neurological disease model wherein malignant cells are created by mutations in genetic pathways that may act in a homologous human disease. By using lineage analysis and cell-type specific markers, neoplastic glial cells presumably originated from committed glial progenitor cells, and not from multipotent neuroblasts. Genetic analyses demonstrated that EGFR-Ras and PI3K induce fly glial neoplasia through activation of a combinatorial genetic network that is partially comprised of other genetic pathways that are also mutated in human glioblastomas. Future research should focus on extensive genetic screens utilizing this model that could reveal new insights into origins and treatments of human glioblastoma.

8. Perspectives on parasitsm, cancer and immunity

For the past half-century, the dominant paradigm of oncogenesis has been mutational changes that disregulate cellular control of proliferation. The growing recognition of the molecular mechanisms of pathogen-induced oncogenesis and the difficulty of generating oncogenic mutations without first having large populations of dysregulated cells, however, suggests that pathogens, particularly viruses, are major initiators of oncogenesis for many if not most cancers, and that the traditional mutation-driven process becomes the dominant process after this initiation. Molecular phylogenies of individual cancers should facilitate testing of this idea and the identification of causal pathogens (Ewald 2009).

9. Pathogen survival in the external enviornment and the evolution of virulence

Recent studies have provided evolutionary explanations for much of the variation in mortality among human infectious diseases. Walther and Ewald's findings bear on several areas of active research and public health policy: (1) many pathogens used in the biological control of insects are potential sit-and-wait pathogens as they combine three attributes that are advantageous for pest control: high virulence, long durability after application, and host specificity; (2) emerging pathogens such as the 'hospital superbug' methicillin-resistant *Staphylococcus aureus* (MRSA) and potential bio-weapons pathogens such as smallpox virus and anthrax that are particularly dangerous can be discerned by quantifying their durability; (3) hospital settings and the AIDS pandemic may provide footholds for emerging sit-and-wait pathogens; and (4) studies on food-borne and insect pathogens point to future research considering the potential evolutionary trade-offs and genetic linkages between virulence and durability (2004).

All evidence indicates that clonal selection is purely a vertebrate strategy and therefore irrelevant to invertebrates. Some views may insist that anthropocentric mammalian immunologists utilized a tool to propel: the universal innate immune system of ubiquitous and plentiful invertebrates as an essential system for vertebrates. Innate immunity should help if there is a failure of the adaptive immune system. Still to be answered are questions concerning immunologic surveillance that includes clonal selection. We can then ask does immunologic surveillance play a role in the survival of invertebrates that most universally seem to not develop cancer at least of the vertebrate type. Perhaps invertebrates with their efficient innate immune system evolved certain "canceling devices" that maintain survival with short life spans, thus precluding their demise by metastasis.

10. Ancient neurons regulate immunity: innate innervation

According to Tracy (2011), the most evolutionarily ancient type of immunity, called "innate," exists in all living multicellular species. When exposed to pathogens or cellular damage, cells of an organism's innate immune system activate responses that coordinate defense against the insult, and enhance the repair of tissue injury. There is a modern-day cost associated with these processes, however, because innate mechanisms can damage normal tissue and organs, potentially killing the host. Human life is a balance between dual threats of insufficient innate immune responses—which would allow pathogens to prevail—and overabundant innate immune responses—which would kill or impair directly. What has been the key to maintaining this balance throughout years of mammalian evolution?

In this study, the nervous system controlled the activity of a noncanonical UPR pathway required for innate immunity in *Caenorhabditis elegans*. OCTR-1, a putative octopamine G protein–coupled catecholamine receptor (GPCR, G protein–coupled receptor), functioned in sensory neurons designated ASH and ASI to actively suppress innate immune responses by down-regulating the expression of noncanonical UPR genes*pqn/abu* in nonneuronal tissues. Findings suggest a molecular mechanism by which the nervous system may sense inflammatory responses and respond by controlling stress-response pathways at the organismal level.

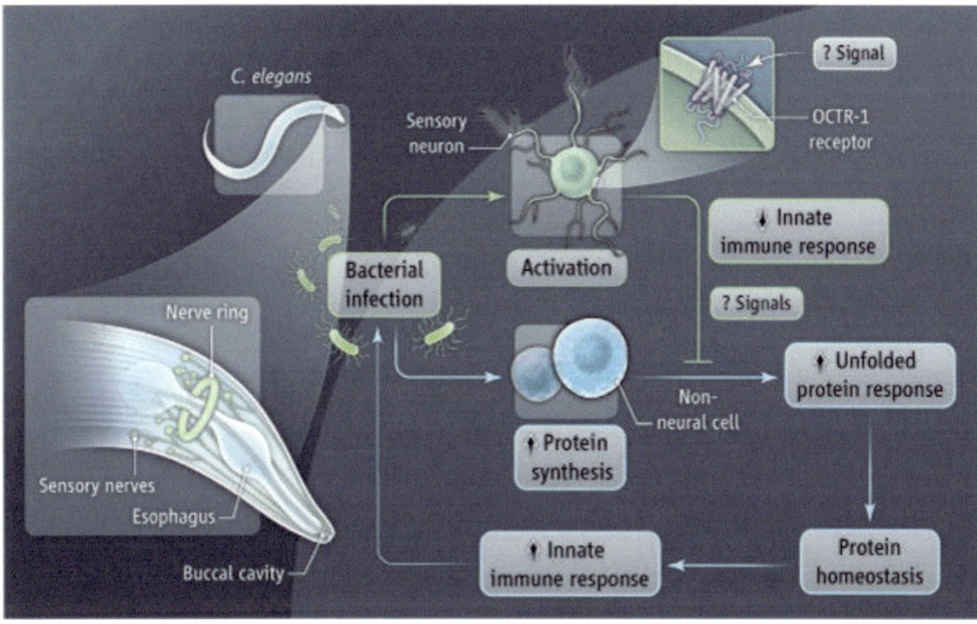

Fig. 7. Infection of *C. elegans* with a pathogen stimulates the innate immune response and activates the synthesis of new proteins, potentially causing the accumulation of unfolded proteins in host cells. (Tracey, 2011) The OCTR-1 receptor in the sensory neurons is required for this effect (figure 5). http://designmatrix.wordpress.com/ 2009/02/03/front-loading-neurons-more-supporting-evidence.

11. Perspectives

Clearly engaging TLRs activates various inflammatory and innate immune responses throughout the animal and plant kingdoms. This is associated with the innate immune system and must depend therefore on the presence, at least for now, of a multicellular system. Thus we would not expect as far as we have current information that prokaryotes would have evolved such a system. At the moment it is even with great difficulty to imagine such. Of course the thrust of this chapter refutes common dogma for it reports the existence of adaptive immunity in prokaryotes! But this impasse has been due to restricted definitions and these in turn due to restricted information based primarily on the dearth of molecular data. Ongoing efforts in many laboratories have led to the identification of TLR-specific signaling components and cellular responses within every major group -setting aside a wealth of new taxonomic data based on TLR. Perhaps this is a turning point in that the existence of TLR is so very basic, it seems inconceivable that investigations will reveal significant departures from what we know already. TLRs function in combination with additional pattern-recognition receptors and co-receptors to add further diversity to their role *in vivo.* How hosts integrate information that is signaled through TLRs and any co-receptors will ultimately control progression of the immune response to pathogens. Understanding this process will surely lead to newer fields that seek to develop novel therapeutics and immune boosting products.

Toll-like receptors (TLRs) are pattern-recognition receptors related to the *Drosophila* Toll protein (Adams 2009). TLR activation alerts the immune system to microbial products and initiates innate and adaptive immune responses. The naturally powerful immunostimulatory property of TLR agonists can be exploited for active immunotherapy against cancer. Antitumor activity has been demonstrated in several cancers, and TLR agonists are now undergoing extensive clinical investigation. Once there is more information, field and will focus on opportunities for clinical development of TLR agonists as single agent immunomodulators, vaccine adjuvants and in combination with conventional cancer therapies.

12. Conclusion

Perlovsky (2010) poses a pervasive and difficult question that challenges the utility of the immune system in relation to survival "Why deadly diseases exist from an evolutionary viewpoint? Some diseases, e.g. Influenza are clear; the disease agents are multiplying inside the host. But why cancer exists? According to surveillance, cancer poses an internal threat, in which cells no longer become recognizable as *self* (self/not self model) and therefore become cancerous and out of control. In this instance, the driving force for evolution of the immune system could be to effectively keep potentially cancerous cells in check, not allowing their uncontrolled metastases.

This review has covered enormous ground with respect to the immune system beginning with the view that microbes possess a form of adaptive immunity for protection against invading viruses. This is an interesting view and renders the immune system more encompassing than previous conceptions. By including the prokaryotes and eukaryotes and analyzing their responses to survival the immune system embraces a newer and broader scope than before when it was restricted to the higher eukaryotes. Gradually we have come to accept the innate immune system that characterizes the armamentarium of plants, invertebrates and vertebrates, it is only the vertebrates which at the moment whose immune system is associated with the appearance of cancer. Now two other points are worthy to raise and may bring us to another level of understanding of the immune system and in this light, I present at least two views concerning living systems in general and the immune system in particular.

In a recent review, the existence of artificial immune systems (AIS) has been presented (Cooper, 2010). Although not clearly defined, it is assumed that the field of AIS concerns an analysis of and development of computationally interesting abstractions of the immune system. Relevant to the current review there is the suggestion that to understand AIS could be inspired from organisms that possess only innate immune system. Moreover there is the suggestion that AISs should employ systemic models of the immune system in order to construct their overall design. For precision AIS should include plant and invertebrate immune systems.

Now we approach a new view presented recently by Bruce Alberts, Editor in Chief of Science (2011). He suggests recently: "A Grand Challenge in Biology" posing several questions and solutions aimed at advancing the field of synthetic biology. He emphasizes the need for basic research aimed at attaining a deep understanding of the chemistry of life. He further urges that a complete catalog of the tens of thousands of different molecules present in a human or mouse cell, along with a map of their myriad mutual interactions, is likely to be obtained with the wide variety of different techniques that are now available. Now, we are even closer to the present chapter and certainly suggestive of relevance to prokaryote immune systems. Albert's suggests: "Because all living things on earth are related through evolution, one can bootstrap one's way to understanding human cells by discovering how simpler cells and organisms work". A detailed study of *Mycoplasma genitalium*, a tiny bacterium that causes human disease, suggests that it can grow and divide with a minimal set of only about 430 genes. This suggests that we may be largely ignorant of some critical functions of proteins, such as their roles in the exquisite spatial organization of the molecules inside cells. (Alberts 2011). Of particular relevance is an article in the news section devoted to virus immunity by George Church, written by Bohannon, J. (2011)

13. Acknowledgements

Acknowledgement: I acknowledge with pleasure the superb assistance of Jesus Heredia and Kyle Hirabayashi.

14. References

Adams S. (2009). Toll-like receptor agonists in cancer therapy. *Immunotherapy*. 2009 , 6, pp.(949-64), 101485158

Janic A, Mendizabal L, Llamazares S, Rossell D & Gonzalez C. (2010). Ectopic expression of germline genes drives malignant brain tumor growth in *Drosophila*. *Science*. 2010 Dec, pp.(1824-1827)

Al-Attar S., Westra E.R., van der Oost J., Brouns S.J. (2011) Clustered regularly interspaced short palindromic repeats (CRISPRs) the hallmark of an ingenious antiviral defense mechanism in prokaryotes. *Biol Chem*, 392, 4, pp. (277-89), 9700112

Alberts B. (2011). A grand challenge in biology. *Science* 333, 2011, pp.(120), 0404511

Barrangou R, Fremaux C, Deveau H, Richards M, Boyaval P, Moineau S, Romero DA & Horvath P. (2007). *CRISPR* provides acquired resistance against viruses in prokaryotes. *Science*. 2007 Mar. pp.(1709-1712)

Besredka A. (1979). *The story of an idea*. Rivenson A, Oestreicher R, Trans.]. Bend, OR: Maverick; 1979

Beutler B, Hoebe K, Du X, Ulevitch RJ: How we detect microbes and respond to them: the Toll-like receptors and their transducers. *J Leukoc Biol*, 74, 4 2003, October, 74 pp.(479–485), 0741-5400

Bonasio R, Lecona E, & Reinberg D. (2010). MBT domain proteins in development and disease.*Semin Cell Dev Biol*. 2010, 2, pp(221-30), 9607332

Bohannon, J. (2011). The Life Hacker. *Science* 333, pp.(1236-1237), 0404511 [

Burnett FM. (1959). The clonal selection theory of acquired immunity. Nasville, Vanderbilt University Press; 1959

Burnet, M. Role of the thymus and related organs in immunity. Br Med J. 1962 Sep 29;2(5308):807-11.

Burnet FM. (1970). *Immunological surveillance*. Oxford: Pergamon; 1970.

Chen G, Zhuchenko O, Kuspa A. (2007). Immune-like phagocyte activity in the social amoeba. *Science*. 2007, 317. pp.(678–81), 0404511

Cooper, E. L. 1969. Neoplasia and transplantation immunity in annelids. J. Nat. Cancer Inst. 31: 655-669.

Cooper EL, Rinkevich B, Uhlenbruck G, Valembois P. (1992). Invertebrate immunity: Another viewpoint. *Scand J Immunol* 1992;35, pp.(247–66), 0323767

Cooper EL. In: Cooper EL, Nisbet-Brown E, editors. *Developmental immunology*. New York: Oxford University Press; 1993. pp. (3–30),

Cooper EL, Kauschke E, Cossarizza A. (2002). Digging for innate immunity since Darwin and Metchnikoff. (2002). *Bioessays*. 2002 Apr;24(4) pp.(319-333) 8510851

Cooper EL, Kvell K, Engelmann P, Nemeth. Still waiting for the toll? P.*Immunol Lett*. 2006, Apr 15, 104, 1 pp,(18-28) , 7910006

Cooper, EL. From Darwin and Metchnikoff to Burnet and beyond. (2008). Contrib Microbiol. 2008, 15. pp(1-11), 1662-291X, 9815689

Cooper, E.L. Evolution of immune systems from self/not self to danger to artificial immune systems (AIS). *Phys Life Rev*. 2010 Mar;7(1):55-78 2009, 101229718

Cooper, E.L. Self/not self, innate immunity, danger, cancer potential. *Phys Life Rev*. 2010. Feb, pp.(85-86) 101229718

Cooper, EL. (2010). Evolution of immune systems from self/not self to danger to artificial immune systems (AIS). *Phys Life Rev. 2010 Mar, pp.(55-78),* 101229718

Cooper, EL. (2010). Self/not self, innate immunity, danger, cancer potential. *Phys Life Rev*. 2010 Feb 1. pp.(55-78) ,101229718

Cossarizza, A. (2010). Know thyself and recognize dangers: An evolutionistic view. Phys Life Rev. 2010 Mar. pp.(81-82), 1873-1457, 101229718

Davidson CR, Best NM, Francis JW, Cooper EL, & Wood TC. (2011). Toll-like receptor genes (TLRs) from *Capitella capitata* and *Helobdella robusta* (Annelida). *Jourl of Biol Chem*. 2011, 284, pp.(608-612), 7708205

Du Pasquier L, & Litman GW. (2000) Origin and evolution of he vertebrate immune system, current topics in microbiology and immunology.2000, Heidelberg, Germany, Springer, 3540664149

Engelmann P. and Nemeth. (2010). Immune evolution and autoimmunity. *Phys life Rev,* 2010. 7, 1, pp.(79-80), 101229718

Ewald PW. (2009). An evolutionary perspective on parasitism as a cause of cancer. *Adv Parasitol*. 2009, 68, pp.(21-43), 0370435

Ferrandon D, Imler JL, Hoffmann JA. Sensing infection in Drosophila: Toll and beyond. *Semi. Immunol*. 2004, 16,. pp.(43-53), 9009458

Franc NC, Dimarcq J-L, Lagueux M, Hoffmann J, & Ezekowitz RAB. (1996). Croquemort, a novel *Drosophila* hemocyte/macrophage receptor that recognizes apoptotic cells. *Immunity*. 1996, 4.5, pp.(431–43), 9432918

Gateff et al 1993. A temperature-sensitive brain tumor suppressor mutation of Drosophila melanogaster: developmental studies and molecular localization of the gene. Mech Dev. 1993 Apr, pp.(15-31),

Grissa I, Bouchon P, Pourcel C & Vergnaud G. (2008). On-line resources for bacterial micro-evolution studies using MLVA or CRISPR typing. *Biochimi*. 2008, April, pp.(660-668)

Hildemann WH, Raison RL, Cheung G, Hull CJ, Akaka L, & Okamoto J.(1977). Immunological specificity and memory in a scleractinian coral. *Nature*. 1977, 270, pp.(219–2230), 0410462

Hoffmann JA. (2004). Primitive Immune Systems., *Immunological Reviews* 2004, 198, pp.(5-9), 1600-065X

Jore, M.M., Lundgren, M., van Duijn, E., Bultema, J.B., Westra, E.R., Waghmare, S.P., Wiedenheft, B., Pul, U., Wurm, R., Wagner, R., Beijer, M.R., Barendregt, A., Zhou, K., Snijders, A.P., Dickman, M.J., Doudna, J.A., Boekema, E.J., Heck, A.J., van der Oost, J., Brouns, S.J. (2011) Structural basis for CRISPR RNA-guided DNA recognition by Cascade. *Nat Struct Mol Biol.* 2011 May, 18, 5, pp.(529-36), 101186374

Kvell K, Cooper EL, Engelmann P, Bovari J, Nemeth. (2007). Blurring borders: innate immunity with adaptive features. (2007). *P.Clin Dev Immunol.* 2007, pp.(1-10), 101183692

Luke A.J. O'Neill. (2011) Innate Immunity in Plants Goes to the PUB. (2011). *Science* 332, 2011, June, pp.(1386-1387), 0404511

Marraffini LA & Sontheimer EJ. (2010). CRISPR interference: RNA-directed adaptive immunity in bacteria and archaea. *Nat Rev Genet.* 2010 Mar, pp.(181-190)

Marraffini LA & Sontheimer EJ. (2010). Self versus non-self discrimination during CRISPR RNA-directed immunity. *Nature* 2010, pp.(568-571)

Medzhitov R, Janeway Jr.C. (2000). The toll receptor family and microbial recognition. *Trends Microbiol* 2000, 10, pp.(452–456), 9310916

Mendizabal JL, LLamazares S, Rossell D, & Gonzalez C. (2010). Ectopic Expression of Germline Genes Drives Malignant Brain Tumor Growth in Drosophila. *Science.* 2010, 330, pp.(1824-1827), 0404511

Miller DJ, Hemmrich G, Ball EE, Hayward DC, Khalturin K, Funayama N, Agata K, Bosch TC. (2007). The innate immune repertoire in cnidaria—ancestral complexity and stochastic gene loss. *Genome Biol* 2007;8. pp.(1–13), 100960660

Ngoi SM, Sylvester FA, & Vella AT. (2011). The role of microbial byproducts in protection against immunological disorders and the hygiene hypothesis. *Discov Med.* 2011, 12.66, pp.(405-12), 101250006

Pancer Z. (2000). Dynamic expression of multiple scavenger receptor cysteine-rich genes in coelomocytes of the purple sea urchin. *Proc Natl Acad Sci.* 2000, 97, pp.(13156–61), 7505876

Parrinello. (2010). "Has innate immunity evolved through different routes?" 85-7. *Phys Life Rev* 2010, 7, pp.(83-84), 101229718

Perlovsky L. 2010; Cooper, E.L. Self/not self, innate immunity, danger, cancer potential. Phys Life Rev, 2010 pp.(55-78), 101229718

Powell AE, Nicotra ML, Moreno MA, Lakkis FG, Dellaporta SL, Buss LW. (2007). Differential effect of allorecognition loci on phenotype in *Hydractinia symbiolongicarpus* (Cnidaria: Hydrozoa). *Genetics.* 2007, 177, pp.(2101-2107) 0374636

Pradeu T. and E.D. Carosella. (2004). Critical analysis of the immunological self/non-self model and of its implicit metaphysical foundations. 2004, 325, 5, pp.(481–492), 101140040

Pradeu T. and E.D. Carosella. (2006). On the definition of a criterion of immunogenicity. *Proc Natl Acad Sci USA,* 2006, 103, 47, pp. (17858–1786), 7505876

Read RD. (2011). Drosophila melanogaster as a model system for human brain cancers. *Glia.* 2011, 59., pp.(1364-76), 8806785

Ribatti D. (2009). Sir Frank Macfarlane Burnet and the clonal selection theory of antibody formation, Clin Exp Med 2009, December, 4, pp.(253-258), 100973405

Riddihough, G. (2011). Structural biology Seahorse Versus Pathogen. *Nat. Struct. Mol. Biol*, 2011, pp.(10), 18, 10.1038/nsmb.2019 (2011).

Sasake Ni, Ogasawara M, Sekiguchi, T, Kusumoto S, & Satake H. (2011). Prototypes with Hybrid Functionalities of Vertebrate Toll-Like Receptors. *Fish Shellfish Immunol.* 2011, 30, pp.(653-660), 2985121R

Silverstein AM. *A history of immunology*. San Diego: Academic Press; 1989.

Sun S-C, Lindstrom I, Boman HG, Faye I, & Schmidt O. (1990). Hemolin: An insect-immune protein belonging to the immunoglobulin superfamily. *Science*. 1990, 250, pp.(1729–32), 0404511

Tauber AI, Chernyak L. (1991). *Metchnikoff and the origins of immunology: From metaphor to theory*. New York: Oxford University Press; 1991.

Theodor JL. (1970). Distinction between "self" and "not-self" in lower invertebrates. *Nature* 1970,227, pp.(690-692), 0410462

Tracey KJ. (2011). Ancient Neurons Regulate Immunity. *Science*. 2011, May, 332, 6030 pp.(673-674), 0404511

Van der Oost J, Jore MM, Westra ER, Lundgren M, Brouns SJ. CRISPR-based adaptive and heritable immunity in prokaryotes. *Trends Biochem Sci*. 2009, Aug, 34, 8, pp.(401-407), 7610674

Walther BA, Ewald PW. Pathogen survival in the external environment and the evolution of virulence. *Biol Rev Camb Philos Soc*. 2004, Nov, 79, 4, pp.(849-869), 0414576

Walker CW, Van Beneden RJ, Muttray AF, Böttger SA, Kelley ML, Tucker AE, & Thomas WK. (2011). Superfamily proteins in marine bivalve cancer and stress biology. *Adv Mar Biol*. 2011, 59, pp.(1-36), 0370431

Watson FL, Püttmann-Holgado R, & Thomas F. (2005). Immunology: Extensive diversity of Ig-superfamily proteins in the immune system of insects. *Science*. 2005, 309. pp.(1874–8), 0404511

Wiedenheft, B., Lander, G.C., Zhou, K., Jore, M.M., Brouns, S.J.J., van der Oost, J., Doudna, J.A., & Nogales E., Structures of the RNA-guided surveillance complex from a bacterial immune system. *Nature* 477, pp.(486–489), 0410462

Wiens M, Korzhev M, Perovic-Ottstadt S, Luthringer B, Brandt D, Klein S, Müller WE: Toll-like receptors are part of the innate immune defense system of sponges (demospongiae: Porifera). *Mol Biol Evol*. 2007, 24. pp.(792–804), 8501455

Wikipedia CRISPR. http://en.wikipedia.org/wiki/CRISPR

Wikipedia Prokaryotes. http://en.wikipedia.org/wiki/Eukaryote

Wu X & Ruykun G. (2010). Cancer. Germ cell genes and cancer..Science. 2010, 330 pp.(1761-1762), 0404511

Zhang S-M, Adema CM, Kepler TB, & Loker ES. (2004). Diversification of Ig superfamily genes in an invertebrate. *Science*. 2004, 305, pp.(251–4). 0404511

Zhang L., Li L., & Zhang G (2011). *Crassostrea gigas* Toll-like receptor and comparative analysis of TLR pathway in invertebrates. *Fish Shellfish Immunol*. 2011, 2, pp.(653-60), 9505220